Statistics for Spatio-Temporal Data

Statistics for Spatio-Temporal Data

NOEL CRESSIE

Department of Statistics
The Ohio State University

CHRISTOPHER K. WIKLE

Department of Statistics
University of Missouri

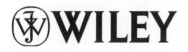

A JOHN WILEY & SONS, INC., PUBLICATION

Published by John Wiley & Sons, Inc., Hoboken, New Jersey
Published simultaneously in Canada

For general information on our other products and services or for technical support, please contact our Customer Care Department within the United States at (800) 762-2974, outside the United States at (317) 572-3993 or fax (317) 572-4002.

Wiley also publishes its books in a variety of electronic formats. Some content that appears in print may not be available in electronic formats. For more information about Wiley products, visit our web site at www.wiley.com.

Library of Congress Cataloging-in-Publication Data:

Cressie, Noel
  Statistics for spatio-temporal data / Noel Cressie, Christopher K. Wikle.
      p. cm.—(Wiley series in probability and statistics)
  Includes bibliographical references and index.
  ISBN 978-0-471-69274-4 (cloth)
  1. Spatial analysis (Statistics) 2. Stochastic processes. 3. Time-series analysis. I. Wikle, Christopher K., 1963– II. Title.
  QA278.2.C754 2011
  519.5–dc22
                              2010033576

10 9 8 7 6 5 4 3 2 1

Contents in Brief

Contents

Preface

Nothing puzzles me more than time and space; and yet nothing troubles me less....

These words, by the English essayist Charles Lamb in his 1810 letter to Thomas Manning, provide a concise summary of this book. Of course, he was not thinking of Statistics, nor Science, nor Statistical Science, rather the more ephemeral notion of space and time. But here, in the physical world, there are scientific questions to resolve and predictions to make, and understanding the effects of dependencies across time and space is a crucial part. Those dependencies are in there somewhere, and we too are puzzled by them.

Up until the mid-twentieth century, Statistics' response to this puzzle was often to ignore the complicated structure, or to find clever ways to remove it. Interestingly, Charles Lamb seemed to be in tune with this, as he finished his sentence by saying, "as I never think about them." As Statistics has progressed through the twentieth century and moved into the twenty-first, spatial and temporal statistical methodology has been incorporated more and more into the scientific models of our world and indeed of our universe. As technology has improved, Statistics has been given a Rosetta Stone to begin to unlock Science's mysteries, from the molecular to the global to the cosmological.

In the beginning, there were data. Then, there were theories, formed from data, and those theories rose and fell according their agreement with new data. Data are central, and they should be cared for accordingly. To do good Science, databases should be fully documented and algorithms ("black boxes") involved in creating them should be in the public domain.

However, data alone do not tell us all that much about our world. When we look at data, how do we know if what we are seeing is "signal" as opposed to "noise"? How do we compare two sources of data—what is the basis of a comparison?

Similarly, theories (or models) by themselves are not often the best descriptions of the real world. What can be said about processes on scales at which there were no observations? What about uncertainties in parameters, or forcings, or interactions with other processes? Indeed, the key is the proper blending of such models and the data. Sometimes this might be done informally, for example, by taking a simulated field, simulated from a mathematical (say) model, and visually comparing it to a field of actual data. From the visual comparison, a deficiency in the model might be obvious, which might lead to a parameter adjustment, or even a new parameter. Then a *new* simulation might be implemented and a new visual comparison made, and so forth. This is one way to combine data and model, but it is not a very efficient way to deal with either. Indeed, the power of Statistical Science is that it provides several frameworks in which to combine data and model, in optimal ways, for the purpose of scientific inference. It might seem strange that there is not just one framework in which to carry out inferences, but even Statistics has its tribes. However, the element that is common to all is an attempt to partition variability and to quantify uncertainty.

In this book, we take the firm stand that the best paradigm (to date) in which to partition variability and quantify uncertainty is the *hierarchical statistical model*. Such a model explicitly acknowledges uncertainty in the data, different from that in the process and parameters, and then it accommodates the uncertainty in the process (and finally in parameters, if necessary). We have used color in key places in our exposition, to distinguish between the parts of the hierarchical model concerned with data (green), with processes (blue) and with parameters (purple).

Hierarchical thinking (i.e., hierarchical modeling) is intimately tied to conditional thinking (i.e., modeling with conditional probabilities). Indeed, it is our perspective that conditional thinking is the aforementioned Rosetta Stone: It allows us to separately partition the effects of measurement error and scales of variability below the resolution of our data, conditioned on the process at possibly some other scale. Similarly, conditional thinking allows us to model a spatio-temporal process as it actually *evolves* through time, as opposed to just accounting for its marginal dependencies. Equally important, it allows us to use spatio-temporal dependencies in errors and/or parameters as a proxy for unknown and unknowable processes. Its impact goes even deeper, in that it allows parameters themselves to be dependent on other processes or other sources of data. Finally, it makes clear that if some components of variability are not interesting for a particular question, then the end result should *not* look like the data. Any unwanted components (e.g., measurement error) are filtered out: What you see (data) is not always what you want to get (process).

Critically, in the presence of data, conditional thinking allows sensible trade-offs to be made between data availability, process complexity, and computational complexity. Combined with the ever-expanding computational tools of the twenty-first century, the hierarchical statistical framework provides the structure to tackle important questions in Energy, Climate, Environment, Food, Finance, and so on. This will be a century of massive (spatio-temporal) datasets collected to answer Society's dominant questions. In this book, we are particularly interested in inference for Climate and the Environment, where processes at small spatio-temporal scales influence those at larger scales, and vice versa. The questions to be resolved are fundamental to sustaining our planet, they involve complex spatio-temporal phenomena, *and* they are inherently statistical.

Our lives are spent marching through a space–time continuum, but space is different from time. We can (and often do) visit the same place over and over but always at different, ordered time points. We can go north, south, east, and west, up and down, but only ever forward from the past to the present and into the future. Any study of a spatio-temporal phenomenon needs to respect this difference. In this book, we have proposed spatio-temporal statistical methodologies that align with the underlying science, and we have found that hierarchical thinking is a natural way to achieve this alignment.

In the pages that follow, we have deliberately tried to build a bridge between the twentieth and twenty-first centuries in our presentation of spatio-temporal statistics. There are strong and powerful traditions that have developed in the last few decades and, even if they are not hierarchical, they provide the tools and motivation that can be used in hierarchical thinking. In some cases, hierarchical approaches that may be appealing in principle may be out of our reach in terms of timely implementation.

The official ftp site associated with the book can be found at:

ftp://ftp.wiley.com/public/sci_tech_med/spatio_temporal_data

In addition to posting errata, we will post supplemental material that we hope will be helpful to the reader.

As mentioned above, we have questions to resolve and predictions to make, so let's get started....

NOEL CRESSIE
CHRISTOPHER K. WIKLE

Columbus, Ohio
Columbia, Missouri
December 2010

Acknowledgments

There are many people to thank, but two are missing. I wish my parents were alive to read this and know how important they are to what I do. I finally have a good answer to Ray's question, "How's the book going?"

My children, Amie and Sean, were only just present for my last book project, and now, as young adults, they are happily cheering on the completion of this one. Everyone has a book in them, and I hope they write theirs.

My dear friends and sibs may not understand all that is on these pages, but they know how important it was for me to "write it down." I would like them to know how important they are to me.

My co-author Chris has been a generous colleague and friend, and I admire enormously his intelligence and erudition. Together, we have been able to write a book that is so much more than what was in each of us; I have learned much from him. The order of authors is simply determined by the alphabet.

I have been taught by co-authors, colleagues, and students, who have shaped the material in this book. Their contributions are there in many, many ways. Some deserve special mention, which can be found in the joint acknowledgment.

The Department of Statistics at The Ohio State University has provided a nurturing environment for the whole lifetime of this book project. As part of my role as Director of the Department's Program in Spatial Statistics and Environmental Statistics, I have relied on my Program Assistant, Terry England, in many ways. This book has been a major project we have shared, and her efforts (which are described in the joint acknowledgment) are deeply appreciated and warmly acknowledged. Paul Brower, our Department Administrative Manager, has been a great supporter of this book project and, more generally, of my attempts to "save the planet." The office staff, the computer-support personnel, and the custodial staff are all warmly thanked for making my working environment in Cockins Hall a place where things get done ... with good cheer.

Finally, it is not lost on me that this book will appear exactly 20 years after an earlier book I authored on spatial data. A lot can happen in two decades....

N. C.

xix

My rather unorthodox training in Statistics and Meteorology would not have been possible without the tremendous support of my advisors, Tsing-Chang (Mike) Chen and Noel Cressie, both of whom set a great example of having mastered the art of teaching and the more elusive skill of mentoring. Mike Chen opened my eyes to the beauty of dynamics through his courses in Dynamic Meteorology and Geophysical Fluid Dynamics (in particular) and his patient one-on-one expositions; he is a master of explaining the "real" meaning behind the mathematics. In addition to teaching these subjects, he taught me the *philosophy of science* and to appreciate the importance of knowing the history of your field. Noel has been an inspirational mentor, collaborator, and friend. In addition to opening my eyes to the beauty of spatial statistics, he has, more than anyone, taught me to think like a statistician, and to stand up for the things in which I believe scientifically. At the time I was choosing an advisor in Statistics, some students warned me that I did not want to work with Noel because he was too "hard." One of the best decisions I ever made professionally was to ignore that advice! If hard means having high expectations, and providing generous advice and support, than I guess he was. Such a mentor has turned into a good friend. Noel mentioned at the beginning of this project how it can be very trying on a friendship to write a book. To be sure, we've had some disagreements, but we have managed quite well and I would not trade this journey for any other professional endeavor. I have learned a tremendous amount from Noel in writing this book, and I believe our friendship is stronger today than it was when we started.

I also want to thank two wonderful mentors with whom I started working when I was a postdoc at the National Center for Atmospheric Research (NCAR), and with whom I have continued to work along the way: Ralph Milliff and Mark Berliner. Ralph is a friend, a mentor, and an inspiration. He is a true scientist and is one of the most generous individuals I have met professionally. On every project in which we work, Ralph reminds me by the example he sets of what it means to be a scientist with integrity. Ralph saw the potential of Bayesian hierarchical modeling (BHM) as a way to manage uncertainty in oceanography before anyone else and, more importantly, he has stuck with it through good times and bad. Although he probably wouldn't admit it, Ralph is indeed an expert in BHM. Mark Berliner probably deserves a special chapter in this book. In fact, the book owes its philosophy to the ideas about hierarchical modeling and science that Mark began promoting when he was the director of the Geophysical Statistics Project (GSP) at NCAR in the mid-1990s. My time in that group was the most stimulating intellectual environment of my career. Mark had a vision of how BHM could be used as a paradigm for Science. Indeed, Mark is a master of weaving Science into the fabric of Statistics; he is always an inspiration! Perhaps more importantly, Mark is a friend and mentor and is one of the truly generous people in Statistics. There is no doubt that I would not be the statistician I am today if it were not for Mark's mentoring and collaborations.

A special thanks to Andy Royle, who was also part of the GSP group. Andy is an amazing statistician, and our interactions and collaborations during my time at NCAR and immediately thereafter were very important in shaping the way in which I envisioned Mark's philosophy playing a role in spatio-temporal statistics. In fact, Andy and I talked about writing a lower-level book on spatio-temporal statistics while we were at NCAR, and we even drafted an outline and a couple of chapters. We both moved in different directions (Andy to ecological statistics in the Fish and Wildlife Service and then to the U.S. Geological Survey, and me to academia), which prevented us from pursuing that project. But, there is no doubt that there is much of Andy in this book.

My path to Statistics was certainly not direct. In fact, the first classes I had in the subject as an undergraduate did little to impress upon me its importance. However, along the way I have had the great fortune of having some fantastic teachers and collaborators. In particular, I would like to thank Peter Sherman and Rol Madden, for introducing me to the power of spectral analysis and its scientific interpretation; and Mark Kaiser, for introducing me to hierarchical modeling in the early 1990s through a wonderful experimental course at Iowa State University. Many other people have influenced me along the way, either through conversations or collaborations. In particular, knowing that I am sure to unintentionally leave someone off of this list, I would like to thank: Chris Anderson, Thomas Bengtsson, Jim Clark, Bob Dorazio, William Dunsmuir, Dave Higdon, Tim Hoar, Dave Larsen, Andy Moore, Doug Nychka, Nadia Pinardi, Yanyan Sheng, Jon Stroud, Joe Tribbia, and Jay Ver Hoef. Of course, there are many others who have influenced me with the quality of their research, their integrity, and through brief discussions at meetings.

I would also like to thank my friends, colleagues, and students at the University of Missouri, past and present. They have been there for me no matter what, and they have made it a pleasure to come to the office. I would like to thank Joe Cavanaugh, Wade Davis, Neil Fox, Scott Holan, Sakis Micheas, Jake Oleson, Larry Ries, Thomas Rose, and Mark Wildhaber, for their much-valued friendship. In particular, the long-standing friendship of Larry Ries and Joe Cavanaugh has been a source of strength and an invaluable outlet; thanks for listening, guys! As a new Assistant Professor, I was so fortunate to have a mentor like Joe, who sets the "gold standard" of what it means to be an academic. Furthermore, I have been fortunate to have a wonderful group of Master's and Ph.D. students over the years, all of whom have contributed to my view of Statistics. My Ph.D. students, past and present, have kept me on my toes, and I value their collaboration and their friendship. Much of what is in this book comes from what we did together. In particular, I would like to acknowledge the implicit contributions of Ali Arab, Mevin Hooten, Yong Song, and Ke (Bill) Xu.

My biggest thanks go to my family! I am eternally grateful to my parents, Bayliss and Irene Wikle, for instilling in me the value of education and for giving me the freedom and support to pursue my dreams. Their support and love has shown me what it means to be a parent. In addition, I want to thank my brothers Shawn, Jeff, and Tim for everything they have done for me through the years. There is no doubt that they got all the brains in the family! I am sure that I continue to benefit in my professional life from the friendly competitions and creative activities that we engaged in, growing up on the "Wikle ancestral compound." In addition, I would like to thank my in-laws, George and MaryIda Heskamp, for their support through the years and for further strengthening my sense of family. Most importantly, I want to thank Carolyn, Olivia, Nathan, and Andrea. Your patience and support while I was working on this project have been a source of strength, and I deeply appreciate it. Olivia, Nathan, and Andrea, you have taught me much more than any book or research paper ever could, and you have provided countless sources of inspiration. Carolyn, you have supported my career unconditionally, and I am so fortunate to be able to share my life and love with you. There is no doubt that I am a better person every single day because of you! Thank you.

C. K. W.

There are many people who deserve our thanks for their direct contributions to this book. At Ohio State and beyond, Rajib Paul has generously prepared many of our figures, well beyond his time as a student; Matthias Katzfuß helped in a pivotal way with his timely reading and editing of most of the chapters; Bethann Pflugeisen was our "reference and editing maven," as well as helping with the rhyme and reason in Chapters 1 and 2; Ana Lucía Ortiz of Universidad Francisco Marroquín helped us obtain permission to use the lienzo shown on the front cover and in Chapter 1; Gardar Johannesson and Desheng Liu made figures in Chapter 4; and Emily Kang made figures in Section 9.2. At Missouri and beyond, Scott Holan gave comments on an early draft of Chapter 3; Sakis Micheas gave comments on Section 4.4.3; Mevin Hooten made figures and gave comments on Section 9.3; Ralph Milliff made figures and gave comments on Section 9.4; Jeremiah Brown, Nadia Pinardi, Alessandro Bonazzi, and the INGV group contributed to figures in Section 9.4; Ali Arab, Rima Dey, Dan Gladish, Mevin Hooten, Bill Leeds, and Wen-Hsi Yang gave general comments on drafts of various chapters; and Mary Peng, Dan Gladish, and Carolyn Wikle helped with the index.

Finally, we wish to give special thanks to Terry England for her invaluable help in typing large portions of the manuscript and for her tremendous LaTeX skills in organizing and typesetting the book. We could not have finished this without her!

At Wiley, the acquisition, production (particularly Lisa Van Horn), and marketing teams have all played a crucial role in taking our idea to write a book on spatio-temporal statistics, all the way to a four-color volume in the Wiley Series in Probability and Statistics. This is a publisher that is committed to getting our ideas into the offices, labs, and libraries of scientists and engineers. We want to change the way they practice Statistics . . . particularly for spatio-temporal data.

N. C.
C. K. W.

CHAPTER 1

Space–Time: The Next Frontier

This book is about the statistical analysis of data... *spatio-temporal* data. By this we mean data to which labels have been added showing where and when they were collected. Good science protocol calls for data records to include place and time of collection. Causation is the "holy grail" of Science, and hence to infer cause–effect relationships (i.e., "why") it is essential to keep track of "when"; a cause always precedes an effect. Keeping track of "where" recognizes the importance of knowing the "lay of the land"; and, quite simply, there would be no History without Geography.

We believe that in order to answer the "why" question, Science should address the "where" and "when" questions. To do that, spatio-temporal datasets are needed. However, spatial datasets that do not have a temporal dimension can occur in many areas of Science, from Archeology to Zoology. The spatial data may be from a "snapshot" in time (e.g., liver-cancer rates in U.S. counties in 2009), or they may be taken from a process that is not evolving in time (e.g., an iron-ore body in the Pilbara region of Australia). Sometimes, the temporal component has simply been discarded, and the same may have happened to the spatial component as well. Also, temporal datasets that do not have a spatial dimension are not unusual, for analogous reasons. For example, two time series, one of monthly mean carbon dioxide measurements from the Mauna Loa Observatory, Hawaii, and the other of monthly surface temperatures averaged across the globe, do not have a spatial dimension (for different reasons).

Spatio-Temporal Data

Spatio-temporal data were essential to the nomadic tribes of early civilization, who used them to return to seasonal hunting grounds. On a grander scale, datasets on location, weather, geology, plants, animals, and indigenous people were collected by early explorers seeking to map new lands and enrich their kings and queens. The conquistadors of Mesoamerica certainly did this for Spain.

Statistics for Spatio-Temporal Data, by Noel Cressie and Christopher K. Wikle
Copyright © 2011 John Wiley & Sons, Inc.

The indigenous people also made their own maps of the Spanish conquest, in the form of a *lienzo*. A lienzo represents a type of historical cartography, a painting on panels of cloth that uses stylized symbols to tell the *history* of a *geographical* region. The *Lienzo de Quauhquechollan* is made up of 15 joined pieces of cotton cloth and is a map that tells the story, from 1527 to 1530, of the Spanish conquest of the region now known as Guatemala. It has been restored digitally in a major project by Exploraciones sobre la Historia at the Universidad Francisco Marroquín (UFM) in Guatemala City (see Figure 1.1). This story of the Spanish conquest in Guatemala is an illustration of complex spatiotemporal interactions. Reading the lienzo and understanding its correspondence with the geography of the region required deciphering; see Asselbergs (2008) for a complete description. The original lienzo dates from about 1530 and represents a spatio-temporal dataset that is almost 500 years old!

In a sense, we are all analyzers of spatial and temporal data. As we plan our futures (economically, socially, academically, etc.), we must take into account the present and seek guidance from the past. As we look at a map to plan a trip, we are letting its spatial abstraction guide us to our destination. The philosopher Ludwig Wittgenstein compared language to a city that has evolved over time (Wittgenstein, 1958): "Our language can be seen as an ancient city: A maze of little streets and squares, of old and new houses, and of houses with additions from various periods; and this surrounded by a multitude of new burroughs with straight and regular streets and uniform houses!"

Graphs of data indexed by time (time series) and remote-sensing images made up of radiances indexed by pixel location (spatial data) show variability at a glance. For example, Figure 1.2 shows the Missouri River *gage-height* levels during the 10-year period, 1988–1997, at Hermann, MO. Figure 1.3 shows two remotely sensed images of the river taken in September 1992, before a major flood event, and in September 1993, after the highest crest ever recorded at Hermann (36.97 ft on July 31, 1993). The top panel of Figure 1.3 shows the town of Gasconade in the middle of the scene, situated in the "V" where the Gasconade River joins the Missouri River; Gasconade is at mile 104.4 and eight miles downstream is the river town of Hermann, visible at the very bottom of the scenes. Notice the intensive agriculture in the river's flood plain in September 1992. The bottom panel of Figure 1.3 shows the same region, one year later, after the severe flooding in the summer of 1993. The inundation of Gasconade, the floodplain, and the environs of Hermann is stunning. There is a multiscale process behind all of this that involves where, when, and how much precipitation occurred upstream, the morphology of the watershed, microphysical soil properties that determine run-off, the U.S. Army Corps of Engineers' construction of levees upstream, and so on. However, by looking only in the spatial dimension, or only in the temporal dimension, we miss the dynamical evolution of the flood event as it progressed downstream. Spatio-temporal data on this portion of the Missouri River, which shows how the river got from "before" to "after," would be best illustrated with a movie, showing a temporal sequence of spatial images before, during, and after the flood.

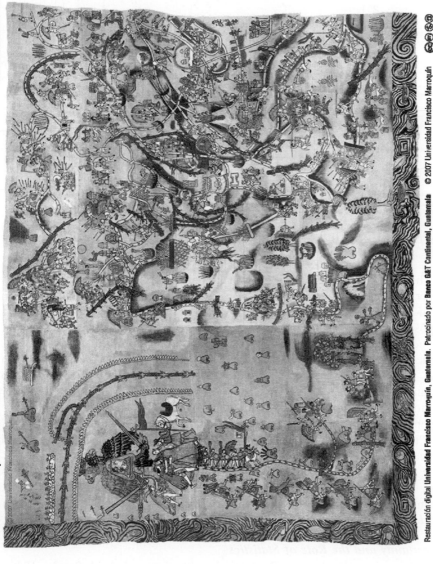

Figure 1.1 Digitally restored Lienzo de Quauhquechollan, whose actual dimensions are 2.45 m in height by 3.20 m in width. [Image is available under the Creative Commons license Attribution-Noncommercial-Share Alike © 2007 Universidad Franc sco Marroquín.]

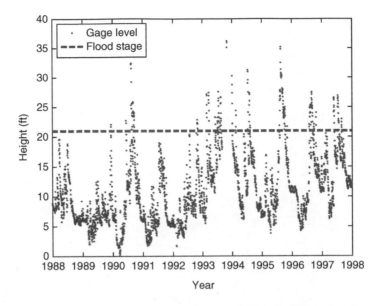

Figure 1.2 Time-series levels of gage height at Hermann, MO (mile 96.5 on the Missouri River) from January 1, 1988 through December 31, 1997. Flood stage is given by the horizontal dashed line. The highest recorded gage height in the 10-year period was 36.97 ft on July 31, 1993.

There is an important statistical characteristic of spatio-temporal data that is very common, namely that nearby (in space and time) observations tend to be more alike than those far apart. However, in the case of "competition," the opposite may happen (e.g., under big trees only small trees can grow), but the general conclusion is nevertheless that spatio-temporal data should *not* be modeled as being statistically independent. [Tobler (1970) called this notion "the first law of Geography."] Even if spatio-temporal trends are used to capture the dependence at large scales, there is typically a cascade of smaller spatio-temporal scales for which a statistical model is needed to capture the dependence. Consequently, an assumption that spatio-temporal data follow the "independent and identically distributed" (*iid*) statistical paradigm should typically be avoided. Paradigms that incorporate dependence are needed: The time series models in Chapter 3 and the spatial process models in Chapter 4 give those paradigms for *temporal data* and *spatial data*, respectively. From Chapter 5 onwards, we are concerned directly with Statistics for *spatio-temporal data*.

Uncertainty and the Role of Statistics
Uncertainty is everywhere; as Benjamin Franklin famously said (Sparks, 1840), "In this world nothing can be said to be certain, except death and taxes." Not only is our world uncertain, our attempts to explain the world (i.e., Science) are uncertain. And our measurements of our (uncertain) world are uncertain. Statistics is the "Science of Uncertainty," and it offers a coherent approach to

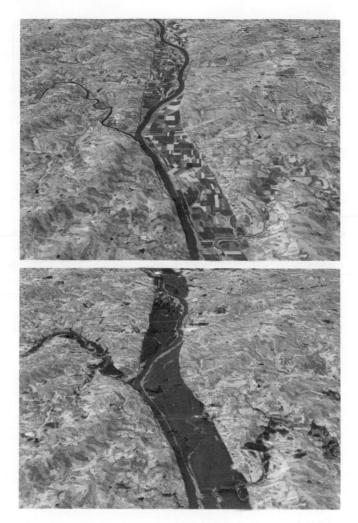

Figure 1.3   Images from NASA's Landsat Thematic Mapper. Each image shows a segment of the Missouri River near Hermann, MO (mile 96.5, at the bottom of the scene), and Gasconade, MO (mile 104.4, in the "V" in the middle of the scene). The river flows from west (top of the scene) to east (bottom of the scene). **Top panel:** September 1992, before a major flood event. **Bottom panel:** September 1993, after a record-breaking flood event in July 1993.

handling the sources of uncertainty referred to above. Indeed, in our work we use the term *Statistical Science* interchangeably with *Statistics* (with a "capital" S); we use *statistics* (with a "small" s) to refer to summaries of the data.

In most of this book, we shall express uncertainty through variability, but we note that other measures (e.g., entropy) could also be used. Just as the physical and biological sciences have the notions of mass balance and energy balance, Statistical Science has a notion of variability balance. The total variability is modeled with variability due to *measurement*, variability due to using a (more-or-less uncertain) *model* of how the world works, and variability due to uncertainty on *parameters* that control the measurement and model variabilities.

Although real-world systems may in principle be partially deterministic, our information is incomplete at each of the stages of observation, summarization, and inference, and thus our understanding is clouded by uncertainty. Consequently, by the time the inference stage is reached, the lack of certainty will influence how much knowledge we can gain from the data. Furthermore, if the dynamics of the system are nonlinear, the processes can exhibit *chaos* (Section 3.2.4), even though the theory is based on *deterministic* dynamical systems. (In Chapters 3 and 7, we show how model uncertainty in these systems naturally leads to *stochastic* dynamical systems that incorporate *system*, or *intrinsic*, noise.)

Data can hold so much potential, but they are an entropic collection of digits or bits unless they can be organized into a database. With the ability in a database to structure, search, filter, query, visualize, and summarize, the data begin to contain *information*. Some of this information comes from judicious use of statistics (i.e., summaries) with a "small s." Then, in going from information to *knowledge*, Science (and, with it, Statistics with a "capital S") takes over. This book makes contributions at all levels of the data–information–knowledge pyramid, but we generally stop short of the summit where knowledge is used to determine policy. The methodology we develop is poised to do so, and we believe that at the interface between Science, Statistics, and Policy there is an enormous need for (spatio-temporal) decision-making in the presence of uncertainty.

In this book, we approach the problem of "scientific understanding in the presence of uncertainty" from a probabilistic viewpoint, which allows us to build useful spatio-temporal statistical models and make scientific inferences for various spatial and temporal scales. Accounting for the uncertainty enables us to look for possible associations within and between variables in the system, with the potential for finding mechanisms that extend, modify, or even disprove a scientific theory.

Uncertainty and Data

Central to the observation, summarization, and inference (including prediction) of spatio-temporal processes are *data*. All data come bundled with error. In particular, along with the obvious errors associated with measuring, manipulating, and archiving, there are other errors, such as discrete spatial and temporal sampling of an inherently continuous system. Consequently, there are always scales of variability that are unresolvable and that will further "contaminate" the observations. For example, in Atmospheric Science, this is considered a form of "turbulence," and it corresponds to the well known aliasing problem in time series analysis (e.g., see Section 3.5.1; Chatfield, 1989, p. 126) and the microscale component of the "nugget effect" in geostatistics [e.g., see the introductory remarks to Chapter 4 and Cressie (1993, p. 59)].

Furthermore, spatio-temporal data are rarely sampled at spatial or temporal locations that are optimal for the analysis of a specific scientific problem. For instance, in environmental studies there is often a bias in data coverage toward areas where population density is large, and within a given area the coverage may be limited by cost. Thus, the location of a measuring site and its temporal sampling frequency may have very little to do with the underlying scientific mechanisms. A scientific study should include the *design* of data locations and sampling frequencies when framing questions, when choosing statistical-analysis techniques, and when interpreting results. This task is complicated, since the data are nearly always statistically dependent in space and time, and hence most of the traditional statistical methods taught in introductory statistics courses (which assume *iid* errors) do not apply or have to be modified.

Uncertainty and Models

Science attempts to *explain* the world in which we live, but that world is very complex. A model is a simplification of some well chosen aspects of the world, where the level of complexity often depends on the question being asked. Pragmatically, the goal of a model is to predict, and at the same time scientists want to incorporate their understanding of how the world works into their models. For example, the motion of a pendulum can be modeled using Newton's second law and the simple gravity pendulum that ignores the effect of friction and air resistance. The model predicts future locations of the pendulum quite well, with smaller-order modifications needed when the pendulum is used for precise time-keeping. Models that are scientifically meaningful, that predict well, and that are conceptually simple are generally preferred. An injudicious application of Occam's razor (or "the law of parsimony") might elevate simplicity over the other two criteria. For example, a statistical model based on correlational associations might be simpler than a model based on scientific theory. The way to bridge this divide is to focus on what is more or less certain in the scientific theory and use *scientific-statistical* relationships to characterize it.

Albert Einstein said: "It can scarcely be denied that the supreme goal of all theory is to make the irreducible basic elements as simple and as few as possible without having to surrender the adequate representation of a single datum of experience," at the Herbert Spencer Lecture delivered at Oxford University on June 10, 1933; see Einstein (1934). Much later, in the October 1977 issue of the *Reader's Digest*, it appears as if Einstein's quote was paraphrased to: "Everything should be made as simple as possible, but not simpler." Statistics and its models, including those involving scientific–statistical relationships, should not be spared from following this advice. Royle and Dorazio (2008, pp. 414–415) give a succinct discussion of this desire for conceptual simplicity in a model. As the data become more expansive, it is natural that they might suggest a more complex model. Clearly, there is a balance to be struck between too much simplicity, and hence failing to recognize an important signal in the data, and too much complexity, which results in a nonexistent signal being "discovered." One might call this desire for balance the *Goldilocks Principle* of modeling. (*Goldilocks and the Three Bears* is a nursery tale about a little girl's discovery of what is "just right.")

It is our belief that statistical models used for describing temporal variability in space should represent the variability dynamically. Models used in Physics, Chemistry, Biology, Economics, and so on, do this all the time with difference equations and differential equations to express the evolutionary mechanisms. Why should this change when the models become statistical? Perhaps it is because there is often an alternative—for example, a model based on autocorrelations that describe the temporal dependence. However, this descriptive approach does not directly involve evolutionary mechanisms and, as a consequence, it pushes understanding of the Physics/Chemistry/Biology/ Economics/etc. into the background. As has been discussed above, there is a way to have both, in the form of a scientific–statistical model that recognizes the dynamical scientific aspects of the phenomenon, with their *uncertainties* expressed through *statistical* models. Descriptive (correlational) statistical models do have a role to play when little is known about the etiology of the phenomenon; this approach is presented in Sections 6.1 and 6.2. Thereafter, this book adopts a dynamical approach to Statistics for spatio-temporal data.

Nearby Things Tend to Be More Alike...

A simple and sometimes effective forecast of tomorrow's weather is to use today's observed weather. This "persistence" forecast is based on observing large autocorrelations between successive days. Such dependence behavior in "nearby" temporal data is also seen in "nearby" spatial data, such as in studies of the environment. Statistics for Spatio-Temporal Data presents the next frontier; this book steps forward into new territories and revisits old ones. It reviews and extends different aspects of statistical methodology based on spatio-temporal dependencies: exploratory data analysis, marginal/conditional models in discrete/continuous time, optimal inference (including parameter estimation and process prediction), model diagnostics and evaluation, and so forth. One fundamental scientific problem that arises is understanding the evolution of processes over time, particularly in environmental studies (e.g., the evolution of sea-ice coverage in the Arctic; changes in sea level; time trends in precipitation). Proper inference to determine if evolutionary components (natural or anthropogenic) are real requires a spatio-temporal *statistical* methodology.

The scientific method involves observation, inspiration, hypothesis generation, experimentation (to support or refute the current scientific hypothesis), inference, more inspiration, more hypothesis generation, and so forth. In a sense, everything begins with observation, but it is quickly apparent to a scientist that unless data are obtained in a more-or-less controlled manner (i.e., using an experimental design), proper inference can be difficult. This is the fundamental difference between "observation" and "experimentation." Understanding the role of dependencies when the data are spatial or temporal, or both, provides an important perspective on working with experimental data versus observational data.

Experimental Data

Earth's population is many billions, and the demand for sustenance is great and continuous. The planet's ability to produce food on a massive scale largely came from fundamental experiments in crop science in the early twentieth century. Fisher (1935) developed a statistical theory of experimental design, based on the three principles of blocking, randomization, and replication, for choosing high-yielding, insect-resistant crops adapted to local conditions. He developed a vocabulary that is used today in scientific experiments of all types: response (e.g., wheat yields), treatments (e.g., varieties of wheat), factors (e.g., soil type, field aspect, growing season), levels of factors (e.g., for the soil-type factor, the levels might be sand, gravel, silt, clay, peat), plot (experimental unit that receives a single treatment), block (collection of plots with the same factor/level combination), randomization (random assignment of treatments to plots), replication (number of responses per treatment), and so on.

Data from designed experiments, when analyzed appropriately, allow stronger (almost) causative inferences, which incubate further scientific inspiration and hypothesis generation, and so forth, through the cycle. In the right hands, and with a component of luck, this cycle leads to great breakthroughs [e.g., the discovery of penicillin in 1928 by Alexander Fleming; see, e.g., Hare (1970)]. Even small breakthroughs are bricks that are laid on the knowledge pyramid.

Space and time are fundamental factors of any experiment. For example, "soil type" is highly spatial and "growing season" is highly temporal. Protocol for any well designed experiment should involve recording the location and time at which each datum was collected, because so many factors (known or unknown) correlate with them. After the experiment has been performed, spatial and temporal information can be used as proxies for unknown, unaccounted-for factors that may later become "known" as the experiment proceeds. From this point of view, the natural place to put spatial and temporal effects in the statistical model is in the mean. But, there is an alternative ....

In R. A. Fisher's pathbreaking work on design of experiments in agricultural science, he wrote (Fisher, 1935, p. 66): "After choosing the area we usually have no guidance beyond the widely verified fact that patches in close proximity are commonly more alike, as judged by the yield of crops, than those which are further apart." Spatial variability, which to Fisher came in the form of plot-to-plot variability, is largely due to physical properties of the soil and environmental properties of the field. Fisher avoided the confounding of treatment effect with plot effect with the inspirational introduction of *randomization* into the scientific method. It was a brilliant insertion of *more* uncertainty into a place in the experiment where uncertainty abounds, leaving the more certain parts of the experiment intact. Fisher's idea has had an enormous effect on all our lives. For example, any medicine we have taken to treat our ailments and illnesses has gone through rigorous testing, to which the *randomized* clinical trial is central (where a "plot" is often the patient).

Randomization comes with a price. It allows valid inference on the treatments through a simple expression for the mean response, but the variances and covariances of the responses are affected too. Under randomization of the assignment of treatments to plots, the notions of "close proximity" and "far apart" have been hustled out the back door. Can we get spatial dependence back into the statistical analysis of responses, resulting in more efficient inferences for treatment effects? The answer to this is a resounding "Yes"; see the introduction to Chapter 4.

Observational Data

Organisms are born, live, reproduce, and die, but they can produce harmful by-products that may threaten their own well-being as well as the well-being of other organisms around them. (The species *Homo sapiens* is unique in many of its abilities, including its ability to have a major impact on all other organisms on Earth.) Variability within organisms can be large (e.g., within *H. sapiens*), as can variability between their environments. Thus, it can be very difficult to conduct controlled experiments on Earth's ecology and environment.

Observational data come from a "wilder side" of Science. The environment (such as climate, air and water quality, radioactive contamination, etc.) is a part of our lives that often will not submit to blocking, randomization, and replication. We cannot control when it rains, nor can we observe two Los Angeles, one with smog and one without. We *can* look for two like communities, one with contaminated water and one without; and we *can* look at health records before and after a toxic emission. However, any inference is tentative because the two factors, space and time, are not controlled for. Collecting samples from ambient air presents a philosophical problem because the parcel of air is unique when it passes the monitoring site; it evolves as the changes in air pressure move it around, and it will never come back to allow us the luxury of obtaining an independent, identically distributed observation. (If these observations are used to study the effect of air quality on human health, there is the further problem that the ambient air is not actually what individuals breathe in their homes or their workplaces; this introduces even more uncertainty into the study.)

In the environmental and life sciences, classical experimental design can struggle to keep up with the questions being asked, but they still need to be answered. And, as we have discussed just above, *uncertainty* is likely to be higher without experimental control. Thus, Statistical Science has a crucial role to play, although it does not fit neatly into the blocking–randomization–replication framework. Even when one is able to "block" the human subjects on age and sex, say, it may be that an unknown genetic factor will determine how a patient responds to a given treatment. (Personalized medicine has as one of its goals to make the unknown genetic factor known.) In epidemiological studies, controls may be randomly matched with cases, but the cases are in no way assigned randomly to neighborhoods. And, although duplicate chemical assays allow for assessment of measurement error in a study on stream pollution, replication of a water parcel from the stream is impossible. In such circumstances, Statistics is even more relevant, and we advocate that the scientific method invoke the principle of *expressing uncertainty through probabilities*.

In the environmental sciences, proximity in space and time is a particularly relevant factor. The word "environ" means "around" in French. While ecology is the study of organisms, the *environment* is the surroundings of organisms. "Nearby" is a relative notion, relative to the spatial and temporal scales of the phenomenon under study. For example, in the spatial case, a toxic-waste-disposal site may directly affect a neighborhood of a few square miles; a coal-burning power plant may directly affect a heavily populated region of many tens of square miles, and an increase in greenhouse gases will affect the whole planet. Clearly, a global effect is felt locally in many ways, from a longer growing season in Alberta, Canada, to a redistribution of beachfront property in Florida, USA. The point we wish to make here is that a quantity like global mean temperature is a largely uninformative summary of how daily lives of a community will be affected by a warmer planet, which means that environmental studies of the globe must recognize the importance of *local* variability. Furthermore, how the spatial variability behaves dynamically (i.e., the spatio-temporal variability) is key to understanding the causes of global warming and what to do about it. Finally, we state the obvious, that political boundaries cannot hold back a one-meter rise in sea level; our environment is ultimately a global resource and its stewardship is an international responsibility.

Einsteinian Physics

Einstein's theory of relativity (e.g., Bergmann, 1976) demonstrated that space and time are interdependent and inseparable. In contrast, our book is almost exclusively concerned with phenomena that reside in a classical Newtonian framework (e.g., Giancoli, 1998). We include a brief discussion of space and time within Einstein's framework, to indicate that modifications would be needed for, say, spatio-temporal astronomical data.

Einstein proposed a "thought experiment," a version of which we now give. Think of a boxcar being pulled by a train traveling at velocity v, and place a source of light at the center of the moving boxcar. An observer on the train sees twin pulses of light arrive at the front and rear end of the boxcar, *simultaneously*. A stationary observer standing by the train tracks sees one pulse arrive at the rear end of the boxcar *before* its twin arrives at the front end. That is, the reference frame of the observer is extremely important to the temporal notions of simultaneity/before/after. What ties together space and time is movement (velocity) of the boxcar.

Einsteinian physics assumes that the velocity of light c, is a universal constant (which is approximately 3×10^5 km/s), regardless of the frame of reference. Thus, for *any* frame of reference, the distance traveled by a pulse of light is equal to the time taken to travel that distance multiplied by c. That this relationship holds under any spatio-temporal coordinate system means that for Einsteinian physics, space and time are inextricably linked. Other physical properties are modified too. The length of an object measured in the moving frame, moving with velocity v, is always smaller than or equal to the length of the object measured in the stationary frame, by a factor of $\{1 - (v/c)^2\}^{1/2}$. A similar factor shortens a time interval in a moving frame, leading to the famous conclusion that the crew of a spaceship flying near the speed of light would return in a few (of *their*) years to find that their generation on Earth had become old.

Einstein's theory of relativity is most certainly important for some phenomena, but in this book we shall stay within scales of space and time where the physical laws of Newton can be assumed. We work with a coordinate system that is a Cartesian product of three-dimensional space and one-dimensional time, while respecting the directionality of the temporal coordinate. Our models of spatio-temporal processes attempt to capture the complex statistical dependencies that can arise from the *evolution* of phenomena at many *spatial and temporal scales*.

Change-of-Support

The global/regional/local scales of spatio-temporal variability lead to a phenomenon we shall call *change-of-support*. In the spatial case, it is known as downscaling/upscaling, or the ecological effect, or the modifiable areal unit problem. It is in fact a manifestation of Simpson's paradox (Simpson, 1951). Simpson's paradox, which has a perfectly rational probabilistic explanation, essentially says the following: In a two-way cross-tabulation, the variables (A and B, say) can exhibit a positive statistical dependence, yet when a third variable (C, say) enters and expands the data to a three-way cross-tabulation, the statistical dependence between A and B can be negative for *each* value of C!

For example, consider the data reported in Charig et al. (1986) and discussed by Meng (2009), on the treatment of kidney stones. *Open surgery* had a success rate of 78%, not as good as the *ultrasound* treatment's success rate of 83%. However, for small stones ($<$2-cm mean diameter), the success rate for open surgery was 93% and that for ultrasound was 87%. That is, open surgery did better than ultrasound for small stones. Surely, for large stones ($\geq$2-cm mean diameter), open surgery would do worse, to account for its inferior success rate based on the results given above for all stones (78% versus ultrasound's 83%). Not so! For large stones, the success rate for open surgery was 73% and that for ultrasound was 69%, *again in favor of open surgery*. This is a sober reminder to all scientists to respect the "lurking variable," manifested here as the size of a patient's kidney stone.

Similarly, in a temporal setting, a causal statistical model built at a 3-monthly scale may have little or no relevance to the mechanisms in play at the daily scale. Day trading on stock markets, based on economic relationships estimated from quarterly trade figures, would probably lead to financial ruin. In a spatial setting, regional climate data may warn, correctly, of a future drought in the Northwest United States (states of Washington and Oregon). However, local orographic effects may favor certain parts of the Willamette Valley in Oregon to the point where above-average rainfall is consistently received there. That is, rather than size of kidney stone, think of Simpson's paradox in terms of size of region (space) or length of period (time). See Cressie (1998a) for a discussion of change-of-support in a spatio-temporal setting.

As we have mentioned, aggregations over time are subject to the change-of-support effect, but there is less discussion of it in the time series literature because time series are often already downscaled to answer the questions of interest. In contrast, spatial aggregation is ubiquitous: In the United States, federal decisions (e.g., carbon "cap and trade") are made at a continental scale, state decisions (e.g., California's clean-air regulations) are made at a regional scale, and city-wide decisions (e.g., the water-conservation policy in the city of Tucson, Arizona) are made at a local scale. These decisions are based on data that come from a variety of spatial scales; however, an inappropriate statistical analysis that does not respect the change-of-support effect could lead to the adoption of inappropriate policies. Our goal in this book is to build spatio-temporal statistical models to *explain* the variability in observable phenomena. While change-of-support should always be respected, there is less of a chance it will cause difficulties when scientifically based dynamical models are used.

Objects in a Dynamical Spatial Environment

There are two major ways to view, and hence to model, the evolving spatial environment in which we live. The *object* view of the world sees individual objects located in a spatial domain and interacting through time with each other, often as a function of their distance apart. Thus, a household and its characteristics make up a unit of interest to census enumerators. This micro-datum is typically unavailable to social scientists, for confidentiality reasons. Consequently, the census data that are released are typically the *number of objects* in small areas, but not their locations. That is, a set of count data from small areas is released, which is simply an aggregated version of the object view of the world. The geographical extent (i.e., spatial support) of a small area can be stored in a Geographical Information System (GIS) as a polygon, and hence the spatial relationships between small areas and their associated counts are preserved in a GIS. [A GIS is a suite of hardware and software tools that feature linked georeferencing in its database management and in its visualization; e.g., Burrough and McDonnell (1998).]

Alternatively, the *field* view of the world loses sight of the objects and potentially has a (multivariate) datum at every spatial location in the domain of interest. Building on the census-enumeration example discussed above, we can define a *field* as the object density, in units of number per unit area, at any location. This is purely a mathematical construct because, at a given location, either there is an object present or there is not. Such a density can be estimated from a moving window, such that at any location the estimated density is the number of objects per unit area in the window at that location.

A useful way to think of the object view versus the field view is to imagine yourself in a helicopter taking off from a clearing in a field of corn. As the helicopter ascends, at some point it is no longer interesting to think of objects (e.g., corn plants), but rather to think of a field, literally and statistically (e.g., in units of bushels per acre). Then the temporal aspect is captured through the field's dynamical evolution during the growing season.

Sometimes the field view is the result of an aggregation of the object view, such as for population-density data. Other times, the field view is all that is of interest, such as for rainfall data where there is typically no interest in the individual raindrops. Again, a GIS is a convenient way to store data for a field, along with the spatial support to which a datum refers. Most of the exposition in this book (with the exception of Sections 4.2, 4.3, 4.4, and Section 6.6) is based on the field view. In general, spatio-temporal data may consist of measurements of both the field type and the object type. Modeling these data with coherent, spatio-temporal, random processes is the next frontier.

Uncertainty and the Role of Conditional Probabilities

The era of building (marginal) probability models directly for the data is coming to a close. A model of this sort defines a likelihood, from which inference on unknown parameters can be made. However, the likelihood does not directly recognize that data are a noisy, incomplete version of the scientific process of interest (see Section 2.1). This can be resolved by building a *conditional probability* model for the data, given the process, and then a separate probability model for the (hidden) process itself. From this perspective, it is clear that the likelihood is based on a *marginal probability* model of the data, where the scientific mechanisms are partially hidden by integration.

A lot of ink has been devoted to whether frequentist or Bayesian probability models are better. We believe that the bigger issue is whether marginal-probability or conditional-probability models should be used, and we are decidedly in the conditional-probability camp. As Statistics has become more a Science than a branch of Mathematics, conditional-probability modeling has shown its power to express uncertainties in all aspects of a scientific investigation. Such models have been called *hierarchical statistical models* (sometimes referred to as latent models or multilevel models); see Section 2.1.

Bayes' Theorem is a fundamental result in probability theory that allows an inverse calculation of the conditional probability of the unknowns (process and parameters) given the data (Bayes, 1763). Inference on the unknowns is based on this conditional probability distribution (called the *posterior distribution*), but the formula depends on a normalizing constant that is typically intractible (see Section 2.1).

Breakthroughs in the last 20 years have shown how an analytical derivation of the normalizing constant can be avoided by a judicious use of, for example, a Monte Carlo sampler from a Markov chain whose stationary distribution is the posterior distribution (see Section 2.3). This has made feasible the statistical analysis of scientific problems in the presence of uncertainty, based on hierarchical statistical models that can be of great complexity. But this comes with great responsibility; just because we can handle a lot of complexity, it does not mean that we should. This echoes our earlier comments at the beginning of this chapter, when discussing the Goldilocks Principle of model building.

Hierarchical Statistical Modeling

Hierarchical statistical modeling represents a way to express uncertainties through well defined levels of conditional probabilities. We follow Berliner's (1996) terminology: At the top level is the *data model*, which expresses the distribution of the data given a hidden process. This hidden process can be thought of as the "true process," uncorrupted by any measurement of it. At the level directly underneath the data model is the *process model,* which models scientific uncertainty in the hidden ("true") process through a probability distribution of the phenomenon of interest. It is quite possible that the process model is itself made up of submodels whose uncertainties are also expressed at sublevels through conditional probabilities. In a sense, the whole approach is a sort of analysis-of-variance decomposition that is more general than the usual additive decomposition given in standard textbooks (e.g., Scheffé, 1959). The result is a *hierarchical model* (HM); see Section 2.1.

The components of a HM are *conditional probability distributions* that, when multiplied together, yield the joint probability distribution of all quantities in the model. The quantities in which we are interested could be as simple as random variables and as complicated as space–time stochastic processes of random sets.

Of course, all the conditional probability distributions specified in the HM typically depend on unknown parameters. If a lower level (underneath the data model and the process model) is established by specifying the joint probability distribution of all the unknown parameters, then the HM qualifies to be called a *Bayesian Hierarachical Model* (BHM). This probability model at the lowest level, which we call the *parameter model*, completes the sequence: data model (top level) followed by process model (second level) followed by parameter model (bottom level); see Section 2.1.1. An alternative approach to specifying the parameter model is to *estimate* the parameters using the data. This might be called an *Empirical Hierarchical Model* (EHM), although historically it has often been called an empirical-Bayesian model; see Section 2.1.2. We prefer the nomenclature EHM, to contrast it with BHM.

Uncertainty and the Role of Statistics, Revisited

It is worth reflecting on how far we have come in this discussion of statistical modeling. We are not rejecting R. A. Fisher's paradigm of controlled scientific experiments; on the contrary, such experiments allow the statistician and scientist to build the suite of conditional probability models needed for hierarchical statistical modeling. For example, when water quality is measured through chemical assays, it is common to send duplicates and "blanks" (i.e., pure water) through the laboratory to gain knowledge about the measurement error in the data model. Furthermore, periodic recalibration of instruments guards against instrument drift over time and possible bias in the measurement errors. In agriculture, uniformity trials (where crops are grown but no treatments are applied to those crops) enable the scientist to build realistic, often spatial, process models. The HM paradigm enables a coherent use of all data and, using models of spatio-temporal statistical dependence, allows inference on parts where there are *no* data at all! Scientific relationships incorporated into the process and parameter models can mitigate the paucity of data. Furthermore, there is a self-correcting mechanism in hierarchical statistical modeling; when there is little known about the scientific relationships or there are poor-quality or few data available, then inferences have very low precision. That is, a signal in the process may be there, but if scientific knowledge or the data are limited, the HM approach will not let us discover it.

Looking at this from another angle, the best scientists collect the best data to build the best (conditional-probability) models to make the most precise inferences in the shortest amount of time. In reality, compromises at every stage may be needed, and we could add that the best scientists make the best compromises!

We conclude by saying that Science cannot be done "by the numbers." Good scientists require just as much inspiration as good artists, and indeed there is a view that they are symbiotic (Shlain, 1991; Osserman, 1995). To this we add Statistics, and particularly hierarchical statistical modeling, where data, Science, and uncertainty join forces.

Summary of the Book
This is a four-color book where not only is color used in the figures, but it is also used strategically in the text. Where appropriate, the data model is in green, the process model is in blue, the parameter model is in purple, and the posterior distribution is in red. Chapter 1 has introduced the broad philosophy of Statistics (with a capital "S") and its role in the scientific method. This is formalized in Chapter 2, where more notation, more methodology, and more statistical concepts are introduced. Readers have a choice at this point. Those unfamiliar with Statistics for temporal data could read Chapter 3, which reviews the fundamentals of temporal processes (i.e., dynamical systems and time series). Those unfamiliar with Statistics for spatial data could read Chapter 4, which reviews the fundamentals of spatial random processes. Those who are familiar with both could "Pass Go" and proceed to Chapter 5.

Chapter 5 introduces spatio-temporal statistical methodology through data, recognizing its roots in Science. Chapter 6 reviews the statistical models that have been used for analyzing spatio-temporal data. This book features dynamical spatio-temporal statistical models (DSTMs), and Chapter 7 gives a comprehensive exposition of them in the context of hierarchical statistical models. Implementation and inference for DSTMs in the hierarchical-modeling framework are presented in Chapter 8. Finally, a number of examples that illustrate Statistics for spatio-temporal data are given in the sections of Chapter 9.

CHAPTER 2

Statistical Preliminaries

In this chapter, we expand on some of the ideas presented in Chapter 1, as well as present some statistical results needed for the rest of the book. We give an overview of how Statistics and Science have related to each other in the past, and we give a viewpoint for how Statistical Science will evolve in the twenty-first century. We are deliberately broad and not overly technical in this chapter, for readers who have not yet had a lot of exposure to Statistics. Here we address general issues to help explain the statistical modeling and inference decisions made in the spatial, temporal, and spatio-temporal contexts of the subsequent chapters.

Several explanations of terminology are needed before we start. Uncertainty in data, processes, or parameters means there will be uncertainty in conclusions. Statisticians call this drawing of conclusions in the presence of uncertainty, *statistical inference* (or just *inference*); in this book, inference will be either *estimation* of fixed but unknown parameters, or *prediction* of unknown random quantities. (Notice that "forecasting," namely concluding something about the future, is a special case of "prediction.")

The terms *normal distribution* and *Gaussian distribution* are synonymous. In this book, we prefer the latter and use the expression $Z \sim Gau(\mu, \sigma^2)$ to denote a random variable Z whose probability distribution is Gaussian (i.e., normal) with mean μ and variance σ^2; it is equivalent to the expression $Z \sim N(\mu, \sigma^2)$, which one might see in other books or articles. The random vector $\mathbf{Z} \equiv (Z_1, \ldots, Z_m)'$ is an m-dimensional column vector, where the symbol "'" means *transpose*. Then $\mathbf{Z} \sim Gau(\boldsymbol{\mu}, \boldsymbol{\Sigma})$ denotes an m-dimensional Gaussian distribution with mean vector $\boldsymbol{\mu}$ and covariance matrix $\boldsymbol{\Sigma}$. The covariance matrix $\boldsymbol{\Sigma}$ (sometimes called a variance matrix or a variance–covariance matrix) is a symmetric, positive-definite (occasionally nonnegative-definite) $m \times m$ matrix whose (i, j)th entry is $cov(Z_i, Z_j)$; $i, j = 1, \ldots, m$.

Statistics for Spatio-Temporal Data, by Noel Cressie and Christopher K. Wikle
Copyright © 2011 John Wiley & Sons, Inc.

Let $[A]$ denote the probability distribution of the random quantity A. For example, the expression, $Z \sim Gau(\mu, \sigma^2)$, is equivalently written as

$$[Z] = \{(2\pi\sigma^2)^{-1/2} \exp[-(1/2)(z - \mu)^2/\sigma^2]: z \in \mathbb{R}\},$$

and $\mathbf{Z} \sim Gau(\boldsymbol{\mu}, \boldsymbol{\Sigma})$, where $\mathbf{Z} = (Z_1, \ldots, Z_m)'$, is written as

$$[\mathbf{Z}] = \{(2\pi)^{-m/2}|\boldsymbol{\Sigma}|^{-1/2} \exp[-(1/2)(\mathbf{Z} - \boldsymbol{\mu})'\boldsymbol{\Sigma}^{-1}(\mathbf{Z} - \boldsymbol{\mu})]: \mathbf{z} \in \mathbb{R}^m\}.$$

If $g(A)$ is a well defined random quantity for some function $g(\cdot)$, then its *expectation*, $E(g(A))$, is equivalently written as $E(g(A)) = \int g(A)[A] \, dA$ in the continuous case, and is written as $E(g(A)) = \Sigma g(A)[A]$ in the discrete case.

Furthermore, let $[A|B]$ denote the conditional distribution of the random quantity A, conditional on specifying a particular value of (the random quantity) B. This is also referred to as the conditional distribution of A given B. For example, the expression, $\mathbf{Z}|\mathbf{Y} = \mathbf{y} \sim Gau(\mathbf{y}, \sigma^2\mathbf{I})$, is equivalently written as

$$[\mathbf{Z}|\mathbf{Y}] = \{(2\pi\sigma^2)^{-m/2} \exp[-(1/2)(\mathbf{z} - \mathbf{y})'(\mathbf{z} - \mathbf{y})/\sigma^2]: \mathbf{z} \in \mathbb{R}^m\},$$

where it is understood that on the left-hand side, $\mathbf{Y} = \mathbf{y}$.

Let the spatial domain of interest be $D_s \subset \mathbb{R}^d$, a subset of d-dimensional Euclidean space, and let the temporal domain of interest be $D_t \subset \mathbb{R}^1$. The spatial index $\mathbf{s}$ (a d-dimensional vector) and the temporal index t (a real number) can vary continuously or discretely over their respective domains, D_s and D_t. This book is concerned, amongst other things, with models for spatio-temporal random processes. When t varies continuously, we write the generic process as $\{Y(\mathbf{s}; t): \mathbf{s} \in D_s, t \in D_t\}$. To follow the usual notational convention for time series, when t varies *discretely*, we write instead $\{Y_t(\mathbf{s}): \mathbf{s} \in D_s, t \in D_t\}$.

Spatial Description and Temporal Dynamics: A Simple Example

The best way to compare space and time in our statistical context is to consider a simple example, where we let $d = 1$, $D_s = \{s_0, s_0 + \Delta, \ldots, s_0 + 24\Delta\}$, and $D_t = \{0, 1, 2, \ldots\}$. Think about D_s as being an east–west transect of regular spacing Δ in a field of wild prairie grass, where the observations on the process $\{Y_{t_0}(s_0), \ldots, Y_{t_0}(s_0 + 24\Delta)\}$ are nondestructive-biomass measurements taken at 25 equally spaced spatial locations $\{s_0, \ldots, s_{24}\} \equiv \{s_0, \ldots, s_0 + 24\Delta\}$, at a fixed point in time $(t = t_0)$: 3 pm on a given day in the middle of a given spring. Compare the spatial process $\{Y_{t_0}(s_0), \ldots, Y_{t_0}(s_0 + 24\Delta)\}$ to the temporal process $\{Y_t(s_0): t = t_0, \ldots, t_0 + 24\}$ of nondestructive-biomass measurements taken at the fixed spatial location $s = s_0$, at 3 pm for each of 25 consecutive days in the middle of the same spring.

Define the *spatial process* at the fixed time point t_0 to be

$$\mathbf{Y}_{t_0} \equiv (Y_{t_0}(s_0), \ldots, Y_{t_0}(s_0 + 24\Delta))',$$

and define the *temporal process* at fixed spatial location s_0 to be

$$\mathbf{Y}(s_0) \equiv (Y_{t_0}(s_0), \dots, Y_{t_0+24}(s_0))'.$$

By comparing spatial statistical models for $\mathbf{Y}_{t_0}$ and time series models for $\mathbf{Y}(s_0)$, we can see to what extent space is modeled differently from time.

A simple departure from independence for a *spatial process* is nearest-neighbor dependence expressed through conditional distributions. Assume, for $i = 1, \dots, 23$, the Gaussian (conditional) distribution

$$Y_{t_0}(s_i) \mid \{Y_{t_0}(s_j): j \neq i\}$$
$$\sim Gau((\phi_{t_0}/(1 + \phi_{t_0}^2))\{Y_{t_0}(s_{i-1}) + Y_{t_0}(s_{i+1})\}, \sigma_{t_0}^2/(1 + \phi_{t_0}^2)), \quad (2.1)$$

where recall that $s_i \equiv s_0 + i\Delta$; $i = 0, \dots, 24$. On the edges of the transect, assume

$$Y_{t_0}(s_0) \mid \{Y_{t_0}(s_j): j \neq 0\} \sim Gau(\phi_{t_0} Y_{t_0}(s_1), \sigma_{t_0}^2),$$
$$Y_{t_0}(s_{24}) \mid \{Y_{t_0}(s_j): j \neq 24\} \sim Gau(\phi_{t_0} Y_{t_0}(s_{23}), \sigma_{t_0}^2).$$

In (2.1), assume that the *spatial-dependence parameter* ϕ_{t_0} satisfies $|\phi_{t_0}| \leq 1$. It can be shown that $E(\mathbf{Y}_{t_0}) = \mathbf{0}$, and the correlation between nearest neighbors is (Section 4.2)

$$\text{corr}(Y_{t_0}(s_i), Y_{t_0}(s_{i-1})) = \phi_{t_0}, \qquad i = 1, \dots, 24.$$

A simple departure from independence for a *time series* is a first-order autoregressive process. Assume that

$$Y_t(s_0) = \phi(s_0) Y_{t-1}(s_0) + \varepsilon_t, \qquad t = t_0 + 1, \dots, t_0 + 24, \qquad (2.2)$$

where ε_t is independent of $Y_{t-1}(s_0)$, and $\varepsilon_t \sim ind. Gau(0, \sigma^2(s_0))$, for $t = t_0, t_0 + 1, \dots, t_0 + 24$. To initialize the process, assume

$$Y_{t_0}(s_0) \sim Gau(0, \sigma^2(s_0)/(1 - \phi(s_0)^2)).$$

In (2.2), we assume that the temporal-dependence parameter $\phi(s_0)$ satisfies $|\phi(s_0)| < 1$. It can be shown that $E(\mathbf{Y}(s_0)) = \mathbf{0}$ and the correlation between two adjacent time points is (Section 3.4.3)

$$\text{corr}(Y_{t-1}(s_0), Y_t(s_0)) = \phi(s_0), \qquad t = t_0 + 1, \dots, t_0 + 24.$$

The process (2.2) is *dynamical* in that it shows how current values are related mechanistically to past values. Generally, the dependence of current values on past values is expressed probabilistically, and (2.2) has an equivalent probabilistic expression:

$$Y_t(s_0)|Y_{t-1}(s_0), \ldots, Y_{t_0}(s_0) \sim Gau(\phi(s_0)Y_{t-1}(s_0), \sigma^2(s_0)).$$

Such time series models are sometimes referred to as causal (Section 3.4.3).

Notice the similarity between the spatial process (2.1) and the time series (2.2). Both are Gaussian, zero mean; and if $\phi_{t_0} = \phi(s_0)$, they imply the *same* correlation between adjacent random variables. In fact, as we show in Section 4.2, if $\phi_{t_0} = \phi(s_0)$, then the processes are probabilistically identical! However, the spatial process (2.1) looks east and west for dependence, in contrast to the time series (2.2), which looks to the past. The example has a cautionary aspect. Clearly, a *description* of the properties of spatial or temporal statistical dependence of the model through just moments or even joint probability distributions can completely miss the genesis of the statistical dependence, such as the *dynamical* structure given by (2.2).

Now, when it comes to considering space and time together, we believe that (whenever possible) the temporal dependence should be expressed dynamically, based on physical/chemical/biological/economic/etc. theory, since here the etiology of the phenomenon is clearest. In a contribution to the Statistics literature that was well ahead of its time, Hotelling (1927) gave various statistical analyses based on stochastic differential equations (albeit without a spatial dimension). Our approach contrasts to that of some others, where time is treated as an extra (although different) dimension, and descriptive expressions of spatial dependencies are modified to account for the temporal dimension; see Section 6.1 for further discussion of the two approaches.

2.1 CONDITIONAL PROBABILITIES AND HIERARCHICAL MODELING (HM)

There is a very general way to express uncertainties coming from different sources, through an approach known as hierarchical (statistical) modeling. Chapter 1 gives a discussion of the HM approach through the introduction of a data model and a process model, where the uncertainties are expressed in terms of *conditional probabilities*. This book is about Statistics for spatio-temporal data, and the quantities we are interested in could be as complicated as spatio-temporal stochastic processes of random variables, random vectors, or random sets.

The conditional-probability distributions specified in the hierarchical model (also abbreviated as HM) typically depend on unknown parameters. If a parameter model is included in the HM, in order to express probabilistically the uncertainty on the parameters, the HM is called a *Bayesian Hierarchical Model* (BHM); see Chapter 1. An alternative approach to specifying a prior distribution is to assume that the parameters are fixed and to estimate them using the data; they are then substituted into the data model and the process model as if they were known. The result is an *Empirical Hierarchical Model* (EHM); also see Chapter 1. We note here (and later in the chapter) that it is possible to put prior distributions on some parameters and to estimate others. In this book, we typically use the term "prior distribution" to be synonymous with "parameter model." However, we recognize that prior information goes into all three components of the hierarchical model. Traditionally, Bayesians have considered what we call the process and parameter distributions to make up the prior distribution. We do not disagree with this but simply prefer to make a distinction between the process and parameters whenever possible.

Consider three generic quantities of interest, Z, Y, and θ, in the HM; for expository purposes we often consider these simply to be random variables. Think of Z as data, Y as a (hidden) process that we wish to predict, and θ as unknown parameters. In a realistic example where Z, Y, and θ are more complicated random quantities, say for spatial statistical mapping of a region's air quality in a given week, Z might be 100-dimensional, Y might be 1000-dimensional, and θ might be five-dimensional. Based on Z, we wish to make inference on Y and θ. That is, in a BHM, we wish to predict both Y and θ; and in an EHM, we wish to predict Y and to estimate/predict θ.

We now give some basic results from probability theory. Recall the notation $[A]$ and $[A|B]$ for marginal and conditional probability distributions, respectively. Then the joint distribution of A and B can be written as

$$[A, B] = [A|B][B], \tag{2.3}$$

and the law of total probability can be written as

$$[A] = \int [A|B][B] \, dB, \tag{2.4}$$

where recall that $\int g(B)[B] \, dB$ denotes the expectation (either an integral or a summation in the case where B is a discrete random quantity) of some function $g(B)$ of B. Finally, in terms of this notation, *Bayes' Theorem* (Bayes, 1763) can be written as

$$[B|A] = \frac{[A|B][B]}{\int [A|B][B] \, dB} = \frac{[A|B][B]}{[A]}. \tag{2.5}$$

2.1.1 Bayesian Hierarchical Modeling (BHM)

The basic representation of a BHM is obtained by splitting up the model into three levels (Berliner, 1996):

Data model: $[Z|Y, \theta]$

Process model: $[Y|\theta]$

Parameter model: $[\theta]$.

Note that sometimes we write $[Z|Y, \theta_D]$ and $[Y|\theta_P]$ to emphasize the data-model parameters θ_D and the process-model parameters θ_P. Then $\theta = \{\theta_D, \theta_P\}$, and the parameter model is $[\theta_D, \theta_P]$.

Now the joint distribution can be decomposed recursively. From (2.3), we have

$$[Z, Y, \theta] = [Z, Y|\theta][\theta]$$

$$= [Z|Y, \theta][Y|\theta][\theta], \tag{2.6}$$

which is simply a product of the data model, the process model, and the parameter model. A special case would be where $\theta = \theta_0$, known, and $[\theta]$ concentrates all its probability at θ_0.

Bayes' Theorem gives the conditional distribution of Y and θ, given the data Z, which is typically called the *posterior distribution*. From (2.5), we obtain

$$[Y, \theta|Z] = \frac{[Z|Y, \theta][Y, \theta]}{\iint [Z|Y, \theta][Y, \theta]\, dY d\theta}$$

$$= \frac{[Z|Y, \theta][Y|\theta][\theta]}{\iint [Z|Y, \theta][Y|\theta][\theta]\, dY d\theta}$$

$$= \frac{[Z|Y, \theta][Y|\theta][\theta]}{[Z]}. \tag{2.7}$$

Within the framework of Bayesian decision theory, all inference on Y and θ in the BHM depends on this distribution.

Suppose that the data come in two "bursts," $Z^{(1)}$ followed by $Z^{(2)}$. After the first burst of data, $Z^{(1)}$, the posterior distribution is

$$[Y, \theta|Z^{(1)}] = [Y|\theta, Z^{(1)}][\theta|Z^{(1)}]; \tag{2.8}$$

think of the two probability distributions on the right-hand side of (2.8) as the "updated" process model and the "updated" parameter model, respectively. The updated probability distributions represent *scientific learning* about Y and θ, respectively. From (2.7) the posterior distribution is proportional to

$$[Z^{(1)}|Y, \theta][Y|\theta][\theta].$$

Now, after the second burst of data, $Z^{(2)}$, the posterior distribution should be recalculated:

$$[Y, \theta|Z^{(1)}, Z^{(2)}] = \frac{[Z^{(1)}, Z^{(2)}|Y, \theta][Y, \theta]}{[Z^{(1)}, Z^{(2)}]}$$

$$= \frac{[Z^{(2)}|Y, \theta, Z^{(1)}][Y, \theta|Z^{(1)}]}{[Z^{(2)}|Z^{(1)}]}, \tag{2.9}$$

which shows how "today's posterior becomes tomorrow's prior." Substituting (2.8) into (2.9) shows that the posterior distribution is proportional to

$$[Z^{(2)}|Y, \theta, Z^{(1)}][Y|\theta, Z^{(1)}][\theta|Z^{(1)}].$$

This expression shows that the posterior distribution is proportional to the product of the updated data model, the updated process model, and the updated parameter model. This is the essence of the sequential implementation given in Section 8.1.1. Furthermore, it is often the case that, given the process Y, $Z^{(1)}$ will not affect the conditional distribution of Y. That is, the first term in this expression often simplies to $[Z^{(2)}|Y, \theta]$.

Since data can come sequentially, these simple calculations are very relevant to how scientists can ascend the knowledge pyramid (see Chapter 1). That is, Bayes' Theorem allows knowledge to be continually improved in a coherent manner.

The numerator in (2.7) is a straightforward product of the individual components of the BHM, but a major problem usually arises when calculating the denominator. The denominator is the normalizing constant that ensures that the posterior distribution has total probability equal to 1. (Because the posterior distribution is conditional on Z, in fact the normalizing "constant" depends on Z.)

When Y and θ are each random variables, the integral in the denominator of (2.7),

$$[Z] = \iint [Z|Y, \theta][Y|\theta][\theta] \, dY \, d\theta,$$

is only two-dimensional and usually quite easy to calculate using numerical quadrature. However, spatio-temporal BHMs can often yield integrals that are of dimensions on the order of thousands (e.g., Wikle, Berliner, and Cressie, 1998). In the last 20 years, computational breakthroughs have been made so that rather than calculating the posterior distribution analytically or numerically, one can often *simulate* from it (Section 2.3). These computational methods, including Markov chain Monte Carlo (MCMC) and importance sampling (IS), have brought HM into the panoply of many statisticians, including those concerned with modeling spatio-temporal data.

2.1.2 Empirical Hierarchical Modeling (EHM)

The following two-level model also qualifies to be called a HM:

Data model: $[Z|Y, \theta]$
Process model: $[Y|\theta]$,

where it is assumed that the parameter θ is *fixed*, but unknown. Formally, one could still consider a third level, but where the parameter model $[\theta]$ concentrates all its probability at the fixed θ. Recall that sometimes we emphasize the data-model parameters as θ_D and the process model parameters as θ_P by writing the two-level model as $[Z|Y, \theta_D]$, $[Y|\theta_P]$, and $\theta = \{\theta_D, \theta_P\}$.

In an EHM, all probability distributions are conditional on θ. Inference on Y depends on the distribution

$$[Y|Z, \theta] = \frac{[Z|Y, \theta][Y|\theta]}{[Z|\theta]}, \tag{2.10}$$

where $[Z|\theta] = \int [Z|Y, \theta][Y|\theta] dY$. Equation (2.10) is sometimes called the *predictive distribution*, but in this book we take some license and continue to call it the posterior distribution. The difference between (2.7) and (2.10) is clear, and which one is used as the posterior distribution depends on the type of HM fitted. Notice that the integral in the denominator of (2.10) is lower dimensional than that in (2.7), but it could still be of a dimension on the order of thousands. The "Empirical" part of the EHM arises from the practice of replacing (2.10) with $[Y|Z, \widehat{\theta}]$, where $\widehat{\theta}$ is an *estimator* of θ (i.e., depends only on the data Z). It is also possible that θ is estimated from an independent study.

Importantly, (2.10) does not require explicit specification of a prior distribution for the parameters, a task that some statisticians are reluctant to do. It can also be the case that (2.10) is faster to compute than (2.7). The price of not specifying uncertainty in the parameter θ is that inferences on Y are generally too liberal, since a simple substitution of $\widehat{\theta}$ for θ does not account for the extra variability associated with the estimation of θ (e.g., Carlin and Louis, 2000, Chapter 4; Kang, Liu, and Cressie, 2009). This can result in misleading inferences for say g(Y), where g(·) is a nonlinear functional (Ghosh, 1992; Stern and Cressie, 1999). Second-order adjustments to these inferences on Y to account for the variability in $\widehat{\theta}$ are available for simple cases (e.g., Rao, 2003, Section 6.2).

We have already noted that some parameters might have a prior distribution specified for them and some might be assumed fixed but unknown and estimated. This is the case in the example that follows, where an EHM was used to search for a missing nuclear submarine.

2.1.3   Search for the USS Scorpion

In late May 1968, for reasons that are still unclear, the USS *Scorpion* (SSN-589), a nuclear submarine, was lost at sea as it was returning to its naval base at Norfolk, Virginia. An official search for the vessel was started in early June of 1968, in an area of the Atlantic Ocean approximately 400 miles southwest of the Azores (Richardson and Stone, 1971). The search was complicated by the remoteness and extreme depth of this part of the ocean, the lack of certainty as to the location of the *Scorpion* when it (presumably) went down, and the cause of its sinking. Because of success in using Bayesian statistical methods to find a hydrogen bomb lost in the Mediterranean Sea in 1966, scientists at the U.S. Naval Research Laboratory (NRL) implemented a hierarchical statistical search procedure to help find the *Scorpion*. This procedure is conceptually simple (but can have practical challenges) and provides an introduction to the power of HM.

The idea is first to define a spatial "grid" and to propose a first guess (prior) of the probabilities that the object in question (here, the *Scorpion*) is located in each of the grid boxes. The prior probabilities suggest which grid box to search first. If the object is not found in that box, the prior probabilities are then updated (yielding the posterior), and the process is repeated until the object is found. This procedure suggests a fairly simple HM.

Assume that the domain of interest is a part of the ocean floor we call D_s, which is made up of n spatial areas (i.e., grid boxes). Let $Y_i = 1$ if the submarine is in the ith grid box, and let $Y_i = 0$ if it is not; $i = 1, \ldots, n$. Now, it is critical to recognize that when a grid box is searched, there is a chance that, even if the submarine is present, it will not be detected. So, let $Z_i = 1$ if the submarine is found in the ith grid box, and $Z_i = 0$ if not. Borrowing from the terminology associated with occupancy modeling in Ecology (e.g., Royle and Dorazio, 2008, p. 100), we distinguish between the *detection probability*,

$$p_i = \Pr(Z_i = 1 | Y_i = 1), \qquad i = 1, \ldots, n,$$

which is a conditional probability, and the *occurrence probability*,

$$\pi_i = \Pr(Y_i = 1), \qquad i = 1, \ldots, n.$$

This suggests an HM of the following form:

Data model: $Z_i | Y_i \sim ind.\ Ber(Y_i p_i), \qquad i = 1, \ldots, n$

Process model: $Y_i \sim ind.\ Ber(\pi_i), \qquad i = 1, \ldots, n,$

where, for now, we assume that $\{p_i\}$ and $\{\pi_i\}$ are known or (more realistically) determined by expert opinion; and $Ber(p)$ denotes the Bernoulli distribution of a binary random variable, where p is the probability of obtaining a "1." Note that this HM suggests that if the submarine is not in the ith grid box (i.e., $Y_i = 0$), then $Z_i = 0$. If it is in the ith grid box, Z_i follows a Bernoulli distribution with (detection) probability p_i.

Now, assume that the ith grid box is searched and the submarine is not found (i.e., $Z_i = 0$). In this case, the probability that the submarine is in the ith grid box (i.e., $Y_i = 1$) is updated using Bayes' Theorem. This yields the posterior probability,

$$
\begin{aligned}
&\Pr(Y_i = 1 | Z_i = 0) \\
&= \frac{\Pr(Z_i = 0 | Y_i = 1)\Pr(Y_i = 1)}{\Pr(Z_i = 0)} \\
&= \frac{\Pr(Z_i = 0 | Y_i = 1)\Pr(Y_i = 1)}{\Pr(Z_i = 0 | Y_i = 1)\Pr(Y_i = 1) + \Pr(Z_i = 0 | Y_i = 0)\Pr(Y_i = 0)} \\
&= \frac{(1 - p_i)\pi_i}{(1 - p_i)\pi_i + (1)(1 - \pi_i)} \\
&= \frac{(1 - p_i)\pi_i}{1 - p_i\pi_i},
\end{aligned}
$$

where we assume that there are no false-positive detections (i.e., $\Pr(Z_i = 0|Y_i = 0) = 1$). Note that the posterior probability of the submarine being in the ith grid box is *less* than or equal to the prior probability π_i, given that the submarine was not observed there.

If the submarine is not detected in the ith grid box, then this should also affect the posterior probability in the other grid boxes. For example, consider the jth grid box, where $j \neq i$. Then,

$$\Pr(Y_j = 1|Z_i = 0) = \frac{\Pr(Z_i = 0|Y_j = 1)\Pr(Y_j = 1)}{\Pr(Z_i = 0)}$$

$$= \frac{\pi_j}{1 - p_i\pi_i},$$

where we further assume that there is only one submarine and, hence, $\Pr(Z_i = 0|Y_j = 1) = 1; \ j \neq i$. Thus, the posterior probability of the submarine being in the jth grid box is *greater* than or equal to the prior probability π_j, given that the submarine is not detected in a different (i.e., the ith) grid box. These new posterior probabilities would then become the prior probabilities in a sequential procedure that would help determine which grid box should be searched next. Recall that "today's posterior becomes tomorrow's prior."

In practice, the parameters $\{p_i\}$ and $\{\pi_i\}$ need to be estimated (EHM), or other information could be used to specify them with more or less uncertainty (BHM). In the actual search for the *Scorpion*, the probabilities $\{\pi_i\}$ were determined from subjective expert opinions and physical/scientific information. NRL scientists Dr. J.P. Craven and Dr. F.A. Andrews considered nine plausible scenarios associated with the (presumed) accident that led to the disappearance of the *Scorpion*. For each of these, they assigned weights, based in part on "the views and opinions of Navy operating personnel as well as the analysis of specialists in many scientific areas" (Richardson and Stone, 1971, p. 144). Basically, for each scenario, "... the movement of the submarine ... [was] then simulated with random numbers drawn as required to represent the uncertainties in course, speed, and position, at the time the emergency occurred, as well as other variables" (Richardson and Stone, 1971, p. 144–145). In the search, a 20×20 grid (i.e., $n = 400$) was considered, and the probabilities $\{\pi_i : i = 1, \dots, 400\}$ were calculated and assigned. The assignment was in no way uniform; in fact, two grid boxes accounted for 23% of the total probability.

A great deal of scientific and engineering expertise went into determining the detection probabilities, $\{p_i\}$, as well. There were multiple instruments used in the search, all with different degrees of detectibility, and operational procedures actually used to conduct the search had to be factored in (Richardson and Stone, 1971). On October 28, 1968, the *Scorpion* was located and its location was within 260 yards of the edge of the grid box with the highest initial prior probability! Unfortunately, it sank in very deep water, its hull was crushed, and all 99 officers and crew were lost.

2.1.4 "Classical" Statistical Modeling

While it might seem unusual, we use "classical" as an adjective here for both frequentist and Bayesian modeling. The HM introduces data Z, process Y, and parameters θ; however, the "classical" model found in the work of Fisher (e.g., Fisher, 1935) has only data Z and parameters θ, as does the contribution of Bayes and many who followed him (e.g., Press, 1989). "Classical" frequentists base their inference on the *likelihood*, $[Z|\theta]$. "Classical" Bayesians base their inferences on the posterior distribution, $[\theta|Z]$, which requires *both* a likelihood and a *prior* (i.e., $[\theta]$) to be specified. Both classical approaches miss the fundamental importance of modeling the process Y, where the Physics/Chemistry/Biology/Economics/etc. typically resides.

To be sure, Statistics has played an important role in Science, but often using blunt instruments, like correlation and regression analyses. Without Y being made explicit in statistical models, Science has often chosen its own statistical path, since it is on Y that scientific theories are postulated. Scientists also know that parameters θ are important; these might be starting values, or boundary conditions, or diffusion constants, or etc. In what follows, we give a deliberately simplistic description of how a scientist might view the role of Statistics, although we note that this is changing fast. One of the goals of this book is to accelerate this change.

Scientific experiments produce data Z, and variability in the data is generally recognized. One approach in Science to analyzing the data (to support, refine, or refute a scientific theory) has been to "smooth" them first. Consider the smoother f and write

$$\widetilde{Y} = f(Z).$$

The scientist might then assume that any (random) variability has been *removed* and that $\widetilde{Y}$ can now be considered the true process with no uncertainty. Less extreme would be to assume that $\widetilde{Y}$ and the true process Y are "close." The scientist might then fit a model for Y using the "data" $\widetilde{Y}$. If the model for Y is $[Y|\theta_P]$, namely a process model that recognizes uncertainty, the scientist might use "classical" Statistics to fit $[Y|\theta_P]$ to $\widetilde{Y}$. Science alert! Control of uncertainty has been lost. While the approach just described can work sometimes, typically when the "signal" is strong, it also has the potential to declare the presence of a "signal" when it may simply be the result of chance fluctuations.

Given the data are to be smoothed, it should be recognized that they are often a combination of raw observations and algorithmic manipulation. The statistician might write instead

$$\widetilde{Z} = f(Z), \tag{2.11}$$

where the notation $\widetilde{Z}$ in (2.11) is used to suggest a fundamental divide between the two approaches.

Now, a hierarchical statistical model can be fitted using the data $\widetilde{Z}$, where the data model $[\widetilde{Z}|Y, \theta_D]$ recognizes any remaining uncertainty in $\widetilde{Z}$. Inference is based on the posterior distribution, which we choose to show here for an EHM:

$$[Y|\widetilde{Z}, \theta_D, \theta_P] \propto [\widetilde{Z}|Y, \theta_D][Y|\theta_P]. \tag{2.12}$$

At first glance, it may seem that thinking of the smoothed data as $\widetilde{Z}$ in (2.11) (rather than as $\widetilde{Y}$) is inconsequential, but we believe that this notational prop guides us (statisticians and scientists, alike) through our "uncertainty audit."

While the picture painted above is simplistic, it does illustrate that Statistics has often failed to establish its proper presence in Science. Scientific interest is in Y, and if a classical frequentist statistician were to fit the scientific model $[Y|\theta_P]$ directly to $\widetilde{Z}$, it should be done through the (marginal) model,

$$[\widetilde{Z}|\theta_D, \theta_P] = \int [\widetilde{Z}|Y, \theta_D][Y|\theta_P]dY.$$

That is, the classical frequentist should integrate out Y; alas, if there is no recognition of Y in the first place, the model chosen to be fitted, $[\widetilde{Z}|\theta]$, may be difficult to interpret scientifically or, worse yet, may be inappropriately interpreted.

In this book, we would like to take Science on a path where original observations Z are used as much as possible, where smoothed data are thought of as $\widetilde{Z}$, where uncertainties are captured in an HM using conditional probabilities, and where inference is based on the posterior distribution, such as (2.12) or its BHM version. This is the statistical tool needed for scientists to ascend the knowledge pyramid (Chapter 1).

2.1.5 Hierarchical Statistical Modeling

The real power of the HM becomes apparent when dependencies become complicated. Each component distribution can be decomposed further if necessary, and they may be simplified with modeling assumptions. In what follows, we give examples and a discussion of HM's strengths and limitations, based on the presentation found in Cressie et al. (2009).

Data Model

Say we are interested in a process Y for which we have several different data sets, Z_1, Z_2, Z_3, all of which measure the process Y with uncertainty, and perhaps they are measured at different spatial or temporal scales. It is often possible in such cases to make the following data-modeling assumption:

$$[Z_1, Z_2, Z_3|Y, \theta_D] = [Z_1|Y, \theta_{D,1}][Z_2|Y, \theta_{D,2}][Z_3|Y, \theta_{D,3}],$$

where the *data-model parameters* θ_D are here given by $\{\theta_{D,1}, \theta_{D,2}, \theta_{D,3}\}$. That is, we might assume that the different datasets are independent, conditional upon the true process. Although such an assumption must be justified, it is often plausible and provides a very convenient approach for synthesizing various types of observations. The parameters in each of the component distributions can accommodate changes of resolution and alignment, as well as different measurement-error characteristics (e.g., Gelfand, Zhu, and Carlin, 2001; Wikle and Berliner, 2005). This is discussed further in Sections 4.1.3 and 7.1.2.

It is also the case that different datasets that correspond to different processes (or parameters) can be combined. For example, assume we have two datasets, Z_1 and Z_2, corresponding to the processes Y_1 and Y_2, respectively, where $Y = (Y_1, Y_2)$. We can often make use of conditional-independence assumptions, as follows:

$$[Z_1, Z_2|Y, \theta_D] = [Z_1|Y_1, \theta_{D,1}][Z_2|Y_2, \theta_{D,2}],$$

where the data-model parameters are here given by $\theta_D = \{\theta_{D,1}, \theta_{D,2}\}$.

Process Model
Decomposition of process-model distributions can also be considered. For example, consider Y to be made up of two subprocesses, Y_1 and Y_2, as in the example just above. We can often make use of conditional-probability modeling in this context:

$$[Y_1, Y_2|\theta_P] = [Y_1|Y_2, \theta_P][Y_2|\theta_P],$$

where θ_P are the *process-model parameters*. That is, it is often possible to simplify the joint interaction of two components of the process by using conditional probabilities.

A well known example of this occurs in a time series model with Markov assumptions (Section 3.4.3). Specifically, consider the time series, $Y_1, Y_2, \ldots, Y_{T-1}, Y_T$; it is often very difficult to specify the joint distribution of all of these random variables. However, consider the conditional-probability factorization:

$$[Y_T, \ldots, Y_1] = [Y_T|Y_{T-1}, \ldots, Y_1][Y_{T-1}|Y_{T-2}, \ldots, Y_1]$$
$$\ldots [Y_2|Y_1][Y_1].$$

This factorization could be simplified, for example, with a first-order Markov assumption, in which the conditional-probability distribution of the process at time t, conditioned on the process at times prior to t, is only dependent on the most recent time. That is, the *first-order Markov* assumption is

$$[Y_t|Y_{t-1}, Y_{t-2}, \ldots, Y_1] = [Y_t|Y_{t-1}].$$

Then, for first-order Markov processes, the joint distribution is

$$[Y_T, Y_{T-1}, \ldots, Y_1] = [Y_T|Y_{T-1}][Y_{T-1}|Y_{T-2}]\ldots[Y_2|Y_1][Y_1]$$

$$= [Y_1]\prod_{i=2}^{T}[Y_i|Y_{i-1}]. \tag{2.13}$$

Notice that the right-hand side now depends only on univariate and bivariate probability distributions, since

$$[Y_i|Y_{i-1}] = [Y_i, Y_{i-1}]/[Y_i].$$

The property (2.13) plays an important role in the updating mechanism that underlies the Kalman filter (Kalman, 1960), which Meinhold and Singpurwalla (1983) demonstrate is the result of optimal prediction of the hidden time series $\{Y_t: t = 1, 2, \ldots\}$ in a temporal HM. When Y_t is a random spatial process, spatio-temporal HMs can be built that result in a spatio-temporal Kalman filter (Huang and Cressie, 1996; Wikle and Cressie, 1999; see also Sections 8.2.1 and 9.2).

Again, these process-model decompositions are attractive because they make use of modeling assumptions that are scientifically plausible. In that way, very complicated joint-probability distributions can be modeled by relatively simple conditional-probability specifications. Often, in the process model, determin-istic models can be reformulated with stochastic components to account for scientific uncertainty. For example, Wikle (2003b) uses a reaction-diffusion partial differential equation to motivate a process model for invasive species.

Of course, it is also possible that the process model can be factorized fur-ther or can be simplified from scientifically based modeling assumptions. For example, Wikle (2003b) specifies the distribution of spatially explicit diffusion-coefficient parameters, conditional on habitat covariates and spatial random fields. The latter processes could then be modeled too (conditional on param-eters), to incorporate sublevels into the process model. HMs can have many levels, so long as there is scientific insight or data upon which to base the decomposition. When there is no longer scientific insight, the BHM typically invokes "noninformative" priors as part of the parameter model.

EHM- and BHM-Based Inferences
Now, if one agrees that the HM approach is reasonable, there remains the question of how to do inference in this setting. Certainly, modeling the uncer-tainty can be carried out at the first two levels: $[Z|Y, \theta_D]$ and $[Y|\theta_P]$, and the parameters $\theta = \{\theta_D, \theta_P\}$ could be considered fixed but unknown. We have seen already that this is the EHM approach. The classical linear mixed model can be thought of as an EHM (e.g., Demidenko, 2004, Chapter 3). In addition, spatial prediction (kriging) fits into this framework (e.g., Cressie, 1988), as do sequential time series methods such as the Kalman filter (e.g., Meinhold and Singpurwalla, 1983; see also Section 8.2.1).

Depending on the complexity of the data model and the process model, it is often possible to use classical statistical estimation approaches to obtain estimates of the parameters θ. Common approaches for estimation in this EHM context include maximum likelihood estimation, the Expectation-Maximization (EM) algorithm, conditional-likelihood and pseudo-likelihood methods, and estimating equations (e.g., Demidenko, 2004), some of which are illustrated in Chapter 8. Although the EHM approach does not explicitly recognize the uncertainty in estimating the parameters, that uncertainty can often be accounted for by resampling and bootstrap procedures (e.g., Stoffer and Wall, 1991; Efron and Tibshirani, 1993; Lahiri, 2003). Bootstrapping (including the parametric bootstrap) in the spatial and temporal context is discussed by Cressie (1993, pp. 492–497). In simple cases, the uncertainty can be accounted for approximately, using statistical perturbation arguments (e.g., Rao, 2003, Section 6.2).

A coherent approach for inference in complicated HMs is to account for the uncertainty in parameter values by adding a parameter model, $[\theta_D, \theta_P]$. We have already seen that this is the BHM approach; recall that inference is based on the posterior distribution of process and parameters, given the data:

$$[Y, \theta_D, \theta_P | Z] \propto [Z | Y, \theta_D][Y | \theta_P][\theta_D, \theta_P].$$

As discussed at the beginning of this section, it is seldom possible to obtain an analytical expression for this posterior distribution. The discovery that *Markov chain Monte Carlo (MCMC)* computational methods could be used to simulate from general BHMs (Gelfand and Smith, 1990) revolutionized Statistical Science and made ever-more-complicated modeling scenarios possible. These computational aspects are discussed initially in Section 2.3 and for spatio-temporal dynamical models in Chapters 8 and 9.

Where, When, and then Why

The problem of determining a causative relationship in a process model can be expressed in terms of conditional probabilities. If Y_1 is a phenomenon that could directly affect Y_2 through a physical/chemical/biological/economic/etc. mechanism, and $[Y_2 | Y_1]$ changes as Y_1 changes, then Y_1 is a candidate to be a cause of Y_2.

However, even the best of theories can miss an important factor (F, say), which might damp down the relationship or yield a negative dependence where there was originally a positive one. We called this Simpson's Paradox and F a "lurking variable" in Chapter 1.

For the simple process, $Y = (Y_1, Y_2, F)$, the process model can be written as

$$[Y] = [Y_1, Y_2 | F][F]$$

$$= [Y_2 | Y_1, F][Y_1 | F][F].$$

Thus, the question, "Why does Y_2 behave as it does?" can be answered, "Because Y_1 causes that behavior, and the *type* of dependence is governed by the factor F." If we mistakenly focused on $[Y_2|Y_1]$ instead of $[Y_2|Y_1, F]$, we may infer incorrect dependencies. When F represents "level of spatial aggregation," these spurious inferences have been called the *ecological fallacy* (Robinson, 1950); a spatial-statistical interpretation of this can be found in Cressie (1996), and it was called change-of-support in Chapter 1.

More generally, many factors have spatial and temporal variability; hence, space and time can act as a *proxy* for F, should the process model fail to account for it. In other words, modeling spatio-temporal variability, along with good experimental design (see Chapter 1), can get us closer to Science's holy grail, namely *causation*.

Additional Remarks

There are many challenges associated with building (Bayesian) hierarchical statistical models and then carrying out valid inferences. A historical criticism of Bayesian methods is that they require "subjective" specification of prior information on the parameters. Of course, there is also subjectivity in the specification of the likelihood in classical marginal probability models. In fact, a broader perspective is that there is subjectivity involved with the specification of *all* model components: data models, process models, and parameter models. However, it isn't always clear what "subjective" means in this context. For example, it might be "subjective" to use deterministic relationships to motivate a stochastic model, such as for tropical winds (e.g., Wikle et al., 2001), yet the science upon which such a model is based comes from Newton's laws of motion! Thus, we believe that it is not helpful to try to classify probability distributions that determine the statistical model, as subjective or objective. Better questions to ask are about the sensitivity of inferences to model choices and whether such choices make sense scientifically.

Given that a modeler brings so much information to the table when developing models, the conditional-probability framework presented earlier can be used to recognize that this information, say I, is part of what is involved in the conditioning. For a BHM, we have

$$[Y, \theta_D, \theta_P|Z, I] \propto [Z|Y, \theta_D, I][Y|\theta_P, I][\theta_D, \theta_P|I].$$

A major challenge in this paradigm is, to the extent possible, appreciation of the importance of this information, I. It is often the case that a team of researchers at the table have a collective "I" that is better quantified and more appropriate than any individual's "I."

In the HM approach, there are certainly cases where models have to be simplified due to practical concerns. Perhaps the computational issues in a given formulation are limiting, which usually leads to a modification of the model. Such practical concerns are not limited to BHM-based or EHM-based inferences, but they concern all statistical inferences in complicated modeling scenarios.

Lastly, it must be recognized that complicated models often take a life of their own; it is the responsibility of the research team to remember the

Goldilocks Principle discussed in Chapter 1 and to keep uppermost the goal of converting data and information to knowledge. To temper the tendency to fit ever-more-complicated models, there are model-selection criteria that could be invoked (e.g., AIC, BIC, DIC, etc.), which concentrate on the twin pillars of *predictability* and *parsimony* (e.g., Spiegelhalter et al., 2002). But they do not address the third pillar, namely *scientific interpretability* (i.e., knowledge). Our approach is to choose, where possible, statistical models based on this third pillar, while not ignoring the other two. As a consequence, we have placed less emphasis on statistical-model-selection criteria in this book.

2.2 INFERENCE AND DIAGNOSTICS

A dataset can be thought of as a window through which knowledge can be obtained, enough to infer answers to the "why" question. What stops a scientist from truly *deducing* answers, rather than inferring them, is the ubiquitous presence of *uncertainty*. Statistics accounts for the uncertainty with a statistical model. Within that framework, statisticians are constantly looking for optimal procedures and then for ways to quantify the uncertainty in those optimal procedures.

In contrast to Statistics, Data Mining does not systematically seek optimality nor quantification of uncertainty. The data miner is often looking for parts of the dataset that are unusual, whereas the statistician is often looking for comprehensive structures that describe the data. Sometimes, the statistician will hold back observations that are unusual, for further study; the data miner tends to focus in on those unusual observations.

The HM approach, when implemented properly, can account for unusual observations in Z through a heterogeneous process Y. In the absence of an HM approach, classical statistical approaches can struggle to account for unusual observations. For example, suppose that precipitation data for a city, say Z_1, shows several extreme values over time. An HM could handle this heterogeneity by modeling the precipitation process, Y_1, to depend on Y_2, say the aerosol content of the atmosphere. That is,

$$[Y_1, Y_2|\theta] = [Y_1|Y_2, \theta][Y_2|\theta].$$

Each component on the right-hand side might be a simple conditional-probability distribution, but their product can yield a complex model. Then the "unusualness" in Z_1 is manifested through the marginal-probability model,

$$[Z_1|\theta] = \iint [Z_1|Y_1, \theta][Y_1|Y_2, \theta][Y_2|\theta]dY_1dY_2.$$

Extreme rainfall values might be due to atmospheric aerosol content on those days. A more classical statistical approach might delete the outliers and fit a time series model or attempt a regression model for $[Z_1|Z_2, \theta]$, where Z_2 are aerosol data, without making the processes Y_1 and Y_2 explicit. The HM gives us a structure to look for reasons for outliers.

A data-mining approach might "tease out" parts of Z_1 that are unusual, often using *ad hoc* (i.e., nonoptimal) methods to find them and often not being able to say what "unusual" means in any consistent way. The particular dataset under study is often the focus. Perhaps a data miner studying the rainfall data Z_1 will think of heterogeneity due to Y_2, perhaps not. Perhaps the "unusual" parts of Z_1 are not actually unusual, and the data miner has found something that is there simply due to chance fluctuations in the data or in the process. We believe that Data Mining has an important place in exploratory data analysis and gives the scientist ideas about how to model the phenomenon (i.e., process) being studied. However, we believe that answering the "why" question (i.e., inference) involves accounting for uncertainty in a coherent way. Statistical modeling and, in particular, HM fulfills this requirement.

Generally speaking, the data model is well defined by the scientist's data-gathering protocol. However, the process model is where the underlying scientific theories, and their uncertainties, are characterized in the form of $[Y|\theta_P]$. Such a theory is often complex, requiring sublevels of conditional-probability models to be defined; examples are given in Chapter 9. These sublevels consist of simpler conditional-probability distributions whose product yields $[Y|\theta_P]$. Consequently, classes of probability distributions developed in the twentieth century, but deemed too simple to model the datasets of the twenty-first century, might in fact have use as simple conditional-probability components of the HM. We shall briefly discuss some of the ideas behind these simple spatial and temporal models.

In the absence of detailed scientific information, simple probability models can provide an initial description of spatio-temporal variability. *Stationarity* in space (time) is a fundamental notion that formally says that a spatial (temporal) process' statistical properties are invariant under translation. Informally, this says that the spatial (temporal) behavior of the process is statistically identical anywhere in D_s (D_t).

Isotropy in space is defined as invariance under rotation about a given spatial location. Consider a "simple" probability distribution for the spatial process Y that is both stationary and isotropic (discussed more fully in Section 4.1). For example, consider the Gaussian process $\{Y(\mathbf{s}): \mathbf{s} \in D_s\}$ whose mean is μ, a constant, and whose *covariance* for any two locations $\mathbf{s} = (s_1, \ldots s_d)'$ and $\mathbf{x} = (x_1, \ldots, x_d)'$ is *stationary*,

$$\text{cov}(Y(\mathbf{s}), Y(\mathbf{x})) = C_Y(\mathbf{s} - \mathbf{x}),$$

and *isotropic*. That is, $C_Y(\mathbf{s} - \mathbf{x})$ is in fact a function of $\|\mathbf{s} - \mathbf{x}\|$, where $\|\mathbf{s} - \mathbf{x}\| \equiv \{(s_1 - x_1)^2 + \cdots + (s_d - x_d)^2\}^{1/2}$. Then it can be shown that the (Gaussian) *process* $Y(\cdot)$ is stationary and isotropic in $\mathbb{R}^d$.

In fact, there are two forms of stationarity in space (and in time). *Strongly stationary* spatial processes have the property that any finite-dimensional joint distribution at spatial locations $\{s_i\}$ is identical to the finite-dimensional joint distribution at the lagged locations, $\{s_i + h\}$, where $h = (h_1, \ldots, h_d)'$. For example, the spatial Gaussian process given just above is strongly stationary, since Gaussian processes are defined uniquely by their means and covariances. There is an obvious, analogous definition of strongly stationary temporal processes, where the spatial lag h is replaced with the temporal lag τ.

The terms *weakly stationary* and *second-order stationary* in space (time) are synonymous. The process $Y(\cdot)$ is second-order stationary if it has finite variance, constant mean, and covariance $C_Y(\cdot)$ that depends only on spatial lag h (or temporal lag τ). Hence, the class of second-order stationary processes contains the class of strongly stationary processes, provided that $C_Y(0) = \sigma_Y^2 < \infty$. Notice that the Gaussian process given just above is not only strongly stationary but also second-order stationary.

Ergodic processes (in space or time) have the property that expectations of functionals of $Y(\cdot)$ are well approximated by spatial or temporal averages, respectively, of the same functional. Ergodic processes are a subset of strongly stationary processes (Cressie, 1993, pp. 53–58).

The covariance function $C_Y(\cdot)$ of a second-order stationary process (in space or time) has a Fourier representation in terms of sines and cosines. The Fourier transform of $C_Y(\cdot)$ defines the (power) spectrum, or spectral density, which is an equivalent way to represent the dependence in the covariance function. Equally, the process itself can be represented as a linear combination of Fourier basis functions (sines and cosines at various frequencies). The frequencies that have large squared coefficients most likely have a physical explanation. Thus, the spectral density is another way to characterize (spatial or temporal) dependence in a second-order stationary process.

Underlying these notions is the concept of information content, and whether more information on parts of Y allows us to decrease our uncertainty. This is a complex issue that has been discussed by Cressie (1993, Section 5.8) using the terminology *infill asymptotics* and *increasing-domain asymptotics*. Lahiri et al. (1999) use *mixed-domain asymptotics*, where the information content is increased by simultaneously allowing the sampling region to grow bigger and the distance between sampling locations to become smaller. In the HM approach, there is rarely need to do asymptotic statistical analysis, but it is still an important notion because, from one extreme point of view, Statistics for spatial, temporal, and spatio-temporal data appears to be *impossible*! The data Z almost never involve replication; Nature does not "do it over" under the same conditions.

Sometimes observations repeated over time, $Z_1, \ldots, Z_T$, can be thought of as comparable and provide a type of pseudo-replication. We saw in Section 2.1 how such data quite often depend on (recent) past values; the first-order Markov assumption is one commonly used model of this temporal dependence. In that case, pseudo-replicates, $Z_1, \ldots, Z_T$, do not have the same information content as a sample of *iid* observations; Cressie (1993, Chapter 1) discussed this from the point of view of "equivalent number of independent observations." Nevertheless, for temporal data, the information content usually grows as $T \to \infty$, in spite of the temporal dependence. Cressie (1993, Section 5.8) called this increasing-domain asymptotics and contrasted it with infill asymptotics (sometimes referred to as fixed-domain asymptotics) that is often more appropriate for spatial data.

Consider the observations Z of a spatial process Y: From an extreme point of view, it is a sample of size 1, from which we wish to make inference! However, this is *not impossible* if there is spatial-dependence structure in the statistical model. We have seen above how that structure might be stationarity and/or isotropy; in an HM it appears as parametric specification of $[Z|Y, \theta_D]$ and $[Y|\theta_P]$. In this new century of very large Z and high-dimensional Y (e.g., spatio-temporal statistical analyses of climate data), invoking stationarity or isotropy assumptions, even within a parametric model, may be inappropriate. We need to look for other ways to avoid tackling an impossible problem, and dimension reduction has proved to be particularly successful; see Sections 3.5.2, 4.1.4, and 7.1.3, and the review by Wikle (2010b). By keeping in mind the notion of information content in Z, one can try to avoid specifying an HM for which inference on unknown quantities can only be weak at best.

2.2.1 Optimal Prediction

Statistical methodology is centered around the notion of optimal inference. Optimal estimators and optimal predictors represent a gold standard, which the collective talents of the Statistics profession have investigated over the last 100 years. These investigations could be classified according to type of inference (Bayesian, frequentist, fiducial, etc.), criteria (bias, variance, efficiency), non/semi/parametric distributional assumptions, exact/approximate/asymptotic optimality, quantification of the optimal estimators'/predictors' uncertainty, and so forth. In this book, our emphasis is on *prediction of random quantities Y* (and θ) in an HM. Estimation of θ is needed for an EHM approach, and we shall leave it as understood that optimal estimators $\widehat{\theta}$ are chosen, to the extent possible; optimal estimation is treated, for example, in great detail in Lehmann (1983).

In what follows, we shall illustrate how to derive optimal predictors of the random quantity Y from the data Z. For the purpose of this presentation, θ will be assumed fixed but unknown (EHM); however, we note that the approach is extendable to the case where both Y and θ are to be predicted (BHM). In the following paragraphs, it is understood that all distributions are conditional on θ.

Let $L(\widehat{Y}, Y)$ denote a loss function that quantifies the consequence of using the predictor $\widehat{Y} = a(Z)$ to make inference on the true value Y. The *optimal predictor* (e.g., DeGroot, 1970) is the $a^*(Z)$ that minimizes $E(L(a(Z), Y))$ with respect to $a(\cdot)$. Consequently, if the loss function L changes, the optimal predictor $a^*(Z)$ changes.

We note that the problem of optimal prediction could be reformulated in terms of a utility function and its maximization with respect to $a(\cdot)$. Loss can be thought of as a negative utility, and hence they give equivalent predictors. It can be shown (e.g., Ferguson, 1967, Chapter 2) that $a^*(\cdot) \in \mathcal{A}$ is the predictor that minimizes the posterior expected loss, where $\mathcal{A}$ is the class of possible predictors. That is, $a^*(\cdot)$ satisfies

$$E\{L(a^*(Z), Y)|Z\} \leq E\{L(a(Z), Y)|Z\}, \qquad \text{for all } a \in \mathcal{A}. \quad (2.14)$$

The derivations below assume that the *predictand* Y and the *predictor* $\widehat{Y}$ are random variables; see, for example, Gotway and Cressie (1993) for derivations when Y and $\widehat{Y}$ are random vectors. We shall consider two examples based on two important loss functions, *squared-error loss* and *0–1 loss*.

Assume squared-error loss:

$$L(\widehat{Y}, Y) = (Y - \widehat{Y})^2,$$

and write $\widehat{Y} = a(Z)$. Then to find the optimal predictor $a^*(\cdot)$,

$$E\{(Y - a(Z))^2|Z\}$$

is minimized with respect to $a(\cdot)$.

In the calculation below, we demonstrate that $a^*(Z) \equiv E(Y|Z)$ is the optimal predictor in an HM. For any $a(\cdot)$, the posterior expected loss is

$$E\{(Y - a(Z))^2|Z\} = E\{(Y - a^*(Z))^2|Z\} + E\{(a^*(Z) - a(Z))^2|Z\}$$
$$+ 2E\{(a^*(Z) - a(Z))(Y - a^*(Z))|Z\}.$$

Now the last term on the right-hand side is zero, since $E\{(Y - a^*(Z))|Z\} = E(Y|Z) - a^*(Z) = 0$. Hence,

$$E\{(Y - a(Z))^2|Z\} \geq E\{(Y - a^*(Z))^2|Z\},$$

which implies that

$$a^*(Z) \equiv E(Y|Z) = mean \text{ of } [Y|Z],$$

is the optimal predictor of Z. We see in Section 4.1 that this optimal predictor is the basis of *kriging*, and we see in Section 8.2 that it is the basis of *smoothing*, *filtering*, and *forecasting*.

One way to quantify the uncertainty in any predictor $a(\cdot)$ is through the expected loss, $E\{L(a(Z), Y)\}$, where here the expectation, $E\{\cdot\}$, is taken over the joint distribution of Y and Z. In the case of squared-error loss, this yields the mean squared prediction error (MSPE),

$$E\{(Y - a(Z))^2\}.$$

For the optimal predictor we have $a^*(Z) = E(Y|Z)$, and hence the *minimized MSPE* is

$$E\{(Y - E(Y|Z))^2\} = E\{\mathrm{var}(Y|Z)\}.$$

The MSPE is the basic quantification of uncertainty in kriging (Chapter 4) and in Kalman smoothing/filtering/forecasting (Chapter 7).

In spite of its optimality, $E(Y|Z)$ has a major weakness. Suppose it is known that Y is binary; that is, $Y \in \{0, 1\}$. However, the optimal predictor is *not* binary: $E(Y|Z) \in [0, 1]$. That is, the optimal predictor takes values *between* 0 and 1, which Y can *never* take. This weakness is apparent when Y is an array of pixels from a black-and-white image, and Z is a noisy gray-scale version of Y. The optimal predictor, $E(Y|Z)$, gives a "smoother" image than Z, as is desired, but it is *not* black-and-white, as is the true image Y. One remedy is to change the loss function. The *0–1 loss function* is often used in statistical image processing.

Assume 0–1 loss:

$$L(\widehat{Y}, Y) = \begin{cases} 0 & \text{if } \widehat{Y} = Y \\ 1 & \text{if } \widehat{Y} \neq Y \end{cases}$$

$$= 1 - I(\widehat{Y} = Y),$$

where $\widehat{Y} = a(Z)$ and $I(\cdot)$ is the indicator function. Then, to find the optimal predictor $a^*(\cdot)$, it is equivalent to minimize

$$E\{1 - I(a(z) = Y)|Z\},$$

with respect to $a(\cdot)$. This is easily seen to be equivalent to *maximizing* $\Pr(Y = a(Z)|Z)$. In other words, the optimal predictor $a^*(Z)$ satisfies

$$[Y|Z]|_{Y = a^*(Z)} \geq [Y|Z],$$

where $[Y|Z]$ is the posterior probability density (or mass function). That is, the optimal predictor is

$$a^*(Z) = mode \text{ of } [Y|Z].$$

This is in contrast to squared-error loss, where the optimal predictor is the *mean* of $[Y|Z]$.

Notice that the weakness of the (posterior) mean is avoided with the (posterior) mode, since it *is* one (actually, the most likely) of the possible values of Y. However, the 0–1 loss function is in some sense uncompromising; in statistical image processing, even one pixel that is incorrect causes a loss of 1, and the loss remains 1 no matter how many additional pixels are incorrect. Finally, there is no agreed-upon measure of uncertainty for the mode of the posterior distribution.

2.2.2   Diagnostics

An HM is formulated from the parametric assumptions $[Z|Y, \theta]$ (data model) and $[Y|\theta]$ (process model). The posterior distribution $[Y|Z, \theta]$ (from the EHM) or $[Y, \theta|Z]$ (from the BHM) is the basis of inference on the random quantities of interest. But, does the HM fit properly?

To answer this question in a complete way would go beyond the scope of this chapter, but we shall present several generic diagnostic procedures to check the fit of an HM. As with all diagnoses, they have the *potential* to eliminate bad theories, but it is quite possible that two models (one good, one bad) could give similar diagnostic results. The aphorism "absence of evidence is not always evidence of absence" should be kept in mind.

Two obvious diagnostic procedures are *validation* and *cross-validation*. Validation involves splitting the data into two parts, $Z = (Z_{obs}, Z_{val})$, where $Z_{val} \equiv \{Z_{val,i}\}$ will be held back for validation. Implicitly, the process is also split into $Y = (Y_{obs}, Y_{val})$. Then the HM is fitted from data Z_{obs}, resulting in the posterior distribution, $[Y|Z_{obs}]$. From this, $[Y_{val}|Z_{obs}]$ is obtained by marginalization and, from this, (optimal) predictors $\hat{Y}_{val} \equiv \{\hat{Y}_{val,i}\}$ are produced.

Furthermore, under the (usual) assumption that Z_{obs} and Z_{val} are conditionally independent given Y, we obtain

$$[Z_{val}|Z_{obs}] = \int [Z_{val}|Y_{val}][Y_{val}|Z_{obs}]dY_{val}.$$

Then simulating Y^*_{val} from $[Y_{val}|Z_{obs}]$, followed by Z^*_{val} from $[Z_{val}|Y^*_{val}]$, yields a simulation from $[Z_{val}|Z_{obs}]$. From this, (optimal) predictors $\hat{Z}_{val} \equiv \{\hat{Z}_{val,i}\}$ are produced. The validation procedure involves "comparing" $\hat{Z}_{val}$ to Z_{val} to see how "close" they are. That measure of closeness is often the empirical mean-squared prediction error,

$$\underset{i}{\text{ave}}\{(Z_{val,i} - \dot{Z}_{val,i})^2\}.$$

A less direct, but commonly used, measure is obtained by replacing $\hat{Z}_{val,i}$ above with $\hat{Y}_{val,i}$.

Cross-validation involves writing $Z = (Z_1, \ldots, Z_m)$; using suggestive notation, we write $Y = (Y_1, \ldots, Y_m, Y_{m+1}, \ldots, Y_n)$, which accounts for the $(n - m)$ missing data. For $i = 1, \ldots, m$, Z_i is deleted, and the posterior distribution $[Y|Z^{(-i)}]$ is obtained, where $Z^{(-i)} \equiv (Z_1, \ldots, Z_{i-1}, Z_{i+1}, \ldots, Z_m)$. In the same manner as for validation, the (optimal) predictors, $\hat{Z}_i^{(-i)}$ and $\hat{Y}_i^{(-i)}$, of Z_i and Y_i, respectively, are produced. Then $\hat{Z}_i^{(-i)}$, or less directly $\hat{Y}_i^{(-i)}$, is compared to Z_i; $i = 1, \ldots, m$. The way the m comparisons are made, individually or *en masse*, is a choice that determines the type of cross-validation diagnostic procedure; for example, Cressie (1993, pp. 101–104) discusses this (in the spatial context) for kriging.

We have already mentioned in Section 2.1 the problem of model selection and the criteria known as AIC, BIC, and DIC (e.g., Spiegelhalter et al., 2002). Another common approach to model selection in a Bayesian statistical context is based on Bayes factors; for example, see the review by Kass and Raftery (1995). In a broad sense, these represent diagnostic procedures also, as does the less-formal strategy for breaking links in the graphical models presented in Section 2.4. In the rest of this section, a diagnostic procedure is presented that is well suited to the HM approach and to prediction as the form of inference. It is based on the *posterior predictive distribution*, and it is at its best when a single model is being fitted. It is similar to a classical significance-testing approach to testing hypotheses, in the sense that a specific alternative model is not specified.

The goal in diagnostics for model fitting is to determine whether the observed data are representative of the type of data expected under the model. In an HM, this can be assessed as follows (presented here for a BHM): Let Z_{rep} denote an independent replicate of the data with the same (unknown) values Y and θ that produced the data Z. The *posterior predictive distribution* (Rubin, 1984; Gelman, Meng, and Stern, 1996) of Z_{rep} is defined as

$$[Z_{rep}|Z] = \iint [Z_{rep}|Y, \theta, Z][Y, \theta|Z] \, dY \, d\theta$$

$$= \iint [Z_{rep}|Y, \theta][Y, \theta|Z] \, dY \, d\theta, \tag{2.15}$$

where the second equality reflects the (conditional) independence of the replicate Z_{rep} produced by the HM. We note that there is another type of diagnostic based on the prior predictive distribution (Box, 1980), $[Z_{rep}] = \int [Z_{rep}|Y, \theta][Y, \theta] \, dY \, d\theta$, but it was developed at a time when simulating from the posterior distribution was usually prohibitive. As we see below, (2.15) involves replicating the entire dataset from a proposed HM and applying the results to rather general discrepancy measures. Other posterior predictive approaches can be found in West (1986) and Gelfand, Dey, and Chang (1992) in settings where, respectively, data are arriving sequentially and cross-validation is being implemented on the existing dataset without the benefit of replicating it.

Gelman, Meng, and Stern (1996) advocate basing inference on replicates from (2.15), as follows: Use the computational devices discussed in Section 2.3 to draw a sample $\{(Y^{(\ell)}, \theta^{(\ell)}): \ell = 1, \ldots, L\}$ from the posterior distribution, $[Y, \theta|Z]$. Then for $\ell = 1, \ldots, L$, $Z_{rep}^{(\ell)}$ is obtained by simulating from the data model, $[Z|Y^{(\ell)}, \theta^{(\ell)}]$. This is also mentioned briefly in Gelfand (1996), although without guidance on how the $\{Z_{rep}^{(\ell)}: \ell = 1, \ldots, L\}$ would be used in a diagnostic procedure.

If the BHM given by the three levels, $[Z|Y, \theta]$, $[Y|\theta]$, and $[\theta]$, is an appropriate model, then the replicates, $\{Z_{rep}^{(1)}, Z_{rep}^{(2)}, \ldots, Z_{rep}^{(L)}\}$, should "look like" the data Z. It is the formalization of this idea that yields *posterior predictive diagnostics*.

To diagnose whether the model fits, we introduce $T(Z; Y, \theta)$ as a "discrepancy measure" that is intended to capture the goodness-of-fit of the model to the data. For example, T may be an overall measure of fit, or it may be a measure designed to tell whether a particular source of variability is adequately addressed by the model. Importantly, T is not restricted to take the form of a test statistic, since it can depend on (Y, θ) as well as on Z. The fit of the model is diagnosed with respect to T by comparing the posterior distribution of $T(Z; Y, \theta)$ to the posterior predictive reference distribution of $T(Z_{rep}; Y, \theta)$.

The joint posterior distribution of $T(Z_{rep}; Y, \theta)$ and $T(Z; Y, \theta)$ can be studied empirically. Recall that $\{(Y^{(\ell)}, \theta^{(\ell)}): \ell = 1, \ldots, L\}$ are L samples from the posterior distribution $[Y, \theta | Z]$. Then, for example, the L pairs of values $\{T(Z_{rep}^{(\ell)}; Y^{(\ell)}, \theta^{(\ell)}), T(Z; Y^{(\ell)}, \theta^{(\ell)}): \ell = 1, \ldots, L\}$ could be displayed in a scatter plot. If the points on the scatter plot are far removed from the 45-degree line, then a lack of model fit would be diagnosed.

One summary of the joint distribution is the *posterior predictive p-value*,

$$\Pr(T(Z_{rep}; Y, \theta) \geq T(Z; Y, \theta) | Z),$$

where the probability is calculated over $[Z_{rep}, Y, \theta | Z]$, a distribution that is easy to compute empirically from posterior samples, $\{(Y^{(\ell)}, \theta^{(\ell)}): \ell = 1, \ldots, L\}$, whose computation is discussed in Section 2.3. Very small posterior predictive p-values would result in rejection of the current model. More moderate values may cast doubt on the model, but whether the model is rejected or not may depend on the ultimate purpose for which it will be used.

One class of discrepancy measures are omnibus measures of fit. An example from this class is the discrepancy based on the usual chi-squared goodness-of-fit measure,

$$T(Z; Y, \theta) = \sum_{i=1}^{m} \frac{(Z_i - E(Z_i | Y, \theta))^2}{\text{var}(Z_i | Y, \theta)}, \tag{2.16}$$

where here the data Z consist of the m individual observations, $Z_1, \ldots, Z_m$, that make up Z. Notice the similarity to classical goodness-of-fit testing when the statistical model is not hierarchical and is simply $[Z | \theta]$. In that case, there is no "Y" in (2.16), and θ is typically replaced with an estimator $\hat{\theta}$ (e.g., the maximum likelihood estimator). For these classical test statistics, there are analytical results establishing their asymptotic distributions as central chi-squared under the null hypothesis of the test. In contrast, the posterior predictive distribution provides a suitable reference distribution for any T and any sample size m, since it is based on (simulating from) the posterior distribution in a BHM.

In the EHM, the posterior distribution is $[Y|Z, \theta]$, and the posterior predictive distribution is

$$[Z_{rep}|Z, \theta] = \int [Z_{rep}|Y, \theta][Y|Z, \theta]\, dY.$$

When a posterior predictive diagnostic is computed, an estimator $\widehat{\theta}$ is substituted for θ throughout the implementation. In the context of an EHM, the discrepancy measure focuses on the appropriateness of the data model and the process model.

To enhance the sensitivity of posterior predictive diagnostics and to make posterior predictive *p*-values uniformly distributed under the assumed model, Bayarri and Berger (2000) developed a related approach based on posterior distributions that condition on only part of the information in the data. However, their approach requires more calculation and can be difficult to apply for complex HMs. Stern and Cressie (2000) combine the ideas of cross-validation and posterior predictive distributions to obtain diagnostics for spatial BHMs on a spatial lattice.

2.3   COMPUTATION OF THE POSTERIOR DISTRIBUTION

Statistics tackles uncertainty directly through the use of (conditional) probability distributions. Let X be a random quantity with *joint* probability distribution $[X]$. For example, suppose $X = (X_1, \ldots, X_n)$ and $\{X_i\}$ are iid $Gau(\mu, \sigma^2)$. Then

$$[X] = \prod_{i=1}^{n}\{(2\pi\sigma^2)^{-1/2}\exp[(-1/2)(x_i - \mu)^2/\sigma^2]: x_i \in \mathbb{R}\}$$

$$= \{(2\pi\sigma^2)^{-n/2}\exp[(-1/2)\sum_{i=1}^{n}(x_i - \mu)^2/\sigma^2]: \mathbf{x} \in \mathbb{R}^n\},$$

where $\mathbf{x} \equiv (x_1, \ldots, x_n)'$. That is, in this case, there is an analytical expression for the joint probability distribution, $[X]$. It would also be possible to calculate all the moments of X_i, $\{E(X_i^k): k = 1, 2, \ldots\}$, and cross-moments are easy too because of the independence between $\{X_i\}$; for example,

$$E(X_1^2 X_2 X_3^4) = E(X_1^2)E(X_2)E(X_3^4).$$

But even in this ideal case, there is one expression that is not available analytically:

$$\Pr(X_1 \leq x) = \int_{-\infty}^{x} [X_1]\, dX_1, \qquad x \in \mathbb{R}.$$

However, as any student in an introductory Statistics class will verify, there are tables available to look up this probability for any x on their exam.

This uneven availability of analytical expressions for densities, moments, sampling distributions, p-values, posterior distributions, and so on, in the twentieth century, was arguably a factor that held back the application of Statistics to complex scientific problems. However, the computing revolution has led to a statistical-modeling revolution! Consider data $Z \equiv (Z_1, \dots, Z_m)$. Then the core model of the twentieth century,

$$Z_1, \dots, Z_m \ iid \ Dist(\theta),$$

where $Dist(\theta)$ is a generic parametric probability distribution with unknown parameters θ, has now been replaced with the core model of the twenty-first century,

$$[Z|Y, \theta],$$

$$[Y|\theta],$$

which is an HM made up of two basic levels of conditional-probability distributions. Recall that $Z = (Z_1, \dots, Z_m)$, and think of $Y = (Y_1, \dots, Y_n)$, where generally m and n are different. Even though the posterior distribution,

$$[Y|Z, \theta] = \frac{[Z|Y, \theta][Y|\theta]}{[Z|\theta]},$$

is not generally analytically tractable (due to the denominator, $[Z|\theta]$), there are now ways to simulate from $[Y|Z, \theta]$.

2.3.1 Simulation-Based Inference

To make the exposition simple, we assume that X is a single random variable and that we wish to evaluate the moment:

$$E(g(X)) = \int g(X)[X]\,dX, \qquad (2.17)$$

where for mathematical correctness, it must be assumed that the moment exists. An example of (2.17) is the cumulative distribution function (CDF):

$$F(x) = \Pr(X \le x) = E(I(X \le x)),$$

where recall that $I(\cdot)$ is the indicator function ($I(A)$ equals 1 if A is true, and it equals 0 if not). The mean of X is the moment $E(X)$, the variance of X is $\text{var}(X) = E(X^2) - (E(X))^2$, and so forth. Indeed, every summary of $[X]$ can be formulated as a moment, $E(g(X))$.

$$[Y|\theta_P, \theta_D, Z],$$

$$[\theta_P|Y, \theta_D, Z],$$

$$[\theta_D|Y, \theta_P, Z],$$

and repeat; at each step, the latest values obtained from the previous steps are used in the conditioning arguments. This defines a *Markov chain* whose stationary distribution is the posterior distribution, $[Y, \theta_P, \theta_D|Z]$.

The conditional distributions in the Gibbs sampler above, are commonly referred to as the *full conditional distributions*. When one of these is difficult to simulate from because it can only be calculated up to a normalizing constant, the simulation in that step can be performed using a Metropolis-type simulation (e.g., Tierney, 1994; Robert and Casella, 2004). For example, consider the first step and suppose that $[Y|\theta_P, \theta_D, Z]$ is given by the density:

$$f(\cdot|\theta_P, \theta_D, Z)/ \int f(y|\theta_P, \theta_D, Z)\,dy,$$

where f is known analytically, but the integral is not. Let Y_{cur} be the *current* value of Y and suppose that Y_{sim} is a simulated random quantity from a distribution centered at Y_{cur} (and satisfying a symmetry property given, e.g., by Robert and Casella, 2004, p. 271). Define the next value of the Markov chain, Y_{nex}, as follows:

$$Y_{nex} \equiv \begin{cases} Y_{sim} \text{ with probability, } \min\{1, f(Y_{sim})/f(Y_{cur})\}, \\ Y_{cur} \text{ with probability, } 1 - \min\{1, f(Y_{sim})/f(Y_{cur})\}. \end{cases}$$

Then Y_{nex} is the updated value of Y (given θ_P, θ_D, Z) in that step of the Gibbs sampler.

The Metropolis algorithm (and its commonly used variant, the Metropolis–Hastings algorithm) can slow up the MCMC procedure; the acceptance probability for Y_{sim} has to be chosen carefully (e.g., 25–30% acceptance rate), so considerable effort is made to avoid using it in the Gibbs sampler. This has perhaps led to (conditional) distributional choices when building the HM that more suit the computational efficiencies than the scientific mechanisms. Clearly, this is a balancing act, and such choices should not have a major impact on the results (see Section 2.5). MCMC algorithms for spatio-temporal HMs are described in Chapter 8.

We now give a similarly simple example for an EHM. In this case, a computational algorithm (e.g., MCMC, Kalman filter) is built to simulate from the posterior distribution, $[Y|Z, \theta]$. Since θ is fixed but unknown, the "empirical" part of the EHM is to substitute in an estimate $\widehat{\theta}$ for θ to simulate from $[Y|Z, \widehat{\theta}]$. In the following paragraph, we give a simple description of the EM estimate $\widehat{\theta}$.

In the HM context, the EM algorithm defined below provides an estimator of θ that attempts to maximize the likelihood, $[Z|\theta]$. It does so by defining the *complete likelihood*, $[Z, Y|\theta]$, which is equal to $[Z|Y, \theta][Y|\theta]$, the product of the data model and the process model. Dempster, Laird, and Rubin (1977) presented the algorithm in terms of successive iterations of an *E*-step and an *M*-step. The ℓth iteration is given by the following:

> *E-step*: Calculate $E(\ln[Z, Y|\theta]|Z = Z_{obs}, \widehat{\theta}^{(\ell-1)}) \equiv q(\theta|\widehat{\theta}^{(\ell-1)})$.
> *M-step*: Find the θ that maximizes $q(\theta|\widehat{\theta}^{(\ell-1)})$; call this $\widehat{\theta}^{(\ell)}$.

With a starting value $\widehat{\theta}^{(0)}$ and repetition of the EM steps, for $\ell = 1, 2, \ldots$, we choose $\widehat{\theta}$ to be the value of $\widehat{\theta}^{(\ell)}$ that satisfies pre-specified convergence criteria. Section 8.3.1 gives an implementation in the spatio-temporal context.

2.3.3 Summaries of the Posterior Distribution

In the case of a BHM, the final result is a simulation, $\{(Y^{(\ell)}, \theta^{(\ell)}): \ell = 1, \ldots, L\}$, from the posterior distribution $[Y, \theta|Z]$. Hence, the optimal predictor $E(Y|Z)$ can be approximated by $\widehat{E}(Y|Z) \equiv (1/L)\sum_{\ell=1}^{L} Y^{(\ell)}$. A measure of its uncertainty, the posterior variance $\text{var}(Y|Z)$, can be approximated by $\widehat{\text{var}}(Y|Z)$. Another measure of uncertainty is the *Bayesian credible interval*,

$$C_{1-\alpha} \equiv \{y: f(y|Z) \geq k_{1-\alpha}\},$$

where $f(y|Z) \equiv dF(y|Z)/dy$, and $k_{1-\alpha}$ is chosen such that

$$\int_{C_{1-\alpha}} f(y|Z)\, dy = 1 - \alpha, \qquad 0 \leq \alpha < 1.$$

Notice that as $\alpha \to 1$, we obtain the posterior mode. Then $\widehat{C}_{1-\alpha}$, the MCMC approximation to $C_{1-\alpha}$, is obtained by replacing $F(\cdot|Z)$ with $\widehat{F}(\cdot|Z)$ above and defining $\widehat{f}(\cdot|Z)$ as the (smoothed) histogram obtained from the CDF $\widehat{F}(\cdot|Z)$. Similar inferences could be obtained for θ.

Notice the advantage of simulating from the joint posterior distribution, $[Y, \theta|Z]$. If one of the quantities (e.g., θ) is not needed, the simulated $\{Y^{(1)}, \ldots, Y^{(L)}\}$ are, *by definition*, distributed according to the marginalized posterior distribution, $\int [Y, \theta|Z]\, d\theta$. Although this might be a difficult integral to obtain analytically, the "law of the unconscious statistician" simply allows us to approximate any moment, $E(g(Y)|Z)$, with $\widehat{E}(g(Y)|Z)$.

2.3.4 Additional Remarks

There is software available to fit HMs using MCMC, the most notable one being BUGS (Spiegelhalter et al., 2010). For the problems we encounter in our research, we have almost exclusively developed our own algorithms and written our own code. This book's emphasis is on the statistical-modeling aspects, but we would like to say that our lesser emphasis here on computations does not reflect our regard for its importance. For example, when developing MCMC algorithms to simulate from the posterior distribution, we take great care in developing full conditional distributions, in looking for ways to increase statistical efficiency (e.g., Rao–Blackwellization) and computational efficiency (e.g., block updating), and in diagnosing the convergence of the Markov chain to its stationary distribution. [More details on MCMC algorithms can be found in the excellent books of Gilks, Richardson, and Spiegelhalter (1996), Gelman et al. (2003), and Robert and Casella (2004).]

We close this section by pointing out that when doing Statistics for temporal, spatial, and spatio-temporal data, the dimensions of Z, Y, and θ can grow fast as the HMs become more complex. The problem becomes particularly acute in the spatio-temporal domain, where the high spatial dimension is combined with a desire to filter the spatial fields as more data arrive. This has led to considerable research in the area of sequential Monte Carlo methods, in particular *particle filtering* (e.g., Doucet, de Freitas, and Gordon, 2001; Andrieu, Doucet, and Holenstein, 2010). We discuss this further in Section 8.4.5.

2.4 GRAPHICAL REPRESENTATIONS OF STATISTICAL DEPENDENCIES

Statistical independence is a property of probability distributions. Two random quantities A and B are (statistically) independent if $[A, B] = [A][B]$. In other words, to know the joint distribution, it is enough to know the marginal distributions and to put the joint distribution equal to their product. *Statistical dependence* is the absence of statistical independence. According to this definition, there are myriad ways that two or more random quantities could be (statistically) dependent. A key component of statistical modeling of complex phenomena is to specify the dependence structure. One way to visualize dependence structures is through a graph.

2.4.1 Directed and Undirected Graphs

Graphs are made up of nodes and edges. If two random quantities A and B are statistically dependent, we could equivalently represent this dependence by a node with label "A," a node with label "B," and an edge (or line) connecting the two nodes. If it is thought that the dependence is causal, namely A causes B, it is sensible to write the dependence in the joint distribution $[A, B]$ as in (2.3):

$$[A, B] = [B|A][A],$$

and the edge between A and B becomes a *directed edge* (or arrow) from A to B. (Of course, the decomposition, $[A, B] = [A|B][B]$, is equally true, but from a modeling point of view it is not a meaningful way to write the joint probability.)

An *undirected graph* consists of two or more *nodes* (appropriately labeled) and *edges* (lines) joining the nodes, where a typical node is joined to only some of the other nodes. A *directed graph* also has nodes, and all edges are replaced with *directed edges* (arrows), where the direction of the arrow is chosen based on the idea that something happening at the arrow-head node has been "caused" by something happening at the arrow-tail node. Figure 2.1 shows both an undirected graph (Figure 2.1a) and a directed graph (Figure 2.1b) for the simple case of two nodes.

An HM can be represented as a directed graph. Figure 2.2a shows the initial node θ, with directed edges from it to nodes Y and Z. There is also a directed edge from node Y to node Z. That is, dependencies in an HM are expressed through the conditional-probability distributions, $[Z|Y, \theta]$ and $[Y|\theta]$. If we split θ up into θ_D and θ_P, so that the BHM is

$$[Z|Y, \theta] = [Z|Y, \theta_D],$$

$$[Y|\theta] = [Y|\theta_P],$$

$$[\theta_D, \theta_P] = [\theta_D][\theta_P],$$

then the independence of θ_D and θ_P yields the directed graph in Figure 2.2b (showing the two "root" nodes θ_D and θ_P with no edge between them). Here, the directed edges from θ_D and Y both go to Z, and the directed edge from θ_P goes to Y. This type of HM is often found in the hierarchical-statistical-modeling literature (e.g., Gelman et al., 2003).

Both undirected and directed graphs can be used to show statistical dependence between random variables, the difference being how that dependence is

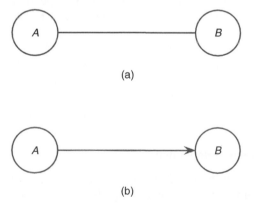

(a)

(b)

Figure 2.1   Graphs with nodes $\{A, B\}$, where A and B are random quantities. (a) Undirected graph showing dependence between A and B, illustrated by an edge (*line*); no line between A and B would illustrate independence. (b) Directed graph showing that B depends on A causally, as illustrated by the directed edge (*arrow*) from A to B.

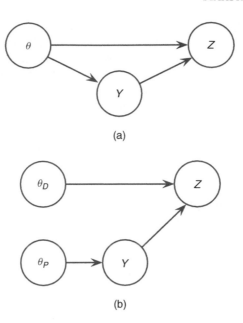

(a)

(b)

Figure 2.2 Hierarchical model represented as a directed graph. (**a**) Generic model showing that Z is (causally) dependent on Y and θ and that Y is (causally) dependent on θ. (**b**) The node θ is separated into two nodes θ_D and θ_P, and θ_D and θ_P are assumed independent (no edge between θ_D and θ_P).

expressed in the statistical model. Graphs can have a combination of undirected and directed edges, and these have been called *chain graphs* (e.g., Lauritzen, 1996, p. 7). Figure 2.3a shows a three-node chain graph where B depends causally on A, but there is a noncausal type of dependence (undirected edge) between B and C. Notice that a directed graph can be obtained by combining nodes B and C and leaving node A where it is; the result is a two-node directed graph shown in Figure 2.3b, deduced from Figure 2.3a. However, Figure 2.3a cannot be recovered from the graph in Figure 2.3b, which illustrates an important point. When building dependence structures, the statistical modeler should try to use as *many* nodes as there are random quantities of interest, but with as *few* edges as there are dependencies between the quantities.

2.4.2 Conditional Independence

Whether the edges in Figure 2.3a are directed or not is immaterial to the next calculation. Assume that there is no edge between A and C, and consider

$$[A, C|B] = [A, B, C]/[B]$$
$$= [A|B, C][B|C][C]/[B]$$
$$= [A|B][B|C][C]/[B],$$

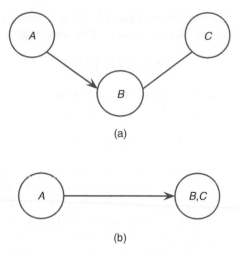

(a)

(b)

Figure 2.3 (a) Chain graph. (b) Directed graph resulting from (a), but showing the dependence structure less precisely.

where we assume the denominator $[B]$ is positive (to keep technicalities to a minimum); the last equality is due to the assumed lack of edge between nodes A and C (see Figure 2.3a). Then from Bayes' Theorem given by (2.5), here applied to B and C,

$$[A, C|B] = [A|B][C|B]. \qquad (2.19)$$

The relation (2.19) is remarkable. The lack of an edge between A and C in Figure 2.3a is expressed in (2.19) in terms of *conditional* independence of A and C given B.

How can conditional independencies be read from a (undirected or directed) graph? The answer is surprisingly simple (e.g., Lauritzen, 1996). If the conditioning nodes (here B) are removed from the graph, and that breaks apart the graph into unconnected graphs, then the random quantities associated with the two graphs (here A and C) are conditionally independent, conditional on those at the removed nodes (here B).

Intuitively, the conditional independence relation (2.19) should imply

$$[A|B, C] = [A|B]; \qquad (2.20)$$

that is, conditional on B, also knowing C should be immaterial to the probability distribution of A. The proof of (2.20) is straightforward:

$$[A|B, C] = [A, C|B]/[C|B],$$

where we assume that the denominator $[C|B]$ is positive (again to keep technicalities to a minimum). Hence, from (2.19), we obtain

$$[A|B, C] = [A|B].$$

It is also straightforward to show that (2.20) implies (2.19). An example of this in a BHM can be deduced from Figure 2.2b:

$$[Z|Y, \theta_D, \theta_P] = [Z|Y, \theta_D]. \tag{2.21}$$

A more complicated example comes from our wish to diagnose (see Section 2.2) whether or not there is a directed edge from Y_1 to Y_2 in the process $Y = (Y_1, Y_2)$. If there is no edge, then $[Y_2|Y_1, \theta_P] = [Y_2|\theta_P]$.

For simplicity of exposition, we use notation that does not show conditioning on the parameters, but they should be thought of as being present. Associated with Y_1 and Y_2 are data Z_1 and Z_2, respectively. The directed graph is

$$Z_1 \leftarrow Y_1 \rightarrow Y_2 \rightarrow Z_2. \tag{2.22}$$

For example, Craigmile et al. (2009) consider Y_1 to be presence of heavy metals in soils, ambient air, and water supply (regional environment), and consider Y_2 to be presence of the same heavy metals in the household environment. In that study, it was of interest to determine whether data Z_1 on the regional environment could help one "learn" what is happening in the household environment. It is not hard to see that if $[Y_2|Y_1] = [Y_2]$ (i.e., no edge), then

$$[Y_2|Z_2, Z_1] = [Y_2|Z_2].$$

That is, there is no learning about Y_2 from Z_1 beyond what can be learned from Z_2. Hence, a diagnosis that the directed edge from Y_1 to Y_2 is needed would come from seeing changes in the posterior of Y_2, depending on whether data Z_2 or data (Z_1, Z_2) are used. Notice that it would be equally appropriate to look for changes in $[Y_1|Z_1]$ in comparison to $[Y_1|Z_1, Z_2]$.

While graphs are a wonderful way to visualize the presence or absence of conditional dependence, they are silent on the actual form of the conditional probability distribution. Thus, the graphical representation should be viewed as a template upon which conditional-probability models are overlaid.

2.4.3 Graphical Models for Temporal, Spatial, and Spatio-Temporal Processes

Time is one-dimensional and ordered, while space is d-dimensional and has no natural ordering. Therefore, directed graphs are natural for time (Section 3.4.6), and undirected graphs are natural for space (Section 4.2.2). Then, chain graphs (i.e., graphs with directed *and* undirected edges) would provide a natural template for expressing spatio-temporal dependencies; see Section 6.4.2.

2.5 DATA/MODEL/COMPUTING COMPROMISES

The modern statistical approach to modeling is fundamentally about capturing uncertainty with HMs and the conditional-probability distributions upon which they are based. While this provides a framework for inference, actually building and implementing an HM involves a number of compromises. First, there is the notion of the data/model compromise. Imagine trying to gain knowledge about a complicated process. With enough noiseless observations at all appropriate temporal and spatial scales, one could in principle re-create the underlying dependence relationships that are inherent in the process. That is, with a fairly generic model structure, the true underlying scientific mechanism that controls the process could be inferred. However, it is never possible to obtain *noiseless* observations, and a process can never be observed at *all* temporal and spatial scales. Thus, inclusion of both a data model and a process model is a way to formalize the data/model compromise and, depending on the nature of the data that is actually present, the process and parameter models can be chosen to show more or less structure. The HM is very flexible, since it allows inclusion of established scientific properties of the process (which to some extent were themselves inferred from historical data analyses). And, since inference for the HM is based on the posterior distribution, this knowledge can compensate for lack of data. However, there is a flip side to this. It might be the case that an established scientific theory suggests a very complex model with multiple levels in the HM (Wikle and Hooten, 2010). When the available data are not rich enough to learn about the processes and parameters of such a model, then a *practical* lack of identifiability (or, lack of learning) may inhibit successfullly fitting the complex HM.

In addition, the practical matter of implementation leads to the computing/model compromise. While advances in statistical computation have allowed HMs to flourish in the last couple of decades, these computational algorithms can be finicky to "tune" and can be quite time consuming to implement. In many cases, one has to recognize the difference between what one *wants to do* and what one *can do*, when it comes to implementation. This can lead to simpler model structure than what is truly desired. The tension between modeling and computing is healthy if one starts with what one wants to do (answer the Science question) and "dials back" to what one can do. Consequently, as new generations of computing technology emerge, harder problems with fewer compromises can be solved.

This book emphasizes modeling, but our experience with implementation and inference for scientific problems has taught us that the "art of compromise" is ever present. In Chapter 9, examples are given that illustrate different aspects of modeling, implementation, and inference.

CHAPTER 3

Fundamentals of Temporal Processes

What do we mean by "the past" or "the future" and what does it mean when things "change in time?" We tend to categorize and define events by notions of order, including *past, present, future*, and *change*. In many respects, it is difficult to imagine a dataset collected in such a way that at least some of these issues are not a factor. The question then is whether the temporal aspect is important to the analysis of the dataset.

Perhaps the easiest way to deal with temporal variability is to assume that it is due to "randomness" and that if enough observations are taken, it will average (in some well defined way) to a central tendency or to a temporal trend. However, it may be that these randomly varying temporal effects are of most interest. Indeed, many environmental, physical, and biological processes are inherently dynamical, and understanding the temporal variability is of primary importance. Statisticians have long been interested in characterizing and modeling such temporal variability, but so has a large community of applied mathematicians, scientists, and engineers.

This chapter provides a very brief introduction to both dynamical systems theory and the statistical analysis of time series. The two areas are related, although the first sometimes takes a deterministic approach and the second a stochastic approach to quantifying temporal variability. Neither is treated comprehensively here, but there is a combined perspective that is very powerful, which we capitalize on in several places in Chapter 7 (where dynamical spatio-temporal models are discussed). By way of a disclaimer, the statistical aspects of time series that we review concentrate on modeling and have less emphasis on inference; for that, there are many excellent texts given in the Bibliographic Notes in Section 3.7.

Traditionally, much of the time series literature has focused on what we describe in Section 2.1 as the "process model." This is a statistical model for a (hidden) process, indexed by time, that is either implicitly or explicitly conditioned on underlying parameters that describe the process evolution and/or dependence structure. However, it is also true that there is a tradition in the time series literature of explicitly recognizing that observations come with measurement error. This recognition leads to what are known as *state-space models* in time series. In the terminology of Section 2.1, there is a *data model* (or *measurement equation*, or *observation model*, etc.) that describes the distribution of the data given the underlying process and given parameters that characterize the measurement process. In addition, there is a *process model* (or *state equation,* or *state process*, etc.) that expresses the distribution of the underlying process, conditional on parameters that characterize the process. This framework is inherently hierarchical, and we refer to such models as *hierarchical statistical models*, abbreviated as HMs (Section 2.1).

The hierarchical statistical modeling framework is very powerful and is the focus of much of this book. However, in the context of an introduction to time series, we first discuss process models for temporal (or time series) processes. This will be followed by a more complete discussion of HMs for time series.

3.1 CHARACTERIZATION OF TEMPORAL PROCESSES

In general, a temporal process model can be written as $Y(\cdot)$ or more completely as

$$\{\mathbf{Y}(r) : r \in D_t\}, \tag{3.1}$$

where r indexes the time of the possibly multivariate process $\mathbf{Y}(\cdot)$ and D_t is a subset of $\mathbb{R}^1$. The process $\mathbf{Y}$ may be *deterministic* or *stochastic*. Furthermore, the model is quite general if we allow the possibility that the index set D_t can be a random set.

For a *continuous-time process*, we assume here that D_t is fixed and has nonzero length in the continuous interval $(-\infty, \infty)$, although we often assume $D_t = [0, \infty)$. Similarly, for a *discrete-time process* (time series) we assume a fixed index set of a finite or countable set of times, $D_t = \{0, \pm1, \pm2, \ldots\}$ (again, we often limit this set to $D_t = \{0, 1, 2, \ldots\}$). A third type of process is a *temporal point process*, where D_t is assumed to be a random set made up of randomly occurring points (events) in $\mathbb{R}^1$. For example, the time of occurrence of a tornado in a given county could be represented by a Poisson process in time. We might also be interested in some attribute of the point process, say the severity of the tornado as measured by its maximum wind speed. In this case, we have a *marked temporal point process* in which the mark (or marks) describe some attribute (or attributes) of the process when it occurs.

It is useful to consider the practical distinction between a continuous-time and discrete-time process and, as will be seen below, we choose to notate them differently. In the *physical* world, it is difficult to think of a truly discrete-time process (except by exogenous aggregation), yet limitations in measurement often force us to consider one. For example, wind speed at a given location in space, considered as a function of time, is an example of a continuous-time process. However, it is not possible to measure such a process continuously, although the temporal resolution can be quite high. Thus, in practice, one might model wind speed as a discrete-time process (e.g., measured hourly). This practical distinction between continuous time and discrete time is common in time series analysis. From a modeling perspective, there are examples where it is important to consider the unobserved (or hidden) process from the continuous-time perspective, even though the observations on that process are taken at discrete times. Many such examples exist in statistical physics and, more recently, in the analysis of financial time series (e.g., Wilmott, Howison, and Dewynne, 1995). In the latter case, if one is interested in trades of some financial instrument at very small time increments, then it makes sense to think about processes with infinitely short time increments, that is, continuous-time processes.

In our notation, we typically refer to a *continuous-time* process with the time index *t in parentheses*, namely $\mathbf{Y}(t)$, and refer to the *discrete-time* process (or time series) with *t as a subscript*, namely $\mathbf{Y}_t$. In this book, we give a lot of attention to discrete-time processes; but, occasionally, to motivate them, we do present discussion of continuous-time processes.

3.1.1 Joint and Conditional Distributions

Typically, when working with real-world temporal processes, we have only one realization of that process; thus, the associated time series can be viewed as just one sample from a *population*. We characterize this population by its *joint distribution*. For example, consider a time series given by $\{Y_t : t = 0, \ldots, T\}$. We denote its joint distribution by

$$[Y_0, Y_1, \ldots, Y_T], \tag{3.2}$$

where recall from Chapter 2 that this is short-hand notation used to represent the (joint) probability distribution of $Y_0, Y_1, \ldots, Y_T$. This notation is described more completely in Chapter 2, including the conditional probability notation, $[A|B]$. In practice, it can be very difficult to fully specify (3.2) because it requires that we specify all possible interactions between $Y_0, \ldots, Y_T$, which can be very problematic in high dimensions. It can often prove useful to think about the joint distribution from a conditional perspective. That is, using basic probability rules (see Chapter 2), we can always rewrite this joint distribution as a product of conditional distributions:

$$[Y_0, \ldots, Y_T] = [Y_T|Y_{T-1}, \ldots, Y_0][Y_{T-1}|Y_{T-2}, \ldots, Y_0] \ldots [Y_1|Y_0][Y_0]. \tag{3.3}$$

However, for practical modeling we still need to make additional assumptions about the components of (3.3). For example, we might assume that the process can be modeled by a first-order Markov property,

$$[Y_t|Y_{t-1}, \ldots, Y_0] = [Y_t|Y_{t-1}], \qquad \text{for all } t = 1, 2, \ldots . \tag{3.4}$$

This property suggests a "lack of memory," so that only the most recent past determines the conditional probabilities about the present given the whole past. In this case, (3.3) becomes

$$[Y_0, \ldots, Y_T] = [Y_0] \prod_{t=1}^{T} [Y_t|Y_{t-1}] . \tag{3.5}$$

The first-order Markov assumption provides a dramatic simplification of the joint distribution, yet the product of these relatively simple conditional distributions can model a process that is quite complicated. Representing complicated joint distributions as a product of conditional distributions is a running theme throughout this book. Although the Markov assumption is very important in time series analysis, there are many other probability models for temporal processes that can be used to simplify joint or conditional distributions.

3.1.2   Deterministic and Stochastic Processes

Although somewhat arbitrary, it is sometimes convenient to characterize temporal processes as either deterministic or stochastic (i.e., random). One might say that for a deterministic process the future is completely determined by the past. For example, a continuous-time process $Y(t)$ might be described via a simple differential equation in which the rate of change of the process Y with time is simply related to a function of the process at time t:

$$\frac{dY(t)}{dt} = f(Y(t)), \qquad t \geq 0, \tag{3.6}$$

where the function f may be linear or nonlinear in $Y(t)$. Thus, given some *initial condition* $Y(0)$, the evolution of the process is completely determined by the function f. Alternatively, if we limit our discussion to only processes at discrete times, then we could write an analogous equation,

$$Y_t = \mathcal{M}(Y_{t-1}), \qquad t = 1, 2, \ldots, \tag{3.7}$$

where the function $\mathcal{M}$ maps the process from the previous time $t-1$ to the current time t. Again, given an initial condition Y_0, the process $\{Y_t : t = 0, 1, 2, \ldots\}$ is completely determined by the function $\mathcal{M}$.

For *stochastic* or *random* processes, we might say that the future is only partially determined from the past. For example, we can add a random "noise" component to equation (3.7):

$$Y_t = \mathcal{M}(Y_{t-1}) + \eta_t, \qquad t = 1, 2, \ldots, \tag{3.8}$$

where $\{\eta_t : t = 1, 2, \ldots\}$ is a mean-zero random process and η_t is statistically independent of Y_{t-1}. This random-noise term implies that the process $\{Y_t\}$ is random as well. Similarly, stochastic differential equations can be formed by the addition of a continuous-time random-noise term to (3.6) (e.g., see the introduction to Chapter 6). The process $\{Y_t : t = 0, 1, \ldots\}$ in (3.8) is an example of what could generally be called a *discrete-time temporal random process*.

Just as the distinction between continuous and discrete time is not always clear, so it is with the difference between deterministic and stochastic processes. For example, consider a *chaotic* process, which is a nonlinear, deterministic temporal process that exhibits sensitivity to initial conditions (e.g., see Section 3.2.4; and Devaney, 2003, p. 50). That is, for nonlinear functions f in (3.6) (or $\mathcal{M}$ in (3.7)), very small changes to the initial condition $Y(0)$ can lead to very different trajectories of the process $Y(t)$. Thus, even though such trajectories are completely determined once the initial condition is known, two slightly different initial conditions can ultimately exhibit sequences that do not appear to be at all related. The practical implication of this is that since there is always some uncertainty in initial conditions for real-world processes (e.g., due to measurement error), nonlinear deterministic processes will ultimately become unpredictable. In fact, when there is this initial-condition uncertainty, one cannot typically distinguish between chaotic uncertainties and uncertainty due to a random process (e.g., see Berliner, 1992; Chan and Tong, 2001; and Section 3.2.2, for more discussion).

The next section gives a brief introduction to *deterministic* dynamical systems. The remainder of the chapter then focuses on random temporal processes.

3.2 INTRODUCTION TO DETERMINISTIC DYNAMICAL SYSTEMS

To facilitate the discussion of statistical models for spatio-temporal dynamical processes, it is necessary to provide some background to deterministic dynamical systems. This discussion is not intended to be a formal treatment of dynamical-systems theory, but rather it is an attempt to provide some definitions and basic concepts in the area. For a detailed and technical overview, the reader is referred to the references in the Bibliographic Notes in Section 3.7.

We say the *state* of a system at time t is described by a set of p_α variables, $\alpha_t = (\alpha_t(1), \ldots, \alpha_t(p_\alpha))'$, which are sometimes known as the *state variables* or, collectively, as the *state process*. In general, state variables may be physical variables (e.g., temperature, pressure, wind components, water vapor, etc., in the atmosphere) defined at specific locations in physical space. From our perspective, any system whose state changes with time is a *dynamical system*. The evolution of the system through *state space* (or, equivalently, *phase space*) is often called a *trajectory*. If the current state of the system, say α_t, uniquely determines the future states $\alpha_{t+\tau}$; $\tau > 0$, the system is referred to as a *deterministic dynamical system*. Correspondingly, if such a unique mapping does not exist, we say the system is a *stochastic dynamical system*.

In general, one might consider discrete-time or continuous-time dynamical systems. In this section, we focus on discrete systems of the form

$$\boldsymbol{\alpha}_t = \mathcal{M}(\boldsymbol{\alpha}_{t-1}; \boldsymbol{\theta}), \qquad t = 1, 2, \ldots, \tag{3.9}$$

where the *mapping* (or *transition*) *function* $\mathcal{M}$, describes the behavior of the state process as time evolves, and $\boldsymbol{\theta}$ is a vector of parameters involved in that description. To complete the definition of the dynamical system, one needs to specify the initial condition, $\boldsymbol{\alpha}_0$, as well as boundary conditions if the elements of $\boldsymbol{\alpha}_t$ depend on boundary values. In the case where the mapping $\mathcal{M}$ varies with time, the system is said to be *nonautonomous*, and where $\mathcal{M}$ does not vary with time, it is said to be *autonomous*. A critical distinction is made between systems in which $\mathcal{M}$ is linear (in the state variables) versus those in which $\mathcal{M}$ is nonlinear. We first consider the case where $\mathcal{M}$ is linear.

3.2.1   Linear Discrete Dynamical Systems

Our discussion of linear discrete dynamical systems follows the introductory treatment in Sandefur (1990).

First-Order Univariate Systems
Initially, we consider the first-order *linear* discrete dynamical system. In general, a univariate first-order system might be written as

$$\alpha_t = \mathcal{M}(\alpha_{t-1}; \boldsymbol{\theta}), \qquad t = 1, 2, \ldots, \tag{3.10}$$

and when $\mathcal{M}$ is linear, it becomes a *first-order affine dynamical system*:

$$\alpha_t = \theta_0 + \theta_1 \alpha_{t-1}, \qquad t = 1, 2, \ldots, \tag{3.11}$$

where θ_0 and θ_1 are parameters. Even such a simple system is useful for establishing some basic definitions and concepts. For example, we say an *equilibrium value* or *fixed point* of the system is a number "a" such that $\alpha_t = a$ for all values of t when $\alpha_0 = a$. That is, for the general formulation (3.10), a is an equilibrium value if and only if $\mathcal{M}(a) = a$. Thus, for the linear system (3.11), the equilibrium value is $a = \theta_0/(1 - \theta_1)$ when $\theta_1 \neq 1$ (if $\theta_1 = 1$, then there is no equilibrium value). Of course, in general, a linear dynamical system can have many different equilibrium values.

Example: Consider a simple example where there is an initial animal population of size α_0 and it is assumed to grow by 5 percent per year. In addition, 30 members of the population are removed each year to supplement smaller populations at other (distinct) locations. A simple linear dynamical system describes how the population varies each year:

$$\alpha_t = 1.05\alpha_{t-1} - 30. \tag{3.12}$$

In this case, the fixed point is $a = 600$; thus, if $\alpha_0 = 600$, the population will stay constant through time ($\alpha_1 = 600, \alpha_2 = 600, \ldots$). If the initial population is fewer than 600, the population will decrease with time, and if the initial population is more than 600, the population will increase with time.

With regard to (3.10), it is interesting to consider what happens as the state of the system nears the equilibrium value. Intuitively, an equilibrium value is said to be *stable* or *attracting* if α_0 "close to" a implies that α_t tends to a (in a limiting sense). The equilibrium value is said to be *unstable or repelling* if, regardless of how close the initial condition α_0 is to a, α_t eventually ends up "far from" a (note that for an unstable equilibrium, the trajectory can come close to a but it cannot stay close). For example, the equilibrium value for the first-order system (3.11) is stable if $|\theta_1| < 1$. However, for $|\theta_1| > 1$, the equilibrium value is unstable ($|\alpha_t|$ tends to infinity for $\alpha_0 \neq a$). For the special case when $\theta_1 = -1$, we see that $\alpha_0 = \alpha_2 = \alpha_4 = \ldots$ and $\alpha_1 = \alpha_3 = \alpha_5 = \ldots$. This type of pattern, often seen in dynamical systems, is known as a *2-cycle*. In this case, since α_t neither converges nor diverges from the equilibrium value, the equilibrium value is said to be *neutral*.

In simple linear systems, for $t = 0, 1, \ldots$, we can obtain solutions of α_t. Consider the first-order dynamical system given in (3.11) but with $\theta_0 = 0$. It is easy to show that the general solution to this system is $\alpha_t = c\theta_1^t$, for $t = 0, 1, \ldots$, where c is a constant. Analogous to differential equations, the particular solution can be found, given α_0, to be $\alpha_t = \alpha_0\theta_1^t$, for $t = 0, 1, \ldots$. The more general affine system (with an additive constant θ_0) given in (3.11) has general solution $\alpha_t = c\theta_1^t + \theta_0/(1 - \theta_1)$, provided $\theta_1 \neq 1$ and for $t = 0, 1, \ldots$. The corresponding particular solution, given α_0, can be shown to be: $\alpha_t = \theta_1^t(\alpha_0 - \theta_0/(1 - \theta_1)) + \theta_0/(1 - \theta_1)$, for $t = 0, 1, \ldots$. The following properties of the solution to the first-order system are useful for describing system behavior:

- If $0 < \theta_1 < 1$, then $\alpha_t \to a$, exponentially.
- If $-1 < \theta_1 < 0$, then α_t oscillates in a dampened manner to a.
- If $|\theta_1| > 1$, then $\alpha_t \to \pm\infty$, exponentially fast; and if $\theta_1 < -1$, then α_t oscillates with increasing amplitude.

Note, for the special case where $\theta_1 = 1$, the general solution is $\alpha_t = c + \theta_0 t$, and if the initial condition is given, the particular solution is, $\alpha_t = \alpha_0 + \theta_0 t$.

Example: Consider the simple system, $\alpha_t = -.7\alpha_{t-1}$, and $\alpha_0 = 12$. Figure 3.1 shows realizations from this system through time $t = 10$. Given

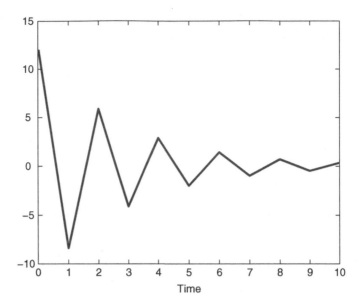

Figure 3.1   The first-order dynamical system: $\alpha_t = -0.7\alpha_{t-1}$, where $\alpha_0 = 12$.

that $-1 < \theta_1 < 0$, we see that the solution is oscillating and decreasing in amplitude over time.

A thorough study of linear dynamical systems considers nonhomogeneous systems such as

$$\alpha_t = \theta_1\alpha_{t-1} + g_{t-1}, \qquad t = 1, 2, \ldots, \qquad (3.13)$$

where typically $\{g_t : t = 0, 1, \ldots\}$ is some deterministic function of t. Such systems do not have equilibrium points. Solutions can be found for specific functional forms for g_t (e.g., when g_t is a polynomial in t or when g_t is an exponential in t). We do not present such systems here, but refer the interested reader to Sandefur (1990).

Second-Order Univariate Systems

The second-order linear discrete homogeneous dynamical system is given by

$$\alpha_t = \theta_1\alpha_{t-1} + \theta_2\alpha_{t-2}, \quad t = 2, 3, \ldots. \qquad (3.14)$$

It is convenient at this point to introduce some notation. We define the *backward-shift operator B* as follows:

$$\alpha_{t-1} = B\alpha_t. \qquad (3.15)$$

Hence,

$$\alpha_{t-2} = B\alpha_{t-1} = BB\alpha_t = B^2\alpha_t, \tag{3.16}$$

and in general,

$$\alpha_{t-p} = B^p\alpha_t. \tag{3.17}$$

Although not considered here, we note that one could use analogous "forward-shift operators" in this context if the general dynamical system is written as $\alpha_{t+1} = \mathcal{M}(\alpha_t; \boldsymbol{\theta})$. Using the backward-shift notation, we can rewrite the dynamical system (3.14) as

$$(1 - \theta_1 B - \theta_2 B^2)\alpha_t = 0, \qquad t = 2, 3, \ldots, \tag{3.18}$$

and we let $1 - \theta_1 z - \theta_2 z^2$ be the *characteristic polynomial* of this system. The behavior of the dynamical system is described by the roots of this polynomial, which we denote by z_1 and z_2. We consider two general cases.

Case 1: $z_1 \neq z_2$. In this case, the general solution of the second-order system is

$$\alpha_t = c_1 z_1^{-t} + c_2 z_2^{-t}, \qquad t = 0, 1, \ldots, \tag{3.19}$$

where the constants c_1 and c_2 depend on the initial conditions, α_0 and α_1:

$$c_1 = \frac{\alpha_1 - \alpha_0 z_2^{-1}}{z_1^{-1} - z_2^{-1}}, \qquad c_2 = \frac{\alpha_1 - \alpha_0 z_1^{-1}}{z_2^{-1} - z_1^{-1}}. \tag{3.20}$$

Before we proceed, it is helpful to recall the following facts concerning complex numbers and sinusoidal processes. Let $h = u + iv$ be a complex number, where $i \equiv \sqrt{-1}$. The complex conjugate is $h = u - iv$, and the modulus is $|h| = \sqrt{u^2 + v^2}$. On occasion, notation is simplified by the *Euler formula*, $\exp(i\gamma) = \cos(\gamma) + i\sin(\gamma)$, or, $\exp(-i\gamma) = \cos(\gamma) - i\sin(\gamma)$. In addition, the *complex plane* is such that the real component (u) is plotted along the horizonal axis and the imaginary component (v) is plotted along the vertical axis. The resulting vector has magnitude given by the modulus $|h|$, and the angle γ between the imaginary and real components is defined such that $\tan(\gamma) = v/u$; thus, $u = |h|\cos(\gamma)$, $v = |h|\sin(\gamma)$, and $h = |h|\exp(i\gamma)$.

In addition, consider a sinusoidal process that is defined in terms of its *amplitude*, *frequency*, and *phase*:

$$Y_t = A\cos(\omega t + \gamma), \tag{3.21}$$

where A is the amplitude, ω is the frequency (in units of radians per time unit), and γ is the phase (in radians). We sometimes refer to γ also as the phase shift.

Using the trigonometric identity, $\cos(\alpha + \beta) = \cos(\alpha)\cos(\beta) - \sin(\alpha)\sin(\beta)$, we can rewrite (3.21) as

$$Y_t = A\cos(\gamma)\cos(\omega t) + (-A\sin(\gamma))\sin(\omega t)$$
$$= a\cos(\omega t) + b\sin(\omega t), \tag{3.22}$$

where $a = A\cos(\gamma)$ and $b = -A\sin(\gamma)$. Thus, if a and b are known, then the amplitude is given by $A = \sqrt{a^2 + b^2}$ and the phase is given by $\gamma = \tan^{-1}(-b/a)$.

Now, for the special case where the two roots, z_1 and z_2, are a complex-conjugate pair, the general solution is still given by (3.19). However, since $z_2 = \bar{z}_1$ and, necessarily, $c_2 = \bar{c}_1$ (since the solution is real), we can write

$$\alpha_t = c_1 z_1^{-t} + \bar{c}_1 \bar{z}_1^{-t}. \tag{3.23}$$

In terms of complex numbers, the components of (3.23) can be written as

$$c_1 = |c_1|\exp(i\psi), \qquad z_1 = |z_1|\exp(i\phi), \tag{3.24}$$

where ψ is the angle between the real and imaginary components of c_1, and ϕ is the angle between the real and imaginary components of z_1. We can write analogous complex notation for the complex conjugates, $\bar{c}_1$ and $\bar{z}_1$. Then the general solution becomes

$$\alpha_t = 2|c_1||z_1|^{-t}\cos(t\phi - \psi), \tag{3.25}$$

where the constants c_1 and ψ must be determined by the initial conditions, α_0 and α_1. The important point to note regarding (3.25) is that the solution exhibits a sinusoidal oscillation with amplitude depending on t and given by $2|c_1||z_1|^{-t}$, frequency given by ϕ, and phase shift given by ψ.

Case 2: $z_1 = z_2(= z_0)$. In this case, the general solution of the second-order system is

$$\alpha_t = (c_1 + c_2 t)z_0^{-t}, \qquad k = 0, 1, \ldots, \tag{3.26}$$

where the constants c_1 and c_2 depend on the initial conditions, α_0 and α_1:

$$c_1 = \alpha_0, \qquad c_2 = \alpha_1 z_0 - \alpha_0. \tag{3.27}$$

Not surprisingly, the behavior of the second-order system relative to its equilibrium value depends on the nature of the roots, z_1 and z_2. First, consider the second-order affine system:

$$\alpha_t = \theta_1 \alpha_{t-1} + \theta_2 \alpha_{t-2} + \theta_0, \qquad t = 2, 3, \ldots. \tag{3.28}$$

The equilibrium value in this case is given by

$$a = \frac{\theta_0}{1 - \theta_1 - \theta_2},$$

(3.29)

provided $\theta_1 + \theta_2 \neq 1$. In the case where z_1 and z_2 are distinct and not equal to 1, the general solution of (3.28) is given by $\alpha_t = c_1 z_1^{-t} + c_2 z_2^{-t} + a$. One can show that if $|z_1| > 1$ and $|z_2| > 1$, then the equilibrium value is attracting (stable). Furthermore, if either $|z_1| < 1$ or $|z_2| < 1$, or both, then the equilibrium value is repelling (unstable).

Example: Consider the dynamical system:

$$\alpha_t = -0.64\alpha_{t-2}, \qquad t = 2, 3, \ldots,$$

(3.30)

with initial conditions $\alpha_0 = 0$ and $\alpha_1 = -5$. The roots of the polynomial, $0.64z^2 + 1 = 0$, are $z_1 = 1.25i$ and $z_2 = -1.25i$. In this case, the general solution is given by (3.25). We also note that $|z_1| = |z_2| = 1.25$, and so the system is stable. In addition, $\phi = \pi/2$ and, given the initial conditions, we find that $\psi = \pi/2$ and $|c_1| = 3.125$, resulting in the solution, $\alpha_t = 6.25(1.25)^{-t}\cos(t\pi/2 + \pi/2)$. This system is shown in Figure 3.2 for time $t = 0, 1, \ldots, 20$, where the damped oscillation is clearly evident.

Linear Dynamical Systems of Several Variables
Consider the p_α-dimensional state process $\{\boldsymbol{\alpha}_t\}$, given by $\boldsymbol{\alpha}_t = (\alpha_t(1), \ldots, \alpha_t(p_\alpha))'$. For example, $\alpha_t(j)$ might represent the temperature at the jth spatial

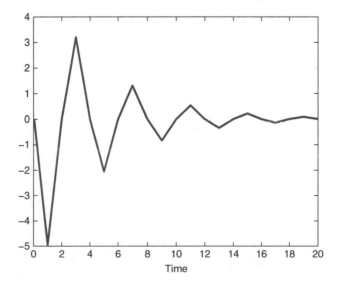

Figure 3.2 The second-order dynamical system: $\alpha_t = -0.64\alpha_{t-2}$, where $\alpha_0 = 0$, $\alpha_1 = -5$.

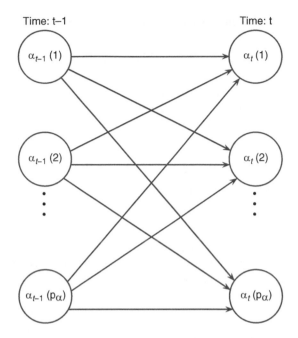

Figure 3.3 Schematic of a p_α-dimensional dynamical system in which each component at time t can be influenced by each component at the previous time, $t - 1$.

location at time t, or the population of the jth species at time t, or the abundance of the jth age class of a species at time t, and so on. Our goal is to describe a system in which the components of this state process interact across time, as shown schematically in Figure 3.3.

In a first-order system, we would have

$$\alpha_t(j) = m_{j1}\alpha_{t-1}(1) + m_{j2}\alpha_{t-1}(2) + \cdots + m_{jp_\alpha}\alpha_{t-1}(p_\alpha), \tag{3.31}$$

for $j = 1, \ldots, p_\alpha$. Thus, $\alpha_t(j)$ is related to itself and the other components of the state process at the previous time, according to the transition coefficients, m_{jk}, $k = 1, \ldots, p_\alpha$. Obviously, the notation will simplify if we write this in an equivalent matrix form:

$$\boldsymbol{\alpha}_t = \mathbf{M}\boldsymbol{\alpha}_{t-1}, \qquad t = 1, 2, \ldots, \tag{3.32}$$

where

$$\mathbf{M} \equiv \begin{pmatrix} m_{11} & m_{12} & \cdots & m_{1p_\alpha} \\ m_{21} & \cdots & & m_{2p_\alpha} \\ \vdots & & & \vdots \\ m_{p_\alpha 1} & \cdots & & m_{p_\alpha p_\alpha} \end{pmatrix}. \tag{3.33}$$

By substitution, the general solution of this system is given by

$$\boldsymbol{\alpha}_t = \mathbf{M}^t \boldsymbol{\alpha}_0, \qquad t = 0, 1, \ldots, \tag{3.34}$$

where $\mathbf{M}^t \equiv \mathbf{MM} \ldots \mathbf{M}$ (t products of the matrix $\mathbf{M}$), and a particular solution is obtained if one specifies the starting value, $\boldsymbol{\alpha}_0$.

One might ask just how general the first-order vector ("multivariate") dynamical system is? In fact, it can be quite general. As an example, consider the second-order univariate system,

$$\beta_t = b_1 \beta_{t-1} + b_2 \beta_{t-2}, \qquad t = 2, 3, \ldots . \tag{3.35}$$

We can rewrite this as a system of equations by defining $\boldsymbol{\alpha}_{t-1} = (\alpha_{t-1}(1), \alpha_{t-1}(2))'$, where $\alpha_{t-1}(1) \equiv \beta_{t-1}$, $\alpha_{t-1}(2) \equiv \beta_{t-2}$. Then, the system (3.35) can be rewritten as

$$\boldsymbol{\alpha}_t = \mathbf{M} \boldsymbol{\alpha}_{t-1}, \tag{3.36}$$

where

$$\mathbf{M} = \begin{pmatrix} b_1 & b_2 \\ 1 & 0 \end{pmatrix}. \tag{3.37}$$

Note that such a reparameterization approach easily extends to higher-order vector systems. For example, for vectors $\{\boldsymbol{\beta}_t\}$, consider the third-order system,

$$\boldsymbol{\beta}_t = \mathbf{G}_1 \boldsymbol{\beta}_{t-1} + \mathbf{G}_2 \boldsymbol{\beta}_{t-2} + \mathbf{G}_3 \boldsymbol{\beta}_{t-3}. \tag{3.38}$$

Then define $\boldsymbol{\alpha}_t \equiv (\boldsymbol{\beta}_t', \boldsymbol{\beta}_{t-1}', \boldsymbol{\beta}_{t-2}')'$, resulting in

$$\boldsymbol{\alpha}_t = \begin{pmatrix} \mathbf{G}_1 & \mathbf{G}_2 & \mathbf{G}_3 \\ \mathbf{I} & 0 & 0 \\ 0 & \mathbf{I} & 0 \end{pmatrix} \boldsymbol{\alpha}_{t-1} \equiv \mathbf{M} \boldsymbol{\alpha}_{t-1}. \tag{3.39}$$

Thus, the first-order vector dynamical system is quite general.

Spectral Representation of the First-Order System

Consider the first-order system (3.32). In general, the matrix $\mathbf{M}$ is nonsymmetric. As shown, for example, by Rao (1965, pp. 38–39), the characteristic equation, $|\mathbf{M} - \lambda \mathbf{I}| = 0$, has p_α roots, some of which may be complex, even if $\mathbf{M}$ is real. Thus, corresponding to each *latent root*, λ_i, there are two vectors, $\mathbf{w}_i$ and $\mathbf{v}_i$, called the right and left *singular vectors*, respectively, such that

$$\mathbf{M} \mathbf{w}_i = \lambda_i \mathbf{w}_i, \tag{3.40}$$

$$\mathbf{M}' \mathbf{v}_i = \lambda_i \mathbf{v}_i, \tag{3.41}$$

for $i = 1, \ldots, p_\alpha$. Then, the following results can be obtained (e.g., Rao, 1965, pp. 38–39):

- The right eigenvectors $\{\mathbf{w}_i\}$ are linearly independent and so are the left eigenvectors $\{\mathbf{v}_i\}$. This implies that $\mathbf{W} \equiv (\mathbf{w}_1, \dots, \mathbf{w}_{p_\alpha})$ and $\mathbf{V} \equiv (\mathbf{v}_1, \dots, \mathbf{v}_{p_\alpha})$ are nonsingular; thus,

$$\mathbf{M} = \mathbf{W}\boldsymbol{\Lambda}\mathbf{W}^{-1} \quad \text{and} \quad \mathbf{M}' = \mathbf{V}\boldsymbol{\Lambda}\mathbf{V}^{-1}, \qquad (3.42)$$

where $\boldsymbol{\Lambda} \equiv \text{diag}(\lambda_1, \dots, \lambda_{p_\alpha})$.
- Orthogonality is of the form, $\mathbf{w}_i'\mathbf{v}_j = 0$ for $i \neq j$ and $\mathbf{w}_i'\mathbf{v}_i \neq 0$ for $i = 1, \dots, p_\alpha$.
- Since $\mathbf{M} = \mathbf{W}\boldsymbol{\Lambda}\mathbf{W}^{-1}$, then $\mathbf{W}^{-1}\mathbf{M} = \boldsymbol{\Lambda}\mathbf{W}^{-1}$, which implies that $\mathbf{W}^{-1} = \mathbf{V}'$; thus, $\mathbf{M} = \mathbf{W}\boldsymbol{\Lambda}\mathbf{V}' = \sum_{i=1}^{p_\alpha} \lambda_i \mathbf{w}_i \mathbf{v}_i'$. *Note*: This assumes that $\mathbf{W}\mathbf{V}' = \mathbf{I}$ (i.e., that the latent roots are normalized). If, in general, $\mathbf{W}\mathbf{V}' = \mathbf{D}$ (where $\mathbf{D}$ is a diagonal matrix, and the singular vectors are chosen so that its diagonal elements are positive), then $\mathbf{M} = \sum_{i=1}^{p_\alpha} (\lambda_i/d_i)\mathbf{w}_i \mathbf{v}_i'$, where d_i is the ith diagonal element of $\mathbf{D}$.

We can use these results to express the solution to the general first-order difference equation in terms of its spectral components $\{(\lambda_i, \mathbf{w}_i, \mathbf{v}_i) : i = 1, \dots, p_\alpha\}$. Using the orthogonality result, one can see that $\mathbf{M}^2 = \mathbf{W}\boldsymbol{\Lambda}\mathbf{V}'\mathbf{W}\boldsymbol{\Lambda}\mathbf{V}' = \mathbf{W}\boldsymbol{\Lambda}^2\mathbf{V}'$. Furthermore, in general, $\mathbf{M}^k = \mathbf{W}\boldsymbol{\Lambda}^k\mathbf{V}'$; $k = 1, 2, \dots$. Thus, we can write the general solution,

$$\boldsymbol{\alpha}_t = \mathbf{M}^t\boldsymbol{\alpha}_0 = \mathbf{W}\boldsymbol{\Lambda}^t\mathbf{V}'\boldsymbol{\alpha}_0 = \sum_{i=1}^{p_\alpha} \lambda_i^t \mathbf{w}_i \mathbf{v}_i'\boldsymbol{\alpha}_0, \qquad t = 0, 1, \dots . \qquad (3.43)$$

Suppose that because of the linear independence of $\{\mathbf{w}_i\}$, we express the initial condition $\boldsymbol{\alpha}_0 = \mathbf{W}\mathbf{c} = \sum_{i=1}^{p_\alpha} c_i \mathbf{w}_i$, for some constants $\mathbf{c} \equiv (c_1, \dots, c_{p_\alpha})'$. Then, it follows that $\mathbf{c} = \mathbf{W}^{-1}\boldsymbol{\alpha}_0 = \mathbf{V}'\boldsymbol{\alpha}_0$, and the particular solution can be written as

$$\boldsymbol{\alpha}_t = \mathbf{W}\boldsymbol{\Lambda}^t\mathbf{c} = \sum_{i=1}^{p_\alpha} c_i \lambda_i^t \mathbf{w}_i, \qquad t = 0, 1, \dots . \qquad (3.44)$$

Now, it is clear that the solution to the linear difference equation is critically dependent on the values of $\{\lambda_i\}$. For example, if $|\lambda_i| < 1$, then $\lim_{t \to \infty} \lambda_i^t = 0$, and thus the ith term in the linear expansion of $\boldsymbol{\alpha}_t$ goes to zero. More generally, let $||\mathbf{M}|| = \max\{|\lambda_i| : i = 1, \dots, p_\alpha\}$. Then, if $||\mathbf{M}|| < 1$, it follows that $\lim_{t \to \infty} \boldsymbol{\alpha}_t = \mathbf{0}$. In this case, the zero vector is a stable equilibrium value. In general, one can show the following:

- If λ_i is real and $\lambda_i > 1$, then the ith component of $\boldsymbol{\alpha}_t$ in the expansion (3.44) exhibits exponential growth.
- If λ_i is real and $0 < \lambda_i < 1$, then the ith component of $\boldsymbol{\alpha}_t$ in the expansion (3.44) exhibits exponential decay.

- If λ_i is real and $-1 < \lambda_i < 0$, then the ith component of $\boldsymbol{\alpha}_t$ in the expansion (3.44) exhibits a damped oscillation with period 2.
- If λ_i is real and $\lambda_i < -1$, then the ith component of $\boldsymbol{\alpha}_t$ in the expansion (3.44) exhibits a divergent oscillation with period 2.
- If λ_i is complex, then there is an associated complex conjugate component in the expansion (3.44). In this case, the associated components of $\boldsymbol{\alpha}_t$ in the expansion (3.44) exhibit oscillations as in the second-order dynamical system (see Section 3.2.1). That is, suppose $\lambda_i = a + b\sqrt{-1}$. Then, using common identities for complex numbers, $\lambda_i^t = |\lambda_i|^t(\cos \phi t + \sqrt{-1} \sin \phi t)$, where $|\lambda_i| = \sqrt{a^2 + b^2}$ is the amplitude and $\phi = \tan^{-1}(b/a)$ is the phase angle formed by λ_i in the complex plane. For a real solution, we must have complex conjugate pairs of eigenvalues, and so

$$\lambda_i^t + \bar{\lambda}_i^t = 2|\lambda_i|^t \cos(\phi t). \tag{3.45}$$

Thus, the amplitude of the oscillation increases or decreases, depending on whether $|\lambda_i|$ is greater or less than 1, respectively. For each unit increase in time, the angle in the complex plane increases by ϕ, and an oscillation is completed with period $2\pi/\phi$.

- If $\lambda_i = 1$ and $|\lambda_j| < 1$, for all $j \neq i$, then $\lim_{t \to \infty} \boldsymbol{\alpha}_t = c_i \mathbf{w}_i$, where the constant c_i depends on the initial condition. We note that this solution is not a stable equilibrium since, depending on the initial condition, the solution will be any multiple of $\mathbf{w}_i$.
- If $\lambda_i = -1$ and $|\lambda_j| < 1$, for all $j \neq i$, then the limiting solution is $\boldsymbol{\alpha}_t = c_i(-1)^t \mathbf{w}_i$, which is a 2-cycle, with the constant c_i determined from the initial condition.
- If $\lambda_i = 1$, $\lambda_j = -1$, $|\lambda_l| < 1$, for all $l \neq i, j$, then the limiting solution is again a 2-cycle: $\boldsymbol{\alpha}_t = c_i \mathbf{w}_i + c_j(-1)^t \mathbf{w}_j$, with c_i, c_j determined by the initial condition.
- If $\lambda_i = a + b\sqrt{-1}$ and $\lambda_j = a - b\sqrt{-1}$, with $a^2 + b^2 = 1$, and $|\lambda_l| < 1$, $l \neq i, j$, then the limiting solution is a constant amplitude oscillation.

It is often useful to examine the sensitivity of the latent roots to changes in the matrix elements m_{qr} through a *sensitivity matrix* (e.g., see Caswell, 2001, Section 9.1). That is, the sensitivity matrix associated with the ith latent root is

$$\mathbf{S}_i \equiv \left(\frac{\partial \lambda_i}{\partial m_{qr}} \right) = \frac{\bar{\mathbf{v}}_i \mathbf{w}_i'}{\mathbf{v}_i' \mathbf{w}_i}. \tag{3.46}$$

Furthermore, given that the latent roots of $\mathbf{M}$ reveal so much about the underlying dynamics of the system, it is often useful to consider the *eigenvalue spectrum* of $\mathbf{M}$, as illustrated below.

Table 3.1   Eigenvalue Spectrum of M

λ_i	$|\lambda_i|$	ϕ/π
1.3070	1.3070	0
$0.8465 + 0.2840\sqrt{-1}$	0.8929	0.1030
$0.8465 - 0.2840\sqrt{-1}$	0.8929	−0.1030

Example: Consider the case where $p_\alpha = 3$ and $\mathbf{M}$ is given by

$$\mathbf{M} = \begin{pmatrix} 1.1 & 0.3 & 0.2 \\ 0.2 & 1.0 & -0.1 \\ -0.2 & 0.4 & 0.9 \end{pmatrix}. \tag{3.47}$$

Then the eigenvalue spectrum is given in Table 3.1.

We can see from this table that there is a dominant mode with $|\lambda_1| = 1.3070 > 1$, implying that α_t will exhibit exponential growth over time. In addition, assuming the time increment is one year, there is a decaying oscillation with period $2\pi/\phi = 19.4$ years. As time increases, this periodic component is dominated by the exponentially growing mode.

The sensitivity matrix for λ_1 in this case is

$$\mathbf{S}_1 = \begin{pmatrix} 0.56 & 0.35 & 0.06 \\ 0.69 & 0.42 & 0.08 \\ 0.11 & 0.07 & 0.01 \end{pmatrix}, \tag{3.48}$$

suggesting that the value of λ_1 is most sensitive to m_{21}, the element of $\mathbf{M}$ in the second row and first column.

The eigenvalue spectrum can be very useful across a wide variety of applications. For example, in ecology and demography, researchers consider so-called "matrix models" [see Caswell (2001)], which are simply discrete linear systems of the structure considered here, where, for example, the components of the state vector might be the number of organisms in different age classes. The transition matrix in that setting then relates the flow of members of the population from one class to another. Another application, more relevant to the spatio-temporal setting of interest here, is to the so-called Principal Oscillation Pattern (POP) analysis. Such analysis considers a spatial process that evolves in time according to a first-order system, such as one might find in meteorology or oceanography. This is considered in detail in Section 5.5.

3.2.2   Nonlinear Discrete Dynamical Systems

Many of the basic concepts defined for linear systems also hold for nonlinear systems, but some modifications and additional concepts must be introduced to describe the more complicated behavior of nonlinear systems. Again, our exposition follows Sandefur (1990), and additional details and examples can be found there and in the Bibliographic Notes in Section 3.7.

We shall motivate our discussion of univariate nonlinear dynamical systems with the basic *logistic equation* or *logistic dynamical system*,

$$\alpha_t = (1 + \theta_1)\alpha_{t-1} - \frac{\theta_1}{\theta_0}\alpha_{t-1}^2, \qquad t = 1, 2, \ldots, \tag{3.49}$$

which is an example of the more general system, $\alpha_t = \mathcal{M}(\alpha_{t-1})$. In population dynamics, (3.49) can be used to model density-dependent population growth. In that case, θ_1 is a growth parameter and θ_0 is the *carrying capacity* of the environment. The set of equilibrium values for the logistic equation is easily found to be $\{0, \theta_0\}$.

As with linear systems, we would like to characterize the system behavior near the equilibrium values. When $\mathcal{M}$ is a differentiable function (with respect to α_{t-1}), one can show that the equilibrium value a is attracting if $|\mathcal{M}^{(\prime)}(a)| < 1$ and is repelling if $|\mathcal{M}^{(\prime)}(a)| > 1$, where the superscript "$(\prime)$" denotes the first derivative with respect to a. Thus, for the logistic equation, $\mathcal{M}^{(\prime)}(a) = 1 + \theta_1 - 2(\theta_1/\theta_0)a$. Then, if $\theta_1 > 0$ or $\theta_1 < -2$, the equilibrium value $a = 0$ is repelling; and if $-2 < \theta_1 < 0$, it is attracting. Similarly, $a = \theta_0$ is repelling if $\theta_1 > 2$ or $\theta_1 < 0$, and it is attracting if $0 < \theta_1 < 2$. Clearly, this suggests that the behavior of the system is quite different, depending on the values of the parameters θ_0 and θ_1. In the context of a population model, a growth parameter θ_1 between 0 and 2 suggests a population that stabilizes at its carrying capacity, whereas a growth parameter value between 0 and -2 suggests a population that eventually becomes extinct (see Figure 3.4). It is then reasonable to ask what the system behavior for other values of these parameters is. In fact, this system can be quite complicated. However, before we give examples, we need a few more concepts.

One has to delve deeper to understand the dynamics at an equilibrium value a when the first derivative is inconclusive (i.e., $|\mathcal{M}^{(\prime)}(a)| = 1$). For example, it can be shown that if $\mathcal{M}^{(\prime)}(a) = 1$ and $\mathcal{M}^{(\prime\prime)}(a) \neq 0$ (where the superscript "$(\prime\prime)$" denotes the second derivative with respect to a), then a is said to be *semistable*. For example, if $\mathcal{M}^{(\prime\prime)}(a) < 0$, we say a is *semistable from above*, which simply means that for values of α_{t-1} greater than a, the process is stable, but is unstable for values of α_{t-1} less than a. Similarly, if $\mathcal{M}^{(\prime\prime)}(a) > 0$, the process is *semistable from below* at a (i.e., stable for values of α_{t-1} less than a and unstable for values of α_{t-1} greater than a). If $\mathcal{M}^{(\prime\prime)}(a) = 0$, one then considers third-derivatives, if possible. The case where $\mathcal{M}^{(\prime)}(a) = -1$ is a little more complicated, but one can in general examine the stability in this case as well, again based on consideration of the second (and third) derivatives of $\mathcal{M}$ at equilibrium value a (e.g., Sandefur, 1990).

As with the linear case, for a first-order nonlinear system, we say that two numbers a_1 and a_2 form a 2-cycle if when $\alpha_t = a_1$, then $\alpha_{t+1} = a_2, \alpha_{t+2} = a_1,$

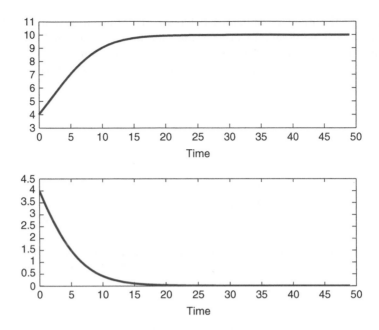

Figure 3.4 The logistic dynamical system (3.49) with starting value $\alpha_0 = 4$. **Top panel:** The case where $\theta_0 = 10$ and $\theta_1 = 0.25$. **Bottom panel:** The case where $\theta_0 = 10$ and $\theta_1 = -0.25$.

etc. In this case, the 2-cycle is stable or attracting if for intervals (γ_1, δ_1) and (γ_2, δ_2) around a_1 and a_2, respectively, the initial condition $a_0 \in (\gamma_1, \delta_1)$ implies that as t increases, the limit of α_{2t} goes to a_1, and the limit of α_{2t+1} goes to a_2; and, if $a_0 \in (\gamma_2, \delta_2)$, then as t increases, the limit of α_{2t} goes to a_2, and the limit of α_{2t+1} goes to a_1. In general, one can have a "k-cycle," consisting of the k values $a_1, \ldots, a_k$, which appear in a repeating sequence as t increases. Such a cycle is stable if $|\mathcal{M}^{(l)}(a_1)\,\mathcal{M}^{(l)}(a_2)\,\ldots\,\mathcal{M}^{(l)}(a_k)|$ is less than one but is unstable if this quantity is greater than one. As before, more complicated behavior occurs in situations where this quantity equals one (e.g., Sandefur, 1990).

3.2.3 Bifurcation

Because it is natural to think linearly, we often believe intuitively that small changes in inputs or parameter values lead to small changes in the behavior of the system. As we have already seen, small changes in parameter values can suggest quite different system behavior. Even more extreme cases exist where, for example, one value of a parameter suggests a completely different set of equilibrium points than a "nearby" value of the same parameter. Thus, the qualitative behavior of the system changes dramatically over relatively small changes in the parameter space. Values of the parameters where this happen are known as *bifurcation values*.

Bifurcations are very important in the study of dynamical systems. Consider a dynamical system that depends on parameter θ. Let n_θ be the number of equilibrium values for the system when the parameter θ takes a particular value. Now, if n_θ is not constant for θ in *any* interval $(\theta_0 - \epsilon, \theta_0 + \epsilon)$, then we say that θ_0 is a *bifurcation value* and the system is said to experience a *bifurcation* at θ_0. One often plots so-called *bifurcation diagrams*, which are plots of all equilibrium values (on the y-axis) as a function of the parameter θ (plotted on the *x*-axis). Different types of bifurcations are defined based on the behavior indicated in these diagrams. As a simple example, consider the one-parameter logistic equation,

$$\alpha_t = \theta\alpha_{t-1}(1 - \alpha_{t-1}), \qquad t = 1, 2, \ldots, \tag{3.50}$$

for $\theta > 0$, which is a special case of (3.49). Then the equilibrium values are $a = 0$ and $a = (\theta - 1)/\theta$. The bifurcation diagram is shown in Figure 3.5. There is a *transcritical bifurcation* at $\theta = 1$ on this diagram (where the two lines intersect). One can show that for this system, $a = 0$ is attracting when $0 < \theta < 1$, semistable from above when $\theta = 1$, and repelling when $\theta > 1$. The critical value $a = (\theta - 1)/\theta$ is attracting when $1 < \theta \leq 3$, and it is repelling when $\theta < 1$ or $\theta > 3$.

Note that when $\theta > 3$, both equilibrium values are repelling. However, the story does not end there, and it is interesting to examine the behavior of the

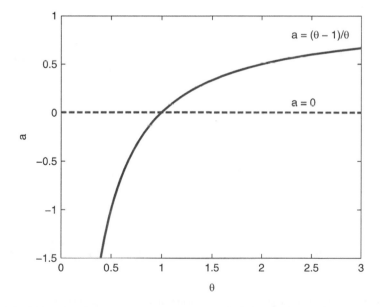

Figure 3.5 Bifurcation diagram for the one-parameter logistic equation (3.50); shown are equilibrium values as a function of θ. The solid blue line corresponds to the equilibrium values $a = (\theta - 1)/\theta$; the dashed blue line corresponds to the constant (as a function of θ) equilibrium value $a = 0$.

system in this case. One can show that for $3 < \theta < 1 + \sqrt{6}$, $\{\alpha_t\}$ behaves as an attracting 2-cycle, with attracting equilibrium values featured in the bifurcation diagram shown in Figure 3.6; the equilibrium values are given by

$$a = \sqrt{\theta + 1}\left(\frac{\sqrt{\theta + 1} \pm \sqrt{\theta - 3}}{2\theta}\right), \tag{3.51}$$

for $3 < \theta < 1 + \sqrt{6} \simeq 3.4495$. That is, there is a *period doubling* (or *pitchfork*) bifurcation at $\theta = 3$. Now, if we increase θ so that $3.45 < \theta < 3.54$, there is an attracting 4-cycle. In fact, there is a sequence of numbers, $\theta_1 < \theta_2 < \ldots < 3.57$, such that when $\theta_n < \theta < \theta_{n+1}$, the dynamical system $\{\alpha_t\}$ exhibits an attracting 2^n-cycle; that is, the system experiences repeated period doublings. For example, for $n = 12$ and $\theta_{12} < \theta < \theta_{13}$, $\{\alpha_t\}$ will exhibit an attracting 4096-cycle! Note that the behavior of $\{\alpha_t\}$ for $\theta > 3.57$ is even more complicated, with continued period-doubling as well as aperiodic behavior. Informally, for a given θ, the set of attracting fixed points (or regions) make up the *attractor*. We say that a dynamical system is *transitive* if, when the initial condition α_0 is "near" some point in the attractor, then for every point in the

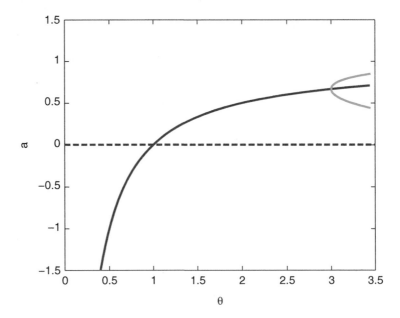

Figure 3.6 Bifurcation diagram for the one-parameter logistic equation (3.50), where now the horizontal axis is extended beyond $\theta = 3$. Shown are equilibrium values as a function of θ. The solid blue line corresponds to the equilibrium values $a = (\theta - 1)/\theta$; the dashed blue line corresponds to the constant (as a function of θ) equilibrium value $a = 0$. The solid green line corresponds to equilibrium values from an attracting 2-cycle, given by (3.51).

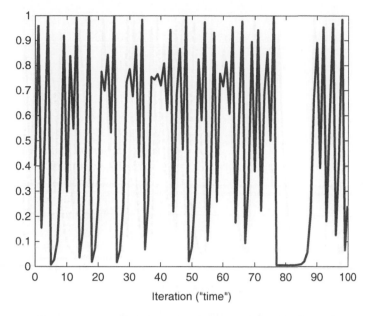

Figure 3.7   Iterations 0–100 of the one-parameter logistic equation (3.50) with $\theta = 4$ and $\alpha_0 = 0.4$.

attractor there is a sequence of values $\{\alpha_t\}$ that converges to that point. Eventually, when $\theta = 4$, the one-parameter logistic equation is said to be "chaotic." Figure 3.7 shows iteration $t = 1$ to $t = 100$ for such a system. Note that the behavior is, to the eye at least, somewhat "random."

3.2.4   Chaos

At this point, it is useful to ask what mathematical chaos is. Unfortunately, there is not a universally accepted definition. So far, we have seen several ways of characterizing complicated systems (e.g., bifurcations, attractors, transitivity). Yet, the colloquial expression of chaos is *sensitivity to initial conditions*. Informally, we say that a dynamical system exhibits sensitivity to initial conditions if, whenever there are two initial values $\alpha_0^{(1)}$ and $\alpha_0^{(2)}$ that are "close" together (i.e., $0 < |\alpha_0^{(1)} - \alpha_0^{(2)}| < \epsilon$, for some arbitrary ϵ), then the associated sequences $\alpha_t^{(1)}$ and $\alpha_t^{(2)}$ eventually get further apart (i.e., $|\alpha_t^{(1)} - \alpha_t^{(2)}| > \epsilon$, for $t > T$).

Consider the one-parameter logistic equation (3.50) with $\theta = 2$ and initial conditions close to the attracting equilibrium value $(\theta - 1)/\theta = 0.5$ (say, $\alpha_0^{(1)} = 0.510$ and $\alpha_0^{(2)} = 0.515$). In this case, there is no sensitivity to initial conditions, as the process is attracted to the equilibrium value, in either case, by the third iteration. Now let $\theta = 4$ with initial conditions, $\alpha_0^{(1)} = .510$ and $\alpha_0^{(2)} = .510001$. Then there is sensitivity to initial conditions as evidenced by the divergence of the realizations shown in Figure 3.8.

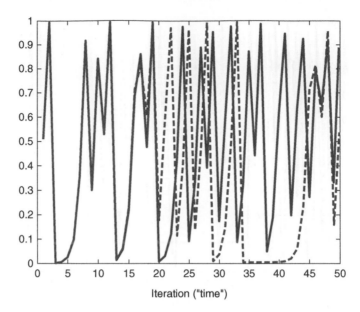

Iteration ("time")

Figure 3.8 Two realizations showing iterations 0–50 of the one-parameter logistic equation (3.50) with $\theta = 4$ and two different starting values: Blue line, $\alpha_0 = 0.51$; red line, $\alpha_0 = 0.510001$.

As another example, consider the simple *linear* system, $\alpha_t = 2.5\alpha_{t-1}$. Clearly, this system shows sensitivity to initial conditions, since $|\alpha_t^{(1)} - \alpha_t^{(2)}| \rightarrow \infty$ for any $\alpha_0^{(1)} \neq \alpha_0^{(2)}$. But, this system does not have an attractor, which suggests that sensitivity to initial conditions is not sufficient to define the notion of chaos. One possible definition of chaos requires that the dynamical system:

- is transitive on its attractor,
- exhibits sensitive dependence on initial conditions,
- has repeating cycles that are "close" to the attractor.

The logistic equation (3.50) with $3.57 < \theta \le 4$ exhibits chaos by this definition.

Consider a simple two-dimensional nonlinear system attributed to Hénon (1976):

$$\alpha_t = 1 + \beta_{t-1} - \theta_1\alpha_{t-1}^2, \tag{3.52}$$

$$\beta_t = \theta_2\alpha_{t-1}; \quad t = 1, 2, \ldots, \tag{3.53}$$

for fixed parameters θ_1 and θ_2. As in Berliner (1992), we let $\theta_1 = 1.4$, $\theta_2 = 0.3$, $\alpha_0 = 0.5$, and $\beta_0 = 0.4$. Figure 3.9 shows a simulation of this system. In addition, the scatter plot of realizations from this system, shown in Figure 3.10, illustrates the *attractor* (i.e., as time increases, the response of the system is

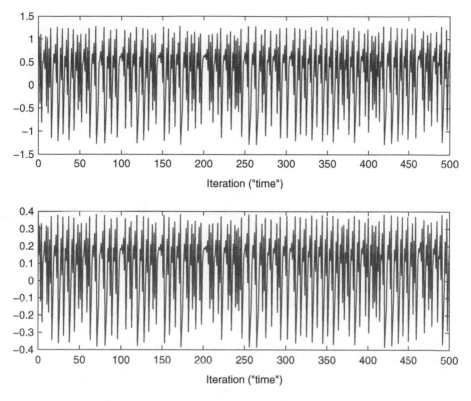

Figure 3.9 The first 500 iterations of the two-dimensional Hénon system (3.52) and (3.53) with $\theta_1 = 1.4$, $\theta_2 = 0.3$, and starting values $\alpha_0 = 0.5$, $\beta_0 = 0.4$. **Top panel:** $\{\alpha_t\}$. **Bottom panel:** $\{\beta_t\}$.

found in patterned geometrical regions of the state space). Clearly, this attractor has a complex geometrical structure and is, in fact, of fractal dimension. Informally, if all volumes in the state space contract as time increases, then the dynamical system is dissipative (i.e., the system will eventually evolve on a reduced set of states given by the attractor). Attractors that arise from chaotic dissipative systems are known as *strange attractors*. In contrast to other attractors, length elements of the geometrical region associated with the attractor will increase for some directions in state space. Yet, if length elements in other directions collapse sufficiently fast, the volume still shrinks overall. As described in Berliner (1992), there are competing mathematical forces at work in this case.

Characterizing Chaos

As we have discussed, sensitivity to initial conditions is a critical component of a chaotic system. However, it is not always so easy to verify such sensitivity. A related idea is the notion of a *Lyapunov exponent* (LE), which can typically be estimated from data. Intuitively, the LE measures the state-space contraction

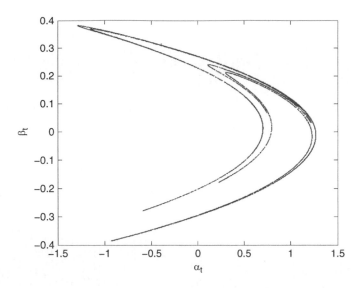

Figure 3.10 Scatterplot of 10,000 iterations of the Hénon system; the horizontal axis corresponds to α_t and the vertical axis corresponds to β_t.

or expansion. For illustration, assume the initial condition is represented by a hypersphere. For example, in two dimensions, (α_0, β_0) can be anywhere on the circle, $\alpha_0^2 + \beta_0^2 = c > 0$. As the system state evolves, the hypersphere transitions into a hyperellipsoid. The way in which the contraction or growth of each dimension (axis) of the ellipsoid relates to the initial condition can be characterized by a single coefficient.

Consider the LE for a scalar process: $\alpha_t = \mathcal{M}(\alpha_{t-1})$, where $\mathcal{M}$ is continuously differentiable with respect to α_{t-1}. Given two initial conditions, α_0 and α_0^*, the separation at time t of the associated states is given by

$$|\alpha_t^* - \alpha_t| = |\mathcal{M}^t(\alpha_0^*) - \mathcal{M}^t(\alpha_0)|, \tag{3.54}$$

where $\mathcal{M}^t(\alpha) \equiv \mathcal{M}(\mathcal{M}(\cdots \mathcal{M}(\alpha)))$. Now, expanding $\mathcal{M}^t(\alpha_0^*) - \mathcal{M}^t(\alpha_0)$ in a Taylor series around $\alpha_0^* = \alpha_0$, one can show that

$$|\alpha_t^* - \alpha_t| \simeq [\mathcal{M}^{(\prime)}(\alpha_0)\mathcal{M}^{(\prime)}(\alpha_1)\dots\mathcal{M}^{(\prime)}(\alpha_{t-1})]|\alpha_0^* - \alpha_0|, \tag{3.55}$$

where $\alpha_t = \mathcal{M}^t(\alpha_0)$. So, by taking appropriate limits, we obtain

$$\lim_{t \to \infty} |\alpha_t^* - \alpha_t| = e^{t\lambda(\alpha_0)}|\alpha_0^* - \alpha_0|, \tag{3.56}$$

where

$$\lambda(\alpha_0) \equiv \lim_{t \to \infty} \frac{1}{t} \sum_{k=0}^{t-1} \ln |\mathcal{M}^{(\prime)}(\alpha_k)| \tag{3.57}$$

is the *Lyapunov exponent*. Thus, one can think of the LE as measuring, on average, the asymptotic (exponential) rate of divergence of orbits with "close" initial conditions. In general, for identifying sensitivity to initial conditions, one looks for $\lambda(\alpha_0) > 0$. In this case, we say $1/\lambda(\alpha_0)$, sometimes known as the *Lyapunov time*, gives an average limit of predictability. However, we note that there can certainly be false indications of chaos in this context. For example, unbounded (periodic) orbits show positive LEs. In addition, it can be the case that orbits diverge, but not exponentially.

We can extend the notion of an LE to higher dimensions, as discussed in the Bibliographic Notes in Section 3.7. Also, we do not discuss the estimation of LEs here. We note that in general we cannot obtain LEs for nonlinear systems exactly, but there are numerical and statistical approaches for their estimation; again, see the Bibliographic Notes in Section 3.7.

3.2.5 State-Space Reconstruction

Consider a set of equations describing a multivariate dynamical system for a state process:

$$\boldsymbol{\alpha}_t = \mathcal{M}(\boldsymbol{\alpha}_{t-1}; \boldsymbol{\theta}), \tag{3.58}$$

where $\mathcal{M}$ is a vector-valued function and $\boldsymbol{\theta}$ is a vector of known parameters. If $\boldsymbol{\alpha}_{t-1}$ completely specifies the state of the system, then exact knowledge of $\boldsymbol{\alpha}_0$, $\mathcal{M}$, and $\boldsymbol{\theta}$ allows the future state to be computed exactly. As we have already seen, lack of perfect knowledge of $\boldsymbol{\alpha}_0$ or $\boldsymbol{\theta}$ can have tremendously important consequences on one's ability to predict the future. What about knowledge of the state itself?

In reality, one would seldom have access to all of the state variables that make up the true state $\boldsymbol{\alpha}_t$. As an extreme case, say we could only measure one component of the system, say Z_t (a scalar), but we measure it perfectly! This leads to a measurement equation,

$$Z_t = h(\boldsymbol{\alpha}_t), \tag{3.59}$$

where h is a measurement function. An impressive result from the theory of dynamical systems suggests that for systems of the form (3.58), we may not need to observe the entire state vector to represent the dynamics, but that noise-free observations of only one component (or some lower-dimensional subset) of the state is enough to reconstruct the system. Specifically, we define a *delay coordinate function* H that constructs an $\mathcal{M}$-dimensional delay vector, $\mathbf{Y}_t \in \mathbb{R}^m$, from $\mathcal{M}$ observations separated by *delay time* τ_d:

$$\begin{aligned} \mathbf{Y}_t &\equiv H(\boldsymbol{\alpha}_t, \boldsymbol{\alpha}_{t-\tau_d}, \ldots, \boldsymbol{\alpha}_{t-(m-1)\tau_d}) \\ &\equiv (h(\boldsymbol{\alpha}_t), h(\boldsymbol{\alpha}_{t-\tau_d}), \ldots, h(\boldsymbol{\alpha}_{t-(m-1)\tau_d}))' \\ &= (Z_t, Z_{t-\tau_d}, \ldots, Z_{t-(m-1)\tau_d})'. \end{aligned} \tag{3.60}$$

Takens (1981) provides the conditions under which such a delay vector can represent the dynamical system. Informally, this suggests that we do not have to measure all of the state variables of a system (which is a good thing, since we typically cannot!), but we can represent the system equivalently by time-lagged scalar noise-free observations of some subset of the system states. Unfortunately, in the real world this is not always practical, because one does not know the form of H, nor is it possible to have truly noise-free observations. So, the conditions of Takens' theorem may not be met in practice. Nevertheless, these ideas can provide useful motivation for building stochastic state-space models and, in some cases, can be used effectively to model real-world time series (e.g., Sugihara and May, 1990). We shall use them in Section 6.6.1 and Chapter 7 when we consider dimension reduction in spatio-temporal statistical models.

3.2.6 The Need for Statistical Models for Dynamical Processes

As we have seen, uncertainty breeds "chaos"; and, given that we always have uncertainty in observations, processes, and parameters, how should we best model real-world processes? Berliner (1992, Section 2.2) provides a nice discussion of randomness and chaos. In particular, he describes how "uncertainty, especially in the presence of complexity, naturally leads to the use of random or probabilistic methods." In essence, the presence of uncertainties in our knowledge of real-world systems, at least at some scales of variability, suggests the need to characterize that uncertainty via probability models. Even if it were possible to know exactly the dynamics of a real-world system, we would still be faced with uncertainties related to our observations of the system, which, of course, lead to issues related to sensitivity to initial conditions. Since it is often not possible to distinguish between such a chaotic effect and true randomness (e.g., a Bernoulli coin toss), one might benefit from modeling a chaotic system as a random system. In fact, a chaotic system such as the logistic map considered in (3.50) can formally be linked to a zero-one process such as the Bernoulli process, thereby creating a zero-one generating mechanism from a deterministic dynamical system that is as rich (and appears as "random") as the Bernoulli process [see Berliner (1992)]. Furthermore, Berliner (1992) discusses the link between *ergodic theory* and chaos.

Although we shall use *notions* from deterministic dynamical-system theory in our discussion of spatio-temporal statistical analysis, modeling of real-world problems involves uncertainty that is best handled in a probability-based framework. Thus, in the rest of this chapter, we consider *stochastic dynamical systems*, which are simply (random) time series.

3.3 TIME SERIES PRELIMINARIES

From the introduction to this chapter, recall that time series models can be viewed as process models for temporal data. Before we discuss them, we must first define some basic functions of a discrete-time sequence of real-valued random variables $\{Y_t : t \in D_t\}$. Henceforth, we assume that $D_t = \{0, 1, \ldots\}$, and we refer to $\{Y_t : t = 0, 1, \ldots\}$ as a *time series*.

The *mean function* is defined as

$$\mu_t \equiv E(Y_t), \qquad t \in D_t, \tag{3.61}$$

which is simply the mean of the process relative to the underlying probability space. Then $\{\mu_t : t = 0, 1, \ldots\}$ is deterministic and it is quite possible that it satisfies a dynamical system of the sort discussed in Section 3.2. Indeed, this will be a key component of certain hierarchical spatio-temporal dynamical models discussed in Chapter 7. However, more typically, we choose simpler models for μ_t and put much of the uncertainty in the remaining stochastic component, $\{Y_t - \mu_t : t = 0, 1, \ldots\}$. This uncertainty can be described through the *autocovariance function* or *covariogram*,

$$C_Y(t, r) = \mathrm{cov}(Y_t, Y_r) = E\{(Y_t - \mu_t)(Y_r - \mu_r)\}, \qquad t, r \in D_t, \tag{3.62}$$

which summarizes how the process co-varies across different time lags, after accounting for the mean function. Notice that $C_Y(t, r) = C_Y(r, t)$ and, furthermore, that the variance is a special case of the autocovariance in which $C_Y(t, t) = \mathrm{var}(Y_t) = \sigma_t^2$. After normalization, one can obtain the *autocorrelation function*, a function that measures linear statistical dependence between different members of the time series:

$$\rho_Y(t, r) \equiv \frac{C_Y(t, r)}{\sqrt{C_Y(t, t) C_Y(r, r)}}, \qquad t, r \in D_t, \tag{3.63}$$

where $\rho_Y(t, r) \in [-1, 1]$. A sufficient condition for (3.62) and (3.63) to exist is $\sigma_t^2 < \infty$, for all D_t.

In Section 2.1, we discussed information content of a dataset and pointed out that, without further assumptions, time series data could be viewed as a sample of size one! One type of assumption commonly made for time series models is that of *stationarity*. There are different forms of stationarity; and to avoid repeating the definitions given in Section 2.2, for d-dimensional space, we simply summarize them here for the special case of one dimension (which here is time). Note that there is further discussion of stationarity in the spatio-temporal context in Section 6.1.2.

Strong stationarity of $\{Y_t\}$ is an assumption that says that any finite collection, $\{Y_{t_1}, \ldots, Y_{t_m}\}$, of random variables from the time series has exactly the same joint distribution as $\{Y_{t_1+\tau}, \ldots, Y_{t_m+\tau}\}$, for any $\tau \in \{0, \pm 1, \pm 2, \ldots\}$. Note that the same definition applies to continuous-time temporal processes $\{Y(t) : t \in D_t\}$, but where the time lag is $\tau \in (-\infty, \infty)$.

Now, it is possible that a probability distribution may not have any moments! For example, the Cauchy distribution has no mean, variance, third moment, etc. Weak stationarity of $\{Y_t\}$ is an assumption that requires initially the *existence* of the second moment (then the first moment automatically exists); that is, assume

$\mathrm{var}(Y_t) \equiv \sigma_t^2 < \infty$, for all $t \in D_t$. Time series whose variances are finite are said to be *second-order stationary* (equivalently, *weakly stationary*) if

(i) $E(Y_t) \equiv \mu$, for all $t \in D_t$.
(ii) $\mathrm{cov}(Y_t, Y_r) \equiv C_Y(t - r)$, for all $t, r \in D_t$.

Second-order stationarity is an assumption that says that any pair, $\{Y_t, Y_r\}$, has exactly the same first and second moments (including the cross-moment, which defines the autocovariance function) as the pair $\{Y_{t+\tau}, Y_{r+\tau}\}$, for any $\tau \in \{0, \pm 1, \ldots\}$. For processes with finite variance, strong stationarity implies second-order stationarity, but not vice versa.

Even if μ_t given by (3.61) is not constant, we can define the *autocovariance function* to be *stationary* if the covariance function given by (3.62) is equal to $C_Y(t - r)$, for all $t, r \in D_t$. Note that the same definitions of second-order stationarity apply to continuous-time temporal processes $\{Y(t)\}$. Finally, a discussion of ergodicity and its relation to strong stationarity is given in Cressie (1993, pp. 53–58).

In addition to characterizing the second-order dependence structure of a time series in terms of a stationary autocovariance (or autocorrelation) function, an equivalent characterization is in terms of a Fourier spectral representation. This formal equivalence is given by the *spectral representation theorem* (e.g., see Shumway and Stoffer, 2006, Appendix C).

In the rest of this chapter, we write the stationary covariance function as $C(\tau)$, rather than $C_Y(\tau)$. Given a second-order stationary time series $\{Y_t\}$ with autocovariance function $C(\tau) \equiv E\{(Y_{t+\tau} - \mu)(Y_t - \mu)\}$, a *spectral distribution function* $F(\omega)$ exists that is monotone, nondecreasing, and bounded for $-1/2 \le \omega \le 1/2$, with $F(-1/2) = 0$, $F(1/2) = C(0)$, such that

$$C(\tau) = \int_{-1/2}^{1/2} \exp\{2\pi i \omega \tau\}\, dF(\omega), \qquad \tau = 0, \pm 1, \pm 2, \ldots . \tag{3.64}$$

For a stationary process with autocovariance function satisfying, $\sum_{\tau=-\infty}^{\infty} |C(\tau)| < \infty$ (absolute summability), the spectral distribution function is absolutely continuous with $dF(\omega) = f(\omega)\, d\omega$, and hence

$$C(\tau) = \int_{-1/2}^{1/2} \exp\{2\pi i \omega \tau\} f(\omega)\, d\omega, \qquad \tau = 0, \pm 1, \pm 2, \ldots . \tag{3.65}$$

Further, the *spectral density function* $f(\omega)$ can be represented as

$$f(\omega) = \sum_{\tau=-\infty}^{\infty} C(\tau) \exp\{-2\pi i \omega \tau\}, \qquad -1/2 \le \omega \le 1/2. \tag{3.66}$$

Note that because time is discrete here, we can interpret the spectral density function (3.66) as the Fourier transform of the autocovariance function and, the autocovariance function (3.65) as the inverse Fourier transform of the spectral density function. Furthermore, the spectral density function is nonnegative over all ω; it is an even function, $f(\omega) = f(-\omega)$; and it has a period of one, $f(\omega) = f(\omega + 1)$.

In the context of a *multivariate* time series $\{\mathbf{Y}_t\}$, we define $\{Y_t^{(i)}\}$, to be the ith time series at time t. Then, in general, we define

$$C_{ij}(t, r) \equiv \text{cov}(Y_t^{(i)}, Y_r^{(j)}), \qquad t, r \in D_t, \qquad (3.67)$$

to be the *cross-covariance function* between the ith time series at time t and the jth time series at time r. A second-order stationarity assumption on the multivariate time series $\{\mathbf{Y}_t\}$ requires that the respective mean functions do not vary with time and that the cross-covariance functions only depend on the lag between times t and r. That is,

$$C_{ij}(\tau) = \text{cov}(Y_t^{(i)}, Y_{t+\tau}^{(j)}), \qquad \tau = 0, \pm 1, \pm 2, \ldots. \qquad (3.68)$$

Note that $C_{ij}(-\tau) = C_{ji}(\tau)$. Furthermore, the *cross-correlation function* is given by

$$\rho_{ij}(\tau) = \frac{C_{ij}(\tau)}{\sqrt{C_{ii}(0)C_{jj}(0)}}, \qquad \tau = 0, \pm 1, \pm 2, \ldots. \qquad (3.69)$$

Empirical Mean and Empirical Covariance Function

Assume that we have a finite sample from a temporal process $\{Y_t\}$, denoted by $Y_1, \ldots, Y_T$, and that there is only this one realization available to summarize the time series. The formulas that follow apply whether $\{Y_t\}$ is deterministic or stochastic, but they have an interpretation as estimators when the time series is second-order stationary.

The *empirical mean* (also called the *sample mean*) of the time series is

$$\hat{\mu} = \frac{1}{T} \sum_{t=1}^{T} Y_t. \qquad (3.70)$$

The empirical (or *sample*) *autocovariance function* is

$$\hat{C}(\tau) \equiv \frac{1}{T} \sum_{t=1}^{T-\tau} (Y_{t+\tau} - \hat{\mu})(Y_t - \hat{\mu}), \qquad \tau = 0, 1, \ldots, T - 1. \qquad (3.71)$$

Note that $\hat{C}(-\tau) = \hat{C}(\tau)$ and $\hat{C}(0)$ is the *empirical* (or *sample*) *variance*. One could divide the sum in (3.71) by $(T - \tau)$ rather than T, and in fact we do this in Chapter 5. Dividing by T in (3.71) guarantees that the empirical autocovariance function is nonnegative definite, which guarantees that the empirical variances of linear combinations of the series, $\{Y_t\}$, will be nonnegative (e.g., Shumway and Stoffer, 2006, Section 1.6). However, (3.71) is clearly biased; and to mitigate this effect for exploratory spatio-temporal data analysis, we divide by $T - \tau$ in Chapter 5. Similarly, the *empirical* (or *sample*) *autocorrelation function* is

$$\hat{\rho}(\tau) \equiv \frac{\hat{C}(\tau)}{\hat{C}(0)}, \qquad \tau = 0, 1, \ldots, T - 1. \tag{3.72}$$

In the multivariate context, assume that we have observations from a process $\{\mathbf{Y}_t\}$; recall that observations on the ith time series are denoted by $Y_1^{(i)}, \ldots, Y_T^{(i)}$. The *empirical* (or *sample*) *cross-covariance function* is

$$\hat{C}_{ij}(\tau) \equiv \frac{1}{T} \sum_{t=1}^{T-\tau} (Y_{t+\tau}^{(i)} - \hat{\mu}_i)(Y_t^{(j)} - \hat{\mu}_j), \qquad \tau = 0, 1, \ldots, T - 1, \tag{3.73}$$

where $\hat{\mu}_i$ is the empirical mean (3.70) for the ith time series and likewise for $\hat{\mu}_j$. Again, the divisor T could be replaced by $T - \tau$ (Chapter 5). We note that $\hat{C}_{ij}(-\tau) = \hat{C}_{ji}(\tau)$. Finally, the empirical cross-correlation function is obtained from (3.69) after substituting the respective empirical covariance and cross-covariance functions from (3.73).

When viewed as estimators, a discussion of the statistical properties of the empirical first and second moments presented here can be found in most advanced time series books. For more details, see the references in the Bibliographic Notes in Section 3.7.

3.4 BASIC TIME SERIES MODELS

In addition to the assumption of stationarity, probabilistic properties of time series are typically specified in order to simplify their characterization. The fact that the time series literature emphasizes such process-model-based descriptions is motivated by Science. This is in contrast to much of the literature in geostatistics (e.g., see Section 4.1), where, for historical reasons, more descriptive (e.g., covariance-based) and less explanatory models are used to represent the data. Geostatistics was originally used in the mining industry for prediction of the mineral content of ore bodies. While the geologist's knowledge is crucial for locating the ore body, geostatistical prediction has typically relied on (spatial) autocovariances, often in the form of variograms, estimated from ore samples. These ideas are taken up in Section 4.1.

Basic process models for time series are described briefly below. Here, we focus only on discrete-time processes, although in most cases analogous models exist for continuous time.

3.4.1 White-Noise Process

We define a *white-noise* process as a discrete-time random process $\{W_t : \ldots, -1, 0, 1, \ldots\}$ whose elements are mutually independent and have a

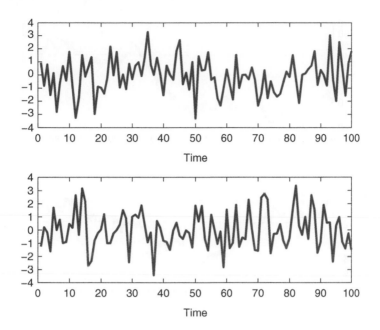

Figure 3.11 Two independent realizations of length 100 of a white-noise process, $W_t \sim iid\ Gau(0, 2)$.

common probability density function (pdf). Typically, its mean μ_w is assumed to be zero, and its autocovariance function is

$$C(\tau) = \begin{cases} \sigma_w^2, & \tau = 0, \\ 0, & \tau = \pm 1, \pm 2, \ldots, \end{cases} \tag{3.74}$$

where $\sigma_w^2 > 0$ is the white-noise variance. From the definition of the spectral density function, (3.66), a white-noise process has, $f(\omega) = \sigma_w^2$, for $-1/2 < \omega < 1/2$. That is, the spectral density is equal for all frequencies, which is analogous to how white light is a mixture of colors with no preference in the color spectrum (hence the name "white noise").

An example of a white-noise process is $W_t \sim iid\ Gau(0, \sigma_w^2)$, for all t. Figure 3.11 shows two (independent) realizations from the same white-noise process with variance $\sigma_w^2 = 2$. Although it is common that a white-noise process is Gaussian, it need not be.

3.4.2 Random-Walk Process

Some processes in the natural world behave in a manner that suggests their value at the current time is simply their value at the previous time plus some noise. More formally, a time series $\{Y_t\}$ is said to be a *random walk* if

$$Y_t = Y_{t-1} + W_t, \qquad t = 1, 2, \ldots, \tag{3.75}$$

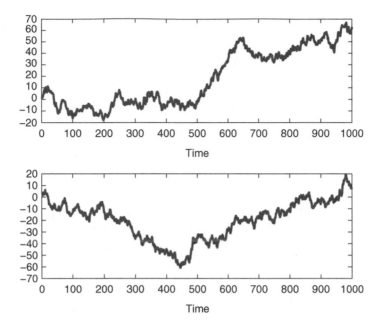

Figure 3.12 Two independent realizations of length 1000 of a random walk process with $Y_0 \equiv 0$, and $W_t \sim iid\ Gau(0, 2)$.

where $\{W_t\}$ is a white-noise process with mean μ_w and variance σ_w^2. One can show that in this case, $E(Y_t) = E(Y_0) + t\mu_w$ and $\mathrm{var}(Y_t) = t\sigma_w^2$. That is, both the mean and variance are functions of time and, thus, the process is nonstationary. Furthermore, $\mathrm{cov}(Y_t, Y_r) = \min(t, r)\sigma_w^2$.

Figure 3.12 shows two independent realizations from the same random-walk process with $W_t \sim iid\ Gau(0, 2)$. Note that such processes exhibit behavior that is "locally smooth" but quite obviously random.

3.4.3 Autoregressive Process

Often, observations of environmental, ecological, biological, and physical processes depend on one or more observations that immediately precede it. A time series that models such structure is the *autoregressive* (or AR) process. A time series $\{Y_t\}$ is said to be an *autoregressive process of order* p, AR(p), if

$$Y_t = m_1Y_{t-1} + m_2Y_{t-2} + \cdots + m_pY_{t-p} + W_t, \quad t = \ldots, -2, -1, 0, 1, 2, \ldots, \tag{3.76}$$

where $\{W_t\}$ is a white-noise process with mean zero and variance σ_w^2, and where $\{m_i : i = 1, \ldots, p\}$, are fixed but unknown parameters.

For example, consider the AR(1) process,

$$Y_t = m_1Y_{t-1} + W_t, \qquad t = \ldots, -2, -1, 0, 1, 2, \ldots, \tag{3.77}$$

where $\{W_t\}$ is white-noise process with mean zero and variance σ_w^2, and we write $\alpha = \alpha_1$ for notational simplicity. By back-substitution, we obtain

$$Y_t = W_t + \alpha W_{t-1} + \alpha^2 W_{t-2} + \alpha^3 W_{t-3} + \cdots$$

$$= \sum_{k=0}^{\infty} \alpha^k W_{t-k}, \tag{3.78}$$

where it is assumed that $|\alpha| < 1$. That is, the AR(1) process can be written as an infinite series of white-noise random variables (i.e., an infinite-order *moving-average process*, as will be discussed in Section 3.4.4). Since $E(W_t) = 0$ and $\text{var}(W_t) = \sigma_w^2$, it follows that $E(Y_t) = 0$ and

$$\text{var}(Y_t) = \sigma_w^2(1 + \alpha^2 + \alpha^4 + \cdots) = \frac{\sigma_w^2}{1 - \alpha^2}, \tag{3.79}$$

which does not depend on t. If the condition $|\alpha| < 1$ is not met, the process is explosive (i.e., the variance of the time series increases exponentially with time). Furthermore, when $\alpha = 1$, the process is a random walk. In the explosive case where $|\alpha| > 1$, one can show that $Y_t = -\sum_{k=1}^{\infty} \alpha^{-k} W_{t+k}$, which is stationary (e.g., Shumway and Stoffer, 2006, Section 3.2). However, such a model requires knowledge of the future and is thus not helpful. We say that a temporal process that does not depend on the future is *causal*.

It is also straightforward to show that for the AR(1) process with $|\alpha| < 1$, the autocorrelation function is given by

$$\rho(\tau) = \alpha^{|\tau|}, \qquad \tau = 0, \pm 1, \pm 2, \ldots . \tag{3.80}$$

Thus, for the AR(1) process, the autocorrelation (i.e., temporal dependence) decreases in magnitude as the time lag τ increases. From (3.66), the spectral density for the AR(1) process is given by

$$f(\omega) = \frac{\sigma_w^2}{1 - 2\alpha \cos(2\pi\omega) + \alpha^2}, \qquad -1/2 < \omega < 1/2. \tag{3.81}$$

When the AR(1) parameter α is greater than 0, the spectral density decreases as $|\omega|$ increases. This is sometimes known as a *red-noise* spectrum, again analogous to the color spectrum. When α is less than 0, the spectrum increases as $|\omega|$ increases, which is sometimes known as a *blue-noise* spectrum. See Figure 3.13 for an illustration of these two cases.

Figure 3.14 shows three realizations of an AR(1) process with different values of α; positive dependence (top panel), negative dependence (middle panel), and explosive growth (bottom panel) are featured.

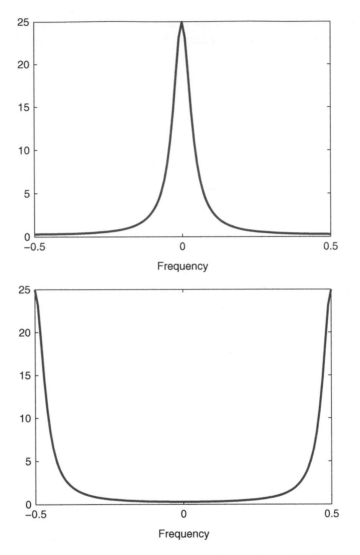

Figure 3.13 AR(1) spectral densities given by (3.81). **Top panel:** $\alpha = 0.8$. **Bottom panel:** $\alpha = -0.8$.

Autocovariance and autocorrelation functions for higher-order causal AR processes can be obtained fairly easily. For example, the AR(2) process,

$$Y_t = \alpha_1 Y_{t-1} + \alpha_2 Y_{t-2} + W_t, \qquad t = 2, 3, \ldots, \qquad (3.82)$$

has an autocorrelation function that satisfies,

$$\rho(\tau) = \alpha_1 \rho(\tau - 1) + \alpha_2 \rho(\tau - 2), \qquad \tau = 1, 2, \ldots, \qquad (3.83)$$

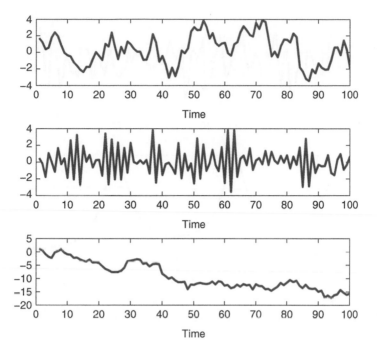

Figure 3.14 AR(1) realizations, defined by (3.77), of length 100. **Top panel:** $m_1 = 0.8$ (analogous to the spectral density in the top panel of Figure 3.13). **Middle panel:** $m_1 = -0.8$ (analogous to the spectral density in the bottom panel of Figure 3.13). **Bottom panel:** $m_1 = 1.01$ (explosive growth). In all cases, $\sigma_w^2 = 1$.

which can be obtained by multiplying both sides of (3.82) by $Y_{t-\tau}$ and taking expectations. One can study the behavior of this function by noting that (3.83) is a second-order deterministic dynamical system (see Section 3.2.1). In particular, given initial conditions, $\rho(0) = 1$ and $\rho(-1) = \alpha_1/(1 - \alpha_2)$, one can show that the autocorrelation function will exhibit exponential decay with increasing lag τ, but may show oscillatory behavior as well (see Section 3.2.1). This behavior is also evident upon examination of the AR(2)'s spectral density function:

$$f(\omega) = \frac{\sigma_w^2}{1 + m_1^2 + m_2^2 - 2m_1(1 - m_2)\cos(2\pi\omega) - 2m_2\cos(4\pi\omega)}, \quad (3.84)$$

for $-1/2 < \omega < 1/2$. Depending on the values of m_1 and m_2, the spectrum can exhibit increased power at the high or low frequencies, similar to the AR(1) process. In addition, as shown in Figure 3.15, the AR(2) spectrum can also accommodate a spectral peak (associated with oscillatory behavior of the process), which suggests that the AR(2) process is quite flexible in its ability to model real-world phenomena.

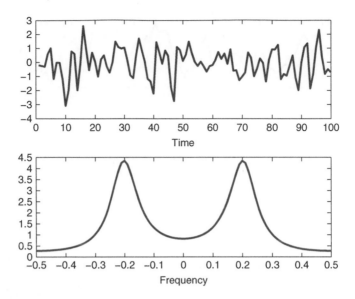

Figure 3.15 Top panel: A realization from an AR(2) process, defined by (3.82), of length 100; $m_1 = .4$, $m_2 = -.5$, and $\sigma_w^2 = 1$. **Bottom panel:** Theoretical spectral density (3.84) for the AR(2) process shown in the top panel.

Parameter Estimation

Given a finite sample $Y_1, \ldots, Y_T$ from (3.76), we could use the empirical covariance function to estimate the parameters of the AR(p) model, namely $m_1, \ldots, m_p$, and σ_w^2. Multiply each side of (3.76) by Y_{t-j}, for $j = 0, \ldots, p$, and take expectations. This results in the set of equations

$$C(0) = m_1 C(1) + \cdots + m_p C(p) + \sigma_w^2 \tag{3.85}$$

$$C(k) = m_1 C(k-1) + \cdots + m_p C(k-p), \qquad k = 1, \ldots, p, \tag{3.86}$$

which are known as the *Yule–Walker equations*. In matrix form, we can write these as

$$\mathbf{C}\mathbf{m} = \mathbf{c} \quad \text{and} \quad \sigma_w^2 = C(0) - \mathbf{m}'\mathbf{c}, \tag{3.87}$$

where $\mathbf{C}$ is a $p \times p$ matrix with (i, j)th element $C(i - j)$, and $\mathbf{m} \equiv (m_1, \ldots, m_p)'$ and $\mathbf{c} \equiv (C(1), \ldots, C(p))'$ are p-dimensional vectors. Method-of-moment estimators for $\mathbf{m}$ are obtained by replacing the autocovariance function $C(\cdot)$ with its empirical version $\hat{C}(\cdot)$ given by (3.71):

$$\hat{\mathbf{m}} \equiv \hat{\mathbf{C}}^{-1}\hat{\mathbf{c}} \tag{3.88}$$

and

$$\hat{\sigma}_w^2 = \hat{C}(0) - \hat{\mathbf{c}}'\hat{\mathbf{C}}^{-1}\hat{\mathbf{c}}. \tag{3.89}$$

Note that the Yule–Walker-based method-of-moments estimators (3.88) and (3.89) can be computed through the Durbin–Levinson algorithm, which does not require inversion of $\mathbf{C}$ (e.g., see Shumway and Stoffer, 2006, Section 3.5).

One can also obtain estimators of AR parameters via ordinary-least-squares and maximum-likelihood procedures. For the causal autoregressive process conditioned on the first p observations, all of these estimators give the same asymptotically normal limiting distribution [e.g., see Brockwell and Davis (1991, Chapter 8) and Fuller (1996, Chapter 8)]. Such results allow one to obtain large-sample confidence regions for model parameters. Note that in practice, a noisy version of the time series $Z_1, \ldots, Z_T$ is observed, where typically $Z_t = Y_t + \varepsilon_t$, with $\{\varepsilon_t\}$ an independent white-noise process, mean 0 and variance σ_ε^2 (see Section 3.6). This requires only slight modification to (3.88) and (3.89), provided that σ_ε^2 is known or estimated from calibration data.

3.4.4   Moving-Average Process

The time series $\{Y_t\}$ is said to be a *moving-average (or MA) process of order q*, or MA(q), if

$$Y_t = W_t + \beta_1 W_{t-1} + \cdots + \beta_q W_{t-q}, \tag{3.90}$$

where $\beta_1, \beta_2, \ldots, \beta_q$ are fixed but unknown parameters, and $\{W_t\}$ is a white-noise process with zero mean and variance σ_w^2. At first glance, this may appear to be similar to a multiple-regression model. However, the key differences are that $\{W_t\}$ are random and, more importantly, they are unobservable!

It follows that for such a model, $E(Y_t) = 0$ and $\mathrm{var}(Y_t) = \sigma_w^2 \sum_{i=0}^{q} \beta_i^2$, which does not depend on t. Furthermore,

$$\rho(\tau) = \begin{cases} 1, & \tau = 0, \\ \sum_{i=0}^{q-\tau} \beta_i \beta_{i+\tau} / \sum_{i=0}^{q} \beta_i^2, & |\tau| = 1, 2, \ldots, q, \\ 0, & |\tau| > q, \end{cases} \tag{3.91}$$

where the process is standardized by setting $\beta_0 = 1$. One can then use (3.66) to obtain the spectral density. For example, the spectral density for the MA(1) process, $Y_t = W_t + \beta W_{t-1}$, is given by

$$f(\omega) = \sigma_w^2 \left(1 + \beta^2 + 2\beta \cos(2\pi\omega)\right), \qquad -1/2 < \omega < 1/2, \tag{3.92}$$

where we write the MA(1) parameter $\beta = \beta_1$, for notational simplicity. The spectral density function is clearly dependent on the value of this parameter. When $\beta < 0$, more power is associated with the higher (in magnitude) frequencies; and when $\beta > 0$, more power is associated with the lower (in magnitude) frequencies (see Figure 3.16).

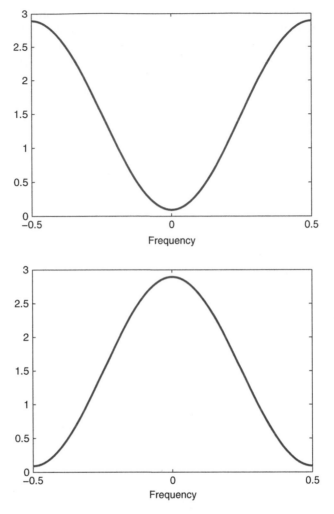

Figure 3.16 MA(1) spectral density given by (3.92). **Top panel:** $\beta = -0.7$. **Bottom panel:** $\beta = 0.7$.

An interesting feature of the MA process is illustrated by considering two different formulations of an MA(1) process (e.g., Chatfield, 1989):

$$Y_t = W_t + \beta W_{t-1}, \tag{3.93}$$

$$Y_t = W_t + \frac{1}{\beta} W_{t-1}. \tag{3.94}$$

From (3.91), it is clear that both models have exactly the same autocorrelation function. Now, from (3.93), we obtain the following representation by back-substitution:

$$W_t = Y_t - \beta Y_{t-1} + \beta^2 Y_{t-2} - \dots, \tag{3.95}$$

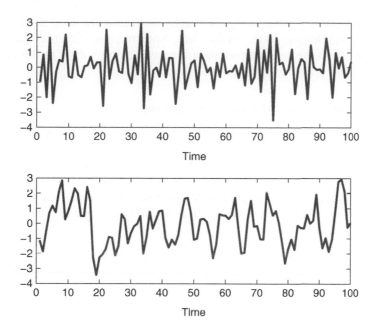

Figure 3.17   Realizations from MA(1) processes defined by (3.90) with $q = 1$. **Top panel:** $\beta = -0.7$. **Bottom panel:** $\beta = 0.7$.

which gives an infinite-order AR process. This converges in mean square if $|\beta| < 1$. However, if we do the same back-substitution for (3.94), the sum does not converge for $|\beta| < 1$. Clearly, an MA(1) cannot always be represented as an infinite-order AR process. We say that the MA(1) given by (3.93) is *invertible* if it can be written as an infinite-order autoregressive process, which occurs if $|\beta| < 1$.

Figure 3.17 shows two realizations from an MA(1) process with different values of β. In the top panel, $\beta = -0.7$, showing more high-frequency behavior. In the bottom panel, $\beta = 0.7$, showing more low-frequency behavior, corresponding to the spectral densities shown in Figure 3.16.

Parameter Estimation

Estimation for the parameters of MA processes is not as straightforward as for those of AR processes, since autocovariances of MA processes are nonlinear in the parameters. One can still use the Yule–Walker equations to obtain estimators, but such estimators are inefficient (e.g., see Brockwell and Davis, 1991, Section 8.5). Just as the Durbin–Levinson algorithm can be used to obtain recursive estimators of AR parameters, the *innovations algorithm* can be used to obtain recursive moment-based estimators of MA parameters (e.g., Brockwell and Davis, 1991, Section 8.3), but they are not in general consistent. For these reasons, maximum-likelihood procedures are typically preferred for estimating MA parameters. However, given the aforementioned nonlinearity in the parameters, explicit solutions are generally not available and the likelihood must be maximized numerically, such as by the Gauss–Newton algorithm (e.g., Shumway and Stoffer, 2006, Section 3.6). Note that it is often reasonable to use the results from the innovations algorithm as starting values in the numerical maximum-likelihood estimation procedure.

3.4.5 Autoregressive Moving-Average Process

We note the duality between the AR and the MA processes described above. That is, an AR(p) process can be written as an infinite-order MA process, and an MA(q) process can be written as an infinite-order AR process. This suggests that a more parsimonious model for many processes might result from a combination of AR and MA processes. The time series $\{Y_t\}$ is said to be an *autoregressive moving-average (ARMA) process of order* (p, q), or ARMA(p, q), if

$$Y_t = \alpha_1 Y_{t-1} + \cdots + \alpha_p Y_{t-p} + W_t + \beta_1 W_{t-1} + \cdots + \beta_q W_{t-q}, \qquad (3.96)$$

where $\alpha_1, \ldots, \alpha_p$, $\beta_1, \ldots, \beta_q$ are fixed but unknown parameters, and $\{W_t\}$ is a white-noise process with zero mean and variance σ_w^2. In the spatio-temporal setting, the analogous processes are called STARMAs (Section 6.4.2).

The properties of ARMA(p, q) processes and estimation of their parameters can be found in most time series textbooks (e.g., see Shumway and Stoffer, 2006, Section 3.2). In addition, many other variations of these models, including, for example, seasonality and differencing, form the foundations of modern parametric time series modeling (Box and Jenkins, 1970; Box, Jenkins, and Reinsel, 2008).

3.4.6 Graphical Models for Time Series

In Section 2.4, we presented directed and undirected graphs as a way to visualize conditional independencies in a joint distribution. Consider this approach applied to time series models for $\{Y_r : r \in D_t\}$. Figure 3.18a shows the directed graph associated with a first-order autoregressive (AR(1)) process, and Figure 3.18b shows the directed graph associated with a second-order autoregressive (AR(2)) process.

In both graphs, consider node t and condition on values associated with all nodes that have arrows between them and t, here node $(t - 1)$ for Figure 3.18a and nodes $\{(t - 2), (t - 1)\}$ for Figure 3.18b. Upon removing these nodes, each respective graph breaks into two unconnected graphs. Using expression (2.20), we see that for the AR(1) time series (Figure 3.18a) we have

$$[Y_t | Y_{t-1}, Y_{t-2}, Y_{t-3}, \ldots] = [Y_t | Y_{t-1}],$$

and for the AR(2) time series (Figure 3.18b) we have

$$[Y_t | Y_{t-1}, Y_{t-2}, Y_{t-3}, \ldots] = [Y_t | Y_{t-1}, Y_{t-2}].$$

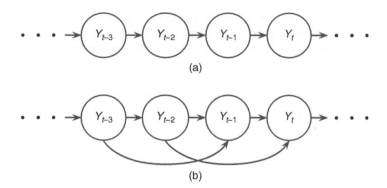

Figure 3.18 (a) Directed graph representing an AR(1) process. (b) Directed graph representing an AR(2) process.

From the directed graphs in Figure 3.18, it is clear that these time series possess a "lack-of-memory" or *Markov*-type property, in that the distribution of the current state, conditional on the past, in fact only depends on the "recent" past.

There are other ways to express temporal dependence that cannot be represented succinctly through a directed graph. For example, the first-order moving average (MA(1)) time series,

$$Y_t = \varepsilon_t + \varepsilon_{t-1} ,$$

where $\{\varepsilon_t\}$ are iid random variables, has a conditional distribution $[Y_t | Y_{t-1}, Y_{t-2}, Y_{t-3}, \ldots]$ that depends on *all* the past values. However, notice that unconditionally there are some very simple *independencies* for the MA(1) time series; for example, $[Y_t, Y_{t+2}] = [Y_t][Y_{t+2}]$.

Another way to express temporal dependence is essentially to ignore the directionality of time and specify only the first two moments of $\{Y_t\}$, namely $E(Y_t)$ and $\mathrm{cov}(Y_t, Y_r)$, for all t and r in the temporal domain of interest D_t. This approach is discussed in some detail in Section 3.3.

3.4.7 Vector Autoregressive Process

It is unusual to find time series in the real world that behave independently of other processes. Thus, it is important to consider several time series simultaneously, which are referred to as *multivariate time series*. As we shall see in Section 6.4, in the spatio-temporal setting it is sometimes useful to think of time series at different spatial locations as multiple (related) time series. We provide here a minimal introduction to some aspects of multivariate discrete time series, and we refer the reader to more advanced treatments (e.g., Lütkepohl, 1993, 2005) for additional discussion and detail.

As with univariate models, there are simple multivariate temporal processes that are useful for modeling many real-world multivariate time series. In this regard, there are analogous models for multivariate white-noise, random walk, autoregressive, moving-average, and ARMA processes. Given its importance to spatio-temporal modeling, we focus here on the *vector autoregressive (VAR) process*.

The VAR process relates the values of the multiple time series at a time t to some linear combination of the multiple time series at previous times. Thus, analogous to the univariate AR case, for a K-variate time series, the VAR(p) process is given by

$$\mathbf{Y}_t = \mathbf{M}_1 \mathbf{Y}_{t-1} + \mathbf{M}_2 \mathbf{Y}_{t-2} + \cdots + \mathbf{M}_p \mathbf{Y}_{t-p} + \mathbf{W}_t, \qquad (3.97)$$

where $\mathbf{Y}_t \equiv (Y_t^{(1)}, \ldots, Y_t^{(K)})'$, $\{\mathbf{M}_l : l = 1, \ldots, p\}$ are $K \times K$ propagator matrices (sometimes referred to as state-transition matrices), and $\{\mathbf{W}_t\}$ is a K-variate white-noise process with mean zero and covariance matrix $\mathbf{Q}$. Typically, this white-noise process is assumed to be Gaussian, in which case $\mathbf{W}_t \sim iid\ Gau(\mathbf{0}, \mathbf{Q})$.

Specifically, for illustration, consider the VAR(1) process,

$$\mathbf{Y}_t = \mathbf{M} \mathbf{Y}_{t-1} + \mathbf{W}_t. \qquad (3.98)$$

Very simply, the ith row of the transition matrix $\mathbf{M}$ contains weights that describe how the multiple time series at time $t - 1$ are linearly combined to influence the i-th time series at time t. For example,

$$Y_t^{(i)} = m_{i,1} Y_{t-1}^{(1)} + m_{i,2} Y_{t-1}^{(2)} + \cdots + m_{i,K} Y_{t-1}^{(K)} + W_t^{(i)}, \qquad (3.99)$$

where $m_{i,j}$ refers to the (i, j)th entry in $\mathbf{M}$, and $W_t^{(i)}$ refers to the ith element of the vector $\mathbf{W}_t$; $i = 1, \ldots, K$. Of course, it is precisely this interaction between the K time series, and between the K potentially correlated noise processes, that can lead to complicated behavior. One can show that the VAR(1) process is causal if the eigenvalues of $\mathbf{M}$ are all less than one in modulus.

Parameter Estimation for the VAR(1) Process

Estimation of the parameter matrices $\mathbf{M}$ and $\mathbf{Q}$ can be obtained via maximum-likelihood (see Lütkepohl, 1993, Chapter 3) or method-of-moments. For illustration, we consider the latter. Assume that the process $\{\mathbf{Y}_t\}$ has mean *zero* and is second-order stationary; that is, all the autocovariance and cross-covariance functions depend only on the lag difference between temporal indices. We then post-multiply both sides of (3.98) by $\mathbf{Y}'_{t-1}$ and take expectations to obtain

$$E(\mathbf{Y}_t \mathbf{Y}'_{t-1}) = \mathbf{M} E(\mathbf{Y}_{t-1} \mathbf{Y}'_{t-1}), \qquad (3.100)$$

or

$$\mathbf{C}_Y^{(1)} = \mathbf{M} \mathbf{C}_Y^{(0)}, \qquad (3.101)$$

where we define $\mathbf{C}_Y^{(\tau)}$ to be the τth lagged covariance matrix of the process $\{\mathbf{Y}_t\}$. Thus, we solve for $\mathbf{M}$ and obtain

$$\mathbf{M} = \mathbf{C}_Y^{(1)}(\mathbf{C}_Y^{(0)})^{-1}. \tag{3.102}$$

Another useful relationship that expresses $\mathbf{C}_Y^{(0)}$ directly in terms of $\mathbf{M}$ and $\mathbf{Q}$ is (Harvey, 1993, Section 7.3)

$$\text{vec}(\mathbf{C}_Y^{(0)}) = [\mathbf{I} - \mathbf{M} \otimes \mathbf{M}]^{-1}\text{vec}(\mathbf{Q}), \tag{3.103}$$

where the symbol $\otimes$ denotes the Kronecker product and the vec($\cdot$) operator stacks the columns of an $a \times b$ matrix to make an $ab \times 1$ column vector (e.g., see Lütkepohl, 1993, for more details).

Then, assuming we have observations $\mathbf{Y}_1, \ldots, \mathbf{Y}_T$, the empirical lagged covariance matrices are

$$\hat{\mathbf{C}}_Y^{(\tau)} = \frac{1}{T} \sum_{t=1}^{T-\tau} (\mathbf{Y}_{t\mid\tau} - \hat{\boldsymbol{\mu}})(\mathbf{Y}_t - \hat{\boldsymbol{\mu}})', \tag{3.104}$$

where the K-dimensional empirical mean is, $\hat{\boldsymbol{\mu}} \equiv \frac{1}{T} \sum_{t=1}^T \mathbf{Y}_t$. As with the univariate case, the divisor T in (3.104) avoids problems with positive-definiteness, but the divisor $(T - \tau)$ mitigates the obvious bias resulting from using T.

It follows from (3.102) that the method-of-moments estimator of $\mathbf{M}$ is given by

$$\hat{\mathbf{M}} = \hat{\mathbf{C}}_Y^{(1)}(\hat{\mathbf{C}}_Y^{(0)})^{-1}, \tag{3.105}$$

where $\hat{\mathbf{C}}_Y^{(0)}$ must be nonsingular. Clearly, it is singular if $T < K$. Although this is not typically the case in multivariate time series analysis, it does become a critical issue in dynamic spatio-temporal models (see Chapter 7). Finally, note that although a zero mean vector was assumed in arriving at (3.105) via (3.104), the estimator $\hat{\mathbf{M}}$ is equally appropriate for $\boldsymbol{\mu} \neq \mathbf{0}$, since there is a correction, $\hat{\boldsymbol{\mu}}$, for $\boldsymbol{\mu}$ in (3.104).

One can obtain an estimator of $\mathbf{Q}$, the white-noise (in time) covariance matrix, in a similar manner. Post-multiply (3.98) by $\mathbf{Y}_t'$ and take expectations of both sides to obtain $\mathbf{Q} = \mathbf{C}_Y^{(0)} - \mathbf{M}\mathbf{C}_Y^{(1)'}$. A method-of-moments estimator is then given by

$$\hat{\mathbf{Q}} = \hat{\mathbf{C}}_Y^{(0)} - \hat{\mathbf{M}}\hat{\mathbf{C}}_Y^{(1)'} \tag{3.106}$$

$$= \hat{\mathbf{C}}_Y^{(0)} - \hat{\mathbf{C}}_Y^{(1)}(\hat{\mathbf{C}}_Y^{(0)})^{-1}\hat{\mathbf{C}}_Y^{(1)'}. \tag{3.107}$$

Maximum-likelihood estimation must generally proceed by numerical maximization of the loglikelihood (e.g., Lütkepohl, 1993). However, if one makes the assumption that $\mathbf{Y}_0$ is known, then maximization of the conditional loglikelihood (conditional on $\mathbf{Y}_0$) can be done analytically. In that case, the maximum-likelihood and the least-squares estimators are equivalent (e.g., Harvey 1993, Section 7.4).

3.4.8 Nonlinear Time-Series Models

As discussed in Section 3.2.2, the behavior of many real-world processes can be characterized by nonlinear dynamical systems. Although it is fairly easy to distinguish between linear and nonlinear processes in the case of deterministic processes, it is not always so easy to distinguish between linear and nonlinear *stochastic* processes. In the case of deterministic processes, nonlinearity is fairly easily characterized by nonlinear interactions in the lagged process state variable. However, in the stochastic setting, nonlinearity can occur from this type of behavior, as well as from parameter interactions and error-process interactions (with white-noise or colored-noise processes and/or state processes.) Furthermore, the characteristics associated with non-Gaussian errors and/or temporal nonstationarity are often indistinguishable from characteristics of nonlinearity (e.g., see Chatfield, 2004, Section 11.1.2 for an excellent overview.) Even with this lack of a clear definition of nonlinearity, there are several model classes in the time-series literature that are commonly viewed as nonlinear. We shall discuss briefly a few of these to facilitate the presentation of spatio-temporal nonlinearity in Chapter 7.

A very general class of nonlinear autoregressive models for the process $\{Y_t\}$ can be written as

$$Y_t = \mathcal{M}(Y_{t-1}, \ldots, Y_{t-p}) + \tau(Y_{t-1}, \ldots, Y_{t-p})\epsilon_t, \qquad t = p, p+1, \ldots, \tag{3.108}$$

where $\{\epsilon_t\}$ are iid with mean 0 and variance 1, and $\mathcal{M}$ and τ are functions of the lagged state process. In general, these functions can be specified parametrically or nonparametrically and can accommodate many different univariate nonlinear time series models as special cases [e.g., see Fan and Yao (2005, Section 1.5.4) for a complete discussion]. We consider briefly a few of these models here, for the special case where $p = 1$. Details and more general forms for these models can be found in the references listed in the Bibliographic Notes in Section 3.7.

Consider the (deceptively simple) first-order autoregression

$$Y_t = \mathcal{M}(Y_{t-1}) + \epsilon_t, \qquad t = 1, 2, \ldots, \tag{3.109}$$

where $\{\epsilon_t\}$ are iid with mean 0 and variance σ_ε^2, $\mathcal{M}$ is some *nonlinear function* of Y_{t-1}, and one can specify various distributions for ϵ_t. Such a model is often referred to as a *functional coefficient autoregressive (FAR)* model (e.g., Fan and Yao, 2005, Section 1.5.4). There are various approaches to specifying the model for $\mathcal{M}$, from fully nonparametric to fully parametric.

Another way to accommodate nonlinearity in autoregressive models is to allow parameters in the linear autoregressive model to vary (randomly) as a function of time. That is,

$$Y_t = a_t Y_{t-1} + \epsilon_t, \qquad t = 1, 2, \ldots, \tag{3.110}$$

where $\{\epsilon_t\}$ are the same as in (3.109). There are several different approaches to modeling this time-varying autoregressive coefficient, depending on what exogenous and endogenous information is available and whether one views a_t as random or not. For example, say there is another (exogenous) process $\{X_t : t = 1, 2, \ldots\}$ available. One might consider the system

$$Y_t = a_t Y_{t-1} + \epsilon_t, \qquad \epsilon_t \sim iid\ (0, \sigma_\varepsilon^2), \tag{3.111}$$

$$a_t = b_0 + b_1 X_t + \gamma_t, \qquad \gamma_t \sim iid\ (0, \sigma_\gamma^2), \tag{3.112}$$

where $\{\epsilon_t\}$ and $\{\gamma_t\}$ are independent, with distributions unspecified. In this case, the nonlinearity is apparent after substituting (3.112) into (3.111) [e.g., see Chatfield (2004, Section 11.2)]. A plot of Y_t versus Y_{t-1} would show both the autoregressive coefficient and the variance changing with time t. Clearly, more complicated relationships (nonlinear, semiparameteric) between X_t and a_t could be specified, and other exogenous variables could be considered. In addition, one might consider $\{X_t\}$ to be a random process. Now, if covariates (or exogenous processes) were not available or considered unimportant, one could consider a simple stochastic time series model for a_t in the system:

$$Y_t = a_t Y_{t-1} + \epsilon_t;\ \epsilon_t \sim iid\ (0, \sigma_\varepsilon^2), \tag{3.113}$$

$$a_t = b_0 + b_1 a_{t-1} + \gamma_t;\ \gamma_t \sim iid\ (0, \sigma_\gamma^2), \tag{3.114}$$

where $\{\epsilon_t\}$ and $\{\gamma_t\}$ are independent. Once again, more complicated models could be considered for $\{a_t\}$. Note that both pairs of equations, (3.111), (3.112) and (3.113), (3.114), are hierarchical representations. If $\{Y_t\}$ is not directly observed (i.e., latent), then a data model could be added to this hierarchy. In addition, the parameters in the models for $\{a_t\}$ could be considered random as well, and time-varying variances could also be included.

A related system assumes that the AR coefficient in (3.110) changes in a more discrete fashion, depending on the value of some exogenous variable, or the present (or past) values of the state itself (Tong, 1990). For example, a simple *threshold autoregression* model can be written as

$$Y_t = \begin{cases} a^{(1)} Y_{t-1} + \epsilon_t^{(1)};\ \epsilon_t^{(1)} \sim iid\ (0, \sigma_1^2), & \text{for } X_t \le c, \\ a^{(2)} Y_{t-1} + \epsilon_t^{(2)};\ \epsilon_t^{(2)} \sim iid\ (0, \sigma_2^2), & \text{for } X_t > c, \end{cases} \tag{3.115}$$

where the model can be extended in an obvious way to account for more than one condition (threshold), c. Thus, there are different linear AR models, depending on how the exogenous variable X_t compares to the corresponding threshold(s). The *state-dependent* version of this threshold autoregression model substitutes Y_{t-1} (or, in general, a function of past values $Y_{t-1}, \ldots, Y_{t-p}$) for X_t, so that the current model depends on some past value of the state process. Now, it could be that X_t is not actually observed, in which case the different regimes are based on a latent process. In addition, one may not actually know the thresholds associated with the regime transition, and thus these might need to be estimated or allowed to be random as well. In general, these models (referred to as *regime-switching* models) can be quite complicated!

As mentioned above, it is certainly possible that the variances in time series models can vary with time as well. In general, models for time-varying variances can be parametric, semiparametric, or nonparametric and can be deterministic or stochastic. In the deterministic parametric context, the classical formulation is the *generalized autoregressive conditional heteroskedastic (GARCH)* model,

$$
\sigma_t^2 = a_0 + \sum_{i=1}^{p} a_i Y_{t-i}^2 + \sum_{j=1}^{q} b_j \sigma_{t-j}^2 , \tag{3.116}
$$

where $a_i, b_j \geq 0$, for all i, j. These models are commonly used in the time series and econometrics literatures. One may also consider a stochastic variance process (i.e., *stochastic volatility*) in which case σ_t^2 (or σ_t) is modeled as a stochastic process. For example, one such (simple) model is given by

$$
\log \sigma_t^2 = b_0 + b_1 \log \sigma_{t-1}^2 + \eta_t, \qquad \eta_t \sim iid\,(0, \sigma_\eta^2), \tag{3.117}
$$

where $\{\eta_t\}$ is independent of the error process $\{\varepsilon_t\}$ in (3.109). Of course, (3.117) may be generalized to have higher-order lags, and the autoregressive function can be nonparametric. We note that the stochastic-volatility formulation fits naturally into the hierarchical statistical modeling framework.

In principle, all of the nonlinear models discussed here can be extended to the multivariate setting (e.g., see Fan and Yao, 2005). Such models rapidly begin to suffer from the "curse of dimensionality," as the number of variables in the state process increases. This makes estimation difficult in general and, typically, one must specify very specific forms for these models. We shall return to this issue when we discuss nonlinear spatio-temporal models in Chapter 7.

3.5 SPECTRAL REPRESENTATION OF TEMPORAL PROCESSES

It is often useful to represent a time series in terms of projections onto a set of underlying spectral basis functions. There are several reasons why we might want to do this. We might be interested in partitioning the overall variability in a time series into different scales of variability. For example, how much variability in the daily-temperature time series at a location can be described by an annual cycle or a semi-annual cycle? In addition, what quasi-periodic phenomena account for the most variability in a physical system? Another reason for thinking about time series projections onto basis functions is that such projections often have much simpler correlation structure than the original series. That is, the transformation into the spectral domain often acts as a decorrelator. It is also the case that some of the projections do not account for much variability and thus can often be ignored without much loss of information. This suggests that lower-dimensional representations of the process can be obtained in the spectral domain than can be obtained in the time domain.

In what follows, we consider a general spectral representation of temporal processes. We do not present many of the technical details; rather, we refer the reader to one of the many more technical books on times series and their spectral representation listed in the Bibliographic Notes in Section 3.7.

3.5.1 Spectral Representations of Continuous-Time Functions via Orthogonal Series

Consider a process that can be written as a function of time, $f(t)$, over the time interval (a, b). We define a sequence of spectral basis functions $\phi_k(t)$; $k = 1, 2, \ldots$, to be *orthogonal* over the interval (a, b) if

$$\int_a^b \phi_k(t)\phi_l(t)\,dt = \begin{cases} 0, & k \neq l, \\ \delta, & k = l, \end{cases} \tag{3.118}$$

where $\delta > 0$. Furthermore, these functions are said to be *orthonormal* if $\delta = 1$.

We now seek to expand $f(t)$ in terms of these functions:

$$f(t) = \sum_{k=1}^{\infty} \alpha_k \phi_k(t), \tag{3.119}$$

where $\{\alpha_k\}$ are the "weights" or *spectral coefficients* of the spectral expansion. If this expansion is possible, then $\{\alpha_k\}$ are given by

$$\alpha_k = \int_a^b f(t)\phi_k(t)\,dt, \qquad k = 1, 2, \ldots. \tag{3.120}$$

That is, the spectral coefficients are simply the projection of $f(t)$ onto the orthogonal basis functions.

In some cases, we may be interested in truncating (3.119) to consider only up to the p_αth function. The *mean squared error* (MSE) of the truncation is then given by

$$\text{MSE} \equiv \int_a^b \left(f(t) - \sum_{k=1}^{p_\alpha} \alpha_k \phi_k(t) \right)^2 dt. \tag{3.121}$$

It can be shown that the MSE is minimized with respect to $\{\alpha_k : k = 1, 2, \ldots, p_\alpha\}$, by the coefficients (3.120).

In addition to the orthogonality property, it is useful to consider one additional property of the basis functions, namely *completeness* (sometimes called L_2-*completeness*). The orthogonal series $\{\phi_k(t)\}$ is complete over the interval (a, b) if, for every piecewise continuous function $f(t)$ on that interval, the MSE (3.121) tends to zero as $p_\alpha \to \infty$ [e.g., see Kaplan (1991, Section 7.11)].

There are many examples of orthogonal basis functions that can be used for temporal processes. Common bases include trigonometric (i.e., Fourier), wavelet, spline, and orthogonal polynomial functions. In the next section, we illustrate the trigonometric case in some detail.

Trigonometric Series Expansion

Consider a function of interest, $f(t)$, defined on the interval $(-1/2, 1/2)$. Let $\{\phi_k(t)\}$ correspond to the trigonometric basis functions, $\sin(2\pi k t)$ and $\cos(2\pi k t)$, for $k = 0, 1, 2, \ldots$. These basis functions are complete and orthogonal. Hence, we can write the function $f(t)$ as

$$f(t) = \frac{a_0}{2} + \sum_{k=1}^{\infty} \{a_k \cos(2\pi k t) + b_k \sin(2\pi k t)\}, \tag{3.122}$$

and the *Fourier coefficients* are

$$a_k = 2 \int_{-\frac{1}{2}}^{\frac{1}{2}} f(t) \cos(2\pi k t) \, dt, \qquad k = 0, 1, \ldots, \tag{3.123}$$

$$b_k = 2 \int_{-\frac{1}{2}}^{\frac{1}{2}} f(t) \sin(2\pi k t) \, dt, \qquad k = 1, \ldots. \tag{3.124}$$

Note that we can make use of Euler's relationship, $e^{\pm i 2\pi k t} \equiv \cos(2\pi k t) \pm i \sin(2\pi k t)$, where $i = \sqrt{-1}$, to simplify the notation (see Section 3.2.1). In this case, we can write (3.122) in its common form:

$$f(t) = \sum_{k=-\infty}^{\infty} \alpha_k e^{i 2\pi k t}, \qquad -1/2 \le t \le 1/2, \tag{3.125}$$

where $\phi_k(t) \equiv e^{i 2\pi k t}$ and $\alpha_k \equiv a_k + i\, b_k$ are both complex functions. The result (3.125) is, of course, just the Fourier transform given in (3.66), and it is known as the *spectral representation theorem* (see Section 3.3).

The coefficients a_k and b_k provide important information regarding the characteristics of the sinusoidal time series, as shown in Section 3.2.1. It follows that when considering (3.122), the coefficients a_k and b_k, $k = 0, 1, 2, \ldots$, have associated amplitude and phase given by $\sqrt{a_k^2 + b_k^2}$ and $\tan^{-1}(-b_k/a_k)$, respectively.

3.5.2 Discrete-Time Spectral Expansion

The trigonometric spectral representation can be applied in the discrete-time setting (i.e., for time series). Let $\{Y_t : t = 1, \ldots, T\}$ be a time series and define $\{\phi_k(t) : t = 1, \ldots, T ; k = 1, \ldots, p_\alpha\}$ to be a complete set of basis functions. Define $\mathbf{Y} \equiv (Y_1, \ldots, Y_T)'$, $\boldsymbol{\alpha} \equiv (\alpha_1, \ldots, \alpha_{p_\alpha})'$, and $\boldsymbol{\Phi} \equiv (\boldsymbol{\phi}_1, \ldots, \boldsymbol{\phi}_{p_\alpha})$, where $\boldsymbol{\phi}_k \equiv (\phi_k(1), \ldots, \phi_k(T))'$. Then, it is convenient to denote the spectral expansion,

$$Y_t = \sum_{k=1}^{p_\alpha} \alpha_k \phi_k(t), \tag{3.126}$$

as

$$\mathbf{Y} = \boldsymbol{\Phi}\boldsymbol{\alpha}. \tag{3.127}$$

Multiply both sides of (3.127) by $\boldsymbol{\Phi}$ to obtain the spectral-coefficient vector,

$$\boldsymbol{\alpha} = (\boldsymbol{\Phi}'\boldsymbol{\Phi})^{-1}\boldsymbol{\Phi}'\mathbf{Y}, \tag{3.128}$$

which is in the form of an ordinary-least-squares estimate. In the case where the basis functions are orthonormal, $\boldsymbol{\Phi}'\boldsymbol{\Phi} = \mathbf{I}$; then (3.128) becomes

$$\boldsymbol{\alpha} = \boldsymbol{\Phi}'\mathbf{Y}. \tag{3.129}$$

Such a projection of data onto discrete basis functions is historically known as *harmonic analysis*, especially in the case where the basis functions are Fourier basis functions. As we shall see, estimation based on (3.128) does not yield consistent estimates of the spectrum, but it does have utility with regard to dimension reduction and decorrelation.

As an example, consider the Fourier series expansion in the discrete-time setting with the series length T an even positive integer (this is not necessary, but makes the notation simpler). Note that the highest frequency we can fit to the data is that corresponding to two measurements per cycle. This is called the *Nyquist frequency*. For example, if we have measurements of temperature at noon each day, we know nothing about what is happening within any day. Thus, the highest frequency we can consider corresponds to one cycle every two days (i.e., 1/2 cycle per day). This is related to another issue in spectral analysis known as *aliasing*, which refers to the presence of incorrect frequencies simply due to the sampling of a series at too slow a rate. For example, if the true-process frequency was 1/2 cycle per day, but we sampled say every third day, we would see (false) evidence of periodic behavior with a period of 6 days per cycle (i.e., a frequency of 1/6 cycle per day). Thus, one should sample a series at a rate of at least two measurements per cycle for the cycle corresponding to the highest conceivable frequency of interest.

In general, for discrete time series, we only need to consider the frequencies,

$$\omega_k = \frac{2\pi k}{T}, \qquad k = 1, \ldots, T/2, \tag{3.130}$$

which are in units of radians per sampling increment. Often, these frequencies are denoted in terms of *cycles* per sampling increment, in which case $\omega_k = k/T$, $k = 1, \ldots, T/2$. In the former case, the Nyquist frequency is $\omega_{T/2} = \pi$ radians per sampling increment, and in the latter case it is $1/2$ cycle per sampling increment. Then the orthonormal basis functions associated with α_k, for $k = 1, \ldots, T/2 - 1$, are given by

$$\phi_k(t) = \sqrt{2/T} \left(\cos\left(\frac{2\pi k}{T}t\right) + i \sin\left(\frac{2\pi k}{T}t\right) \right), \qquad t = 1, \ldots, T. \tag{3.131}$$

In addition, $\phi_k(t)$ for $k = 0$ and $k = T/2$ are given by

$$\phi_0(t) = \sqrt{1/T}, \qquad t = 1, \ldots, T, \tag{3.132}$$

and

$$\phi_{T/2}(t) = \sqrt{1/T} \cos(\pi t), \qquad t = 1, \ldots, T. \tag{3.133}$$

Thus, for each of the $T/2 - 1$ basis functions given by (3.131), $\alpha_k = a_k + i\, b_k$ is complex and represents the contribution associated with the kth basis function (which contains k cycles over the series of length T). Some practitioners prefer to consider the analysis without the use of the complex-number notation. In that case, one can simply define T basis functions corresponding to a_k and b_k as follows:

$$\phi_{a_0}(t) \equiv \sqrt{1/T} \tag{3.134}$$

$$\phi_{a_k}(t) \equiv \sqrt{2/T} \cos\left(\frac{2\pi k}{T}t\right) \tag{3.135}$$

$$\phi_{b_k}(t) \equiv \sqrt{2/T} \sin\left(\frac{2\pi k}{T}t\right) \tag{3.136}$$

$$\phi_{a_{T/2}}(t) \equiv \sqrt{1/T} \cos(\pi t), \tag{3.137}$$

where $t = 1, \ldots, T$ and $k = 1, \ldots, T/2 - 1$; it is clear from the complex representation above that we do not need a basis function corresponding to b_0 or $b_{T/2}$; we can think of $b_0 = b_{T/2} = 0$. Thus, in this formulation, there are T basis functions, and they can be used to construct the $T \times T$ matrix, $\boldsymbol{\Phi}$, defined at the beginning of this subsection.

Consider the simple example where we have a time series of length $T = 6$ given by

$$\mathbf{Y} = (-.0831, \ .7187, \ .2182, \ .3068, \ -.9568, \ -.4170)'. \quad (3.138)$$

This series is plotted in Figure 3.19. It is evident from this plot that most of the variability is occurring at a frequency of approximately one cycle per six time increments. We can construct the following basis functions:

$$\phi_{a_0}(t) = \frac{1}{\sqrt{6}} \quad (3.139)$$

$$\phi_{a_1}(t) = \sqrt{2/6} \cos\left(\frac{2\pi}{6}t\right) \quad (3.140)$$

$$\phi_{b_1}(t) = \sqrt{2/6} \sin\left(\frac{2\pi}{6}t\right) \quad (3.141)$$

$$\phi_{a_2}(t) = \sqrt{2/6} \cos\left(\frac{4\pi}{6}t\right) \quad (3.142)$$

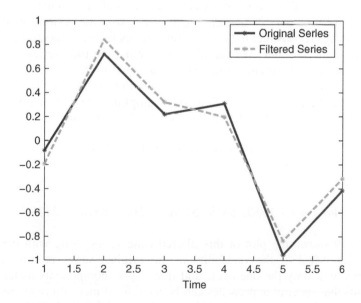

Figure 3.19 Original time series given by (3.138) (solid blue line) and filtered representation given by (3.139) (dashed green line).

$$\phi_{b_2}(t) = \sqrt{2/6} \sin\left(\frac{4\pi}{6} t\right) \tag{3.143}$$

$$\phi_{a_3}(t) = \sqrt{1/6} \cos(\pi t), \tag{3.144}$$

for $t \in \{1, 2, \ldots, 6\}$. Letting $\boldsymbol{\Phi} = [\boldsymbol{\phi}_{a_0} \ \boldsymbol{\phi}_{a_1} \ \boldsymbol{\phi}_{b_1} \ \boldsymbol{\phi}_{a_2} \ \boldsymbol{\phi}_{b_2} \ \boldsymbol{\phi}_{a_3}]$, we obtain

$$\boldsymbol{\Phi} = \begin{bmatrix} .4082 & .2887 & .5000 & -.2887 & .5000 & -.4082 \\ .4082 & -.2887 & .5000 & -.2887 & -.5000 & .4082 \\ .4082 & -.5774 & .0000 & .5774 & .0000 & -.4082 \\ .4082 & -.2887 & -.5000 & -.2887 & .5000 & .4082 \\ .4082 & .2887 & -.5000 & -.2887 & -.5000 & -.4082 \\ .4082 & .5774 & .0000 & .5774 & .0000 & .4082 \end{bmatrix}. \tag{3.145}$$

Write $\boldsymbol{\alpha} = (\tilde{a}_0, \tilde{a}_1, \tilde{b}_1, \tilde{a}_2, \tilde{b}_2, \tilde{a}_3)'$, where

$$\boldsymbol{\alpha} = \boldsymbol{\Phi}'\mathbf{Y} = (-.0871, -.9630, .6428, -.1106, .2309, .5839)'. \tag{3.146}$$

The amplitudes associated with the orthonormal eigenfunctions (3.139)–(3.144) are then given by $A_k \equiv \sqrt{\tilde{a}_k^2 + \tilde{b}_k^2}$, where $\tilde{b}_0 \equiv 0$. Hence,

$$A_0 = .09, \qquad A_1 = 1.16, \qquad A_2 = .26, \qquad A_3 = .58. \tag{3.147}$$

Thus, the most dominant cycles (i.e., frequencies corresponding to the most variation) in this time series correspond to A_1 and A_3, which represent one cycle per six time periods and three cycles per six time periods, respectively. We can always reconstruct the original time series from the spectral coefficients by the formula $\mathbf{Y} = \boldsymbol{\Phi}\boldsymbol{\alpha}$. We can also reconstruct the time series after setting some of the less important coefficients in $\boldsymbol{\alpha}$ equal to zero (i.e., *filtering*). For example, assume a threshold value corresponding to an amplitude of 0.5, so that any coefficients corresponding to an amplitude less than 0.5 are set to zero. Thus, we obtain the filtered time series, $\mathbf{Y}_R$, from the vector,

$$\boldsymbol{\alpha}_R = (0, -.9630, .6428, 0, 0, .5839)', \tag{3.148}$$

as follows:

$$\mathbf{Y}_R \equiv \boldsymbol{\Phi}\boldsymbol{\alpha}_R = (-.1950, .8378, .3176, .1950, -.8378, -.3176)'. \tag{3.149}$$

Figure 3.19 shows the plot of this filtered time series along with the original time series. Most of the variability in the original series is still evident in the series with only the one-cycle and three-cycle components included. This illustrates that spectral approaches can be used for dimension reduction; in this case, we can characterize most of the variability with only half the number of parameters (i.e., $\tilde{a}_1$, $\tilde{b}_1$, and $\tilde{a}_3$). However, note that such a filtering approach is quite naive, and more sophisticated approaches are used in practice (e.g., Shumway and Stoffer, 2006, Chapter 4).

In practice, one does not typically form the matrix $\boldsymbol{\Phi}$ as shown in this example, since for time series of even moderate length, the dimensionality of $\boldsymbol{\Phi}$ is prohibitive, from a computational and storage perspective. Fortunately, this matrix does not have to be formed directly. Rather, the *Fast Fourier Transform* (FFT) algorithm (Cooley and Tukey, 1965) can be used to obtain the spectral coefficients in a very efficient manner. Thus, the operation $\boldsymbol{\Phi}'\mathbf{Y}$ can be carried out using the FFT algorithm, and the operation $\boldsymbol{\Phi}\boldsymbol{\alpha}$ can be carried out by the inverse FFT algorithm. Similar computational efficiencies can be obtained for other basis functions. For example, the multiresolution algorithm of Mallat (1989) can be used when the basis functions are wavelets. However, there are examples where one still must form the matrix $\boldsymbol{\Phi}$ and compute the matrix multiplications directly. Examples include empirical basis functions (e.g., see the discussion of EOFs in Section 5.3) or theoretical basis functions suggested by the normal modes of some natural system (e.g., Wikle et al., 2001).

In addition to dimension reduction, the spectral decomposition also has a decorrelating effect on the original time series. For example, if the process is second-order stationary, then in the spectral domain,

$$\text{var}(\boldsymbol{\alpha}) \simeq \text{diag}(\mathbf{d}), \tag{3.150}$$

where $\mathbf{d}$ is a vector containing the variances of the spectral coefficients $\{\alpha_i\}$. That is, α_i and α_j are asymptotically independent (e.g., Shumway and Stoffer, 2006, Appendix C). This can simplify models dramatically. For example, assume that $\mathbf{Y} \sim Gau(\mathbf{0}, \boldsymbol{\Sigma})$, $\{\phi_k(\cdot)\}$ are orthonormal, and we have $\mathbf{Y} = \boldsymbol{\Phi}\boldsymbol{\alpha}$, or equivalently, $\boldsymbol{\alpha} = \boldsymbol{\Phi}'\mathbf{Y}$. Thus, using basic properties of the multivariate Gaussian distribution, we obtain $\boldsymbol{\alpha} \sim Gau(\mathbf{0}, \boldsymbol{\Phi}'\boldsymbol{\Sigma}\boldsymbol{\Phi})$. When $\boldsymbol{\Phi}$ are Fourier basis functions and $\mathbf{Y}$ comes from a stationary times series, it follows that $\boldsymbol{\Phi}'\boldsymbol{\Sigma}\boldsymbol{\Phi} \simeq \text{diag}(\mathbf{d})$. Hence, from a modeling perspective, it is much easier to work with the process $\boldsymbol{\alpha}$ than the process $\mathbf{Y}$, since its dependence structure is much simpler.

3.5.3 Univariate Spectral Analysis

In the case of discrete Fourier basis functions, the coefficients $\{\alpha_k\}$ in the expansion (3.126) can be written in terms of the frequencies $\{\omega_k\}$: $\alpha(\omega_k) \equiv \alpha_k$, where recall from (3.130) that $\omega_k = 2\pi k/T$; $k = 0, \ldots, T/2$. In this case, the Fourier basis functions are complex, and (3.129) is modified to

$$\alpha(\omega_k) = \sum_{t=1}^{T} Y_t \overline{\phi}_k(t), \tag{3.151}$$

where recall that $\{Y_t: t = 1, \ldots, T\}$ is a time series, and the overbar indicates the complex conjugate of the Fourier basis functions given in (3.131), (3.132), and (3.133). We can then define the *periodogram* as the squared modulus of $\alpha(\omega_k)$:

$$\hat{I}(\omega_k) \equiv \alpha(\omega_k)\overline{\alpha}(\omega_k) = |\alpha(\omega_k)|^2, \qquad k = 0, \ldots, T/2, \qquad (3.152)$$

which correspond to the "amplitudes" for the frequencies $\{\omega_k\}$ discussed in the example of the previous section. One can also define the periodogram as the discrete version of (3.66), with $C(\tau)$ replaced with the empirical autocovariance function (3.71). Thus, the periodogram can be thought of as an estimator of the spectrum of $\{Y_t\}$.

As an estimator of the spectrum, the periodogram has some problems. Although the periodogram is asymptotically unbiased for stationary processes, for finite sample sizes there may in fact be large biases, and the periodogram is not a consistent estimator of the spectrum (e.g., Chatfield, 1989, Section 7.3.2). Thus, we seek an estimator that reduces bias as well as variance. Of course (as is always the case in statistical estimation), there is a trade-off between bias reduction and variance reduction. We discuss briefly below some approaches that seek to deal with this trade-off. Although the topic is too extensive to cover in detail here, the Bibliographic Notes in Section 3.7 include resources for such details.

When the bias is asymptotically zero, one obvious way to reduce it is to use more data. Typically, that is not a viable option. Another option for bias reduction is *data tapering* (or *data windowing*), where each Y_t is replaced with a weighted version, $Y_t w_t$, where the weights $\{w_t\}$ typically taper to zero at the endpoints of the data and are equal to one in the middle. For example, a common data window is the cosine bell taper (e.g., Bloomfield, 2000, Section 6.2),

$$w_t = \frac{1}{2}\left[1 - \cos\left(\frac{2\pi(t - .5)}{T}\right)\right], \qquad t = 1, \ldots, T. \qquad (3.153)$$

Such data tapering is most useful when there are large differences between the beginning and end portions of the time series, or when certain frequency components contain much more variance than adjacent frequencies (e.g., Shumway and Stoffer, 2006, Section 4.5). Alternatively, we may *pre-whiten* the data. In this case, we filter the data initially (e.g., consider $U_t \equiv Y_t - Y_{t-1}$), perform the spectral analysis on the filtered data $\{U_t\}$, and then *post-color* the spectral estimate by accounting for the spectrum of the filter. (Note that in the frequency domain, this is a simple multiplication for each frequency.) This is described, for example, in Percival and Walden (1993, Section 6.5).

There are several alternatives when it comes to variance reduction. A common approach is to smooth the periodogram, whereby a moving average of the periodogram is calculated (Daniell, 1946):

$$\hat{f}(\omega_k) \equiv \frac{1}{2P + 1} \sum_{j = k-P}^{k+P} \hat{I}(\omega_j). \qquad (3.154)$$

Clearly, the spectral estimate at frequencies within P frequencies from the ends of the spectrum cannot be obtained with this estimator. As this approach amounts to low-pass filtering of the periodogram, we could easily pick other averaging approaches (filters) as well, and typically this is considered in the context of windows applied to the autocovariance function [e.g., see Chatfield (1989, Section 7.6) for a concise discussion]. By smoothing the periodogram estimates (which are essentially uncorrelated), we reduce the variance by order $1/P$, but at the expense of introducing a bias (and correlation). Clearly, the choice of P is critical in this regard. Chatfield (1989, Section 7.4.4) suggests choosing a P on the order of $T/40$, but then some additional trial-and-error is needed to balance the desire for smoothness versus identification of sharp spectral peaks.

Another approach to averaging the periodogram was proposed by Bartlett (1948), and it consists of splitting the data into segments, calculating the periodogram for each segment, and then averaging these multiple periodograms at each frequency. Welch (1967) extended this approach so that the segments overlap, thereby reducing the bias. So-called *multitaper* methods, which use a family of tapers (typically, "discrete prolate spheroidal sequences") have been shown to be a convenient way to manage effectively the trade-off between bias and variance reduction in nonparametric spectral estimation (Thomson, 1982; Percival and Walden, 1993). The statistical properties of the various estimators have been well studied; see the Bibliographic Notes in Section 3.7.

Finally, we note that a parametric approach can be taken to spectral estimation, whereby a model (typically an ARMA model) is specified for which we know the theoretical spectral density in terms of the model parameters. The model is fitted to $\{Y_1, \ldots, Y_T\}$ (e.g., Sections 3.4.3, 3.4.4, and 3.4.5), and the parameter estimates are substituted into the theoretical spectral density to obtain the spectral-density estimate. For more discussion of this approach, see, for example, Percival and Walden (1993, Chapter 9).

Example: The foundation of the theory of equatorial waves in the atmosphere was elegantly described in the landmark paper of Matsuno (1966). Matsuno showed, using a simplified set of hydrodynamical equations, that propagating waves were theoretically possible in tropical regions. Shortly thereafter, such waves were discovered in upper-level (rawinsonde) data, and their study has been of significant interest in the atmospheric sciences ever since. As an example, consider data for the north/south component of the upper (70-hPa)-level wind measured by rawinsondes daily at Chuuk (formerly Truk) Island in the tropical Pacific from 1964 to 1994, as described in Wikle, Madden, and Chen (1997). A smoothed-periodogram spectral analysis was performed on these 11,323 observations, after application of a split-cosine bell taper (10% on each end; e.g., see Bloomfield, 2000, Section 6.2). The spectral estimate was obtained from (3.154) with smoothing parameter $P = 50$. For comparison, an AR(24) spectral estimate was also obtained and both estimates are shown in Figure 3.20. Note that there are several spectral peaks associated

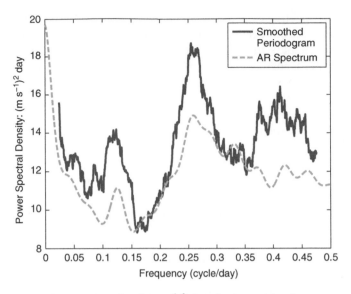

Figure 3.20   Spectral density (in units of $(m\ s^{-1})^2\ day$) for the north/south component of the 70-hPa-level wind at Chuuk (formerly Truk) Island based on daily observations from 1964 to 1994. The smoothed periodogram estimate is given by the red solid line and the AR(24) spectral estimate is given by the dashed green line.

with these spectral estimates. Of particular interest, meteorologically, is the peak from about 0.22–0.33 cycles per day (corresponding to waves with periods of 3–4.5 days). As shown in Wikle, Madden, and Chen (1997), these are likely to correspond to the so-called "mixed-Rossby gravity waves" suggested by Matsuno's theory and originally discovered in observations by Yanai and Maruyama (1966).

3.5.4   Bivariate Spectral Analysis

Recall that for jointly second-order stationary processes, $\{Y_t^{(1)}\}$ and $\{Y_t^{(2)}\}$, the cross-covariance function is given by $C_{12}(\tau)$, as defined in (3.68). If $\sum_{\tau=-\infty}^{\infty} |C_{12}(\tau)| < \infty$, then the *cross-spectrum* is defined as

$$f_{12}(\omega) \equiv \sum_{\tau=-\infty}^{\infty} C_{12}(\tau)\exp\{-2\pi i \omega \tau\}, \tag{3.155}$$

$$\equiv c_{12}(\omega) - i\ q_{12}(\omega), \qquad -1/2 \le \omega \le 1/2, \tag{3.156}$$

where $f_{12}(\omega)$ is a complex-valued function, the real part, $c_{12}(\omega)$, is known as the *co-spectrum*, and the imaginary part, $q_{12}(\omega)$, is known as the *quadrature spectrum*. We can then define two useful quantities. The first is the *squared coherence function* (sometimes known as the *magnitude squared coherence*), which is given by

$$\text{coh}_{12}^2(\omega) \equiv \frac{|f_{12}(\omega)|^2}{f_1(\omega) f_2(\omega)} = \frac{c_{12}^2(\omega) + q_{12}^2(\omega)}{f_1(\omega) f_2(\omega)}, \qquad -1/2 \le \omega \le 1/2,$$

$$(3.157)$$

where $f_i(\omega)$ refers to the spectral density of $\{Y_t^{(i)}\}$; $i = 1, 2$. The squared coherence is analogous to the usual squared correlation coefficient, in that $0 \le \text{coh}_{12}^2(\omega) \le 1$; it measures the square of the linear association between the components of the two processes at frequency ω.

In addition, we can define the *phase spectrum*, which is given by

$$\theta_{12}(\omega) \equiv \tan^{-1} \left(\frac{-q_{12}(\omega)}{c_{12}(\omega)} \right), \qquad -1/2 \le \omega \le 1/2, \qquad (3.158)$$

and varies between $-\pi$ and π. In conjunction with the squared coherence function, the phase spectrum is useful for establishing linear relationships between components of time series in the frequency domain. In particular, a constant phase together with a peak in the squared coherence suggests that one series leads/lags the other by the amount given by the phase. The example given at the end of this subsection will demonstrate how this works for bivariate time series data.

Let $\{\alpha^{(i)}(\omega_k)\}$ be the discrete Fourier transform (3.151) of series $\{Y_t^{(i)}\}$. Then, the *cross-periodogram* is defined as

$$I_{12}(\omega_k) \equiv \alpha^{(1)}(\omega_k) \bar{\alpha}^{(2)}(\omega_k), \qquad (3.159)$$

where again the overbar indicates the complex conjugate. As an estimate of the cross-spectrum, the cross-periodogram suffers from the same problems (i.e., bias and lack of consistency) as the univariate periodogram. As in (3.154), we could smooth across frequencies:

$$\hat{f}_{12}(\omega_k) \equiv \frac{1}{2P + 1} \sum_{j=k-P}^{k+P} \hat{I}_{12}(\omega_j). \qquad (3.160)$$

Given this estimate of the cross-spectrum and estimates of the individual spectra, $\hat{f}_1(\omega_k)$ and $\hat{f}_2(\omega_k)$, one can obtain estimates of the co-spectrum and quadrature spectrum, the magnitude squared coherence, and the phase spectrum by simply substituting these into their respective definitions, (3.156), (3.157), and (3.158). The statistical properties of these estimators are well known and are described in the Bibliographic Notes in Section 3.7.

Example: Continuing the example presented in Section 3.5.3, we consider the east/west upper level (70-hPa) wind component at Chuuk Island, in addition to the north/south component. Figure 3.21 shows the smoothed

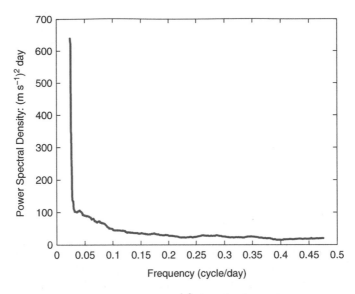

Figure 3.21   Spectral density (in units of $(m\ s^{-1})^2\ day$) for the east/west component of the 70-hPa-level wind at Chuuk (formerly Truk) Island based on daily observations from 1964 to 1994. The smoothed periodogram estimate is shown, analogous to that for the north/south component shown in Figure 3.20.

periodogram estimate of the spectrum of this east/west wind component. Note that this spectrum is much more "red" than that for the north/south component shown in Figure 3.20; that is, it has much more power at lower frequencies. Clearly, the mixed-Rossby gravity wave frequencies are not as dominant in the east/west-wind-component observations. However, this does not mean they are not present. Consider the cross-spectral analysis of these two wind components. In particular, Figure 3.22 shows the magnitude squared coherence function and the phase spectrum estimates (using the same smoothed periodogram estimates as for Figure 3.21). There are substantial peaks in the squared coherence across several frequency bands. In particular, note that in the mixed-Rossby gravity wave frequency band (0.22–0.33 cycles per day) mentioned in Section 3.5.3, there is strong coherence, and the phase is close to $-\pi/2$ in this range, indicating that the north/south wind component leads the east/west wind component by a quarter of a cycle. This is precisely what was predicted by Matsuno's (1966) theory for such waves. Wikle, Madden, and Chen (1997) discuss the likely wave types associated with other parts of the spectrum using a variety of cross-spectral analyses and multiple tropical stations (see also Section 5.2).

3.6   HIERARCHICAL MODELING OF TIME SERIES

As discussed in Chapter 2, hierarchical modeling (HM) is just the re-expression of a joint distribution of data, process, and parameters into a series of conditional models. Recall from basic probability that

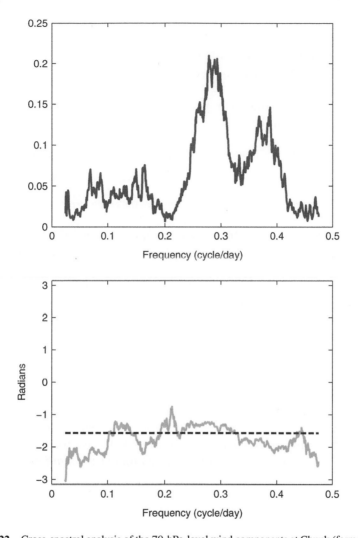

Figure 3.22 Cross-spectral analysis of the 70-hPa-level wind components at Chuuk (formerly Truk) Island based on daily observations from 1964 to 1994. **Top panel:** Estimate of the magnitude squared coherence function between the east/west and north/south wind components obtained from the smoothed periodogram estimates. **Bottom panel:** Estimate of the phase spectrum (in radians) associated with the magnitude squared coherence estimates in the top panel. The dashed black line is a reference line associated with a frequency of $-\pi/2$ radians. Note that a negative phase indicates that the north/south wind component leads the east/west component.

$[A, B, C] = [A|B, C][B|C][C]$. That is, the joint distribution of (say) three random variables, A, B, C, can always be factored into two conditional distributions and a marginal distribution. Thus, for complicated models for which there are data, a (hidden) process, and parameters involved, all known with more-or-less uncertainty, we consider the following general, three-stage factorization of [data, process, parameters] suggested by Berliner (1996):

Data model: [data|process, parameters]
Process Model: [process|parameters]
Parameter Model: [parameters]

In general, Bayes' rule then gives the posterior distribution of the process and parameters given the data:

$$[process, parameters|data] \propto [data|process, parameters]$$

$$\times[process|parameters]$$

$$\times [parameters].$$

In this general case, where the parameters are assigned prior distributions and hence are part of posterior inference, the model is referred to as a *Bayesian hierarchical model* (BHM).

In the case where the parameters are known or estimated from the data (traditionally known as *empirical Bayes*), the parameter model is dropped; we refer to this hierarchical model as an *empirical hierarchical model* (EHM). The general hierarchical model is discussed in Section 2.1; in this section, we are concerned with its use in Statistics for temporal data.

Data Models

A key idea behind the HM approach is that measurements of a process always occur with noise. Therefore, the parameter estimation presented in Sections 3.4.3–3.4.7 and 3.5.3–3.5.4 was under the ideal scenario of no measurement error. In general, it is not possible to observe the true state of a system. We might write this heuristically as follows: *Conditional* on the state process,

$$observation\ process = state\ process + error\ process, \qquad (3.161)$$

where the state process describes the state of the system and is of primary interest. Because of the conditioning, the structure of the error process can be quite simple. Then we concentrate our (temporal) modeling effort on the state process at a lower level of the hierarchy. The advantages of this hierchical modeling approach are discussed in Section 2.1.5.

Consider a data (or measurement) model often used in multivariate time series analysis:

$$\mathbf{Z}_t = \mathcal{H}(\mathbf{Y}_t) + \boldsymbol{\varepsilon}_t, \qquad t = 0, 1, \ldots, \qquad (3.162)$$

where $\mathbf{Z}_t$ is an m_t-dimensional vector of observations at time t, $\mathbf{Y}_t$ is the corresponding n-dimensional vector representing the unobservable state process, $\mathcal{H}$ is a measurement function that relates the observation vector to the state vector (often assumed to be known), and $\boldsymbol{\varepsilon}_t$ is the corresponding m_t-dimensional vector of observation errors, usually assumed to be independent in time. The classical data model assumes a *linear* measurement function $\mathcal{H}$ and independent Gaussian errors for $\{\boldsymbol{\varepsilon}_t\}$. That is,

$$\mathbf{Z}_t = \mathbf{H}_t \mathbf{Y}_t + \boldsymbol{\varepsilon}_t \; ; \; \boldsymbol{\varepsilon}_t \sim ind. \, Gau(\mathbf{0}, \mathbf{R}_t),$$

where $\mathbf{H}_t$ is an $m_t \times n$ matrix (of parameters), and $\mathbf{R}_t$ is an $m_t \times m_t$ error covariance matrix. The matrix $\mathbf{R}_t$ is also a source of parameters in the measurement model. From Chapter 2, we call the collection of unknown parameters $\boldsymbol{\theta}_D$.

Process Models

Process models describe the underlying scientific process of interest, $\{Y_t\}$. They are also often factored further into a series of conditional models: Let $\mathbf{Y}_t = (Y_t^{(1)}, Y_t^{(2)})'$; $t = 0, 1, \ldots$, denote a two-dimensional vector time series; then their joint probability can be written as

$$[Y_t^{(1)}, Y_t^{(2)} | \theta_P] = [Y_t^{(1)} | Y_t^{(2)}, \theta_P][Y_t^{(2)} | \theta_P].$$

For example, if $Y_t^{(1)}$ corresponds to a process Y at time t and $Y^{(2)}$ corresponds to the *same* process Y but at time $t - 1$, then this is just a model for Markovian evolution structure (e.g., AR(1)), as discussed in Section 3.4.7. In general, such factorizations are also important for simplifying multivariate processes. For example, Berliner, Milliff, and Wikle (2003) consider such a conditional framework for modeling the time-varying ocean conditioned on the time-varying atmosphere (see Section 7.4.3).

In so-called "state-space" modeling in time series analysis, a general evolution model for the process might be written as

$$\mathbf{Y}_t = \mathcal{M}(\mathbf{Y}_{t-1}) + \boldsymbol{\eta}_t, \tag{3.163}$$

where $\mathcal{M}$ is the transition function that describes the one-step evolution of the state process, and $\boldsymbol{\eta}_t$ is independent of $\mathbf{Y}_{t-1}$. A typical form of the model assumes this evolution function is *linear* (i.e., VAR(1)), such that $\mathbf{Y}_t = \mathbf{M}_t \mathbf{Y}_{t-1} + \boldsymbol{\eta}_t$, where in general the $n \times n$ propagator (or transition) matrix $\mathbf{M}_t$ can be time-varying. Furthermore, the error process $\{\boldsymbol{\eta}_t\}$ is white noise in time and, typically, $\boldsymbol{\eta}_t \sim Gau(\mathbf{0}, \mathbf{Q}_t)$, where the covariance matrix $\mathbf{Q}_t$ can also be time-varying. We write this as $\boldsymbol{\eta}_t \sim ind. \, Gau(\mathbf{0}, \mathbf{Q}_t)$.

One can make various inferences on $\mathbf{Y}_t$, given the data. For observations $\mathbf{Z}_1, \ldots, \mathbf{Z}_T$ and index $t \in \{1, \ldots, T-1\}$, a *filtered* estimate of $\mathbf{Y}_t$ is given by $E(\mathbf{Y}_t | \mathbf{Z}_1, \ldots, \mathbf{Z}_t)$; a *smoothed* estimate is given by $E(\mathbf{Y}_t | \mathbf{Z}_1, \ldots, \mathbf{Z}_T)$; and a *forecast* estimate is given by $E(\mathbf{Y}_{T+\tau} | \mathbf{Z}_1, \ldots, \mathbf{Z}_T)$, for $\tau > 0$. Section 8.2 can be consulted for further details on filtering, smoothing, and forecasting.

Parameter Models

In the case where the parameters in the data and process models are known, we obviously do not need to specify parameter models. Similarly, in cases where these parameters are estimated from the data, the HM has no parameter model. This is an EHM and more akin to the traditional state-space estimation in time series. In contrast, under a BHM scenario, we specify models (distributions) for the various parameters appearing in the previous levels of hierarchy. Like before, parameter models from each stage can also be factored into subcomponents. For example, we often assume independence:

$$[\theta_D, \theta_P] = [\theta_D][\theta_P].$$

Furthermore, scientific insight and previous studies can facilitate the specification of $[\theta_D]$ and $[\theta_P]$. For example, measurement-error parameters in θ_D can often be obtained from previous studies that focus on such issues (this is typically the case for environmental variables and some ecological data). Certainly, process parameters in θ_P often carry scientific insight as well (e.g., Wikle et al., 2001; Wikle, 2003b).

In the specific data model (3.162) and process model (3.163) given above, if the parameters are known, then relatively computationally efficient estimates of the state process can be obtained if the functions $\mathcal{M}$ and $\mathcal{H}$ are linear and the error distributions are Gaussian. However, most commonly, the parameters are not known. Chapters 8 and 9 describe implementation and inference for EHMs and BHMs fitted to spatio-temporal data.

3.7   BIBLIOGRAPHIC NOTES

General Time Series

There are many excellent books on statistical time series analysis, including those for both the time domain and the frequency domain. These books provide a much more thorough background of the theory and application of time series than presented in this relatively brief overview chapter. A partial list of such books that we have found particularly helpful in writing this chapter are: Box and Jenkins (1970), Chatfield (1989), Brockwell and Davis (1991), Harvey (1993), Lütkepohl (1993, 2005), Fuller (1996), West and Harrison (1997), Bloomfield (2000), Shumway and Stoffer (2000, 2006), Durbin and Koopman (2001), Kitagawa (2010), and Prado and West (2011). Chandler and Scott (2010) present time series methods for trend detection and analysis, especially for environmental processes.

Dynamical Systems

A search of any academic library will provide many excellent references on dynamical systems, linear systems theory, and nonlinear dynamics. The discipline has progressed to the point where one can find such references at all levels of technical sophistication. General texts that we have found particularly helpful are Sandefur (1990), Lorenz (1993), and Devaney (2003). For a statistical perspective, we highly recommend the paper by Bartlett (1990), the review paper by Berliner (1992), and the references therein, as well as the article by Wolff (1998) and the texts by Tong (1990) and Chan and Tong (2001). We have also found Caswell (2001) to be excellent in its discussion of multivariate linear systems. Some classical works in the area that we have found helpful include Lorenz (1963), Hénon (1976), Mandelbrot (1982), Takens (1981, 1985), and Gleick (1987). A classical text on random continuous-time processes is Srinivasan and Vasudevan (1971). The monographs by Majda, Abramov, and Grote (2005) and Majda and Wong (2006) provide a nice exposition of nonlinear dynamical systems for geophysical processes.

Nonlinear Time Series

Classical references for statistical nonlinear time series include Priestley (1988) and Tong (1990). These are invaluable introductions to a technically demanding subject that is growing in importance. A more-recent text with a nonparametric emphasis is Fan and Yao (2005). In addition, many general time series texts include at least a chapter on nonlinear aspects of time series; an excellent example is found in Chatfield (2004, Chapter 11). Furthermore, many of the general time series texts include discussion of GARCH and stochastic-volatility models. Books in financial econometrics also include a discussion of nonlinear time series (e.g., Tsay, 2005). Although not considered in this book, we note that there is also an extensive literature on neural network methods for analyzing nonlinear behavior in time series (e.g., Kay and Titterington, 2000).

Spectral Representations/Analysis

The basic background of spectral analysis and spectral representations can often be found in most of the texts on statistical time series analysis cited above. In addition, we have found the book by Walter (1994) to be an excellent source for general spectral decompositions, and the books by Marple (1987) and Percival and Walden (1993) are particularly helpful in applications of spectral analysis. In addition, we recommend the classic papers by Daniell (1946), Bartlett (1948), Cooley and Tukey (1965), Welch (1967), Thomson (1982), and Mallat (1989). We have also made reference to examples found in Wikle, Madden, and Chen (1997) and Wikle et al. (2001). Background material on equatorial waves and their observation can be found in Matsuno (1966) and Yanai and Maruyama (1966).

Hierarchical Statistical Methods

The notion of hierarchical statistical modeling has been around for quite some time (see the Bibliographic Note in Gelman et al., 2003, Section 5.7). A general discussion can also be found in Sections 2.1–2.3. Indeed, almost any modern text in Bayesian theory, methods, or applications will have a substantial discussion of hierarchical statistical modeling. Gelman et al. (2003) is an excellent place to start. For an empirical hierarchical modeling (i.e., empirical-Bayes) approach, see Carlin and Louis (2000). Banerjee, Carlin, and Gelfand (2004) discuss the BHM approach for spatial models.

The more modern texts in time series analysis contain material on hierarchical Bayesian analysis (e.g., West and Harrison, 1997; Shumway and Stoffer, 2000, 2006). An important paper on Bayesian estimation of nonlinear time series is Carlin, Polson, and Stoffer (1992). Our perspective is shaped significantly by the paper of Berliner (1996). This approach is further outlined in the book by Royle and Dorazio (2008) as well as in papers by Wikle, Berliner, and Cressie (1998), Berliner, Wikle, and Cressie (2000), Wikle et al. (2001), Berliner, Milliff, and Wikle (2003), and Wikle (2003a,b), among many others discussed here and in later chapters.

General References:

We have found excellent background material related to basis functions in Kaplan (1991). General background on statistical theory and matrix identities can be found in Rao (1965). Background on the theory of financial temporal processes can be found in Tsay (2005) and Wilmott, Howison, and Dewynne (1995).

CHAPTER 4

Fundamentals of Spatial Random Processes

You are here. What happens north, south, east, or west of you is very likely to be (positively) dependent on what is happening here. This expresses a "law of Geography" that says nearby things tend to be more alike than those far apart. Why? Because there is a flux of causal relationships in the space–time continuum that, when integrated out over time or captured in a micro-instant of time, shows neighboring values to be more highly correlated. A caveat that should be mentioned is that physical barriers like rivers and mountains can affect what is meant by "nearby" or "neighboring." Also, the presence of competition can lead to correlations that are negative; to put a biological face on the point, under big trees only small trees can grow.

A spatial process can be a temporal snapshot, a temporal aggregation, or a temporally frozen state of a space–time process. The snapshot may actually be the result of aggregation over a very short time scale, resulting in "instantaneous" spatial dependence (e.g., contiguous scenes from a series of remotely sensed images). Aggregation over longer time scales occurs in studies of climate; climate is sometimes characterized as a long-term average of daily weather (i.e., climate is what you expect, weather is what you get!), although we prefer to think of it as a long-term statistical distribution. Finally, an ore deposit deep underground represents a temporally "frozen" state in the evolution of its mineralization.

In this chapter, we shall review the ways that spatial dependence has been incorporated into spatial statistical models, the eventual goal being to incorporate them into hierarchical statistical models. Spatial statistics is a relatively new development within Statistics; ironically, Fisher (1935) was well aware of potential complications from the spatial component in agricultural experiments but, as explained in Chapter 1, he used *randomization* to neutralize its effect (and to control for bias in the assignment of treatments to experimental units).

In 1938, Fairfield Smith wrote an article (Fairfield Smith, 1938) showing empirically that, as plot size increased, the variance of the average yield computed from his crop data decreased, but beyond a particular plot size the decrease was negligible. Clearly, this cannot happen if the data are uncorrelated, so that Fairfield Smith's study indirectly recognized the presence of spatial correlation; it has only been recently that a spatial statistical model has been developed that is consistent with Fairfield Smith's observations (McCullagh and Clifford, 2006).

Papadakis (1937) and Bartlett (1938) gave spatial analyses for data from agricultural field trials, but *spatial statistical models* for such phenomena did not begin to appear until much later (e.g., Whittle, 1954; Besag, 1974). It has become clear in the last two decades that spatial statistical analyses do not usurp the standard designs and analyses of variance proposed by Fisher, but they can augment them to yield more efficient inferences and hence shorter, less costly experiments (e.g., Gotway and Cressie, 1990; Grondona and Cressie, 1991, 1993; Brownie and Gumpertz, 1997; Federer, Newton, and Altman, 1997; Legendre et al., 2004).

Like Chapter 3, this chapter does not attempt to review the whole field. Our goal is to establish enough spatial statistical methodology so that our subsequent expositions on spatio-temporal statistical methodology can be adequately explained. In some sections, we have added a subsection of "Other Topics" that represent areas of special interest. By no means do these topics cover the explosion of spatial statistical research seen in the last twenty years. An excellent reference for that is the *Handbook of Spatial Statistics*, edited by Gelfand, Diggle, Fuentes, and Guttorp (2010).

Spatial Hierarchical Statistical Models

In this chapter, we continue with our emphasis on process modeling within hierarchical statistical models (HMs), here for *spatial* data. To provide context, the data model is considered along with the process model, but we discuss in less depth the treatment of the unknown parameters. Recall that a Bayesian hierarchical model (BHM) results from modeling uncertainty of parameters at a parameter-model level, and an empirical hierarchical model (EHM) results from estimating the parameters directly from the data and "plugging" them back into the model. Statistical inference in this chapter, for both the EHM and the BHM, is primarily concerned with prediction of the spatial random process, given the data. (In the case of an EHM, the variability of the estimated parameter values is typically, but not always, ignored.) Inference on the parameters themselves can also be of scientific interest.

Accounting for Measurement Error

A lot of the earlier literature in spatial statistics did not explicitly specify, nor did it disentangle, the variability from two important sources. One of the sources is due to the *measurement* of the phenomenon of interest, and the other is due to *incomplete knowledge* of the phenomenon. In a time-series context, Berliner (1996) called these the "data model" and the "process model," respectively; in this book, we shall also use this terminology. This is most straightforwardly seen in the geostatistics literature, where the nugget effect is defined as being equal to the discontinuity of the variogram at the origin (e.g., Journel and Huijbregts, 1978, pp. 151–152). Although it is sometimes recognized by geostatisticians that this discontinuity can be made up of *both* measurement error *and* spatial dependence at scales smaller than the available distances between observations, subsequent kriging (i.e., optimal spatial prediction) has often ignored the difference between these two sources of variability. Cressie (1988) derived optimal spatial prediction (kriging) in the presence of measurement error. When using geostatistical software, caution is advised, since many kriging algorithms fail to filter out the variability due to measurement error. In Section 4.1, we put measurement error, spatial prediction, and related issues into an HM context.

In Chapter 3, HMs are temporal; in this chapter, HMs are spatial; and in Chapters 6 and 7, HMs are spatio-temporal. The articles by Besag, York, and Mollié (1991) and by Diggle, Tawn, and Moyeed (1998) show the power of spatial HMs in diverse settings, albeit with considerable computational demands, and the book by Banerjee, Carlin, and Gelfand (2004) gives a modern perspective on spatial HMs.

Consider the basic *geostatistical* problem of *kriging* (i.e., spatial prediction) of, say, an unobserved climate variable such as temperature, at a known location, from observed temperatures at known locations throughout the region of interest $D_s \subset \mathbb{R}^d$. Let $Y(\cdot) \equiv \{Y(\mathbf{s}): \mathbf{s} \in D_s\}$ be the true temperature. The observations are "noisy" versions of the true temperatures at known locations $\{\mathbf{s}_1, \ldots, \mathbf{s}_m\}$; assuming additive measurement error, write the observations as,

$$Z(\mathbf{s}_i) = Y(\mathbf{s}_i) + \varepsilon(\mathbf{s}_i), \qquad i = 1, \ldots, m,$$

where, independently of $Y(\cdot)$, $\varepsilon(\cdot) \equiv \{\varepsilon(\mathbf{s}): \mathbf{s} \in D_s\}$ is a white-noise process with mean zero and variance $\sigma_\varepsilon^2 \geq 0$. Figure 4.1 shows $D_s \subset \mathbb{R}^2$ and data location(s) of temperature changes from the 1980s to the 1990s, produced by a model developed by the National Center for Atmospheric Research (NCAR); the temperature-change data are considered in Section 4.1.1.

From Section 2.2.1, an optimal spatial predictor of $Y(\mathbf{s}_0)$ at known location $\mathbf{s}_0$, based on squared error loss and data,

$$\mathbf{Z} \equiv (Z(\mathbf{s}_1), \ldots, Z(\mathbf{s}_m))',$$

is

$$E(Y(\mathbf{s}_0)|\mathbf{Z}).$$

Different loss functions imply different optimal summaries of the posterior distribution. For example, to make inference on exceedances and exceedance regions of $Y(\cdot)$, Zhang, Craigmile, and Cressie (2008) use a *weighted ranks* squared error loss function [adapted from Wright, Stern, and Cressie (2003)] and Baddeley's distance between binary images.

Notice that $E(Y(\mathbf{s}_0)|\mathbf{Z})$ is different from the quantity $E(Z(\mathbf{s}_0)|\mathbf{Z})$, which is the optimal predictor of the noisy (scientifically less relevant quantity) $Z(\mathbf{s}_0)$. There *are* instances where one might be interested in predicting the data process, $Z(\cdot)$, from observations (see Section 2.2.2). In cross-validation,

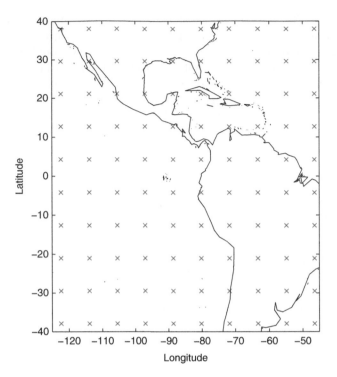

Figure 4.1 Data locations of temperature change for the Americas; "×" represents a sampled grid cell whose resolution is $2.8° \times 2.8°$. The whole map is made up of 28×28 grid cells and the 10×10 sampled grid cells are shown.

$Z(\mathbf{s}_i)$ is deleted, so that logically it should be compared to the optimal spatial predictor of $Z(\mathbf{s}_i)$ (not $Y(\mathbf{s}_i)$), given

$$\mathbf{Z}^{(-i)} \equiv (Z(\mathbf{s}_1), \ldots, Z(\mathbf{s}_{i-1}), Z(\mathbf{s}_{i+1}), \ldots, Z(\mathbf{s}_m))' .$$

That is, $E(Z(\mathbf{s}_i)|\mathbf{Z}^{(-i)})$ is computed and compared to $Z(\mathbf{s}_i)$; $i = 1, \ldots, m$. In a similar vein, suppose we generate a sample from the posterior distribution, $Y(\cdot)|\mathbf{Z}$, and then use the resulting $\mathbf{Y} \equiv (Y(\mathbf{s}_1), \ldots, Y(\mathbf{s}_n))'$ to generate a sample, $\mathbf{Z}_{rep}$, from the conditional distribution of $\mathbf{Z}|\mathbf{Y}$ (see Section 2.2.2). If this is repeated many times, one obtains a sample $\mathbf{Z}_{rep}^{(1)}, \mathbf{Z}_{rep}^{(2)}, \ldots$ from the *posterior predictive distribution*, $[\mathbf{Z}_{rep}|\mathbf{Z}]$ (e.g., Gelman et al., 2003, Chapter 6), which, like cross-validation, can be used to check the fit of the HM.

A Spatial Hierarchical Model to Explain the Nugget Effect

For simplicity, we assume here that $Y(\cdot)$ and $\varepsilon(\cdot)$ in $Z(\cdot) = Y(\cdot) + \varepsilon(\cdot)$, are independent Gaussian processes, and hence only the first two moments are needed to characterize completely the probability distributions. A further assumption of second-order stationarity (see Section 4.1.6) allows us to define

$$C_Y(\mathbf{h}) \equiv \operatorname{cov}(Y(\mathbf{s}), Y(\mathbf{s} + \mathbf{h})), \qquad \text{for all } \mathbf{s}, \mathbf{s} + \mathbf{h} \in D_s .$$

Define $\sigma_Y^2 \equiv C_Y(\mathbf{0})$, and

$$\lim_{\mathbf{h} \to \mathbf{0}} (C_Y(\mathbf{0}) - C_Y(\mathbf{h})) \equiv C_Y(\mathbf{0}+) \equiv \sigma_0^2 \geq 0,$$

where $\sigma_0^2 \leq \sigma_Y^2$. Then σ_0^2 represents the variance of the microscale component of the process $Y(\cdot)$. Recall that $\operatorname{var}(\varepsilon(\mathbf{s})) = \sigma_\varepsilon^2$. Hence,

$$\operatorname{cov}(Z(\mathbf{s}), Z(\mathbf{s} + \mathbf{h})) \equiv C_Z(\mathbf{h}) = \begin{cases} \sigma_Y^2 + \sigma_\varepsilon^2, & \mathbf{h} = \mathbf{0}, \\ C_Y(\mathbf{h}), & \mathbf{h} \neq \mathbf{0}, \end{cases}$$

which implies that

$$\lim_{\mathbf{h} \to \mathbf{0}} (C_Z(\mathbf{0}) - C_Z(\mathbf{h})) \equiv C_Z(\mathbf{0}+) - \sigma_0^2 + \sigma_\varepsilon^2 \equiv c_0 \geq 0.$$

It is this quantity, c_0, that has been called the *nugget effect* in the geostatistics literature (e.g., Journel and Huijbregts, 1978, p. 151), but we see that it is made up of *two* nonnegative components, σ_0^2 (the microscale variance of $Y(\cdot)$) and σ_ε^2 (the measurement-error variance of $Z(\cdot)$).

Optimal spatial prediction should filter out the measurement-error variability $\varepsilon(\cdot)$ and predict $Y(\mathbf{s}_0)$, just as algorithms such as the Kalman filter (Kalman, 1960) smooth, filter, or forecast past, present, or future signals, respectively, in the time domain (Section 8.2). However, much of the geostatistics literature has formulated spatial prediction (kriging) inappropriately in terms of predicting $Z(\mathbf{s}_0)$, not $Y(\mathbf{s}_0)$. This makes scientific sense if in fact $\sigma_\varepsilon^2 = 0$ and hence $Z(\cdot) \equiv Y(\cdot)$.

It is implicit in a lot of the geostatistics literature, that measurements are made perfectly, without error, and hence the nugget effect c_0 is made up of only microscale variance: $c_0 = \sigma_0^2$. Even the etiology of the term "nugget effect"—variability due to small discrete nuggets (of gold) surrounded by dross—only refers to the microscale variability. To sum up, the correct way to formulate kriging is that of optimal (linear) spatial prediction of $Y(\mathbf{s}_0)$ based on noisy data $Z(\mathbf{s}_1), \ldots, Z(\mathbf{s}_m)$ (Section 4.1.2).

The simple geostatistical model on $D_s \subset \mathbb{R}^d$ that we have just described, can be written hierarchically as follows.

Data model: Conditional on σ_ε^2, and for $i = 1, \ldots, m$,

$$Z(\mathbf{s}_i) | Y(\mathbf{s}_i), \sigma_\varepsilon^2 \sim \mathit{ind}.\, Gau(Y(\mathbf{s}_i), \sigma_\varepsilon^2).$$

Process model: Conditional on μ and C_Y, $Y(\cdot)$ is a stationary Gaussian process with mean μ and covariance function $C_Y(\mathbf{h})$; $\mathbf{h} \in \mathbb{R}^d$.

For optimal spatial prediction, Geostatistics has traditionally taken an EHM approach, estimating unknown parameters of the HM (e.g., σ_ε^2, μ, C_Y) from the empirical variogram (Section 4.1.1). In contrast, contributions by Diggle, Tawn, and Moyeed (1998), Banerjee, Carlin, and Gelfand (2004), Le and Zidek (2006), and Diggle and Ribeiro (2007), among others, give a BHM approach to these geostatistical prediction problems.

In this chapter, we present the spatial models that we think are the most important and most relevant to the spatio-temporal models presented and discussed in Chapters 6 and 7. Other topics of special interest to us are included, and broad coverage of recent developments in spatial statistics is given in the Bibliographic Notes in Section 4.5. Our presentation is divided into several sections, presenting spatial process models based on geostatistical processes (Section 4.1), lattice processes (Section 4.2), spatial point processes (Section 4.3), and random-set processes (Section 4.4). General references to each are found in the Bibliographic Notes in Section 4.5.

4.1 GEOSTATISTICAL PROCESSES

The prefix *geo* in geostatistics originally implied Statistics pertaining to the Earth (see Matheron, 1962, 1963). However, more recently, Geostatistics has been used in a variety of disciplines from Agriculture to Zoology. [Within Meteorology, a virtually identical theory called *objective analysis* was developed by Gandin (1963).] It is known for its applicability under rather mild assumptions about the mean and covariance function of the phenomenon of interest. Less well known is its ability to incorporate the known action of scientific processes (e.g., a transport model for aerosol on continental scales might be used to define the mean function, with residual uncertainty represented by random spatial variability).

Geostatistical processes are spatial random processes defined on $D_s \subset \mathbb{R}^d$ whose parameters are defined directly through first and second moments (means, variances, and covariances). Often, although not always, D_s has positive d-dimensional volume. To see how a geostatistical process can be used as a process model in an HM, consider the following generalization of the simple HM given above.

Data model: Conditional on σ_ε^2, and for $i = 1, \ldots, m$,

$$Z(\mathbf{s}_i)|Y(\mathbf{s}_i), \sigma_\varepsilon^2 \sim ind. Gau(Y(\mathbf{s}_i), \sigma_\varepsilon^2).$$

Process model: Conditional on the p-dimensional vector $\boldsymbol{\beta}$ and C_Y, $Y(\cdot)$ is a Gaussian process with the following properties: For $\mathbf{s} \in D_s$, $\mathbf{h} \in \mathbb{R}^d$,

$$\begin{pmatrix} Y(\mathbf{s}) \\ Y(\mathbf{s}+\mathbf{h}) \end{pmatrix} \Bigg| \ \boldsymbol{\beta}, C_Y(\cdot)$$

$$\sim Gau\left(\begin{pmatrix} \mathbf{x}(\mathbf{s})' \\ \mathbf{x}(\mathbf{s}+\mathbf{h})' \end{pmatrix} \boldsymbol{\beta}, \boldsymbol{\Sigma}_2(\mathbf{h}) \right),$$

where $\mathbf{x}(\cdot)$ is a p-dimensional vector of covariates that is potentially available at every location in D_s, $\boldsymbol{\Sigma}_2(\mathbf{h})$ is a 2×2 covariance matrix whose two diagonal elements are both σ_Y^2 and whose off-diagonal element is $C_Y(\mathbf{h})$; and C_Y is a positive-definite function on $\mathbb{R}^d$ with $C_Y(\mathbf{0}) = \sigma_Y^2 < \infty$.

An equivalent way to write this process model is

$$Y(\mathbf{s}) = \mathbf{x}(\mathbf{s})'\boldsymbol{\beta} + \delta(\mathbf{s}), \qquad \mathbf{s} \in D_s, \tag{4.1}$$

where $\delta(\cdot)$ is a mean-zero Gaussian process with stationary covariance function C_Y. Then, for the observation locations, $\{\mathbf{s}_1, \ldots, \mathbf{s}_m\}$, we can write $\mathbf{Y} \equiv (Y(\mathbf{s}_1), \ldots, Y(\mathbf{s}_m))'$ according to the linear mixed model:

$$\mathbf{Y} = \mathbf{X}\boldsymbol{\beta} + \boldsymbol{\delta}, \tag{4.2}$$

where $\boldsymbol{\beta}$ is a p-dimensional *fixed* effect, $\mathbf{X} \equiv (x_j(\mathbf{s}_i))$ is a known $m \times p$ matrix ($p < m$) of covariates, $\boldsymbol{\delta}$ is a (spatial) *random* effect, and var($\boldsymbol{\delta}$) $\equiv (C_Y(\mathbf{s}_i - \mathbf{s}_j))$ is an $m \times m$ positive-definite matrix. Furthermore, the data model can be written as (conditional on $\{Y(\mathbf{s}_i)\}$):

$$Z(\mathbf{s}_i) = Y(\mathbf{s}_i) + \varepsilon(\mathbf{s}_i), \qquad i = 1, \ldots, m, \tag{4.3}$$

where $\{\varepsilon(\mathbf{s}_i)\}$ are iid $Gau(0, \sigma_\varepsilon^2)$ and independent from $Y(\cdot)$.

The geostatistical model that is equivalent to the HM given just above is obtained from interpreting (4.3) unconditionally, where $Y(\cdot)$ is defined by (4.1). Consequently,

$$\mathrm{var}(Z(\mathbf{s})) \equiv \sigma_Z^2 = \sigma_Y^2 + \sigma_\varepsilon^2, \qquad \mathbf{s} \in D_s,$$

which is referred to as the *sill* in the geostatistics literature. We have already seen in the introduction to this chapter that the *nugget effect* is,

$$c_0 = \sigma_0^2 + \sigma_\epsilon^2,$$

where $\sigma_0^2 \equiv C_Y(\mathbf{0}+)$.

Geostatistics is mostly concerned with building models of spatial dependence and with predicting (some functional of) the spatial process optimally. The emphasis in this section will be on the spatial-dependence models (based on the variogram or the covariance function) and on a spatial-prediction method known as *kriging*, viewed in the context of hierarchical modeling.

4.1.1 The Variogram and the Covariance Function

First, we present a model-based measure of the spatial statistical dependence in a geostatistical process, called the *variogram*. In Chapter 3, we saw that time series analysts have traditionally expressed temporal dependence through the *covariance function* and the mathematically equivalent power spectrum, and in Yaglom (1962, 1987) analogous measures of spatial dependence are developed. In fact, the class of processes with a stationary variogram contains the class of processes with a stationary covariance function, and optimal linear prediction can be carried out on a wider class of processes than the second-order stationary class traditionally used in Statistics (Matheron, 1963; Cressie, 1993, Section 2.3.2). It should be noted that early papers by Kolmogorov (1941) and Jowett (1952) defined and used the variogram in one dimension. (Kolmogorov called it the *structure function* and Jowett called it the *mean-squared difference*.)

Stationary Variogram

Let $\{Y(\mathbf{s}): \mathbf{s} \in D_s \subset \mathbb{R}^d\}$ be a real-valued spatial process defined on a domain D_s of the d-dimensional Euclidean space $\mathbb{R}^d$, and suppose that differences of variables displaced $\mathbf{h}$-apart vary in a way that depends only on $\mathbf{h}$. Specifically, suppose that

$$\text{var}(Y(\mathbf{s}+\mathbf{h}) - Y(\mathbf{s})) = 2\gamma_Y(\mathbf{h}), \qquad \text{for all } \mathbf{s}, \mathbf{s}+\mathbf{h} \in D_s. \tag{4.4}$$

The quantity $2\gamma_Y(\cdot)$, which is a function only of the *difference* between the spatial locations $\mathbf{s}$ and $(\mathbf{s}+\mathbf{h})$, is called the stationary *variogram*. The variogram must satisfy the conditional-nonpositive-definiteness condition,

$$\sum_{i=1}^{k} \sum_{j=1}^{k} \alpha_i \overline{\alpha}_j 2\gamma_Y(\mathbf{s}_i - \mathbf{s}_j) \leq 0, \tag{4.5}$$

for any positive integer k, any set of spatial locations $\{\mathbf{s}_i : i = 1, \ldots, k\}$, and any set of complex numbers $\{\alpha_i : i = 1, \ldots, k\}$ satisfying $\sum_{i=1}^{k} \alpha_i = 0$. (If α is a complex number, then recall that $\overline{\alpha}$ denotes its complex conjugate.) The condition (4.5) is extremely important, because it guarantees that all model-based variances are nonnegative (e.g., Cressie, 1993, Section 2.5.2). Any variogram that satisfies (4.5) is referred to as *valid*.

When $2\gamma_Y(\mathbf{h})$ can be written as a function of $\|\mathbf{h}\|$, for $\mathbf{h} = (h_1, \ldots, h_d)' \in \mathbb{R}^d$, where $\|\mathbf{h}\| \equiv (h_1^2 + \cdots + h_d^2)^{1/2}$, the variogram is said to be *isotropic*; otherwise it is said to be *anisotropic*. When clarity demands it, we write an isotropic semivariogram as, $\gamma_Y(\mathbf{h}) = \gamma_Y^o(\|\mathbf{h}\|)$, where γ_Y^o has domain $\mathbb{R}$. Figure 4.4 shows a commonly used isotropic (semi)variogram exponential model $\gamma_Y^o(\cdot)$. Note the discontinuity at the origin (which is due to the microscale variation, σ_0^2, discussed in the introduction to this chapter).

Variogram models that depend on only a few parameters, $\boldsymbol{\theta}$, can be used as succinct summaries of the spatial dependence. Variograms are an important component of optimal spatial linear prediction (kriging), as we shall see later in Section 4.1.2. For example, the *Matérn semivariogram* is

$$\gamma_Y(\mathbf{h}; \boldsymbol{\theta}) = C_Y(\mathbf{0}; \boldsymbol{\theta}) - C_Y(\mathbf{h}; \boldsymbol{\theta}); \qquad \mathbf{h} \in \mathbb{R}^d,$$

where

$$C_Y(\mathbf{h}; \boldsymbol{\theta}) = \sigma_0^2 I(\|\mathbf{h}\| = 0) + \sigma_1^2 \{2^{\theta_2-1}\Gamma(\theta_2)\}^{-1} \{\|\mathbf{h}\|/\theta_1\}^{\theta_2} K_{\theta_2}(\|\mathbf{h}\|/\theta_1) \tag{4.6}$$

is the Matérn covariance function (Stein, 1999, p. 31)). In (4.6), $C_Y(\mathbf{0}; \boldsymbol{\theta}) = \sigma_0^2 + \sigma_1^2$, K_{θ_2} is a modified Bessel function of the second

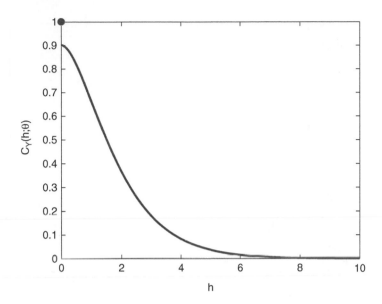

Figure 4.2 Matérn covariance function with scale parameter $\theta_1 = 1$ and smoothness parameter $\theta_2 = 1.5$; the nugget effect is 10% of the total variance.

kind of order θ_2 (e.g., Abramowitz and Stegun, 1964, pp. 374–379), and $\boldsymbol{\theta} \in \{(\theta_1, \theta_2, \sigma_0^2, \sigma_1^2)': \theta_1 > 0, \theta_2 > 0, \sigma_0^2 \geq 0, \sigma_1^2 \geq 0\}$. Figure 4.2 shows a plot of (4.6) versus $\|\mathbf{h}\|$, for the particular case of $\boldsymbol{\theta} = (1, 1.5, 0.1, 0.9)'$. Its corresponding semivariogram is

$$\gamma_Y(\mathbf{h}) = (0.1)I(\|\mathbf{h}\| \neq 0) + (0.9) - (0.9)e^{-\|\mathbf{h}\|}(1 + \|\mathbf{h}\|), \qquad \mathbf{h} \in \mathbb{R}^d .$$

Another common isotropic semivariogram used is the *powered-exponential*,

$$\gamma_Y(\mathbf{h}; \boldsymbol{\theta}) = C_Y(\mathbf{0}; \boldsymbol{\theta}) - C_Y(\mathbf{h}; \boldsymbol{\theta}) ,$$

where

$$C_Y(\mathbf{h}; \boldsymbol{\theta}) = \sigma_0^2 I(\|\mathbf{h}\| = 0) + \sigma_1^2 \exp\{-(\|\mathbf{h}\|/\theta_1)^{\theta_2}\}, \qquad \mathbf{h} \in \mathbb{R}^d , \qquad (4.7)$$

and $\boldsymbol{\theta} \in \{(\theta_1, \theta_2, \sigma_0^2, \sigma_1^2)': \theta_1 > 0, 0 < \theta_2 \leq 2, \sigma_0^2 \geq 0, \sigma_1^2 \geq 0\}$. The powered-exponential covariance function (4.7) is discussed, for example, in Diggle and Ribeiro (2007, Section 3.4.2). The most familiar member of the class is the exponential covariance function, obtained when $\theta_2 = 1$:

$$C_Y(\mathbf{h}; \boldsymbol{\theta}) = \sigma_0^2 I(\|\mathbf{h}\| = 0) + \sigma_1^2 \exp\{-\|\mathbf{h}\|/\theta_1\}, \qquad \mathbf{h} \in \mathbb{R}^d . \qquad (4.8)$$

Figure 4.3 shows the particular case of (4.7) with $\boldsymbol{\theta} = (1, 1, 0.1, 0.9)'$; that is, it is a plot of the exponential covariance function, $(0.1)I(\|\mathbf{h}\| = 0) +$

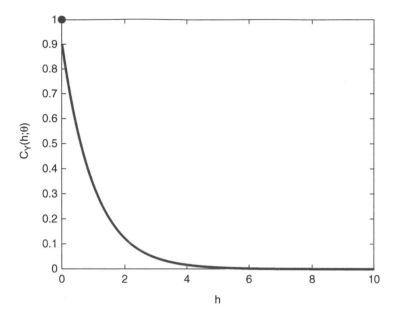

Figure 4.3 Powered exponential covariance function with scale parameter $\theta_1 = 1$ and power parameter $\theta_2 = 1$; the nugget effect is 10% of the total variance.

$(0.9)e^{-\|\mathbf{h}\|}$, versus $\|\mathbf{h}\|$. Further details on the powered-exponential class given by (4.7) can be found in Yaglom (1987, Vol. II, pp. 48–49). Figure 4.4 shows a plot of the corresponding *exponential semivariogram* given by

$$\gamma_Y(\mathbf{h}) = (0.1)I(\|\mathbf{h}\| \neq 0) + (0.9) - (0.9)e^{-\|\mathbf{h}\|}, \qquad \mathbf{h} \in \mathbb{R}^d,$$

versus $\|\mathbf{h}\|$. Other models, such as the spherical, the rational-quadratic, the wave, the linear, and the power semivariograms, are discussed, for example, in Cressie (1993, pp. 61–63).

When the variogram is anisotropic, it is no longer a function purely of distance between the two spatial locations. Anisotropies are caused by the underlying physical process evolving differentially in space. That is, different (temporal) dynamics in different directions can cause the process to be anisotropic in space. Sometimes the anisotropy can be corrected by an invertible linear transformation of the lag vector $\mathbf{h}$. If $2\gamma_Y(\cdot)$ can be written as

$$2\gamma_Y(\mathbf{h}) = 2\gamma_Y^\circ(\|\mathbf{A}\mathbf{h}\|), \qquad \mathbf{h} \in \mathbb{R}^d, \tag{4.9}$$

where $\mathbf{A}$ is an invertible $d \times d$ matrix and γ_Y° has domain $\mathbb{R}$, it is said to be *geometrically anisotropic*.

In the paragraphs that follow, it will be seen that stationary variogram models are more general than stationary covariance-function models.

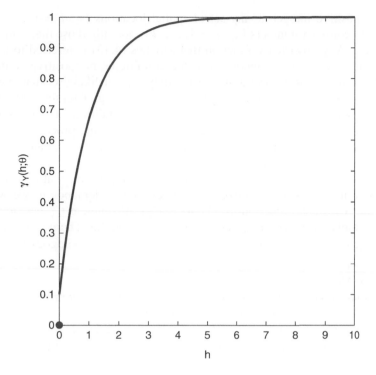

Figure 4.4 Exponential semivariogram with scale parameter $\theta_1 = 1$; the nugget effect is 10% of the total variance (sill).

Stationary Covariance Function

Replace (4.4) with the (stronger) assumption,

$$\text{cov}(Y(\mathbf{s} + \mathbf{h}), Y(\mathbf{s})) = C_Y(\mathbf{h}), \qquad \text{for all } \mathbf{s}, \mathbf{s} + \mathbf{h} \in D_s, \qquad (4.10)$$

and specify the mean function to be constant; that is,

$$E(Y(\mathbf{s})) = \mu, \qquad \text{for all } \mathbf{s} \in D_s. \qquad (4.11)$$

Then, restrictions (4.10) and (4.11) define the class of *second-order* (or weakly) *stationary* processes in D_s, with stationary *covariance function* $C_Y(\cdot)$. Time series analysts often assume the temporal analogue of (4.10) and work with the correlation function,

$$\rho_Y(\cdot) \equiv C_Y(\cdot)/C_Y(\mathbf{0}). \qquad (4.12)$$

The quantity $C_Y(\cdot)$ is called the (stationary) covariance function, which must satisfy the nonnegative-definiteness condition,

$$\sum_{i=1}^{k} \sum_{j=1}^{k} \alpha_i \overline{\alpha}_j C_Y(\mathbf{s}_i - \mathbf{s}_j) \geq 0, \qquad (4.13)$$

for any positive integer k, any set of spatial locations $\{\mathbf{s}_i : i = 1, \ldots, k\}$, and any set of complex numbers $\{\alpha_i : i = 1, \ldots, k\}$ (not only those that sum to zero; see (4.5)). Any covariance function that satisfies (4.13) is referred to as *valid*. The condition (4.13) is analogous to the conditional-nonpositive-definiteness condition (4.5) that a variogram must satisfy, and it likewise guarantees that model-based prediction variances are nonnegative (e.g., Cressie, 1993, Section 2.5.1). Notice that the nonnegative-definiteness condition (4.13) has to hold for *all* complex numbers $\{\alpha_i\}$. Hence, there will be some processes with valid stationary variograms that do not have valid stationary covariance functions (e.g., Cressie, 1993, p. 68).

When $C_Y(\mathbf{h})$ can be written as a function of $\|\mathbf{h}\|$, we say that it is *isotropic*; otherwise it is said to be *anisotropic*. When clarity demands it, we write an isotropic covariance function as, $C_Y(\mathbf{h}) = C_Y^o(\|\mathbf{h}\|)$, where C_Y^o has domain $\mathbb{R}$. Two examples of $C_Y^o(\cdot)$ are given in Figures 4.2 and 4.3. There is also a notion of geometric anisotropy, $C_Y(\mathbf{h}) = C_Y^o(\|\mathbf{A}\mathbf{h}\|)$; $\mathbf{h} \in \mathbb{R}^d$, analogous to (4.9).

Intrinsic Stationarity

Conditions (4.4) and (4.11) define the class of *intrinsically stationary* processes, which we now show contains the class of second-order stationary processes. Assuming only the existence of the stationary covariance function given by (4.10), the *semivariogram* (i.e., one half the variogram) of $Y(\cdot)$ exists and is given by

$$\gamma_Y(\mathbf{h}) = C_Y(\mathbf{0}) - C_Y(\mathbf{h}), \quad \mathbf{h} \in \mathbb{R}^d. \tag{4.14}$$

As an example, see Figure 4.3, which shows an exponential covariance function, and Figure 4.4, which shows the corresponding exponential semivariogram. Equation (4.14) is easy to prove and establishes that a second-order stationary process is always intrinsically stationary. To see that the converse is *not* true, consider a one-dimensional standard Wiener process $\{W(s): s \geq 0\}$. Here, $2\gamma_W(h) = -|h|$ (where $-\infty < h < \infty$), but $\mathrm{cov}(W(s), W(u)) = \min(s, u)$, which is *not* a function of $|s - u|$; an analogous result is true in $\mathbb{R}^d$ (e.g., Cressie, 1993, p. 62). Thus, since the constant-mean assumption (4.11) is common to both, the class of second-order stationary processes is *strictly* contained in the class of intrinsically stationary processes. In other words, intrinsic stationarity holds (and hence the stationary variogram exists) for a larger class of processes.

Spectral Representation

Both the variogram and the covariance function have a representation in terms of a (power) spectral density, under appropriate regularity conditions. We present the result here for the more familiar case of the covariance function; the result for the variogram can be found in, for example, Cressie (1993, Section 2.5).

Theorem 4.1 (Bochner, 1955). If $\int_{-\infty}^{\infty} \cdots \int_{-\infty}^{\infty} |C_Y(\mathbf{h})| d\mathbf{h} < \infty$, then a valid, real-valued covariance function can be written as

$$C_Y(\mathbf{h}) = \int_{-\infty}^{\infty} \cdots \int_{-\infty}^{\infty} \cos(\boldsymbol{\omega}'\mathbf{h}) f_Y(\boldsymbol{\omega}) d\boldsymbol{\omega}, \qquad (4.15)$$

where $f_Y(\boldsymbol{\omega}) \geq 0$ is symmetric about $\boldsymbol{\omega} = \mathbf{0}$.

The quantity $f_Y(\cdot)$ is called the *spectral density* of $C_Y(\cdot)$, and it partitions the total variation through $\sigma_Y^2 = C_Y(\mathbf{0}) = \int_{\mathbb{R}^d} f(\boldsymbol{\omega}) d\boldsymbol{\omega}$. It is the nonnegativity of the spectral density that guarantees nonnegative-definiteness of the covariance function, and vice versa. Consequently, substituting any absolutely integrable, nonnegative, symmetric function $f(\cdot)$ into (4.15) generates a valid, real-valued covariance function; further details on these constructions can be found in Cressie (1993, pp. 84–86). Sometimes the spectral density has a more succinct representation than the covariance function; such is the case with the Matérn covariance function (Stein, 1991; Fuentes, Chen, and Davis, 2008).

As we noticed above, the nonnegative-definiteness condition (4.13) for $C_Y(\cdot)$ is stronger than the *conditional* nonpositive-definiteness condition (4.5) for $\gamma_Y(\cdot)$. However, not surprisingly, $\gamma_Y(\cdot)$ has a spectral representation analogous to Theorem 4.1 (e.g., Cressie, 1993, p. 87).

The Variogram (Covariance Function) is a Parameter

There has been some confusion in the geostatistics literature whether the variogram is something computed from spatial data $\mathbf{Z} = (Z(\mathbf{s}_1), \ldots, Z(\mathbf{s}_m))'$, or whether it is a theoretical function. We would like to think of the variogram as a (infinite-dimensional) parameter in the space of all conditionally negative-definite functions, and then we refer to the *empirical variogram* as the quantity computed from the data:

$$2\widehat{\gamma}_Z^o(h) \equiv \text{ave}\{(Z(\mathbf{s}_i) - Z(\mathbf{s}_j))^2 : \|\mathbf{s}_i - \mathbf{s}_j\| \in T(h) ; i, j = 1, \ldots, m\}, \quad (4.16)$$

where $T(h)$ is a tolerance region around h (such as $h \pm \Delta$, Δ small). The *empirical semivariogram* is $\widehat{\gamma}_Z^o(\cdot)$. For (4.16) to be an *appropriate estimator* of the parameter $2\gamma_Y(\cdot)$, the isotropy assumption that $2\gamma_Y(\mathbf{h}) \equiv 2\gamma_Y^o(\|\mathbf{h}\|)$ has to be made; the mean of $Z(\cdot)$ and of $Y(\cdot)$ has to be assumed constant; and the measurement-error variance component $2\sigma_\varepsilon^2$ has to be subtracted from (4.16).

Initially, we wish to test the null hypothesis, H_0: $Y(\cdot)$ has *no* spatial dependence. This initial test is important to carry out, to avoid modeling spatial structure that is not actually there. Consider the test statistic

$$F \equiv \widehat{\gamma}_Z^o(h_1)/\widehat{\sigma}_Z^2,$$

where $\widehat{\sigma}_Z^2 \equiv \sum_{i=1}^{m}(Z(\mathbf{s}_i) - \widehat{\mu}_Z)^2/(m-1)$, $\widehat{\mu}_Z \equiv \sum_{i=1}^{m} Z(\mathbf{s}_i)/m$, and h_1 is the smallest lag from all possible lags $h_1, \ldots, h_L$. We reject H_0 for $|F - 1|$ large.

A permutation-based test of H_0 does not make any distributional assumptions about $\mathbf{Z}$; the data locations are permuted and F is recomputed for all possible permutations (or for a computer-generated sample of random permutations). If the observed F is above the 97.5 percentile or below the 2.5 percentile of the permutation distribution, then reject H_0 (at a 5% level of significance). If we make the additional assumption that $Y(\cdot)$ is a Gaussian process and the measurement-error process $\varepsilon(\cdot)$ is Gaussian, then H_0 can be tested based on the percentiles of the ratio of two quadratic forms (cf. Moran's I statistic discussed at the beginning of Section 4.2).

The variogram, $2\gamma_Y(\cdot)$, is generally an unknown quantity, for which statistical inference, based on spatial data $\mathbf{Z} \equiv (Z(\mathbf{s}_1), \ldots, Z(\mathbf{s}_m))'$, is needed. As we discussed above, the process $Z(\cdot)$ is not the same as the process $Y(\cdot)$, but they are related quite simply through (4.3), where the measurement-error variance is defined to be σ_ε^2. It is straightforward to show that

$$2\gamma_Z(\mathbf{h}) = 2\gamma_Y(\mathbf{h}) + 2\sigma_\varepsilon^2 I(\mathbf{h} \neq \mathbf{0}), \quad \mathbf{h} \in \mathbb{R}^d,$$

and

$$C_Z(\mathbf{h}) = C_Y(\mathbf{h}) + \sigma_\varepsilon^2 I(\mathbf{h} = \mathbf{0}), \quad \mathbf{h} \in \mathbb{R}^d.$$

Assuming isotropy, analogous relations are available between $2\gamma_Z^o(\cdot)$, $2\gamma_Y^o(\cdot)$, $C_Z^o(\cdot)$, and $C_Y^o(\cdot)$.

From the point of view of the HM outlined in Section 2.1, the variogram (or the covariance function) could be thought of as a parameter. Thus, its estimation and subsequent use in optimal spatial prediction (kriging) could be viewed as working within the framework of an empirical hierarchical model (EHM). Specifically, the estimate is "plugged" into optimal-spatial-prediction equations (Section 4.1.2). Putter and Young (2001) show that, for Gaussian processes, the effect of this estimation is negligible under continuity conditions for the estimated and true Gaussian probability measures. Variogram-model fitting using several different criteria, including maximum likelihood, REML, and weighted least squares, is considered in Cressie (1993, Section 2.6), for a data model that assumes additive measurement error. Having more general data models (e.g., Diggle, Tawn, and Moyeed, 1998) requires rethinking some of these estimators. The composite-likelihood approach of Vecchia (1988) is one possibility, and EM estimation is another (Zhu, Gu, and Peterson, 2007).

Ecker and Gelfand (1997) consider inference on the variogram in the context of a Bayesian hierarchical model (BHM) and give the posterior (conditional on the data $\mathbf{Z}$) distribution of the variogram parameters. Daniels and Cressie (2001) give inference on a stationary covariance function in an HM setting (in one dimension). Assuming a BHM, inference on model parameters $\boldsymbol{\theta}$ and process $Y(\cdot)$ is based on the posterior distribution $[Y(\cdot), \boldsymbol{\theta}|\mathbf{Z}]$; see Diggle and Ribeiro (2007, Chapter 7) for a discussion of analytical and Monte Carlo methods for obtaining the posterior distribution. Omre and Tjelmeland (1997) and Diggle, Tawn, and Moyeed (1998) show how to carry out this inference, particularly

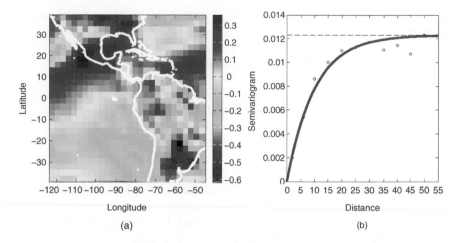

Figure 4.5 (a) Temperature change (1990s minus 1980s) in 28 × 28 grid cells over the Americas. The values were originally produced by an NCAR model, and they represent "the truth." (b) Empirical and fitted (exponential model) semivariogram after the values in (a) were detrended by latitude and longitude. Units on the horizontal axis are the same as those given in (a).

on $Y(\cdot)$, based on MCMC. In a sense, inference in an EHM is simpler, in that once an estimator of θ is obtained, say $\widehat{\theta}(\mathbf{Z})$, inference on $Y(\cdot)$ is based on the posterior distribution $[Y(\cdot)|\mathbf{Z}, \theta]$, with $\widehat{\theta}(\mathbf{Z})$ substituted for θ in that posterior. However, inference in an EHM is often overly liberal in finite samples, since the variability in the estimator $\widehat{\theta}(\mathbf{Z})$ is not accounted for.

Having considered the variogram as a parameter, we now turn to inference on the process $Y(\cdot)$; that is, we turn to spatial prediction. One commonly used Bayes estimator is $E(Y(\cdot)|\mathbf{Z})$ in a BHM, or $E(Y(\cdot)|\mathbf{Z}, \widehat{\theta})$ in an EHM. In the small example that follows, we assume Gaussian distributions for $Y(\cdot)$ and $\epsilon(\cdot)$, and we motivate optimal spatial prediction through a series of figures showing the results of (simple) kriging.

Decadal Temperature Differences over the Americas

The basis of this illustrative example is output from the Climate System Model at the National Center for Atmospheric Research (NCAR) in Boulder, CO. The output is monthly temperature on longitude–latitude grid cells, each of which is roughly 2.8° longitude by 2.8° latitude. We have chosen to concentrate on a region over the Americas made up of 28 × 28 grid cells. Monthly temperatures for the 1980s were averaged for each grid cell and likewise for the 1990s. Consider these two averages in grid cell centered at $\mathbf{s} \in D_s \subset \mathbb{R}^2$, and define $Y(\mathbf{s}) \equiv$ 1990s average − 1980s average. The values of $Y(\cdot)$ are shown in Figure 4.5a.

Although $Y(\cdot)$ was produced by a deterministic model, in this example we think of it as the "truth," and we model it statistically as a random process defined on the 28 × 28 grid centers, D_s. After exploratory spatial data analysis,

Zhang, Craigmile, and Cressie (2008) found the following spatial model to provide a good fit:

$$Y(\mathbf{s}) = \mathbf{x}(\mathbf{s})'\boldsymbol{\beta} + \delta(\mathbf{s}), \qquad \mathbf{s} \in D_s,$$

where for $\mathbf{s} = (s_1, s_2)'$, $\mathbf{x}(\mathbf{s}) = (1, s_1, s_2, s_2^2, s_2^3)'$, and $\boldsymbol{\beta} \equiv (\beta_0, \beta_1, \beta_2, \beta_3, \beta_4)'$ $= (-.1419, -.0020, .0091, -.000087, -.0000051)'$. The component process $\delta(\cdot)$ is second-order stationary with mean zero and exponential covariance function, $C_Y(\mathbf{h}; \boldsymbol{\theta})$, given by (4.8), with parameters $(\theta_1, \sigma_0^2, \sigma_1^2) = (10.0284, 0, 0.0123)$. Its fit to the empirical semivariogram [see (4.16)] of the detrended temperature differences is excellent, as can be seen in Figure 4.5b. Notice that all 28×28 values of $Y(\cdot)$ were used to fit this model; for the purposes of this example, we shall consider the fitted parameter values as *known* and proceed to introduce optimal spatial prediction (here, simple kriging), to motivate the next subsection.

We now "corrupt" $Y(\cdot)$ by subsampling only a 10×10 subset and adding random noise $\varepsilon(\cdot)$ (with known σ_ε^2) to it. By doing this, we can see how well simple kriging recovers the true process $Y(\cdot)$ at all 28×28 locations. Following Zhang, Craigmile, and Cressie (2008), we choose to sample at 10×10 spatially regular locations illustrated by the crosses in Figure 4.1. That is, the spatial dataset we shall consider has $m = 100$, and

$$Z(\mathbf{s}_i) = Y(\mathbf{s}_i) + \varepsilon(\mathbf{s}_i), \qquad i = 1, \ldots, 100,$$

where $\{\mathbf{s}_i : i = 1, \ldots, 100\}$ are the grid cells defined by the crosses in Figure 4.1, and $\varepsilon(\cdot)$ is a white-noise process with mean zero and variance $\sigma_\varepsilon^2 = 0.00615$. Our goal is to make inference on $\{Y(\mathbf{s}): \mathbf{s} \in D_s\}$ based on noisy and incomplete data $\mathbf{Z} \equiv (Z(\mathbf{s}_1), \ldots, Z(\mathbf{s}_{100}))'$. This includes not only predicting $Y(\mathbf{s}_0)$, but also providing a measure of uncertainty associated with that prediction.

Using the theory presented in Section 4.1.2, we use formula (4.28) to produce the optimal spatial predictor,

$$\{Y^*(\mathbf{s}_0): \mathbf{s}_0 \in D_s\},$$

and formula (4.26) to produce the associated measure of uncertainty,

$$\{\sigma_{Y,sk}(\mathbf{s}_0): \mathbf{s}_0 \in D_s\}.$$

The former is called the (simple) *kriging predictor*, and the latter is called the (simple) *kriging standard error*. Figure 4.6 illustrates all this through a sequence of maps: Figure 4.6a shows the smooth, complete $Y(\cdot)$ that we have called the "truth" (it is identical to the map shown in Figure 4.5a). Figure 4.6b shows the noisy, corrupted data $\mathbf{Z}$ from which we intend to recover $Y(\cdot)$.

Figure 4.6c shows the optimal (simple kriging) predictor, which should be compared directly to the map above it in Figure 4.6a. Based on a data fraction of

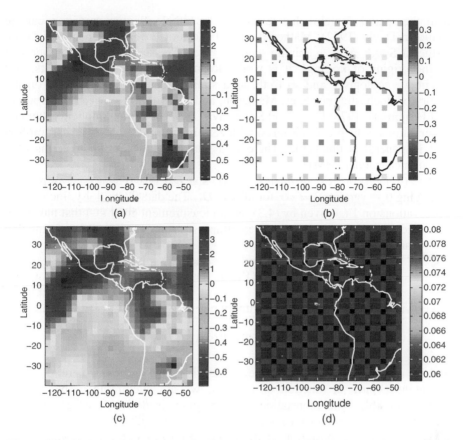

Figure 4.6 (a) Same plot as Figure 4.5a: Temperature change (1990s minus 1980s); the 28×28 values represent "the truth." (b) The 10×10 observations are obtained by subsampling "the truth" and adding mean-zero Gaussian noise. (c) Simple kriging predictor obtained from the missing and noisy data in (b). (d) Kriging standard error corresponding to simple kriging; the pattern is expected due to regular sampling in (b).

only $(10 \times 10)/(28 \times 28) = 13\%$, the reconstruction of $Y(\cdot)$ given by $Y^*(\cdot)$ in Figure 4.6c is visually very good, albeit somewhat "smoother" than the original $Y(\cdot)$ in Figure 4.6a. The map in Figure 4.6d shows how good we expect $Y^*(\cdot)$ to be based on the covariance function C_Y and the 100 data locations $\{s_i\}$. Its patterned appearance is not surprising due to the regular spatial locations of the data, and the uncertainty of $Y^*(s_0)$ increases the further s_0 is from a data location (as expected).

4.1.2 Kriging (Optimal Spatial Prediction)

Kriging is a spatial prediction methodology due to Matheron (1963), with roots in the geodesy work of Gauss carried out early in the nineteenth century. A very early derivation of optimal prediction (in the temporal domain rather than the spatial domain) that results in the simple kriging predictor, can be found in Davis (1952). Matheron coined the term *kriging* in honor of D. G. Krige, a South African mining engineer [see Cressie (1990) for an account of the origins of kriging]. It is well known to geologists, hydrologists, soil scientists, ecologists, and so forth, as a statistical methodology based on the theory of stochastic processes. Matheron, and many that followed (e.g., Journel and Huijbregts, 1978; Isaaks and Srivastava, 1989), assumed implicitly that any observation on the process is taken with zero measurement error, an assumption that in general is untenable. There is a way to view kriging in terms of a hierarchical model (HM).

The (hidden) process of interest $\{Y(s): s \in D_s\}$ is a spatial random process satisfying $0 < \text{var}(Y(s)) < \infty$, for all $s \in D_s$. The data $\mathbf{Z}$ are noisy, incomplete observations on $Y(\cdot)$ given by (4.3), with measurement error $\varepsilon(\cdot)$ that has mean zero and variance $\sigma_\varepsilon^2 \in [0, \infty)$. It is simplest to assume for the moment that the mean function,

$$\mu_Y(s) \equiv E(Y(s)), \qquad s \in D_s, \tag{4.17}$$

is known and that the covariance function,

$$C_Y(\mathbf{u}, \mathbf{v}) \equiv \text{cov}(Y(\mathbf{u}), Y(\mathbf{v})), \qquad \mathbf{u}, s \in D_s, \tag{4.18}$$

and the measurement-error variance, σ_ε^2, are known. Notice that here, $C_Y(\mathbf{u}, \mathbf{v})$ is not necessarily a function of $(\mathbf{u} - \mathbf{v})$; we are attempting to be as general as possible. The (nonstationary) variogram is derivable as $2\gamma_Y(\mathbf{u}, \mathbf{v}) \equiv \text{var}(Y(\mathbf{u}) - Y(\mathbf{v})) = C_Y(\mathbf{u}, \mathbf{u}) + C_Y(\mathbf{v}, \mathbf{v}) - 2C_Y(\mathbf{u}, \mathbf{v})$.

We require the posterior distribution, $[Y(\cdot)|\mathbf{Z}, \mu_Y, C_Y, \sigma_\varepsilon^2]$, where $\mathbf{Z} \equiv (Z(s_1), \ldots, Z(s_m))'$, to make inference on $Y(\cdot)$. This is obtained in an HM setting from (*i*) a data model, $[\mathbf{Z}|Y(\cdot), \sigma_\varepsilon^2]$, and (*ii*) a process model, $[Y(\cdot)|\mu_Y, C_Y]$. However, in its original formulation, geostatistics eschewed distributional assumptions. Diggle, Tawn, and Moyeed (1998) coined the term *model-based geostatistics* to describe a BHM formulation of kriging with the distributional assumptions needed to derive the posterior distribution. In the rest of this section, we present the original formulation of kriging *first* and *then* compare it to an EHM and a BHM formulation of the same.

Simple Kriging

The methodology known as *simple kriging* looks in the class of all heterogeneously linear predictors, $\{\boldsymbol{\ell}'\mathbf{Z} + k: \boldsymbol{\ell} \in \mathbb{R}^m, k \in \mathbb{R}\}$, to obtain an optimal spatial predictor of $Y(s_0)$; $s_0 \in D_s$. Recall from Section 2.2 that $E(Y(s_0)|\mathbf{Z})$ is optimal in terms of minimizing the mean squared prediction error. Likewise, the simple kriging predictor is the heterogeneously linear combination of the data that minimizes the mean squared prediction error,

$$\text{MSPE}(\boldsymbol{\ell}, k) \equiv E(Y(s_0) - \boldsymbol{\ell}'\mathbf{Z} - k)^2, \tag{4.19}$$

with respect to $\boldsymbol{\ell}$ and k. It is generally *not* appropriate to minimize $E(Z(\mathbf{s}_0) - \boldsymbol{\ell}'\mathbf{Z} - k)^2$, as one often sees in the geostatistics literature; from an HM point of view, this ignores the data model and implicitly assumes that $\sigma_\varepsilon^2 = 0$. One could look upon the derivations we give below as "kriging done right," under the general assumption that $\sigma_\varepsilon^2 \geq 0$.

Write

$$\mathrm{MSPE}(\boldsymbol{\ell}, k) = \mathrm{var}(Y(\mathbf{s}_0) - \boldsymbol{\ell}'\mathbf{Z} - k) + \{E(Y(\mathbf{s}_0) - \boldsymbol{\ell}'\mathbf{Z} - k)\}^2.$$

The second term is $\{\mu_Y(\mathbf{s}_0) - \boldsymbol{\ell}'\boldsymbol{\mu}_Y - k\}^2$, where $\boldsymbol{\mu}_Y \equiv (\mu_Y(\mathbf{s}_1), \ldots, \mu_Y(\mathbf{s}_m))'$, which is minimized (in fact, is equal to 0) if k satisfies

$$k = \mu_Y(\mathbf{s}_0) - \boldsymbol{\ell}'\boldsymbol{\mu}_Y. \tag{4.20}$$

Now, since k is not random, the first term is

$$C_Y(\mathbf{s}_0, \mathbf{s}_0) - 2\boldsymbol{\ell}'\mathrm{cov}(Y(\mathbf{s}_0), \mathbf{Z})' + \boldsymbol{\ell}'\mathbf{C}_Z\boldsymbol{\ell}, \tag{4.21}$$

where the $m \times m$ covariance matrix is given by $\mathbf{C}_Z \equiv (C_Z(\mathbf{s}_i, \mathbf{s}_j))$;

$$C_Z(\mathbf{u}, \mathbf{v}) \equiv \begin{cases} C_Y(\mathbf{v}, \mathbf{v}) + \sigma_\varepsilon^2, & \mathbf{u} = \mathbf{v}, \\ C_Y(\mathbf{u}, \mathbf{v}), & \mathbf{u} \neq \mathbf{v}; \end{cases} \tag{4.22}$$

and

$$\mathrm{cov}(Y(\mathbf{s}_0), \mathbf{Z}) = (C_Y(\mathbf{s}_0, \mathbf{s}_1), \ldots, C_Y(\mathbf{s}_0, \mathbf{s}_m))$$

$$\equiv \mathbf{c}_Y(\mathbf{s}_0)'. \tag{4.23}$$

Unless $\sigma_\varepsilon^2 = 0$, there is a non-zero difference between $\mathbf{c}_Y(\mathbf{s}_0)$ in (4.23) and $\mathbf{c}_Z(\mathbf{s}_0)' \equiv \mathrm{cov}(Z(\mathbf{s}_0), \mathbf{Z}) = (C_Z(\mathbf{s}_0, \mathbf{s}_1), \ldots, C_Z(\mathbf{s}_0, \mathbf{s}_m))$, the latter quantity being the one used incorrectly in some classical geostatistics kriging equations.

Upon differentiating (4.21) with respect to $\boldsymbol{\ell}$ and setting the result equal to $\mathbf{0}$, we obtain

$$-2\mathbf{c}_Y(\mathbf{s}_0) + 2\mathbf{C}_Z\boldsymbol{\ell} = \mathbf{0}; \tag{4.24}$$

that is, the optimal coefficients are given by $\boldsymbol{\ell}^* \equiv \mathbf{C}_Z^{-1}\mathbf{c}_Y(\mathbf{s}_0)$, and hence the optimal constant term is, $k^* \equiv \mu_Y(\mathbf{s}_0) - \mathbf{c}_Y(\mathbf{s}_0)'\mathbf{C}_Z^{-1}\boldsymbol{\mu}_Y$. Finally then, the simple-kriging predictor is

$$Y^*(\mathbf{s}_0) \equiv \mu_Y(\mathbf{s}_0) + \mathbf{c}_Y(\mathbf{s}_0)'\mathbf{C}_Z^{-1}(\mathbf{Z} - \boldsymbol{\mu}_Y), \tag{4.25}$$

where $\mathbf{c}_Y(\mathbf{s}_0)'$ is given by (4.23). Furthermore, upon substituting (4.20) and (4.24) into (4.19), the minimized mean squared prediction error, often called the (simple) kriging variance, is

$$\sigma_{Y,sk}^2(\mathbf{s}_0) \equiv \mathrm{MSPE}(\boldsymbol{\ell}^*, k^*) = C_Y(\mathbf{s}_0, \mathbf{s}_0) - \mathbf{c}_Y(\mathbf{s}_0)'\mathbf{C}_Z^{-1}\mathbf{c}_Y(\mathbf{s}_0), \tag{4.26}$$

where the subscript "*sk*" on the left-hand side denotes *simple kriging*. When $\sigma_\varepsilon^2 = 0$, these formulas are the same as those found in, for example, Journel and Huijbregts (1978, p. 562).

As an example, consider the linear model (4.1), where

$$\mu_Y(\mathbf{s}) = \mathbf{x}(\mathbf{s})'\boldsymbol{\beta}, \qquad \mathbf{s} \in D_s, \tag{4.27}$$

for $\mathbf{x}(\mathbf{s}) \equiv (x_1(\mathbf{s}), \ldots, x_p(\mathbf{s}))'$, a p-dimensional vector of known covariates, and for $\boldsymbol{\beta} \equiv (\beta_1, \ldots, \beta_p)'$, a p-dimensional vector of (for the moment, *known*) regression parameters. Traditional choices in geostatistics are, for example in $\mathbb{R}^2$, the spatial covariates $x_1(\mathbf{s}) = 1$, $x_2(\mathbf{s}) = s_1$, $x_3(\mathbf{s}) = s_2$, $x_4(\mathbf{s}) = s_1^2, \ldots$, where $\mathbf{s} \equiv (s_1, s_2)'$. Polynomials, splines, and wavelets are special cases of spatial covariates (sometimes called basis functions). Basis functions model trend terms, but it should be realized that they can be augmented by or replaced with other covariates that attempt to explain directly the underlying physical/chemical/biological/economic/etc. mechanisms of the process $Y(\cdot)$. The principal requirement of a covariate $x_j(\mathbf{s})$ is that it is known at *all* $\mathbf{s} \in D_s$. Substituting (4.27) into (4.25), the simple-kriging predictor is

$$Y^*(\mathbf{s}_0) = \mathbf{x}(\mathbf{s}_0)'\boldsymbol{\beta} + \mathbf{c}_Y(\mathbf{s}_0)'\mathbf{C}_Z^{-1}(\mathbf{Z} - \mathbf{X}\boldsymbol{\beta}), \tag{4.28}$$

where $\mathbf{c}_Y(\mathbf{s}_0)$ is given by (4.23), $\mathbf{C}_Z = \text{var}(\mathbf{Z})$, and recall from (4.2) that $\mathbf{X} \equiv (x_j(\mathbf{s}_i))$ is an $m \times p$ matrix of covariate values at the locations where the data $\mathbf{Z}$ are observed. The simple-kriging variance for the predictor (4.28) is still given by (4.26); it does not involve the covariates, since $\boldsymbol{\beta}$ is assumed (for the moment) known.

A small example is illustrative of the calculations that are involved in (4.25) and (4.26). First, let the known mean $\mu_Y(\mathbf{s}) \equiv 18$; $\mathbf{s} \in D_s$, which is everywhere constant, and let the variance, $\text{var}(Y(\mathbf{s})) = 1$; $\mathbf{s} \in D_s$. Suppose $m = 2$; then $\boldsymbol{\mu}_Y = (18, 18)'$. Regarding the covariances, $C_Y(\mathbf{s}_0, \mathbf{s}_1)$, $C_Y(\mathbf{s}_0, \mathbf{s}_2)$, and $C_Y(\mathbf{s}_1, \mathbf{s}_2)$, we suppose that prediction location $\mathbf{s}_0$ is different from $\mathbf{s}_1$ and $\mathbf{s}_2$, that $\mathbf{s}_1$ is closer to $\mathbf{s}_0$ than is $\mathbf{s}_2$, and that $\sigma_\varepsilon^2 = 0.5$. We assume an exponential covariance function that results in

$$\mathbf{c}_Y(\mathbf{s}_0) = (C_Y(\mathbf{s}_0, \mathbf{s}_1), C_Y(\mathbf{s}_0, \mathbf{s}_2))' \equiv (0.61, 0.22)',$$

$$\mathbf{C}_Z = \begin{bmatrix} C_Y(\mathbf{s}_1, \mathbf{s}_1) & C_Y(\mathbf{s}_2, \mathbf{s}_1) \\ C_Y(\mathbf{s}_1, \mathbf{s}_2) & C_Y(\mathbf{s}_2, \mathbf{s}_2) \end{bmatrix} + \sigma_\varepsilon^2 \mathbf{I}$$

$$\equiv \begin{bmatrix} 1 & 0.37 \\ 0.37 & 1 \end{bmatrix} + 0.5 \begin{bmatrix} 1 & 0 \\ 0 & 1 \end{bmatrix} = \begin{bmatrix} 1.5 & 0.37 \\ 0.37 & 1.5 \end{bmatrix},$$

and

$$Y^*(\mathbf{s}_0) = 18 + (0.61, 0.22) \begin{bmatrix} 1.5 & 0.37 \\ 0.37 & 1.5 \end{bmatrix}^{-1} (\mathbf{Z} - (18, 18)')$$

$$= 18 + 0.3945\{Z(\mathbf{s}_1) - 18\} + 0.0494\{Z(\mathbf{s}_2) - 18\},$$

$$\sigma_{Y,sk}^2(s_0) = 1 - (0.61, 0.22) \begin{bmatrix} 1.5 & 0.37 \\ 0.37 & 1.5 \end{bmatrix}^{-1} (0.61, 0.22)'$$

$$= 0.7485.$$

Notice that $Z(s_1)$ has a larger simple-kriging coefficient ($\ell_1^* = 0.395$) than $Z(s_2)$ ($\ell_2^* = 0.049$) because s_1 is closer to s_0 than is s_2. Notice also that $\sigma_{Y,sk}^2(s_0)$ does not depend on the data $\mathbf{Z}$, and it is less than $\text{var}(Y(s_0)) = 1$.

The Hierarchical Model (HM) and Simple Kriging

We now return to the HM formulation given at the beginning of Section 4.1. Recall that both the data model and the process model assumed Gaussian processes; but, in deriving the kriging equations (4.25) and (4.26), we avoided model assumptions and instead made assumptions about linearity of the predictor. We now provide the connection between the two approaches. The earlier data model is repeated here.

Data model: Conditional on σ_ε^2, and for $i = 1, \ldots, m$,

$$Z(s_i) | Y(s_i), \sigma_\varepsilon^2 \sim ind. \, Gau(Y(s_i), \sigma_\varepsilon^2).$$

Recall that $\mathbf{Z} \equiv (Z(s_1), \ldots, Z(s_m))'$. Now the earlier process model is generalized slightly to allow for nonstationary covariances.

Process model: Conditional on $\boldsymbol{\beta}$ and $C_Y(\cdot, \cdot)$, $Y(\cdot)$ is a Gaussian process with the following properties:

$$E(Y(\cdot)) = \mathbf{x}(\cdot)'\boldsymbol{\beta}, \text{ and we write } \text{cov}(Y(\mathbf{u}), Y(\mathbf{v})) \equiv C_Y(\mathbf{u}, \mathbf{v}).$$

Because all joint and conditional distributions are Gaussian, the optimal spatial predictor $E(Y(s_0)|\mathbf{Z}, \boldsymbol{\beta}, C_Y(\cdot, \cdot), \sigma_\varepsilon^2)$ is (heterogeneously) linear in the data. Consequently, the Gaussian assumptions imply that the simple-kriging predictor (4.28) is exactly the optimal spatial predictor in the class of all measurable functions of $\mathbf{Z}$.

We now demonstrate this equivalence algebraically, because it is illustrative of what can be done with more complicated spatial HMs. Based on the data model and the process model given just above, we seek the posterior distribution of $Y(s_0)$ given $\mathbf{Z}$. It is implicit that any unknown parameters are given too; recall we are assuming that $\boldsymbol{\beta}$, $C_Y(\cdot, \cdot)$, and σ_ε^2 are known, and hence for the algebra that follows we can drop them from the notation. Then,

$$Y(s_0)|\mathbf{Z} \sim Gau(E(Y(s_0)|\mathbf{Z}), \text{var}(Y(s_0)|\mathbf{Z})), \tag{4.29}$$

where the conditional mean and conditional variance are given, for example, by Rencher (2002, p. 88):

$$E(Y(s_0)|\mathbf{Z}) = \mathbf{x}(s_0)'\boldsymbol{\beta} + \mathbf{c}_Y(s_0)'\mathbf{C}_Z^{-1}(\mathbf{Z} - \mathbf{X}\boldsymbol{\beta}) \tag{4.30}$$

$$\text{var}(Y(s_0)|\mathbf{Z}) = C_Y(s_0, s_0) - \mathbf{c}_Y(s_0)'\mathbf{C}_Z^{-1}\mathbf{c}_Y(s_0).$$

It is illustrative in this rather simple HM to derive the formulas (4.29) and (4.30) from first principles. Associated with the data vector $\mathbf{Z}$ is the vector $\mathbf{Y}$, obtained from the hidden process:

$$\mathbf{Y} \equiv (Y(\mathbf{s}_1), \ldots, Y(\mathbf{s}_m))' . \tag{4.31}$$

Then the data model implies that $\mathbf{Z}|\mathbf{Y} \sim Gau(\mathbf{Y}, \sigma_\varepsilon^2 \mathbf{I})$. From the process model given just above, we obtain

$$\begin{bmatrix} Y(\mathbf{s}_0) \\ \mathbf{Y} \end{bmatrix} \sim Gau \left(\begin{bmatrix} \mathbf{x}(\mathbf{s}_0)' \\ \mathbf{X} \end{bmatrix} \boldsymbol{\beta} , \begin{bmatrix} C_Y(\mathbf{s}_0, \mathbf{s}_0) & \mathbf{c}_Y(\mathbf{s}_0)' \\ \mathbf{c}_Y(\mathbf{s}_0) & \boldsymbol{\Sigma}_Y \end{bmatrix} \right) , \tag{4.32}$$

where $\boldsymbol{\Sigma}_Y \equiv var(\mathbf{Y})$. Standard results for the multivariate Gaussian distribution yield

$$Y(\mathbf{s}_0)|\mathbf{Y} \sim Gau(\mathbf{x}(\mathbf{s}_0)'\boldsymbol{\beta} + \mathbf{c}_Y(\mathbf{s}_0)'\boldsymbol{\Sigma}_Y^{-1}(\mathbf{Y} - \mathbf{X}\boldsymbol{\beta}), C_Y(\mathbf{s}_0, \mathbf{s}_0)$$

$$- \mathbf{c}_Y(\mathbf{s}_0)'\boldsymbol{\Sigma}_Y^{-1}\mathbf{c}_Y(\mathbf{s}_0)) , \tag{4.33}$$

and $\mathbf{Y} \sim Gau(\mathbf{X}\boldsymbol{\beta}, \boldsymbol{\Sigma}_Y)$.

Our interest is in the posterior distribution, $[\mathbf{Y}|\mathbf{Z}]$. Bayes' Theorem gives

$$[\mathbf{Y}|\mathbf{Z}] \propto [\mathbf{Z}|\mathbf{Y}][\mathbf{Y}] ,$$

and hence from the HM, and after some algebra, we derive

$$\mathbf{Y}|\mathbf{Z} \sim Gau((\sigma_\varepsilon^{-2}\mathbf{I} + \boldsymbol{\Sigma}_Y^{-1})^{-1}(\sigma_\varepsilon^{-2}\mathbf{Z} + \boldsymbol{\Sigma}_Y^{-1}\mathbf{X}\boldsymbol{\beta}), (\sigma_\varepsilon^{-2}\mathbf{I} + \boldsymbol{\Sigma}_Y^{-1})^{-1}) . \tag{4.34}$$

Using well known Sherman-Morrison-Woodbury matrix identities,

$$(\mathbf{A}'\mathbf{B}^{-1}\mathbf{A} + \mathbf{D}^{-1})^{-1} = \mathbf{D} - \mathbf{D}\mathbf{A}'(\mathbf{A}\mathbf{D}\mathbf{A}' + \mathbf{B})^{-1}\mathbf{A}\mathbf{D}$$

$$(\mathbf{A}'\mathbf{B}^{-1}\mathbf{A} + \mathbf{D}^{-1})^{-1}\mathbf{A}'\mathbf{B} = \mathbf{D}\mathbf{A}'(\mathbf{B} + \mathbf{A}\mathbf{D}\mathbf{A}')^{-1} ,$$

we can write

$$E(\mathbf{Y}|\mathbf{Z}) = \mathbf{X}\boldsymbol{\beta} + \mathbf{K}(\mathbf{Z} - \mathbf{X}\boldsymbol{\beta}) \tag{4.35}$$

$$var(\mathbf{Y}|\mathbf{Z}) = (\mathbf{I} - \mathbf{K})\boldsymbol{\Sigma}_Y , \tag{4.36}$$

where $\mathbf{K}$ is the "gain,"

$$\mathbf{K} \equiv \boldsymbol{\Sigma}_Y(\sigma_\varepsilon^2 \mathbf{I} + \boldsymbol{\Sigma}_Y)^{-1} . \tag{4.37}$$

Now we return to prediction of $Y(\mathbf{s}_0)$. In general, the posterior distribution of $Y(\mathbf{s}_0)$ can be obtained from

$$[Y(\mathbf{s}_0)|\mathbf{Z}] = \int [Y(\mathbf{s}_0)|\mathbf{Y}][\mathbf{Y}|\mathbf{Z}] \, d\mathbf{Y} . \tag{4.38}$$

In the Gaussian case, the components of the integrand are given by (4.33) and (4.34). More directly, $[Y(\mathbf{s}_0)|\mathbf{Z}]$ is Gaussian, and hence one only has to derive the first two (posterior) moments to characterize the distribution. The posterior mean can be derived as follows:

$$E(Y(\mathbf{s}_0)|\mathbf{Z}) = E\{E(Y(\mathbf{s}_0)|\mathbf{Y}, \mathbf{Z})|\mathbf{Z}\}$$
$$= E\{\mathbf{x}(\mathbf{s}_0)'\boldsymbol{\beta} + \mathbf{c}_Y(\mathbf{s}_0)'\boldsymbol{\Sigma}_Y^{-1}(\mathbf{Y} - \mathbf{X}\boldsymbol{\beta})|\mathbf{Z}\},$$

since $[Y(\mathbf{s}_0)|\mathbf{Y}, \mathbf{Z}] = [Y(\mathbf{s}_0)|\mathbf{Y}]$. Hence, from (4.35) and (4.37), we obtain

$$E(Y(\mathbf{s}_0)|\mathbf{Z}) = \mathbf{x}(\mathbf{s}_0)'\boldsymbol{\beta} + \mathbf{c}_Y(\mathbf{s}_0)'\boldsymbol{\Sigma}_Y^{-1}\mathbf{K}(\mathbf{Z} - \mathbf{X}\boldsymbol{\beta})$$
$$= \mathbf{x}(\mathbf{s}_0)'\boldsymbol{\beta} + \mathbf{c}_Y(\mathbf{s}_0)'(\sigma_\varepsilon^2\mathbf{I} + \boldsymbol{\Sigma}_Y)^{-1}(\mathbf{Z} - \mathbf{X}\boldsymbol{\beta})$$
$$= Y^*(\mathbf{s}_0), \tag{4.39}$$

since $\mathbf{C}_Z = \boldsymbol{\Sigma}_Y + \sigma_\varepsilon^2\mathbf{I}$.

From (4.33), (4.36), and (4.37), the posterior variance can be derived as follows:

$$\mathrm{var}(Y(\mathbf{s}_0)|\mathbf{Z}) = E\{\mathrm{var}(Y(\mathbf{s}_0)|\mathbf{Y})|\mathbf{Z}\} + \mathrm{var}\{E(Y(\mathbf{s}_0)|\mathbf{Y})|\mathbf{Z}\}$$
$$= C_Y(\mathbf{s}_0, \mathbf{s}_0) - \mathbf{c}_Y(\mathbf{s}_0)'\boldsymbol{\Sigma}_Y^{-1}\mathbf{c}_Y(\mathbf{s}_0) + \mathrm{var}\{\mathbf{c}_Y(\mathbf{s}_0)'\boldsymbol{\Sigma}_Y^{-1}\mathbf{Y}|\mathbf{Z}\}$$
$$= C_Y(\mathbf{s}_0, \mathbf{s}_0) - \mathbf{c}_Y(\mathbf{s}_0)'\boldsymbol{\Sigma}_Y^{-1}\mathbf{K}\mathbf{c}_Y(\mathbf{s}_0)$$
$$= C_Y(\mathbf{s}_0, \mathbf{s}_0) - \mathbf{c}_Y(\mathbf{s}_0)'(\sigma_\varepsilon^2\mathbf{I} + \boldsymbol{\Sigma}_Y)^{-1}\mathbf{c}_Y(\mathbf{s}_0)$$
$$= \sigma_{Y,sk}^2(\mathbf{s}_0), \tag{4.40}$$

again since $\mathbf{C}_Z = \boldsymbol{\Sigma}_Y + \sigma_\varepsilon^2\mathbf{I}$. The result (4.40) should not be surprising because, assuming the HM given just above, we obtain

$$\sigma_{Y,sk}^2(\mathbf{s}_0) = E(Y(\mathbf{s}_0) - Y^*(\mathbf{s}_0))^2$$
$$= E\{(Y(\mathbf{s}_0) - E(Y(\mathbf{s}_0)|\mathbf{Z}))^2|\mathbf{Z}\}$$
$$= E\{\mathrm{var}(Y(\mathbf{s}_0)|\mathbf{Z})\}$$
$$= \mathrm{var}(Y(\mathbf{s}_0)|\mathbf{Z});$$

the last equality is a consequence of the Gaussian assumptions in the HM, which imply that the posterior variance does *not* depend on $\mathbf{Z}$.

In summary, the simple-kriging predictor given by (4.28), and the simple-kriging variance given by (4.26), can equally be derived from the HM given just above.

In the case where two (or more) values, $Y(\mathbf{s}_{0,1})$ and $Y(\mathbf{s}_{0,2})$, are to be predicted, the optimal predictors are still $Y^*(\mathbf{s}_{0,1})$ and $Y^*(\mathbf{s}_{0,2})$, respectively.

As well as calculating the mean squared prediction errors, $\sigma^2_{Y,sk}(\mathbf{s}_{0,1})$ and $\sigma^2_{Y,sk}(\mathbf{s}_{0,2})$, the mean cross-prediction errors can be calculated and shown to satisfy

$$E\{(Y(\mathbf{s}_{0,1}) - Y^*(\mathbf{s}_{0,1}))(Y(\mathbf{s}_{0,2}) - Y^*(\mathbf{s}_{0,2}))\} = E\{\text{cov}(Y(\mathbf{s}_{0,1}), Y(\mathbf{s}_{0,2})|\mathbf{Z})\}.$$

In Section 4.1.1, we gave a motivating example of simple kriging based on decadal temperature differences over the Americas. In fact, the original data (see Figure 4.6a) were produced from NCAR's Climate System Model, to which we deliberately added measurement error after subsampling. Figure 4.6b shows the noisy, corrupted data $\mathbf{Z}$ to which we applied simple kriging. Figures 4.6c and 4.6d show the simple kriging predictor $Y^*(\cdot)$ given by (4.28) and the simple kriging prediction standard error $\sigma_{Y,sk}(\cdot)$ obtained from (4.26), respectively.

Non-Gaussian Geostatistical Models

The HM given just above (4.29) has both a Gaussian data model and a Gaussian process model. As a consequence, the joint distribution of $\mathbf{Z}$ and $Y(\cdot)$ is Gaussian, as is the posterior distribution, $Y(\cdot)|\mathbf{Z}$ (assuming all parameters are known). We saw above that, in this case, to obtain the posterior distribution, we only need to calculate posterior means, variances, and covariances.

When the data $\mathbf{Z}$ are binary or are counts, a Gaussian data model is inappropriate. Diggle, Tawn, and Moyeed (1998) proposed that the *Gaussian* data model be replaced with an *exponential-family* data model. Let a random variable Z have density from the exponential family given by

$$\exp\{(z\eta - b(\eta))/a(\theta_1) + c(z, \theta_1)\}, \tag{4.41}$$

where, for the moment, θ_1 is considered to be known, and η is often referred to as the canonical parameter of the *exponential-family model (EFM)*. For example, if $Z \sim Gau(\eta, \sigma^2_\varepsilon)$, then $\theta_1 = \sigma^2_\varepsilon$, $a(\theta_1) = \theta_1$, $b(\eta) = \eta^2/2$, and $c(z, \theta_1) = (-1/2)\{z^2/\theta_1 + \log(2\pi\theta_1)\}$; and if $Z \sim Poi(\exp(\eta))$, then there is no nuisance parameter θ_1, $a = 1$, $b(\eta) = \exp(\eta)$, and $c(z) = -\log(z!)$. Other exponential-family models include the binomial distribution, the gamma distribution, and the inverse-Gaussian distribution (e.g., McCullagh and Nelder, 1989, p. 30).

Now define $\mu \equiv E(Z)$, which in general depends on η. Assuming the EFM, then it can be shown that (e.g., McCullagh and Nelder, 1989)

$$\mu(\eta) = b^{(\prime)}(\eta), \tag{4.42}$$

and $\text{var}(Z) = b^{(\prime\prime)}(\eta)a(\theta_1)$, where the superscripts denote first and second derivatives with respect to η. The canonical link function, $g(\mu)$, has the property that

$$g(\mu(\eta)) = \eta. \tag{4.43}$$

For example, if $Z \sim Gau(\eta, \sigma_\varepsilon^2)$, then it can be verified that $g(\mu) = \mu$, the identity link; and if $Z \sim Poi(\exp(\eta))$, then $g(\mu) = \log \mu$, the log link. It is important to know this link because the *generalized linear model* defines the dependence of μ on covariates $\mathbf{x} \equiv (x_1, \ldots, x_p)'$ through

$$\eta = g(\mu) = \mathbf{x}' \boldsymbol{\beta}, \tag{4.44}$$

where $\boldsymbol{\beta} \equiv (\beta_1, \ldots, \beta_p)'$ are regression parameters.

We are now ready to define a non-Gaussian geostatistical model, using an HM.

Data model: Conditional on θ_1, and for $i = 1, \ldots, m$,

$$Z(\mathbf{s}_i)|Y(\mathbf{s}_i), \theta_1 \sim ind.\, EFM,$$

with canonical parameter $Y(\mathbf{s}_i)$ and functions $a(\theta_1)$, $b(Y(\mathbf{s}_i))$, and $c(Z(\mathbf{s}_i), \theta_1)$ in (4.41).

Process model: Conditional on $\boldsymbol{\beta}$ and $C_Y(\cdot, \cdot)$, $Y(\cdot)$ is a Gaussian process with the following properties:

$$E(Y(\cdot)) = \mathbf{x}(\cdot)' \boldsymbol{\beta}, \text{ and we write } \operatorname{cov}(Y(\mathbf{u}), Y(\mathbf{v})) \equiv C_Y(\mathbf{u}, \mathbf{v}).$$

A special case of the process model is where $Y(\cdot)$ has *no random variability*, and hence $Y(\mathbf{s}) = \mathbf{x}(\mathbf{s})' \boldsymbol{\beta}$; then the HM reduces to a model where the elements of $\mathbf{Z} \equiv (Z(\mathbf{s}_1), \ldots, Z(\mathbf{s}_m))'$ are independently sampled from a generalized linear model. With random spatial variability in $Y(\cdot)$, the HM allows the introduction of spatial dependence in a natural way through the canonical parameter of the EFM.

We have already seen that, in the special case of a Gaussian data model and Gaussian process model, the posterior distribution is Gaussian and the posterior means and variances can be calculated in closed form (assuming all parameters are known). We referred to these as the simple-kriging predictor and the simple-kriging (prediction) variance, respectively. For the more general HM with an EFM data model, the posterior distribution is not available in closed form, and a Monte Carlo algorithm is needed to obtain the posterior distribution. Cressie (2000) gives the MCMC algorithms for the HM given just above. Diggle, Tawn, and Moyeed (1998) add a parameter model to the HM and develop MCMC algorithms for the resulting BHM, and Wikle (2010a) discusses computational issues associated with non-Gaussian BHMs.

Another way to define *non-Gaussian* geostatistical models is to modify the *process model* in the HM. Suppose we write the covariance function C_Y as

$$C_Y(\mathbf{u}, \mathbf{v}) = \sigma(\mathbf{u})\sigma(\mathbf{v})\rho_Y(\mathbf{u}, \mathbf{v}), \qquad \mathbf{u}, \mathbf{v} \in \mathbb{R}^d, \tag{4.45}$$

where $\rho_Y(\mathbf{u}, \mathbf{u}) \equiv 1$, and hence $C_Y(\mathbf{u}, \mathbf{u}) \equiv \sigma^2(\mathbf{u})$, for $\mathbf{u} \in \mathbb{R}^d$. Palacios and Steel (2006) suggest that $\sigma(\cdot)$ might be further modeled as a spatial process.

Using appropriate conditional distributions, the following HM results in non-Gaussian (but continuous) behavior for $Z(\cdot)$.

Data model: Conditional on σ_ε^2, and for $i = 1, \ldots, m$,

$$Z(\mathbf{s}_i)|Y(\mathbf{s}_i), \sigma_\varepsilon^2 \sim ind.\, Gau(Y(\mathbf{s}_i), \sigma_\varepsilon^2).$$

Process model 1:   Conditional on $\boldsymbol{\beta}$, $\sigma^2(\cdot)$, and $\rho_Y(\cdot, \cdot)$, $Y(\cdot)$ is a Gaussian process with the following properties:

$E(Y(\cdot)) = \mathbf{x}(\cdot)'\boldsymbol{\beta}$, and we write $cov(Y(\mathbf{u}), Y(\mathbf{v})) \equiv \sigma(\mathbf{u})\sigma(\mathbf{v})\rho_Y(\mathbf{u}, \mathbf{v})$.

Process model 2:   Conditional on $C_\omega(\cdot, \cdot)$, $\sigma(\cdot)$ is a log Gaussian process with the following properties:

$E(\sigma(\mathbf{s})) \equiv 1$, and we write $cov(\sigma(\mathbf{u}), \sigma(\mathbf{v})) \equiv \exp(C_\omega(\mathbf{u}, \mathbf{v}) - 1)$, where $C_\omega(\cdot, \cdot)$ is the covariance function for $\omega(\cdot) \equiv \log \sigma(\cdot)$.

Notice that $\omega(\cdot) \equiv \log \sigma(\cdot)$ is a Gaussian process, and if we put $E(\omega(\mathbf{s})) = (-1/2)C_\omega(\mathbf{s}, \mathbf{s})$, $\mathbf{s} \in D$, then on the exponential scale the process $\sigma(\cdot) \equiv \exp(\omega(\cdot))$ does have mean 1, as specified in process model 2. Hence, if the Gaussian process $\omega(\cdot)$ is chosen to have constant variance σ_ω^2, then $E(\omega(\mathbf{s})) \equiv (-1/2)\sigma_\omega^2$, a constant.

We note that some modelers may wish to consider the model on $\sigma(\cdot)$, given in process model 2, in a parameter level of the HM. Indeed this illustrates how one person's processes are another's parameters. At this point, the choice is somewhat semantic, but we wish to emphasize that $Y(\cdot)$ is conditioned on $\sigma(\cdot)$, and we are using the spatial variability of $\sigma(\cdot)$ simply to generate a non-Gaussian process. Hence, we leave it in the process model in this example.

Implementation of HMs with a geostatistical process model typically involves discretizing D_s onto a fine grid of n cells, resulting in a process that can be written as the n-dimensional vector $\mathbf{Y}$ (e.g., Figure 4.5a). Consequently, the data model may involve an incidence matrix $\mathbf{H}$ that assigns each $Z(\mathbf{s}_0)$ to one of the n cells. Then a statistical analysis often proceeds through an MCMC algorithm (e.g., Cressie, 2000; Wikle, 2010a).

The Kriging Predictor

We have already seen that nonparametric assumptions of the sort made in classical geostatistics produce a simple-kriging predictor and a kriging variance that can be interpreted as the posterior mean and posterior variance, respectively, in a Gaussian–Gaussian HM. We now take a small detour away from HMs to derive more general versions of kriging under different nonparametric assumptions. We shall then return to consider a BHM to show that these various kriging predictors can be obtained from the posterior distribution.

Observe two things from (4.25) and (4.27). First, the mean of the process $Y(\cdot)$ cannot be computed if the regression parameter vector $\boldsymbol{\beta}$ is unknown.

(We assume in the rest of this presentation of kriging that the covariance function $C_Y(\cdot, \cdot)$ is known.) Second, the simple kriging predictor $Y^*(s_0)$ satisfies $E(Y^*(s_0)) = E(Y(s_0)) = \mathbf{x}(s_0)'\boldsymbol{\beta}$, for all possible values of $\boldsymbol{\beta} \in \mathbb{R}^p$. We refer to this property as (*uniform*) *unbiasedness* of the predictor $Y^*(s_0)$. The two observations are related. Typically, $\boldsymbol{\beta}$ is unknown, making the simple kriging predictor, $Y^*(s_0) \equiv \boldsymbol{\ell}^*\mathbf{Z} + k^*$, given by (4.28), unusable. But notice that $\boldsymbol{\beta}$ only appears in the optimal constant term, k^*. So, if we change from the class of heterogeneously linear predictors, $\{\boldsymbol{\ell}'\mathbf{Z} + k : \boldsymbol{\ell} \in \mathbb{R}^m, k \in \mathbb{R}\}$, to the class of homogeneously linear predictors, $\{\boldsymbol{\lambda}'\mathbf{Z} : \boldsymbol{\lambda} \in \mathbb{R}^m\}$, and *impose* unbiasedness, then there may be a computable optimal spatial predictor that is usable. In fact there is, and it is called the *universal kriging predictor*. [The word "universal" was used by Matheron and his school of geostatisticians to denote the generalization from assuming a known mean to assuming (4.27), where the regression parameter $\boldsymbol{\beta} \in \mathbb{R}^p$ is fixed but unknown.]

Ordinary Kriging
In what is to follow, we give the derivation of kriging assuming the special case (4.11), namely $E(Y(s)) = \mu$, for all $s \in D_s$, which is a special case of (4.27) with $p = 1$, $\mathbf{x}(\cdot) = 1$, and $\boldsymbol{\beta} = \mu$. This is known as *ordinary kriging* in the geostatistics literature. (Universal kriging is also discussed below, but without derivation.) Here, we derive ordinary kriging of $Y(s_0)$ in terms of covariance functions, and we just state the formulas in terms of semivariograms. The ordinary-kriging predictor is the homogeneously linear combination of the data $\mathbf{Z}$ that minimizes the mean squared prediction error,

$$\text{MSPE}(\boldsymbol{\lambda}) \equiv E(Y(s_0) - \boldsymbol{\lambda}'\mathbf{Z})^2, \tag{4.46}$$

with respect to coefficients $\boldsymbol{\lambda}$, *subject to* the unbiasedness condition, $E(\boldsymbol{\lambda}'\mathbf{Z}) = E(Y(s_0)) = \mu$, for all $\mu \in \mathbb{R}$.

Since $E(Z(s)) = E(Y(s)) = \mu$, then $E(\mathbf{Z}) = \mu\mathbf{1}$, where $\mathbf{1} \equiv (1, \ldots, 1)'$ is the m-dimensional vector of 1s. Hence, the unbiasedness condition is equivalent to

$$\boldsymbol{\lambda}'\mathbf{1} = 1; \tag{4.47}$$

that is, the sum of the ordinary-kriging coefficients is 1. Sometimes $\lambda_1, \ldots, \lambda_m$ are referred to as kriging weights, but we find this misleading since they can be positive *or* negative; we refer to them as kriging *coefficients*.

Using the method of Lagrange multipliers to incorporate the constraint (4.47), we minimize the objective function,

$$\text{MSPE}(\boldsymbol{\lambda}) - 2\kappa(\boldsymbol{\lambda}'\mathbf{1} - 1), \tag{4.48}$$

with respect to $\boldsymbol{\lambda}$ and the Lagrange multiplier κ. Evaluating (4.48), we obtain

$$C_Y(s_0, s_0) - 2\boldsymbol{\lambda}'\mathbf{c}_Y(s_0) + \boldsymbol{\lambda}'\mathbf{C}_Z\boldsymbol{\lambda} - 2\kappa(\boldsymbol{\lambda}'\mathbf{1} - 1), \tag{4.49}$$

whose partial derivative with respect to λ and κ, set equal to zero, results in

$$-\mathbf{c}_Y(\mathbf{s}_0) + \mathbf{C}_Z\lambda = \kappa\mathbf{1}$$
$$\lambda'\mathbf{1} = 1. \tag{4.50}$$

Recall that $\mathbf{C}_Z \equiv \text{var}(\mathbf{Z})$ and $\mathbf{c}_Y(\mathbf{s}_0)$ is given by (4.23).

Let the solution to (4.50) be λ^* and κ^*. Then, from the first equation, we obtain

$$\lambda^* = \mathbf{C}_Z^{-1}(\mathbf{c}_Y(\mathbf{s}_0) + \kappa^*\mathbf{1}),$$

and, from the second equation, $\kappa^* = (1 - \mathbf{1}'\mathbf{C}_Z^{-1}\mathbf{c}_Y(\mathbf{s}_0))/(\mathbf{1}'\mathbf{C}_Z^{-1}\mathbf{1})$. Finally, the *ordinary-kriging predictor* is

$$\widehat{Y}(\mathbf{s}_0) \equiv \{\mathbf{c}_Y(\mathbf{s}_0) + \mathbf{1}(1 - \mathbf{1}'\mathbf{C}_Z^{-1}\mathbf{c}_Y(\mathbf{s}_0))/(\mathbf{1}'\mathbf{C}_Z^{-1}\mathbf{1})\}'\mathbf{C}_Z^{-1}\mathbf{Z} \equiv (\lambda^*)'\mathbf{Z}. \tag{4.51}$$

The minimized mean squared prediction error, often called the *(ordinary) kriging variance*, is obtained by substituting λ^* into (4.46):

$$\sigma_{Y,ok}^2(\mathbf{s}_0) \equiv \text{MSPE}(\lambda^*)$$
$$= C_Y(\mathbf{s}_0, \mathbf{s}_0) - \mathbf{c}_Y(\mathbf{s}_0)'\mathbf{C}_Z^{-1}\mathbf{c}_Y(\mathbf{s}_0)$$
$$+ (1 - \mathbf{1}'\mathbf{C}_Z^{-1}\mathbf{c}_Y(\mathbf{s}_0))^2/(\mathbf{1}'\mathbf{C}_Z^{-1}\mathbf{1}), \tag{4.52}$$

where the subscript "*ok*" on the left-hand side of (4.52) denotes ordinary kriging. Comparing (4.52) to (4.26), we see that the unbiasedness restriction in ordinary kriging results in $\sigma_{Y,ok}^2(\mathbf{s}_0) \geq \sigma_{Y,sk}^2(\mathbf{s}_0)$. This is intuitively reasonable, since for ordinary kriging μ is unknown, which leads to greater prediction uncertainty.

Ordinary-kriging prediction intervals can also be computed from (4.51) and (4.52), although their accuracy is in doubt when the data are non-Gaussian. Schelin and Sjöstedt-de Luna (2010) give kriging prediction intervals based on a semiparametric bootstrap.

While it is not obvious, it is seen below that (4.51) can be written equivalently as

$$\widehat{Y}(\mathbf{s}_0) = \widehat{\mu}_{gls} + \mathbf{c}_Y(\mathbf{s}_0)'\mathbf{C}_Z^{-1}(\mathbf{Z} - \widehat{\mu}_{gls}\mathbf{1}), \tag{4.53}$$

where $\widehat{\mu}_{gls}$ is the generalized-least-squares estimator of μ, namely

$$\widehat{\mu}_{gls} \equiv (\mathbf{1}'\mathbf{C}_Z^{-1}\mathbf{Z})/(\mathbf{1}'\mathbf{C}_Z^{-1}\mathbf{1}). \tag{4.54}$$

By comparing (4.53) with the simple kriging predictor (4.25), where $\mu_Y(\cdot) \equiv \mu$, it is clear that ordinary kriging is just simple kriging with the optimal (generalized-least-squares) estimator $\widehat{\mu}_{gls}$ substituted for μ.

The expression (4.53) is no accident; the result is due to Goldberger (1962) and (in the spatial context) Gotway and Cressie (1993), who show that for any linear estimator, $\overline{\mu} \equiv \mathbf{a}'\mathbf{Z}$, the linear predictor, $\overline{Y}(\mathbf{s}_0) \equiv \overline{\mu} + \mathbf{c}_Y(\mathbf{s}_0)'\mathbf{C}_Z^{-1}(\mathbf{Z} - \overline{\mu}\mathbf{1})$, satisfies

$$E(Y(\mathbf{s}_0) - \overline{Y}(\mathbf{s}_0))^2 = \text{MSPE}(\boldsymbol{\ell}^*, k^*) + (1 - \mathbf{1}'\mathbf{C}_Z^{-1}\mathbf{c}_Y(\mathbf{s}_0))^2 E(\mu - \overline{\mu})^2 .$$

Gotway and Cressie also show that there always exists a $\overline{\mu}$ ($= \mathbf{a}'\mathbf{Z}$, for some $\mathbf{a}$) such that *any* homogeneously linear predictor can be written as $\overline{Y}(\mathbf{s}_0)$. Hence, $\overline{Y}(\mathbf{s}_0)$ is an unbiased predictor of $Y(\mathbf{s}_0)$, if and only if $\overline{\mu}$ is an unbiased estimator of μ. Furthermore, the optimal homogeneously linear (ordinary-kriging) predictor results from choosing the $\overline{\mu}$ that minimizes $E(\mu - \overline{\mu})^2$. Provided $\overline{\mu}$ is unbiased, $E(\mu - \overline{\mu})^2 = \text{var}(\overline{\mu}) = \mathbf{a}'\mathbf{C}_Z\mathbf{a}$. It is a well known result from estimation theory that this *best* linear unbiased estimator (BLUE) of μ is the generalized-least-squares estimator, $\widehat{\mu}_{gls}$, given by (4.54). That is, once the simple-kriging coefficients $\mathbf{c}_Y(\mathbf{s}_0)'\mathbf{C}_Z^{-1}$ are chosen, the *optimality* of the (homogeneously) linear spatial *predictor* is in one-to-one correspondence with the *optimality* of the linear *estimator* of the mean. By giving up both linearity and unbiasedness of the predictor, it is possible to find a predictor whose mean squared prediction error is *smaller* than the ordinary-kriging variance (Gotway and Cressie, 1993).

So far, we have presented simple kriging and ordinary kriging in terms of the covariance function $C_Y(\cdot, \cdot)$. There is an equivalent formulation of ordinary kriging (but not of simple kriging) in terms of the semivariogram,

$$\gamma_Y(\mathbf{u}, \mathbf{v}) = (1/2)\{C_Y(\mathbf{u}, \mathbf{u}) + C_Y(\mathbf{v}, \mathbf{v}) - 2C_Y(\mathbf{u}, \mathbf{v})\} . \tag{4.55}$$

In terms of semivariograms, we have

$$\text{MSPE}(\boldsymbol{\lambda}) = 2\boldsymbol{\lambda}'\widetilde{\boldsymbol{\gamma}}_Y(\mathbf{s}_0) - \boldsymbol{\lambda}'\boldsymbol{\Gamma}_Z\boldsymbol{\lambda} , \tag{4.56}$$

where the $m \times m$ matrix $\boldsymbol{\Gamma}_Z \equiv (\gamma_Z(\mathbf{s}_i, \mathbf{s}_j))$;

$$\gamma_Z(\mathbf{u}, \mathbf{v}) = \gamma_Y(\mathbf{u}, \mathbf{v}) + \sigma_\varepsilon^2 I(\mathbf{u} \neq \mathbf{v}) ;$$

and $\widetilde{\boldsymbol{\gamma}}_Y(\mathbf{s}_0) \equiv (\gamma_Y(\mathbf{s}_0, \mathbf{s}_1) + \sigma_\varepsilon^2/2, \ldots, \gamma_Y(\mathbf{s}_0, \mathbf{s}_m) + \sigma_\varepsilon^2/2)'$; see Cressie (1993, Section 3.2.1).

Again, using the method of Lagrange multipliers to impose the restriction $\boldsymbol{\lambda}'\mathbf{1} = 1$, we wish to minimize (4.48) with respect to $\boldsymbol{\lambda}$ and κ. Using (4.56) in (4.48) and setting the partial derivatives with respect to $\boldsymbol{\lambda}$ and κ equal to zero, we obtain equivalent ordinary-kriging equations in terms of the semivariogram:

$$\widehat{Y}(\mathbf{s}_0) = \{\widetilde{\boldsymbol{\gamma}}_Y(\mathbf{s}_0) + \mathbf{1}(1 - \mathbf{1}'\boldsymbol{\Gamma}_Z^{-1}\widetilde{\boldsymbol{\gamma}}_Y(\mathbf{s}_0))/(\mathbf{1}'\boldsymbol{\Gamma}_Z^{-1}\mathbf{1})\}'\boldsymbol{\Gamma}_Z^{-1}\mathbf{Z}, \tag{4.57}$$

$$\sigma_{Y,ok}^2(\mathbf{s}_0) = \widetilde{\boldsymbol{\gamma}}_Y(\mathbf{s}_0)'\boldsymbol{\Gamma}_Z^{-1}\widetilde{\boldsymbol{\gamma}}_Y(\mathbf{s}_0) - (1 - \mathbf{1}'\boldsymbol{\Gamma}_Z^{-1}\widetilde{\boldsymbol{\gamma}}_Y(\mathbf{s}_0))^2/(\mathbf{1}'\boldsymbol{\Gamma}_Z^{-1}\mathbf{1}) . \tag{4.58}$$

Notice that simple kriging and ordinary kriging require either the covariance function or the semivariogram to be known. In practice, they have to be estimated, which means that, strictly speaking, they no longer yield optimal predictors.

Universal Kriging

When the constant-mean assumption (4.11) is generalized to the linear-model assumption (4.27), namely $E(Y(\cdot)) = \mathbf{x}(\cdot)'\boldsymbol{\beta}$, we have already noted that optimal (homogeneously) linear spatial prediction is known as *universal kriging* in the geostatistics literature. Recall from (4.28) the definitions of $\mathbf{X}$, $\mathbf{C}_Z$, and $\mathbf{c}_Y(\mathbf{s}_0)$. Then, it is straightforward to show that the universal-kriging predictor of $Y(\mathbf{s}_0)$ is

$$\widehat{Y}(\mathbf{s}_0) = \mathbf{x}(\mathbf{s}_0)'\widehat{\boldsymbol{\beta}}_{gls} + \mathbf{c}_Y(\mathbf{s}_0)'\mathbf{C}_Z^{-1}(\mathbf{Z} - \mathbf{X}\widehat{\boldsymbol{\beta}}_{gls}), \qquad (4.59)$$

where $\widehat{\boldsymbol{\beta}}_{gls} \equiv (\mathbf{X}'\mathbf{C}_Z^{-1}\mathbf{X})^{-1}\mathbf{X}'\mathbf{C}_Z^{-1}\mathbf{Z}$, is the generalized-least-squares estimator of $\boldsymbol{\beta}$. The result is analogous to (4.53) and a direct consequence of a decomposition of the mean squared prediction error for the linear-model case (see, e.g., Cressie, 1993, p. 174). The decomposition also implies that the (universal) kriging variance is

$$\sigma^2_{Y,uk}(\mathbf{s}_0) = C_Y(\mathbf{s}_0, \mathbf{s}_0) - \mathbf{c}_Y(\mathbf{s}_0)'\mathbf{C}_Z^{-1}\mathbf{c}_Y(\mathbf{s}_0) + (\mathbf{x}(\mathbf{s}_0)$$
$$-\mathbf{X}'\mathbf{C}_Z^{-1}\mathbf{c}_Y(\mathbf{s}_0))'(\mathbf{X}'\mathbf{C}_Z^{-1}\mathbf{X})^{-1}(\mathbf{x}(\mathbf{s}_0) - \mathbf{X}'\mathbf{C}_Z^{-1}\mathbf{c}_Y(\mathbf{s}_0)). \quad (4.60)$$

The equivalent formulation of universal kriging in terms of the semivariogram only holds if $\mathbf{x}(\cdot)'\boldsymbol{\beta}$ has an intercept term (i.e., $x_1(\mathbf{s}) \equiv 1$). In that case, simply replace $\mathbf{c}_Y(\mathbf{s}_0)$ with $-\widetilde{\boldsymbol{\gamma}}_Y(\mathbf{s}_0)$ and $\mathbf{C}_Z$ with $-\boldsymbol{\Gamma}_Z$ in (4.59) and (4.60), to obtain formulas for $\widehat{Y}(\mathbf{s}_0)$ and $\sigma^2_{Y,uk}(\mathbf{s}_0)$, respectively.

BHM and Kriging

There is a BHM that yields the universal kriging predictor, $\widehat{Y}(\mathbf{s}_0)$. Let a BHM be defined by the Gaussian data model and the Gaussian process model given at the beginning of this section (Section 4.1). The HM becomes Bayesian by specifying a parameter model. Here we specify an improper distribution for $\boldsymbol{\beta}$; we continue to assume that variances and covariances are known.

Parameter model: $\boldsymbol{\beta} \sim U((-\infty, \infty)^p)$, which is an improper uniform distribution on $\mathbb{R}^p$. (Parameters C_Y and σ^2_ε are assumed known.)

Then, $E(Y(\mathbf{s}_0)|\mathbf{Z}) = \widehat{Y}(\mathbf{s}_0)$, and $\mathrm{var}(Y(\mathbf{s}_0)|\mathbf{Z}) = \sigma^2_{Y,uk}(\mathbf{s}_0)$, are the relevant universal-kriging quantities (Omre and Halvorsen, 1989).

As a special case, ordinary kriging is obtained from the following parameter model.

Parameter model: $\mu \sim U(-\infty, \infty)$, which is an improper uniform distribution on $\mathbb{R}$. (Parameters C_Y and σ_ε^2 are assumed known.)

Other, more general parameter models that put (prior) distributions on β and on covariance parameters θ can be specified. Early examples can be found in Kitanidis (1986) and in Diggle, Tawn, and Moyeed (1998); Banerjee, Carlin, and Gelfand (2004) and Wikle (2010a) can be consulted for more recent developments.

The simple-, ordinary-, and universal-kriging formulas are all given above in terms of nonstationary covariance functions (and semivariograms); hence they are appropriate for a stationary covariance function, $C_Y(\mathbf{h})$, or a stationary semivariogram, $\gamma_Y(\mathbf{h})$. Stationarity is not a requirement for a BHM, but it can be important for an EHM, which is the approach typically used in geostatistical analyses. Stationarity provides a type of pseudo-replication of dependencies at given spatial lags $\mathbf{h}$, from which C_Y (and γ_Y) can be estimated (e.g., Cressie, 1993, Chapter 2).

Splines and Kriging

There is a close relationship between the universal-kriging predictor and thin-plate smoothing splines. This is made most transparent through the dual kriging equations; see the discussion given by Cressie (1993, pp. 180–183) and Kent and Mardia (1994). Both presentations adopt an EHM approach to inference. From the point of view of kriging, thin-plate smoothing splines *pre-select* a particular semivariogram (or more generally a generalized covariance function) without letting the data decide which semivariogram gives the best fit (in contrast to kriging; e.g., see Figure 4.5b). When using an approach based on thin-plate smoothing splines, the data are used to determine the size of a measurement-error variance, which is classically assumed to be the only source of randomness. The use of splines as smoothers, rather than as predictors, means that there is no analogous notion to the kriging variance, although Wahba (1983) did give a Bayesian interpretation of smoothing splines (from which posterior variances could be calculated). Of course, different spline basis functions could be used as spatial basis functions in the Spatial Random Effects model (4.79) below.

4.1.3   Change-of-Support

The support of

$$Y(B) \equiv (1/|B|) \int_B Y(\mathbf{u}) \, d\mathbf{u},$$

is simply B, the region over which $Y(\cdot)$ is averaged, where $|B| > 0$ is the d-dimensional volume of B. The quantity on the right-hand side is a stochastic integral, and it may be interpreted in terms of an integral of each realization coming from the probability space that defines the stochastic process $Y(\cdot)$. Alternatively, a finite collection $\{Y(\mathbf{s}_{0,j})\}$ defined on $\{\mathbf{s}_{0,j}\}$ has a multivariate distribution; an appropriately weighted sum, converging in mean square to a limiting random variable, defines the right-hand side (Yaglom, 1962, p. 23). The notion of *support* is an extremely important one in modeling a physical process; one can think of $|B|$ as the spatial resolution at which the phenomenon is being studied, although data often come as $\mathbf{Z} = (Z(\mathbf{s}_1), \ldots, Z(\mathbf{s}_m))'$, at point support (or more generally at *different* supports). In Chapter 1, we noted that change-of-support is analogous to Simpson's Paradox, and sometimes it helps to think of it this way (e.g., Ma, 2009).

In this section, as previously, we give some classical geostatistical approaches to this problem, followed by a formulation in terms of a BHM. Kriging adapts very easily to accommodate the change from predicting $Y(\mathbf{s}_0)$ with point support $\mathbf{s}_0$, to predicting $Y(B)$ with block support B. For example, in the formulas (4.28) and (4.51) for kriging predictors of $Y(\mathbf{s}_0)$, $\mathbf{x}(\mathbf{s}_0)$, and $\mathbf{c}_Y(\mathbf{s}_0)$ are modified very simply to

$$\mathbf{x}(B) \equiv (1/|B|)\left(\int_B x_1(\mathbf{u})\,d\mathbf{u}, \ldots, \int_B x_p(\mathbf{u})\,d\mathbf{u}\right)'$$

and

$$\mathbf{c}_Y(B) \equiv (1/|B|)\left(\int_B C_Y(\mathbf{u}, \mathbf{s}_1)\,d\mathbf{u}, \ldots, \int_B C_Y(\mathbf{u}, \mathbf{s}_m)\,d\mathbf{u}\right)',$$

respectively, resulting in the simple-kriging predictor $Y^*(B)$ and the ordinary-kriging predictor $\widehat{Y}(B)$. The same modification is made in (4.26) and (4.52), and $C_Y(\mathbf{s}_0, \mathbf{s}_0)$ is replaced with $C(B, B) \equiv (1/|B|)^2 \int_B \int_B C_Y(\mathbf{u}, \mathbf{v})\,d\mathbf{u}d\mathbf{v}$, to yield $\sigma^2_{Y,sk}(B)$ and $\sigma^2_{Y,ok}(B)$, respectively. For more details, see Cressie (1993, pp. 172–173).

Now consider the prediction of $g(Y(B))$, where g is a nonlinear function. Then the essential quantity we need is the conditional distribution, $Pr(Y(B) \le y|\mathbf{Z})$, which is the posterior distribution of $Y(B)$; any optimal predictor of $g(Y(B))$ is obtained from it. Disjunctive kriging and indicator kriging attempt to estimate a similar quantity, $\Pr(Z(B) \le z|\mathbf{Z})$, based on bivariate distributional properties of the (possibly transformed) process; see Cressie (1993, Section 5.2). However, these methods have serious drawbacks, associated with failing to distinguish between $Z(B)$ and $Y(B)$, and with difficulty in estimating block-to-block and point-to-block spatial dependencies of indicator variables from the point-to-point spatial dependencies indicated by the data.

Aldworth and Cressie (2003) present a methodology they call *covariance-matching constrained kriging (CMCK)*. Write the predictand as $\mathbf{Y(B)} \equiv (Y(B_1), \ldots, Y(B_m))'$, where $\mathbf{B} \equiv \{B_1, \ldots, B_m\}$. Then CMCK looks for an optimal homogeneously linear predictor, $\mathbf{Y}^@(\mathbf{B}) \equiv (Y^@(B_1), \ldots, Y^@(B_m))' \equiv \mathbf{AZ}$, of $\mathbf{Y}(\mathbf{B})$ with constraints:

$$E(\mathbf{Y}^@(\mathbf{B})) = E(\mathbf{Y}(\mathbf{B})) \qquad (4.61)$$

$$\text{var}(\mathbf{Y}^@(\mathbf{B})) = \text{var}(\mathbf{Y}(\mathbf{B})) ; \qquad (4.62)$$

there are conditions to check that guarantee CMCK is a solution to the constrained optimization problem. This has strong similarities to the constrained empirical Bayes estimators introduced by Louis (1984) and extended by Ghosh (1992). The CMCK predictor of $\mathbf{g}(\mathbf{Y}(\mathbf{B}))$ is defined to be $\mathbf{g}(\mathbf{Y}^@(\mathbf{B}))$, for any vector function $\mathbf{g}(\cdot)$, and it is *approximately* unbiased.

The traditional change-of-support problem that has been formulated in the geostatistics literature (e.g., Journel and Huijbregts, 1978, Chapter VI) is to make inference on $\mathbf{Z}(\mathbf{B})$ from observations $\mathbf{Z}$, which, from our discussion in Section 4.1.2, does not recognize the general goal of filtering out measurement error. Generally, inference should be on $\mathbf{Y}(\mathbf{B})$ rather than on $\mathbf{Z}(\mathbf{B})$. Traditional approaches also assume that trend parameters and covariance parameters are fixed but unknown, and they effectively adopt an EHM. Gelfand, Zhu, and Carlin (2001) give one way to modify the traditional EHM approach by showing how a BHM can be used to make inference on $\mathbf{Z}(\mathbf{B})$ from observations $\mathbf{Z}$; they do *not* discuss inference on $\mathbf{Y}(\mathbf{B})$.

Wikle and Berliner (2005) have formulated the change-of-support problem using a BHM that includes measurement error. Inference is on $\mathbf{Y}(\mathbf{B})$, based on data at levels of aggregation different from $\mathbf{B} = \{B_j\}$ (finer *or* coarser), say $\mathbf{Z}(\mathbf{A})$ and $\mathbf{Z}(\mathbf{C})$. They assume that for any $\mathbf{s} \in D_s$, there is some $B_j \subset D_s$ such that $Y(\mathbf{s}) = Y(B_j) + \zeta(\mathbf{s})$, where $\zeta(\cdot)$ is a spatial process with covariance function, $C_\zeta(\mathbf{u}, \mathbf{v})$, and the distribution of $\zeta(\mathbf{s})$ does not depend on $\{Y(B_j)\}$. For the finer-scale process, they derive

$$Y(A_i) = \mathbf{G}(A_i)'\mathbf{Y}(\mathbf{B}) + (1/|A_i|) \int_{A_i} \zeta(\mathbf{u}) \, d\mathbf{u} , \qquad (4.63)$$

where the jth element of $\mathbf{G}(A_i)$ is $|B_j \cap A_i|/|A_i|$; $j = 1, \ldots, n$. Notice that

$$\text{cov}(Y(A_i), Y(A_{i'})|\mathbf{Y}(\mathbf{B})) = (|A_i||A_{i'}|)^{-1} \int_{A_i} \int_{A_{i'}} C_\zeta(\mathbf{u}, \mathbf{v}) \, d\mathbf{u}d\mathbf{v} , \qquad (4.64)$$

which results in covariance matrix $\mathbf{C}_\zeta^A$. Observations $\mathbf{Z}(\mathbf{A})$ at the finer scale are made with measurement error; Wikle and Berliner assume that, conditional on $\mathbf{Y}(\mathbf{A})$, $\mathbf{Z}(\mathbf{A})$ has mean $\mathbf{Y}(\mathbf{A})$ and measurement-error covariance matrix $\mathbf{C}_\varepsilon^A$. This, along with (4.63) and (4.64), leads to the following BHM based on data $\mathbf{Z}(\mathbf{A})$:

Data model: Conditional on $\mathbf{Y(B)}$ and variance–covariance parameters, the data vector $\mathbf{Z(A)}$ has mean

$$\mathbf{G(A)'Y(B)},$$

where the ith row of $\mathbf{G(A)}$ is $\mathbf{G}(A_i)$; and $\mathbf{Z(A)}$ has covariance matrix,

$$\mathbf{C}_Z^A = \mathbf{C}_\zeta^A + \mathbf{C}_\varepsilon^A.$$

The conditional distribution is specified (e.g., a joint Gaussian distribution).

Process model: Conditional on process-model parameters, the joint distribution of $\mathbf{Y(B)}$ is specified (e.g., a joint Gaussian distribution).

Parameter model: The joint distribution of all unknown parameters is specified.

   The distributions in the data model and the process model are often assumed to be Gaussian, but they do not have to be; this hierarchical formulation of change-of-support allows more flexibility in modeling, because (fully specified) non-Gaussian distributions are just as welcome, provided they adapt well to obtaining the posterior distribution (e.g., through simulating full conditional distributions in an MCMC algorithm). Once the conditional distributions in the BHM above are specified, an MCMC algorithm can be derived and implemented. After "burn in," the MCMC yields realizations $\{\mathbf{Y(B)}^{(\ell)}: \ell = 1, \ldots, L\}$ from the posterior distribution,

$$[\mathbf{Y(B)}|\mathbf{Z(A)}],$$

and inference on nonlinear $\mathbf{g(Y(B))}$ is straightforward. For example, the conditional distribution,

$$[\exp\{Y(B_1)\}|\mathbf{Z(A)}],$$

is obtained simply by computing histograms from $\{\exp\{Y(B_1)^{(\ell)}\}: \ell = 1, \ldots, L\}$. Wikle and Berliner (2005) give the BHM for the general case where both finer-scale and coarser-scale data are available, and they use MCMC to simulate from the posterior distribution, $[\mathbf{Y(B)}|\mathbf{Z(A)}, \mathbf{Z(C)}]$.

4.1.4 Spatial Moving Average (SMA) Models

This section on geostatistical processes centers around modeling the covariance function or the variogram of a spatial process. Covariance functions sometimes come from physical processes, such as the exponential covariance function that is based on a proportional growth process, or the spherical covariance function that is based on the volume of intersecting spheres of equal radius, or the linear variogram that is based on Brownian motion (of gas molecules). When building HMs, it is very useful to have flexible classes of models at hand that exhibit spatial dependence.

In either a classical geostatistical setting or an HM setting, spatial statistical dependence is ubiquitously captured by the covariance function. Let $\{Y(\mathbf{s}): \mathbf{s} \in D_s \subset \mathbb{R}^d\}$ be a spatial process, where $\text{var}(Y(\mathbf{s})) < \infty; \mathbf{s} \in D_s$. Recall that $C_Y(\mathbf{s}, \mathbf{x}) = \text{cov}(Y(\mathbf{s}), Y(\mathbf{x}))$ or, in the second-order-stationary case, $C_Y(\mathbf{h}) = \text{cov}(Y(\mathbf{s}), Y(\mathbf{s} + \mathbf{h}))$. The semivariogram is $\gamma_Y(\mathbf{s}, \mathbf{x}) = (1/2)\text{var}(Y(\mathbf{s}) - Y(\mathbf{x}))$ or, in the intrinsically stationary case, $\gamma_Y(\mathbf{h}) = (1/2)\text{var}(Y(\mathbf{s} + \mathbf{h}) - Y(\mathbf{s}))$.

Recall that both $C_Y(\cdot)$ and $\gamma_Y(\cdot)$ have a spectral representation. Thus, by generating classes of models for the spectral distribution, we can generate classes of models for $C_Y(\cdot)$ or $\gamma_Y(\cdot)$ by inverting a Fourier transform. For example, the Matérn covariance function given by (4.6) with $\sigma_0^2 = 0$ and $\sigma_1^2 = 1$, has spectral density given by

$$f_Y(\boldsymbol{\omega}) = (\theta_1/\pi^{1/2})^d (\Gamma(\theta_2 + d/2)/\Gamma(\theta_2))(1 + \theta_1^2\|\boldsymbol{\omega}\|^2)^{-(\theta_2 + d/2)}, \quad (4.65)$$

where $\int f_Y(\boldsymbol{\omega}) \, d\boldsymbol{\omega} = 1$. Now the spectral representation of a covariance function is a decomposition of the covariation into an integral of the spectral density f_Y, weighted by cosines at various frequencies; see (4.15). Furthermore, the infinitesimal quantity $f_Y(\boldsymbol{\omega}) \, d\boldsymbol{\omega}$ can be attributed to an infinitesimal orthogonal random component. That is, in two dimensions, consider the spatial process defined by

$$Y(\mathbf{s}) = \int_{-\infty}^{\infty} \int_{-\infty}^{\infty} e^{i\boldsymbol{\omega}'\mathbf{s}} V_Y(d\boldsymbol{\omega}), \quad \mathbf{s} \in \mathbb{R}^2, \quad (4.66)$$

where $V_Y(\cdot)$ is a complex-valued random process with independent increments, $E(|V_Y(d\boldsymbol{\omega})|^2) = F_Y(d\boldsymbol{\omega})$, and $F_Y(d\boldsymbol{\omega}) = f_Y(\boldsymbol{\omega}) \, d\boldsymbol{\omega}$. Then $Y(\cdot)$ has stationary covariance function $C_Y(\cdot)$ given by (4.15).

The Spatial Moving Average (SMA) models use (4.66) to *motivate* the following construction of spatial dependence in a spatial process in $\mathbb{R}^d$. Consider starting directly with standard zero-mean, d-dimensional Brownian motion, $W(\cdot)$, and define the process,

$$Y(\mathbf{s}) \equiv \int k(\mathbf{s}, \mathbf{u}) W(d\mathbf{u}), \quad \mathbf{s} \in D_s, \quad (4.67)$$

where the kernel $k(\cdot, \cdot)$ satisfies $\int k(\mathbf{s}, \mathbf{u})^2 d\mathbf{u} < \infty$ for all $\mathbf{s} \in D_s$. We say that $Y(\cdot)$ defined by (4.67) is a *spatial moving average* with kernel $k(\cdot, \cdot)$.

Notice that $W(\cdot)$ is a (Gaussian) process with independent increments and $E(\{W(d\mathbf{u})\}^2) = d\mathbf{u}$, which, as is seen below, makes computation of the covariance function $C_Y(\cdot, \cdot)$ straightforward.

To explain "SMA," recall from Section 3.4.4 the Moving Average (MA) time-series model,

$$Y_t = \sum_{i=1}^{\infty} a_i \varepsilon_{t-i+1} ,$$

which is a linear combination of *iid* (Gaussian) random variables $\{\varepsilon_j\}$. Now, a discretized version of (4.67) is

$$Y(\mathbf{s}) = \sum_{i=1}^{\infty} k(\mathbf{s}, \mathbf{u}_i) \varepsilon(\mathbf{u}_i),$$

where $\{\mathbf{u}_i\}$ is a dense grid of spatial locations on D_s and $\varepsilon(\cdot)$ is a (Gaussian) white-noise process. Both the MA time series and the SMA spatial process are linear combinations of *iid* random variables. Notice that, in general, they *cannot* be written in terms of a Markov random field with sparse neighborhood structure (Section 4.2.2). In Section 4.2.8, we make the comment that SMA models align more naturally with geostatistical models than CAR or SAR models.

The representation (4.67) has also been called a *process convolution (PC)*; see Higdon (1998). Recall that the convolution $a \circ b$ of two functions a and b is defined as

$$(a \circ b)(\mathbf{s}) \equiv \int a(\mathbf{u}) b(\mathbf{s} - \mathbf{u}) \, d\mathbf{u}, \qquad \mathbf{s} \in \mathbb{R}^d .$$

We see that (4.67) is a slightly more general *random* version of this. The advantage of having $k(\mathbf{s}, \mathbf{u})$ not be a function of $(\mathbf{s} - \mathbf{u})$ is obvious, since (4.67) can generate larger, nonstationary classes of (Gaussian) processes.

In this section, we have paid particular attention to covariance properties of various $Y(\cdot)$. From (4.67), spatial covariances for SMA models can be easily calculated:

$$C_Y(\mathbf{s}, \mathbf{x}) \equiv \text{cov}(Y(\mathbf{s}), Y(\mathbf{x})) = \int \int k(\mathbf{s}, \mathbf{u}) k(\mathbf{x}, \mathbf{v}) E(W(d\mathbf{u}) W(d\mathbf{v}))$$

$$= \int k(\mathbf{s}, \mathbf{u}) k(\mathbf{x}, \mathbf{u}) \, d\mathbf{u}, \tag{4.68}$$

because of orthogonality of the increments of $W(\cdot)$. In general, this is *not* a function of $(\mathbf{s} - \mathbf{x})$. Furthermore, the semivariogram is

$$\gamma(\mathbf{s}, \mathbf{x}) = (1/2)C_Y(\mathbf{s}, \mathbf{s}) + (1/2)C_Y(\mathbf{x}, \mathbf{x}) - C_Y(\mathbf{s}, \mathbf{x}), \tag{4.69}$$

which, in general, is not a function of $(\mathbf{s} - \mathbf{x})$ either. That is, in general, SMA models are *not* stationary. Higdon, Swall, and Kern (1999) give examples of kernels $k(\cdot, \cdot)$ that lead to nonstationary spatial models. The kernel $k(\cdot, \cdot)$ can be parameterized, which in turn leads to a parametric form for the covariance function (4.68) and its associated semivariogram (4.69). Alternatively, specifying the kernel in terms of support points leads to a "predictive process" approach (Banerjee et al., 2008, Finley et al. 2009).

Recall that classical geostatistics is often involved with building models of stationary covariance functions or stationary semivariograms. Are there choices of kernels $k(\cdot, \cdot)$ that yield these classical geostatistical models? For example, can (4.68) be used to obtain the spherical covariance function referred to in Section 4.1.1? In general, it cannot, although Cressie and Pavlicova (2002) show how a $k(\cdot, \cdot)$ can be chosen so that (4.68) is stationary and has the same range, sill, and derivative at the origin as the spherical covariance function. When simulating geostatistical models, the advantage of using the SMA model (4.67) is immediately obvious: Classical geostatistical simulations are much more cumbersome [e.g., the turning-bands method due to Matheron (1973); or Gaussian sequential simulation due to Deutsch and Journel (1992)] than SMA-based simulations.

If we assume that the kernel $k(\cdot, \cdot)$ in (4.67) is continuous and square integrable on $\mathbb{R}^d \times \mathbb{R}^d$, then, from Wahba (1990, p. 3), it can be written as

$$k(\mathbf{s}, \mathbf{u}) = \sum_{j=1}^{\infty} v_j \phi_j(\mathbf{s}) \phi_j(\mathbf{u}), \tag{4.70}$$

where $v_1 \geq v_2 \geq \cdots$ are eigenvalues and $\{\phi_j(\cdot) : j = 1, 2, \ldots\}$ are orthonormal eigenvectors (i.e., $\int \phi_j(\mathbf{u}) \phi_k(\mathbf{u}) d\mathbf{u} = I(j = k)$) that solve the Fredholm integral equation:

$$\int k(\mathbf{s}, \mathbf{u}) \phi_j(\mathbf{u}) \, d\mathbf{u} = v_j \phi_j(\mathbf{s}), \qquad j = 1, 2, \ldots. \tag{4.71}$$

From (4.67),

$$Y(\mathbf{s}) = \sum_{j=1}^{\infty} v_j \phi_j(\mathbf{s}) \int \phi_j(\mathbf{u}) W(d\mathbf{u})$$

$$\equiv \sum_{j=1}^{\infty} v_j V_j \phi_j(\mathbf{s}), \tag{4.72}$$

where $\{V_j\}$ are zero-mean orthonormal random variables, as we now demonstrate:

$$E(V_j \cdot V_k) = \int \int \phi_j(\mathbf{u}) \phi_k(\mathbf{v}) E(dW(\mathbf{u}) \cdot dW(\mathbf{v}))$$

$$= \int \phi_j(\mathbf{u}) \phi_k(\mathbf{u}) \, d\mathbf{u}$$

$$= I(j = k). \tag{4.73}$$

Furthermore, because $W(\cdot)$ is Brownian motion, $\{V_j\}$ in (4.72) is a sequence of *iid* standard Gaussian random variables. If we write (4.72) as

$$Y(\mathbf{s}) = \sum_{j=1}^{\infty} \alpha_j \phi_j(\mathbf{s}),$$

where $\alpha_j \equiv v_j V_j$, then $\{\alpha_j\}$ are independent random variables such that $\mathrm{var}(\alpha_j) = v_j^2$. Notice that the orthonormal eigenvectors $\{\phi_j(\cdot)\}$ capture the spatial structure directly.

Due to the orthonormality given by (4.73), the covariance function of $Y(\cdot)$ defined by (4.67) or (4.72) follows easily as

$$C_Y(\mathbf{s}, \mathbf{x}) = \sum_{j=1}^{\infty} v_j^2 \phi_j(\mathbf{s}) \phi_j(\mathbf{x}), \tag{4.74}$$

which is often referred to as a Karhunen–Loéve expansion. Now, any positive-definite function that is continuous and square integrable on $\mathbb{R}^d \times \mathbb{R}^d$ has a Karhunen–Loéve expansion with nonnegative eigenvalues (e.g., Papoulis, 1965, pp. 457–461). Through (4.67), we have shown that such covariance functions can be obtained from a process $Y(\cdot)$ that is a spatial moving average of Brownian motion.

The result (4.74) is a consequence of Mercer's Theorem: For any positive-definite function $C(\mathbf{s}, \mathbf{x})$, there are *nonnegative* eigenvalues $\{\kappa_j : j = 1, 2, \ldots\}$ and eigenfunctions $\{\phi_j(\cdot) : j = 1, 2, \ldots\}$ corresponding to the eigensystem, $\int C(s, x)\phi(s)\,ds = \kappa \phi(x)$, such that $C(\mathbf{s}, \mathbf{x}) = \sum_{j=1}^{\infty} \kappa_j \phi_j(s)\phi_j(x)$, where the domain is $a \leq x, s \leq b$, for $a < b$.

The representation (4.72) is interesting in its own right. Notice that $Y(\cdot)$ is a linear combination of deterministic basis functions $\{\phi_j(\cdot) : j = 1, 2, \ldots\}$; the randomness in the process $Y(\cdot)$ comes from the randomness in the *coefficients* $\{\alpha_j = v_j V_j : j = 1, \ldots, n\}$, which do not depend on spatial location.

Let $\{\mathbf{s}_1, \ldots, \mathbf{s}_n\}$ be a set of n sites, at which $Y(\cdot)$ is evaluated. The resulting vector $\mathbf{Y} \equiv (Y(\mathbf{s}_1), \ldots, Y(\mathbf{s}_n))'$ has covariance matrix, $\boldsymbol{\Sigma}_Y \equiv \mathrm{var}(\mathbf{Y})$. Now, a principal components analysis yields

$$\boldsymbol{\Sigma}_Y = \boldsymbol{\Psi} \, \mathrm{diag}(\lambda_1, \ldots, \lambda_n) \, \boldsymbol{\Psi}', \qquad \boldsymbol{\Psi}'\boldsymbol{\Psi} = \mathbf{I} = \boldsymbol{\Psi}\boldsymbol{\Psi}', \tag{4.75}$$

where $\lambda_1 \geq \lambda_2 \geq \cdots \geq \lambda_n \geq 0$. Write $\boldsymbol{\Psi} = (\boldsymbol{\psi}_1, \ldots, \boldsymbol{\psi}_n)$ and the kth column of $\boldsymbol{\Psi}$ as

$$\boldsymbol{\psi}_k = (\psi_k(\mathbf{s}_1), \ldots, \psi_k(\mathbf{s}_n))', \qquad k = 1, \ldots, n. \tag{4.76}$$

The vectors $\{\boldsymbol{\psi}_1, \ldots, \boldsymbol{\psi}_n\}$ are sometimes referred to as the *empirical orthogonal functions (EOFs)*, although strictly speaking the orthogonal functions should not be called "empirical" until an estimate $\widehat{\boldsymbol{\Sigma}}_Y$ is used in place of $\boldsymbol{\Sigma}_Y$

above (Section 5.3). Define $a_k \equiv \boldsymbol{\psi}_k' \mathbf{Y}$, $k = 1, \ldots, n$. Then the orthogonality allows us to write

$$Y(\mathbf{s}_i) = \sum_{k=1}^{n} a_k \psi_k(\mathbf{s}_i), \qquad i = 1, \ldots, n, \tag{4.77}$$

where $a_1, \ldots, a_n$ are uncorrelated with variances given by $\lambda_1, \ldots, \lambda_n$, respectively. Again, we see that $\mathbf{Y}$ is a random linear combination of basis vectors $\{\boldsymbol{\psi}_j : j = 1, \ldots, n\}$. That is, the decomposition in (4.77) of $\{Y(\mathbf{s}_i)\}$ in terms of EOFs is a finite-spatial-location version of the expressions (4.67) or (4.72).

Consider the general spectral expansion,

$$Y(\mathbf{s}_i) = \sum_{k=1}^{n} \alpha_k \phi_k(\mathbf{s}_i), \qquad i = 1, \ldots, n, \tag{4.78}$$

where $\{\phi_k(\cdot)\}$ are complete and orthonormal on $\{\mathbf{s}_1, \ldots, \mathbf{s}_n\}$. As discussed in Section 3.5.2, one distinct advantage of such a spectral decomposition is the decorrelation it induces. For example, recall that if $\{\phi_k(\mathbf{s}_i)\}$ are Fourier basis functions, then $\{\alpha_k\}$ are approximately uncorrelated. This property can be used to perform efficient spatial prediction on a discrete lattice for very large n. Consider $\mathbf{Y} \sim Gau(\mathbf{0}, \boldsymbol{\Sigma}_Y)$, where $\mathbf{Y}$ is an n-dimensional vector. Given that $\mathbf{Y} = \boldsymbol{\Phi}\boldsymbol{\alpha}$ and $\boldsymbol{\alpha} = \boldsymbol{\Phi}'\mathbf{Y}$, we note that $\boldsymbol{\alpha} \sim Gau(\mathbf{0}, \boldsymbol{\Sigma}_\alpha)$, where $\boldsymbol{\Sigma}_\alpha \equiv \boldsymbol{\Phi}'\boldsymbol{\Sigma}_Y\boldsymbol{\Phi}$. With the choice of basis functions such that $\boldsymbol{\Sigma}_\alpha$ is diagonal (or reasonably approximated by a diagonal) matrix, say $\mathbf{D}$, one can show that the matrix inverses used in the kriging formulations only require the inverse of a diagonal matrix, *greatly* simplifying computations. In addition, for the case where $\boldsymbol{\Phi}$ is made up of discrete Fourier basis functions or certain classes of wavelet basis functions, then discrete Fourier transforms or multiresolution transforms (or their associated inverse transforms) can be used in place of matrix multiplication involving $\boldsymbol{\Phi}$ (or $\boldsymbol{\Phi}'$), so that $\boldsymbol{\Phi}$ need not actually be stored. This allows the spectral approach to spatial prediction to be used on *very large* spatial domains.

The spectral approach to spatial prediction can be used when the form of the covariance function is known and stationary (e.g., Wikle, 2002b; Royle and Wikle, 2005; Paciorek, 2007; Lindgren et al., 2011) or when it is unknown and/or nonstationary (e.g., Davis, 1952; Nychka, Wikle, and Royle, 2002; Pavlicova, Santner, and Cressie, 2008; Yue and Speckman, 2010). For example, in the case of the former, assume that a Matérn covariance structure is specified, in which case $\boldsymbol{\Sigma}_Y$ will depend on parameters $\boldsymbol{\theta}$ as shown in (4.6). In this case, if $\boldsymbol{\Phi}$ is made up of Fourier basis functions, then the diagonal matrix $\mathbf{D}$ is also parameterized in terms of the same parameters by using the spectral representation of the Matérn covariance function (e.g., see Royle and Wikle, 2005). Perhaps more importantly, in the BHM framework, such spectral parameterizations can be used in the process model when one has non-Gaussian data models (Wikle, 2002b; Hooten, Larsen, and Wikle, 2003; Royle and Wikle, 2005; Paciorek, 2007). This is a theme we pick up again in the dynamical spatio-temporal setting (Section 7.1.3).

Return to the case where spatial index $\mathbf{s} \in D_s$; one possible parameterization of $k(\mathbf{s}, \mathbf{u})$ in (4.67) might be to restrict $v_{p+1} = v_{p+2} = \cdots = 0$, resulting in

$$k(\mathbf{s}, \mathbf{u}) = \sum_{j=1}^{p} v_j \phi_j(\mathbf{s}) \phi_j(\mathbf{u}) \quad \text{and} \quad Y(\mathbf{s}) = \sum_{j=1}^{p} v_j V_j \phi_j(\mathbf{s}) . \tag{4.79}$$

This generates a class of *models* whose parameter space is defined by the integer p and positive real numbers $\{v_j : j = 1, \ldots, p\}$. The randomness in $Y(\cdot)$ comes from (4.79). The model (4.79) should *not* be confused with (4.75) and (4.77), which give the EOF *representation* obtained from the covariance matrix $\mathbf{\Sigma}_Y$.

Finally, we emphasize that SMA models, or their discrete versions, are usually defined as moving averages of *uncorrelated* random variables. By reducing the number of random variables but allowing them to be correlated, a low-dimensional but highly flexible class of spatial processes can be generated.

Let $\boldsymbol{\alpha} \equiv (\alpha_1, \ldots, \alpha_{p_\alpha})'$ be a p_α-dimensional random vector with $\text{var}(\boldsymbol{\alpha}) = \mathbf{\Sigma}_\alpha$. Then the smooth *Spatial Random Effects* model is

$$Y(\mathbf{s}) = \sum_{i=1}^{p_\alpha} \phi_i(\mathbf{s}) \alpha_i = \boldsymbol{\phi}(\mathbf{s})' \boldsymbol{\alpha}, \qquad \mathbf{s} \in D_s , \tag{4.80}$$

for $\boldsymbol{\phi}(\cdot) \equiv (\phi_i(\cdot) : i = 1, \ldots, p_\alpha)'$ a p_α-dimensional vector of specified basis functions (which may or may not be orthogonal). In this book, we continue to call (4.80) a spectral decomposition, even though the basis functions may no longer be orthogonal and $\{\alpha_i\}$ may no longer be independent.

The covariance function of $Y(\cdot)$ is nonstationary and given by

$$C_Y(\mathbf{s}, \mathbf{x}) = \boldsymbol{\phi}(\mathbf{s})' \mathbf{\Sigma}_\alpha \boldsymbol{\phi}(\mathbf{x}) . \tag{4.81}$$

This spatial covariance model (with bisquare spatial basis functions) was used by Cressie and Johannesson (2006, 2008) for kriging of very large datasets, resulting in a methodology they called *Fixed Rank Kriging*. Optimal spatial prediction (Section 4.1.2) based on the covariance function (4.81) is computationally efficient, representing an improvement in order of computation over covariance tapering (Furrer, Genton, and Nychka, 2006). For discussion on various choices of basis functions, see Wikle (2010b).

4.1.5 Multivariate Geostatistical Processes

So far, this chapter has concentrated on a univariate spatial process $Y(\cdot)$. Phenomena typically do not act alone, although they might be studied in isolation. There have been two paths taken to model multivariate spatial data: The *joint-distribution path* has predominated, but we believe that the *conditional-distribution path* comes closer to modeling the etiology of how phenomena interact.

Let $\mathbf{Y}(\cdot) \equiv (Y_1(\cdot), \ldots, Y_K(\cdot))'$ denote a vector of K spatial processes observed over the same spatial domain D_s. The joint-distribution path involves defining and estimating measures of cross-dependence, such as the cross-variogram, the pseudo-cross-variogram, the cross-covariance function, and the generalized cross-covariance function. Künsch, Papritz, and Bassi (1997) are the clearest on the relationship between these measures, showing that the most satisfactory summary is the generalized cross-covariance function.

The conditional-distribution path is natural when one has scientific knowledge about how $Y_2(\cdot)$ behaves given knowledge about $Y_1(\cdot)$, where for illustration we have considered the case $K = 2$. Then, because of the probability decomposition, $[Y_1(\cdot), Y_2(\cdot)] = [Y_2(\cdot)|Y_1(\cdot)][Y_1(\cdot)]$, it is more natural to model $Y_2(\cdot)$ *conditionally* on $Y_1(\cdot)$ rather than jointly with $Y_1(\cdot)$. Royle and Berliner (1999) propose this approach and it is discussed further in the paper by Gelfand et al. (2004). We would like to return to this discussion and offer a fresh perspective on it.

A basic goal of spatial statistical modeling in a multivariate setting is the specification of a *valid* model for $\mathbf{Y}(\cdot)$ based on first and second moments. That is, for *any* positive integer n_k and locations $\{\mathbf{s}_{k1}, \ldots, \mathbf{s}_{kn_k}\}$, $k = 1, \ldots, K$, the $(\sum_{k=1}^{K} n_k) \times (\sum_{k=1}^{K} n_k)$ covariance matrix,

$$\text{var}(Y_1(\mathbf{s}_{11}), \ldots, Y_1(\mathbf{s}_{1n_1}), \ldots, Y_K(\mathbf{s}_{K1}), \ldots, Y_K(\mathbf{s}_{Kn_K})),$$

is *always* positive-definite. Any multivariate spatial model must achieve this. Only then can the model be compared to others, based on such criteria as interpretability, simplicity, and ease of use in inference (including ease of computing). A major problem with the joint-distribution path has been the difficulty in specifying parametric models of between-variable spatial dependence that result in a valid multivariate spatial model for $\mathbf{Y}(\cdot)$. Ver Hoef and Barry (1998) and Ver Hoef, Cressie, and Barry (2004) achieve this through spatial moving average (SMA) models (Section 4.1.4). Banerjee, Carlin, and Gelfand (2004, Chapter 7) and Gelfand et al. (2004) achieve this through the Linear Model of Coregionalization (LMC), given here for $K = 2$. Define

$$\mathbf{Y}(\mathbf{s}) = \mathbf{A}\mathbf{W}(\mathbf{s}) \equiv (\mathbf{a}_1 \ \mathbf{a}_2) \begin{pmatrix} W_1(\mathbf{s}) \\ W_2(\mathbf{s}) \end{pmatrix}, \qquad \mathbf{s} \in D_s, \qquad (4.82)$$

where $\mathbf{Y}(\cdot) \equiv (Y_1(\cdot), Y_2(\cdot))'$, $\mathbf{A} \equiv (\mathbf{a}_1, \mathbf{a}_2)$ is a 2×2 matrix, and $W_1(\cdot)$ and $W_2(\cdot)$ are two independent stationary random processes with mean 0 and variance 1. Consequently,

$$\text{cov}(\mathbf{Y}(\mathbf{s}), \mathbf{Y}(\mathbf{x})) = \mathbf{a}_1\mathbf{a}_1'\rho_1(\mathbf{s} - \mathbf{x}) + \mathbf{a}_2\mathbf{a}_2'\rho_2(\mathbf{s} - \mathbf{x}),$$

where $\rho_k(\cdot)$ is the correlation (also covariance) function associated with $W_k(\cdot)$; $k = 1, 2$.

From the expression above, it is easy to see that the LMC has a very strong symmetry assumption, namely,

$$\text{cov}(Y_1(\mathbf{s}), Y_2(\mathbf{x})) = \text{cov}(Y_1(\mathbf{x}), Y_2(\mathbf{s})).$$

For example, when applied to (the average maximum and minimum) temperature and precipitation on a given day, this assumption says that the covariance of temperature in St. Louis, MO, with precipitation in Columbus, OH, is *equal to* the covariance of precipitation in St Louis, MO, with temperature in Columbus, OH. This is a strong constraint to put on the joint distribution, and it limits the modeler's ability to capture properly the between-variable spatial dependence. Gelfand et al. (2004) emphasize the LMC's computational advantages in a BHM.

The conditional-distribution path has a distinct advantage over the joint-distribution path, since it allows a valid spatial multivariate model to be built with relative ease, as we set out below. We choose $K = 2$, and hence $\mathbf{Y}(\mathbf{s}) \equiv (Y_1(\mathbf{s}), Y_2(\mathbf{s}))'$; $\mathbf{s} \in D_s$, since the exposition is clearest in this case. Then, from scientific considerations, there is often a natural ordering for conditioning. Here we model the process $Y_1(\cdot)$ given $Y_2(\cdot)$ for illustration, although if there is no natural ordering, one could simply be chosen. Now consider the processes defined on the discretized finite grid, $\{\mathbf{s}_1, \ldots, \mathbf{s}_n\}$, and write $\mathbf{Y}_k \equiv (Y_k(\mathbf{s}_1), \ldots, Y_k(\mathbf{s}_n))'$; $k = 1, 2$. The conditional-probability path is based on the decomposition,

$$[\mathbf{Y}_1, \mathbf{Y}_2] = [\mathbf{Y}_2 | \mathbf{Y}_1][\mathbf{Y}_1],$$

where for the purposes of illustration we assume the left-hand side has a joint Gaussian distribution with mean zero. Hence,

$$\mathbf{Y}_2 | \mathbf{Y}_1 \sim Gau(\mathbf{BY}_1, \boldsymbol{\Sigma}_{2|1})$$
$$\mathbf{Y}_1 \sim Gau(\mathbf{0}, \boldsymbol{\Sigma}_{11}).$$

$$(4.83)$$

The *mechanistic* model of $\mathbf{Y}_2 | \mathbf{Y}_1$ determines the form of $\mathbf{B}$ (which is any $n \times n$ matrix) and $\boldsymbol{\Sigma}_{2|1}$ (which is any $n \times n$ symmetric positive-definite matrix). Finally, $\boldsymbol{\Sigma}_{11}$ is specified (as any $n \times n$ positive-definite matrix) to complete the model.

We wish to emphasize that (4.83) requires specification of only two positive-definite matrices, something that spatial statistical modelers are very experienced with. There is *no* requirement of specifying any cross-dependence, since it is already captured in the regression relationship, $E(\mathbf{Y}_2 | \mathbf{Y}_1) = \mathbf{BY}_1$, and $\mathbf{B}$ is completely general. This is key, since validity of the joint model is guaranteed no matter how $\mathbf{B}$ is chosen. In fact, from (4.83), the joint model's moments follow straightforwardly as

$$\text{var}(\mathbf{Y}_2) = \boldsymbol{\Sigma}_{2|1} + \mathbf{B}\boldsymbol{\Sigma}_{11}\mathbf{B}',$$
$$\text{var}(\mathbf{Y}_1) = \boldsymbol{\Sigma}_{11},$$

and

$$\text{cov}(\mathbf{Y}_1, \mathbf{Y}_2) = \mathbf{B}\boldsymbol{\Sigma}_{11}.$$

It is this last quantity, $\operatorname{cov}(\mathbf{Y}_1, \mathbf{Y}_2)$ that causes modelers taking the joint-probability path so much trouble. They, too, have to specify two positive-definite matrices ($\operatorname{var}(\mathbf{Y}_1)$ and $\operatorname{var}(\mathbf{Y}_2)$), but whatever model they choose for $\operatorname{cov}(Y_1(\cdot), Y_2(\cdot))$, the $2n \times 2n$ matrix,

$$
\begin{bmatrix}
\operatorname{var}(\mathbf{Y}_1) & \operatorname{cov}(\mathbf{Y}_1, \mathbf{Y}_2) \\
\operatorname{cov}(\mathbf{Y}_2, \mathbf{Y}_1) & \operatorname{var}(\mathbf{Y}_2)
\end{bmatrix}
$$

has to be symmetric and positive-definite for the model to be valid. Notice that after choosing two positive-definite matrices, the conditional-distribution path (4.83) results in a bivariate model that is automatically valid, no matter what $\mathbf{B}$ is chosen. See the Bibliographic Notes in Section 4.5 for further discussion.

4.1.6 Other Topics

Change-of-Resolution Spatial Models

In this topic, we present an example of a spatial HM that has strong computational and change-of-support features. Our goal is to illustrate the breadth of the hierarchical-modeling approach. Geostatistical processes can be aggregated from the point level to regions; Section 4.1.3 shows how the mean and covariance functions of the regions are determined by the point-level geostatistical model. In practice, computational problems can arise when data are massive and there are change-of-support issues associated with data being of differing resolutions than that of the process to be predicted. Multiresolution models give a consistent way to build the process model over partitions of the spatial region $D_s \subset \mathbb{R}^d$, that nest successively within each other. Multiresolutional models are a powerful way to look at data with different spatial scales of variation (e.g., Ferreira and Lee, 2007; Gramacy and Lee, 2008; Pasanen and Holmström, 2008; Jansen, Nason, and Silverman, 2009).

The following exposition is adapted from Huang, Cressie, and Gabrosek (2002). Let $\{D(i, r): i = 1, \ldots, n_r\}$, for *each* resolution-index $r = 0, \ldots, R$, be a family of *disjoint partitions* of D_s such that

$$
D(i, r) = \bigcup_{j=1}^{m_r} D(ch_j(i, r)), \qquad (i, r) \in \mathcal{N}_{R-1},
$$

where $\{ch_j(i, r): j = 1, \ldots, m_r\}$ indexes the m_r *children cells* of $D(i, r)$; $m_0, \ldots, m_{R-1}$ are the *aperture (i.e., resolution) changes*; and $\mathcal{N}_k \equiv \{(i, r): i = 1, \ldots, n_r, r = 0, \ldots, k\}$. Hence, there are multiresolution partitions of D_s with a tree-structured parent–children relationship between cells (pixels) at adjacent resolutions.

Let $\{Y(\mathbf{s}): \mathbf{s} \in D_s\}$ be a real-valued univariate spatial process (i.e., a geostatistical process) that is defined on D_s. Based on the partitioning $\{D(i, r)\}$, define the multiresolution, aggregated Y-process as

$$
Y(i, r) \equiv \frac{1}{v(i, r)} \int_{D(i,r)} Y(\mathbf{s}) \, d\mathbf{s}, \qquad (i, r) \in \mathcal{N}_R,
$$

where $v(i, r) \equiv |D(i, r)|$ is the volume of $D(i,r)$. Hence, $\{Y(\cdot, r)\}$ represents the resolution-r values associated with the process $Y(\cdot)$; $r = 0, \ldots, R$. Furthermore, denote by

$$\mathbf{Y}(ch(i, r)) \equiv (Y(ch_1(i, r)), \ldots, Y(ch_{m_r}(i, r)))', \qquad (i, r) \in \mathcal{N}_{R-1},$$

the vector of the aggregated process on the children cells of *(i,r)*, which are values defined at resolution *(r + 1)*. The vector of all resolution-r values is denoted by

$$\mathbf{Y}(r) \equiv (Y(1, r), \ldots, Y(n_r, r))', \qquad r = 0, \ldots, R.$$

In what follows, we define the *data model* via a linear statistical relationship between data and the hidden process Y, and we define the *process model* as a coarse-to-fine, change-of-resolution autoregression in Y.

At each resolution *(r + 1)*, we have (potentially) observed data $\{\mathbf{Z}(ch(i, r))\}$ that are assumed to be related to the process Y at resolution *(r + 1)*, according to an additive-measurement-error model.

Data model: Conditional on σ^2, $\mathbf{V}(ch(i, r))$, and $\mathbf{Y}(ch(i, r))$,

$$\mathbf{Z}(ch(i, r)) = \mathbf{H}(ch(i, r))\mathbf{Y}(ch(i, r)) + \boldsymbol{v}(ch(i, r)),$$

$(i, r) \in \mathcal{V} \subseteq \mathcal{N}_{R-1}$, where $\mathbf{H}(ch(i, r))$ is a known incidence matrix and $\boldsymbol{v}(ch(i, r)) \sim ind. Gau(\mathbf{0}, \sigma^2 \mathbf{V}(ch(i, r)))$, independently of $\mathbf{Y}(\cdot)$.

The data vector $\mathbf{Z}(ch(i, r))$ is sometimes the same length as $\mathbf{Y}(ch(i, r))$, with each element being a direct measurement of the corresponding element of $\mathbf{Y}(ch(i, r))$; in that case, $\mathbf{H}(ch(i, r)) = \mathbf{I}$. However, $\mathbf{Z}(ch(i, r))$ may have some missing data (i.e., some of the elements of $\mathbf{Y}(ch(i, r))$ may be unobserved); in that case, $\mathbf{H}(ch(i, r))$ is an incidence matrix of zeros and ones that matches each of the observed elements of $\mathbf{Z}(ch(i, r))$ to its corresponding element of $\mathbf{Y}(ch(i, r))$. The measurement-error covariance matrices $\{\sigma^2 \mathbf{V}(ch(i, r))\}$ are typically diagonal, corresponding to independent measurement errors.

Instead of specifying the spatial covariance structure of $Y(\cdot)$ directly, spatial dependence is introduced in the process model indirectly through the following coarse-to-fine-resolution model:

Process model: Conditional on $\mathbf{W}(ch(i, r))$,

$$\mathbf{Y}(ch(i, r)) = Y(i, r)\mathbf{1} + \boldsymbol{\omega}(ch(i, r)); \quad (i, r) \in \mathcal{N}_{R-1},$$

where $\boldsymbol{\omega}(ch(i, r)) \sim ind. Gau(\mathbf{0}, \sigma^2 \mathbf{W}(ch(i, r)))$, independently of $Y(i,r)$.

The spatial dependence in $\mathbf{Y}(\cdot)$ depends on the variation in the process-model errors $\{\boldsymbol{\omega}(ch(i, r))\}$, where smaller variation results in stronger spatial dependence. As such, the spatial dependence is indirectly specified through the covariance matrices $\{\sigma^2 \mathbf{W}(ch(i, r))\}$; while σ^2 is known through the data model, the elements of $\mathbf{W}$ contain parameters that require estimation (EHM) or a prior distribution (BHM). The process model is then fully specified, once a distribution is specified at the coarsest resolution.

Process model, ctd: Conditional on $\mathbf{a}(0)$, σ^2, and $\mathbf{R}(0)$,

$$\mathbf{Y}(0) \sim Gau(\mathbf{a}(0), \sigma^2 \mathbf{R}(0)).$$

This resolution-0 process model, along with a recursive use of the coarse-to-fine-resolution process model, yields the distribution of Y (at all aggregated resolutions) to be multivariate Gaussian:

$$\mathbf{Y}(ch(i, r)) \sim Gau(\mathbf{a}(ch(i, r)), \sigma^2 \mathbf{R}(ch(i, r))), \quad (i, r) \in \mathcal{N}_{R-1},$$

where $\mathbf{a}(ch(i, r))$ and $\mathbf{R}(ch(i, r))$ are derived via successive application of the coarse-to-fine-resolution process model just above. Given the data $\{\mathbf{Z}(ch(i, r))\}$, we are able to derive the *posterior distribution* of Y at *all* resolutions using a change-of-resolution Kalman filter (Chou, Willsky, and Nikoukhah, 1994). The derivation consists of two steps, the leaves-to-root filtering step and the root-to-leaves smoothing step (Huang, Cressie, and Gabrosek, 2002). In a sense, the change-of-resolution in the process model sets up an ordering in space to which a type of Kalman filter can be applied. A spatio-temporal version of the multiresolution model presented below can be found in Section 7.2.7.

Example: Total Column Ozone

Total column ozone (TCO) data from the Total Ozone Mapping Spectrometer (TOMS) instrument from October 5, 1998 are shown in Figure 4.7. These data are part of a spatio-temporal dataset analyzed by Johannesson, Cressie, and Huang (2007); the figure shows a considerable amount of missing data associated with different orbits of the satellite on that day.

At the very finest resolution (resolution R), the pixels are $1°$ latitude $\times 1.25°$ longitude; thus, there are $n_R = 288 \times 180 = 51,840$ pixels that cover the globe. The (level 3) data released by the U.S. National Aeronautics and Space Administration (NASA) are at this resolution; there is none at any coarser resolutions $R - 1, \ldots, 0$. Thus, the data model above is quite simple: It is only nontrivial at resolution R, where the matrix $\mathbf{H}$ serves to annihilate pixels whose data are missing.

The posterior mean of Y at resolution R is shown in the top panel of Figure 4.8, and the corresponding posterior standard deviation is shown in the bottom panel of Figure 4.8. (Parameter estimates are "plugged into" the posterior mean and standard deviation.)

Parameters specified in the process model are estimated using composite-likelihood methods, and hence this multiresolution modeling takes an EHM

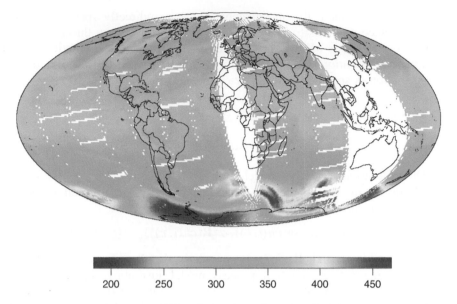

200   250   300   350   400   450

Figure 4.7 Total column ozone (TCO) data retrieved from the TOMS instrument on October 5, 1988. Regions of the globe in white depict places where no data were retrieved. Low (high) TCO values are shown in blue (red).

approach. More details of the model and the computational algorithms associated with it can be found in Huang, Cressie, and Gabrosek (2002), Tzeng, Huang, and Cressie (2005), and Johannesson, Cressie, and Huang (2007).

What makes this EHM particularly attractive is its computational advantage; the computational cost of deriving the posterior distribution is linear in the number of parent cells, namely $O(\sum_{r=0}^{R-1} m_r^3 n_r)$. Fixed Rank Kriging referred to in Section 4.1.4 is also linear in the data size, namely $O(n_R)$. These are in contrast to many traditional spatial modeling approaches, for example, classical kriging presented in Section 4.1.2, where the computational cost is cubic in the size of the data, namely $O(n_R^3)$.

Spatial Sampling Design
Fedorov (1972) is an early reference to research carried out in spatial sampling design; it has become an area of considerable activity in the last ten years. The monograph by Müller (2000) gives a snapshot of the literature at the beginning of the period, and Le and Zidek (2006, Chapter 11) is devoted to environmental network design. Two comprehensive articles should be consulted for different approaches, one taking a design-based approach (Stevens and Olsen, 2004) and the other taking a model-based approach (Diggle, Menezes, and Su, 2010) to spatial sampling. There have been many articles in the last 20 years, including Cressie, Gotway, and Grondona (1990), Overton and Stehman (1996), Brus and de Gruijter (1997), Cressie (1998b), Aldworth and Cressie (1999), Berliner, Lu, and Snyder (1999), Wikle and Royle (1999), Martin (2001), Thompson (2002),

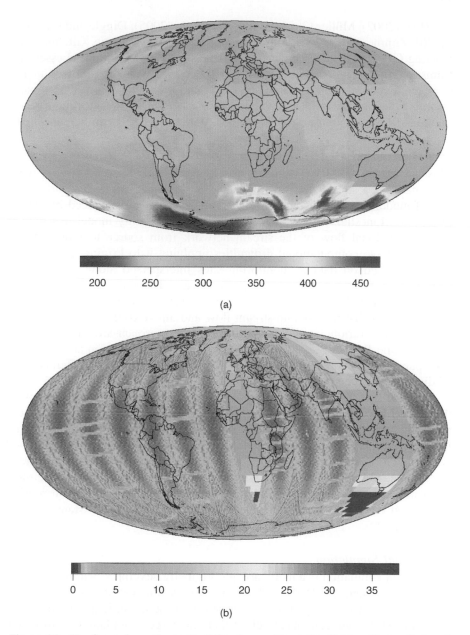

(a)

(b)

Figure 4.8 The figure shows the result of the change-of-resolution Kalman filter applied to the TOMS data retrieved on October 5, 1988, shown in Figure 4.7. **Top panel:** Posterior mean of the latent process Y at its finest possible resolution. **Bottom panel:** Posterior standard deviation of the latent process Y; notice large standard deviations in regions of the globe where data are missing.

Ver Hoef (2002), Müller (2005), Wikle and Royle (2005), Diggle and Lophaven (2006), Zimmerman (2006), Marchant and Lark (2007), Irvine, Gitelman, and Hoeting (2007), Dobbie, Henderson, and Stevens (2008), Munoz, Lesser, and Ramsay (2008), Müller and Stehlík (2010), and Nowak (2010). The area of computer experiments has a large literature that is very closely related to spatial sampling design. An early review paper is Sacks et al. (1989); for more recent literature, the book by Santner, Notz, and Williams (2003) can be consulted.

Spatial Statistical Models on Stream Networks and the Sphere

Most spatial models have spatial index in Euclidean space. However, when the "space" is a stream network, statistical dependence can be directional and spatial models are needed where Euclidean distances are replaced by stream distances. Monestiez et al. (2005) developed a probability model that reflects the unidirectional flow of the stream network from source to mouth. However, they have computational difficulties applying it to kriging at all stream locations based on data at monitoring sites interspersed along the network. Cressie et al. (2006) and Ver Hoef, Peterson, and Theobald (2006) use spatial moving average (SMA) models on a generic stream network to define valid spatial models that incorporate stream flow and allow kriging in a straightforward manner. Various applications of the SMA approach are summarized in Ver Hoef and Peterson (2010) and the accompanying discussion and rejoinder. That paper also features models of spatial dependence involving different types of directional dependence; fish can swim upstream

Banerjee (2005) and Jun and Stein (2008) consider covariance functions on the sphere. Distances that are no longer Euclidean require special care because a simple substitution into a (Euclidean-distance) isotropic covariance function can yield invalid models; for example, the validity of the spatio-temporal covariance function used by Cressie and Majure (1997) was assumed but may not be true. Curriero (2006) discusses the use of non-Euclidean distance measures in geostatistics; even in Euclidean space, anisotropy of a spatial process might lead one to use non-Euclidean distances (e.g., Boisvert, Manchuk, and Beutsch, 2009).

Conditional Simulation

Conditional simulation is a methodology originally developed within geostatistics (e.g., Journel, 1974) that allows one to see the variability of a spatial process at locations between the observations. In a sense, it is now obsolete, since the HM approach makes clear that the target simulation is from the posterior distribution $[Y(\mathbf{s}_0)|\mathbf{Z}, \boldsymbol{\theta}]$ or $[Z(\mathbf{s}_0)|\mathbf{Z}, \boldsymbol{\theta}]$.

In its simplest form, conditional simulation relies on an *orthogonal* decomposition of the spatial process into the kriging predictor plus the residual process (e.g., Cressie, 1993, Section 3.6.2). There is an implicit assumption that the process being simulated is Gaussian, since if it were not, then the conditionally simulated quantity is *not* the posterior distribution. In spite of these limitations, conditional simulation has been developed (in largely *ad hoc* ways) to handle ever more complex problems; the software GSLIB (Deutsch and Journel, 1992, and later versions and editions) and SGeMS (Remy, Boucher, and Wu, 2009) depend on stochastic simulation algorithms that will almost certainly not yield the posterior distributions of the unobserved parts of the spatial process, and they do not account for the measurement error in the observed parts. Recent research in conditional simulation tends to ignore the desirability of the posterior distribution; for example, Emery (2005) develops a conditional-simulation algorithm for a bivariate gamma isofactorial model, and Strebelle (2002) introduces the notion of multiple-point statistics to improve conditional simulation for non-Gaussian processes by modeling the process' moments beyond the covariance function (in his terminology, the covariance is a two-point statistic).

4.2 LATTICE PROCESSES

Recall that lattice processes $\{Y(\mathbf{s}) : \mathbf{s} \in D_s\}$ are defined on a finite or countable subset D_s of $\mathbb{R}^d$. They are used to model lattice data, $\mathbf{Z} \equiv (Z(\mathbf{s}_1), \ldots, Z(\mathbf{s}_m))'$, where $\{\mathbf{s}_1, \ldots, \mathbf{s}_m\}$ are reference locations for data defined on discrete spatial features (e.g., grid nodes, pixels, small areas). Define the spatial-neighborhood matrix $\mathbf{W} \equiv (w_{ij})$ as an $m \times m$ matrix with zero down the diagonals and $w_{ij} = 1$ if location $\mathbf{s}_j$ is considered "close to" location $\mathbf{s}_i$. Here, the definition of "close to" is made specific by the modeler; for example, it might be whenever $\|\mathbf{s}_i - \mathbf{s}_j\| \leq r$, for some specified "radius of influence" $r > 0$.

Moran (1950) considered the simple case of $\mathbb{R}^1$, $s_i = i$; $i = 1, \ldots, m$, and $w_{ij} = w_{ji} = 1$ if $0 < |s_i - s_j| \leq 1$. Then for detrended data $\mathbf{Z}$ satisfying $E(\mathbf{Z}) = \mathbf{0}$, he defined the statistic,

$$I \equiv \mathbf{Z}'\mathbf{W}\mathbf{Z}/\mathbf{Z}'\mathbf{Z},$$

which he used to test the null hypothesis that $Z(\mathbf{s}_1), \ldots, Z(\mathbf{s}_m)$ are *iid*. Cliff and Ord (1981) proposed the use of more general $\mathbf{W}$, where $\mathbf{W}$ does not have to be symmetric and off-diagonal elements do not have to be 1, and named the statistic Moran's I. This has become a ubiquitous statistic for testing the null hypothesis of the absence of spatial autocorrelation in $\mathbf{Z}$, although a more powerful alternative has recently been suggested (Li, Calder, and Cressie, 2007).

The statistic I is directly analogous to the statistic F defined in terms of the empirical semivariogram in Section 4.1.1. Under the null hypothesis, both statistics have a permutation distribution or an asymptotic distribution that allows an initial check to see whether the spatial data warrant spatial modeling. Figure 4.9 is a plot of cantons and their reference locations (centroids) $\{\mathbf{s}_i : i = 1, \ldots, 268\}$ in the Midi-Pyrénées region of south-west France. Define $w_{ij} = 1$ if and only if canton i shares a boundary with canton j. In this case, the data are prescription amounts per doctor consultation for each canton. With or without detrending, a test based on Moran's I rejects the null hypothesis of independence.

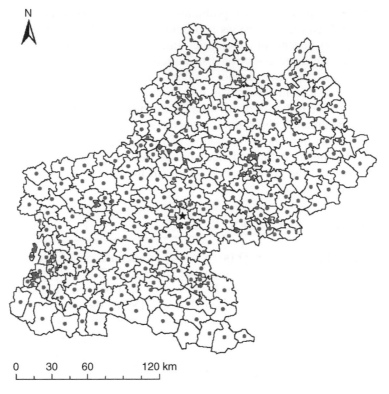

Figure 4.9 Boundaries and spatial locations of cantons in the Midi-Pyrénées region of southwest France. The "star" denotes the canton containing Toulouse.

A spatial lattice in $\mathbb{R}^d$ is made up of a finite or countable number of locations $D_s \equiv \{s_1, s_2, \dots\}$. Figure 4.9 is an example of an irregular spatial lattice. Regular spatial lattices are often achieved by discretization or aggregation of a continuous spatial domain; for example, see Figure 4.5a, or consider pixelization of an image. In the rest of this section, we assume $|D_s| < \infty$, and we build lattice models for the second level (i.e., the process-model level) of the hierarchy.

A Markov Model in One Dimension

Spatial processes in two or higher dimensions are fundamentally different from those in one dimension. The difference arises because it is easy to completely order elements in $\mathbb{R}^1$, but in $\mathbb{R}^d$, for $d \geq 2$, complete orderings are not as natural. Even partial orderings are difficult to motivate when modeling purely spatial data; we shall return to partial orderings in Section 4.2.8.

We now introduce spatial dependence in $\mathbb{R}^1$ and discuss the extent to which it can be generalized to lattice processes in $\mathbb{R}^d$. Any two elements $a, b \in \mathbb{R}^1$ are always related through the (complete) ordering, "$\leq$" ("less than or equal to").

If $a \leq b$ but $a \neq b$, then we write $a < b$ to mean that a is (strictly) less than b. We can use this complete ordering when defining a random process on $\mathbb{R}^1$. For mathematical simplicity, we shall consider the finite subset $D_s = \{1, 2, \ldots, n\}$ consisting of the first n integers of $\mathbb{R}^1$ and define the process $\{Y(s) : s \in D_s\}$.

Suppose that we specify the distribution of $Y(s)$ in terms of values of Y at locations *less than* s. For example, consider the first-order *unilateral* spatial process,

$$Y(s) = \phi Y(s - 1) + \varepsilon(s), \qquad s = 2, \ldots, n, \tag{4.84}$$

where $|\phi| < 1$; $\varepsilon(s)$ is independent of $Y(s - 1)$, for $s = 2, \ldots, n$; and $\varepsilon(s) \sim iid\, Gau(0, \sigma^2)$. Finally, assume

$$Y(1) \sim Gau(0, \sigma^2/(1 - \phi^2)), \tag{4.85}$$

to obtain a stationary Gaussian process on $\{1, 2, \ldots, n\}$. This simple example was already considered in the introduction to Chapter 2, and it has a well known covariance function, $\text{cov}(Y(s), Y(s + h)) \propto \phi^h$. (The analogous temporal process is called a first-order autoregressive process; see Section 3.4.3.) It is not difficult to show that (4.84) and (4.85) imply that $\mathbf{Y} \equiv (Y(1), \ldots, Y(n))'$ is jointly Gaussian with $E(\mathbf{Y}) = \mathbf{0}$,

$$\text{var}(\mathbf{Y}) = (\sigma^2/(1 - \phi^2)) \cdot \begin{bmatrix} 1 & \phi & \cdots & \phi^{n-1} \\ \phi & 1 & \cdots & \phi^{n-2} \\ \vdots & \vdots & & \vdots \\ \phi^{n-1} & \phi^{n-2} & \cdots & 1 \end{bmatrix}, \tag{4.86}$$

and $\text{corr}(Y(s), Y(s + 1)) = \phi$.

There is an equivalent way to specify the model (4.84), although *a priori* it is not clear that they do result in the same probability distribution; the equivalence is demonstrated using the result (4.96) below. For $s = 2, \ldots, n - 1$, assume

$$Y(s)|Y(1), \ldots, Y(s - 1), Y(s + 1), \ldots, Y(n)$$
$$\sim Gau((\phi/(1 + \phi^2))(Y(s - 1) + Y(s + 1)), \sigma^2/(1 + \phi^2)), \tag{4.87}$$

and

$$Y(1)|Y(2), \ldots, Y(n) \sim Gau(\phi Y(2), \sigma^2), \tag{4.88}$$

$$Y(n)|Y(1), \ldots, Y(n - 1) \sim Gau(\phi Y(n - 1), \sigma^2), \tag{4.89}$$

where $|\phi| < 1$. That is, apart from the edge locations $s = 1$ and $s = n$, the conditional distributions are Gaussian with a mean determined by the sum of the two values of Y at the neighboring locations. The equivalence between

(4.87)–(4.89) and (a temporal version of) (4.84)–(4.85) has already been discussed in Chapter 2. We have a different point to make in comparing the two *spatial* lattice processes.

Based on the theory given below for Markov random fields, in particular for the conditional autoregressive (CAR) models in Section 4.2.5, (4.87)–(4.89) imply that $\mathbf{Y}$ is jointly Gaussian with $E(\mathbf{Y}) = \mathbf{0}$ and

$$(\text{var}(\mathbf{Y}))^{-1}$$

$$= (1/\sigma^2) \begin{bmatrix} 1 & -\phi & 0 & 0 & \cdots & 0 & 0 & 0 \\ -\phi & 1+\phi^2 & -\phi & 0 & \cdots & 0 & 0 & 0 \\ 0 & -\phi & 1+\phi^2 & -\phi & \cdots & 0 & 0 & 0 \\ \vdots & \vdots & \vdots & \vdots & & \vdots & \vdots & \vdots \\ 0 & 0 & 0 & 0 & \cdots & -\phi & 1+\phi^2 & -\phi \\ 0 & 0 & 0 & 0 & \cdots & 0 & -\phi & 1 \end{bmatrix}.$$

This shows that the *inverse* of the covariance matrix, var($\mathbf{Y}$), is sparse, which is typical for a CAR model. For this particular model defined on $\{1, \ldots, n\} \subset \mathbb{R}^1$, it is possible to find an exact expression for the inverse of $(\text{var}(\mathbf{Y}))^{-1}$. Then,

$$\{(\text{var}(\mathbf{Y}))^{-1}\}^{-1} = \text{right-hand side of (4.86)},$$

which can be verified by multiplying both matrices to obtain the $n \times n$ identity matrix. Hence, although specified completely differently, both the first-order unilateral spatial process (4.84) and (4.85) and the CAR model (4.87)–(4.89) are the *same* statistical model. (They are both Gaussian with mean zero and the same covariance matrix.) Thus, seemingly different conditional probability specifications can lead to equivalent lattice models; more general results of this nature are given in Section 4.2.8.

Still in one-dimensional space, it is straightforward to show that the Markov chain defined by

$$[Y(s)|Y(1), \ldots, Y(s-1)] = [Y(s)|Y(s-1)], \qquad s = 2, 3, \ldots, \qquad (4.90)$$

and $[Y(1)]$, can be equivalently characterized by

$$[Y(2), \ldots, Y(s)|Y(1)] = \prod_{i=2}^{s} P_i(Y(i), Y(i-1)), \qquad s = 2, 3, \ldots, \qquad (4.91)$$

and $[Y(1)]$; in (4.91), P_i is a function that depends only on $Y(i)$ and $Y(i-1)$. Furthermore, a special case of Result 2 in Cressie and Davidson (1998) shows that the model defined by (4.90) on $\{1, 2, \ldots, n\}$ can be written as a random process on $\{1, 2, \ldots, n\}$, characterized by

$$[Y(s)|\{Y(j): j = 1, \ldots, n, j \neq s\}]$$
$$= [Y(s)|Y(s-1), Y(s+1)], \qquad s = 2, \ldots, n-1, \qquad (4.92)$$

$[Y(1)|Y(2)]$, and $[Y(n)|Y(n-1)]$. That is, in one-dimensional space, the Markov assumption (4.90) implies (4.91) and (4.92), and either (4.91) or (4.92) implies (4.90).

In two or more dimensions, the locations are no longer completely ordered, and it is not *a priori* clear how to generalize the "lack of memory" assumption (4.90), nor whether there are Markov notions analogous to (4.91) and (4.92). This is taken up in Sections 4.2.1–4.2.5 and 4.2.8.

4.2.1 Markov-Type Models in Space

In looking for Markov-type models in space, in particular on the two-dimensional integer lattice, various authors have attempted to generalize (4.90) or (4.91). Undoubtedly, the most successful generalization has been of (4.90), where the notion of (Markov) neighborhoods is critical (Besag, 1974); for continuous, non-skewed data, the CAR models (Section 4.2.5) are a popular choice. In Section 4.2.2 below, we give a probabilistic definition of the lattice models in $\mathbb{R}^d$ that are called *Markov random fields* (MRFs).

Alternatively, Whittle (1963) attempted a generalization of (4.91); however, the class of *partially ordered Markov models (POMMs)* developed by Cressie and Davidson (1998) turns out to be the appropriate generalization of (4.91). Its probabilistic definition requires a *partial* order on the spatial locations D_s. A brief discussion of POMMs is given in Section 4.2.8.

In another generalization, this time of (4.84), Whittle (1954) gave a simultaneous specification of a spatial process that under Gaussian assumptions has been called a *simultaneous autoregressive (SAR) model* (e.g., Anselin, 1988). We give a brief discussion of such models, including unilateral versions, in Section 4.2.7.

As an illustration of an MRF, we define here (briefly) the *CAR model* on $D_s = \{s_1, \ldots, s_n\} \subset \mathbb{R}^d$: Let the sequence of conditional distributions $\{[Y(s_i)|Y_{-i}]: i = 1, \ldots, n\}$ each be Gaussian with mean and variance,

$$E(Y(s_i)|\mathbf{Y}_{-i}) = \sum_{s_j \in N(s_i)} c_{ij} Y(s_j), \qquad (4.93)$$

$$\text{var}(Y(s_i)|\mathbf{Y}_{-i}) = \tau_i^2, \qquad (4.94)$$

where $\mathbf{Y}_{-i} \equiv (Y(s_1), \ldots, Y(s_{i-1}), Y(s_{i+1}), \ldots, Y(s_n))'$, and $N(s_i)$ is a set of prespecified locations that define the *neighborhood* of s_i, $i = 1, \ldots, n$. Inspection of (4.93) shows from where the CAR model gets its name; a detailed treatment is given in Section 4.2.5.

Notice from (4.93) and (4.94) that the conditional distribution, $[Y(s_i)|\mathbf{Y}_{-i}]$, depends functionally on $\{Y(s_j): s_j \in N(s_i)\}$, which is a Markov-type property in space defined in terms of the neighborhood $N(s_i)$. This Markov property is discussed in considerable detail in Section 4.2.2. Notice that specifying $[Y(s_i)|\mathbf{Y}_{-i}]$, $i = 1, \ldots, n$, as Gaussian with mean (4.93) and variance (4.94), does *not guarantee existence* of the joint distribution $[\mathbf{Y}]$. For example, consider the homogeneous case of $\tau_1^2 = \ldots = \tau_n^2$ in (4.94); then it only takes specifying $c_{12} \neq c_{21}$ in (4.93) for there to be *no* joint distribution $[\mathbf{Y}]$. Regularity conditions on $\{c_{ij}\}$ and $\{\tau_i^2\}$ that do guarantee existence are given in Section 4.2.5.

Because $N(\mathbf{s}_i)$ does not include the location $\mathbf{s}_i$, it makes sense in (4.93) to define $c_{ii} = 0$. Furthermore, if we define $c_{ij} = 0$, for $\mathbf{s}_j \notin N(\mathbf{s}_i)$; $i = 1, \ldots, n$, then we can write

$$E(Y(\mathbf{s}_i)|\mathbf{Y}_{-i}) = \sum_{j=1}^{n} c_{ij} Y(\mathbf{s}_j), \qquad i = 1, \ldots, n. \tag{4.95}$$

Define the $n \times n$ matrix $\mathbf{C} \equiv (c_{ij})$, whose (i,j)th element is c_{ij}; and define the $n \times n$ diagonal matrix $\mathbf{M} \equiv \text{diag}(\tau_1^2, \ldots, \tau_n^2)$. Besag (1974) shows that if $\mathbf{M}^{-1}(\mathbf{I} - \mathbf{C})$ is symmetric and positive-definite, then the joint distribution of the CAR model is

$$\mathbf{Y} \sim Gau(\mathbf{0}, (\mathbf{I} - \mathbf{C})^{-1}\mathbf{M}). \tag{4.96}$$

Notice that $\text{var}(\mathbf{Y})^{-1} = \mathbf{M}^{-1}(\mathbf{I} - \mathbf{C})$, which is sparse (i.e., few nonzero elements) if $\mathbf{C}$ is sparse. Modelers typically choose c_{ij} to be nonzero for $\mathbf{s}_j$ "close to" $\mathbf{s}_i$; otherwise it is zero. (This is in contrast to the geostatistical models presented in Section 4.1, where $\text{var}(\mathbf{Y})$ is often sparse.)

To see how a Gaussian MRF (or CAR) model could be used as a *process model* in an HM, consider the following example (often used in small-area estimation; see Section 4.2.6).

Data model: For $i = 1, \ldots, n$,

$$Z(\mathbf{s}_i)|Y(\mathbf{s}_i) \sim ind. Poi(\exp\{Y(\mathbf{s}_i)\}),$$

where $Poi(v)$ denotes a Poisson distribution with mean v.

Process model: Conditional on $\boldsymbol{\beta}$, τ^2, ϕ, and for $\mathbf{Y} \equiv (Y(\mathbf{s}_1), \ldots, Y(\mathbf{s}_n))'$,

$$\mathbf{Y}|\boldsymbol{\beta}, \tau^2, \phi \sim Gau(\mathbf{X}\boldsymbol{\beta}, \tau^2(\mathbf{I} - \phi\mathbf{H})^{-1}),$$

where $\mathbf{X} \equiv (x_j(\mathbf{s}_i))$ is an $n \times p$ matrix derived from the p-dimensional covariate $\mathbf{x}(\mathbf{s}_i)$ at location $\mathbf{s}_i$, $i = 1, \ldots, n$; $\mathbf{H}$ is a known matrix with zeros down the diagonal that is often the spatial neighborhood matrix (i.e., $h_{ij} = 1$ iff $\mathbf{s}_j \in N(\mathbf{s}_i)$, equivalently iff $\mathbf{s}_i \in N(\mathbf{s}_j)$); and the parameter space of ϕ ensures that the matrix inverse exists.

Clearly, the process-model variance is a special case of that in (4.96).

Another way to write the process model is

$$\mathbf{Y} = \mathbf{X}\boldsymbol{\beta} + \boldsymbol{\delta}, \tag{4.97}$$

where $\boldsymbol{\beta}$ is fixed but unknown, and $\boldsymbol{\delta}|\tau^2, \phi \sim Gau(\mathbf{0}, \tau^2(\mathbf{I} - \phi\mathbf{H})^{-1})$. Notice that this is a particular case of a general linear model with $\text{var}(\boldsymbol{\delta}) = \tau^2(\mathbf{I} - \phi\mathbf{H})^{-1}$. However, we prefer the specification through $[\mathbf{Y}|\boldsymbol{\beta}, \tau^2, \phi]$ rather than (4.97), since the former generalizes easily to more complex, nonadditive decompositions of variation. More general HMs (not necessarily Poisson distributions in the data model and not necessarily Gaussian distributions in the process model) can be found in Sections 4.2.2 and 4.2.6.

Inference for the HM given above is mostly concerned with prediction of $\mathbf{Y}$ from data $\mathbf{Z}$, and inference on parameters $\boldsymbol{\beta}$, τ^2, and ϕ. Consider the EHM, where point estimators of $\boldsymbol{\beta}$, τ^2, and ϕ are sought. The marginal likelihood is

$$\mathcal{L}(\boldsymbol{\beta}, \tau^2, \phi) \equiv [\mathbf{Z}|\boldsymbol{\beta}, \tau^2, \phi] = \int [\mathbf{Z}|\mathbf{Y}][\mathbf{Y}|\boldsymbol{\beta}, \tau^2, \phi]\, d\mathbf{Y};$$

however, the integration is most often analytically intractible. Maximum likelihood estimates $\widehat{\boldsymbol{\theta}}$ of $\boldsymbol{\theta} \equiv (\boldsymbol{\beta}, \tau^2, \phi)'$ have been developed by simulating from the HM and simultaneously optimizing the likelihood (e.g., Geyer and Thompson, 1992; Lee, Kaiser, and Cressie, 2001). These estimates can then be substituted into the EHM's posterior distribution. For example, the (squared-error-loss) optimal predictor of the true rate $\exp\{Y(\mathbf{s}_1)\}$ at location $\mathbf{s}_1$ is $E(\exp\{Y(\mathbf{s}_1)\}|\mathbf{Z}, \boldsymbol{\beta}, \tau^2, \phi)$, which is estimated by $E(\exp\{Y(\mathbf{s}_1)\}|\mathbf{Z}, \widehat{\boldsymbol{\beta}}, \widehat{\tau^2}, \widehat{\phi})$. Unfortunately, the posterior expectation is not known in closed form, and this is typical for all HMs that do not have a Gaussian data model and a Gaussian process model; Clayton and Kaldor (1987) and Breslow and Clayton (1993) give useful approximations.

Suppose that the parameter estimate $\widehat{\boldsymbol{\theta}}$ is obtained from the data $\mathbf{Z}$ and substituted in place of $\boldsymbol{\theta}$ in the posterior distribution, resulting in $[\mathbf{Y}|\mathbf{Z}, \widehat{\boldsymbol{\theta}}]$; see Section 2.1.2. Cressie (2000) discusses MCMC algorithms that produce realizations $\mathbf{Y}^{(1)}, \ldots, \mathbf{Y}^{(L)}$ from $[\mathbf{Y}|\mathbf{Z}, \widehat{\boldsymbol{\theta}}]$, where the process model in the HM is a MRF. Then, to finish the example introduced in the previous paragraph, the (estimated) optimal spatial predictor of the true rate at $\mathbf{s}_1$ is approximated by

$$(1/L) \sum_{\ell=1}^{L} \exp\{Y(\mathbf{s}_1)^{(\ell)}\},$$

and this approximation improves as L increases (Section 2.3).

In contrast, the BHM requires specification of another level, namely the parameter model. For example, consider the parameter model used by Stern and Cressie (2000) in a disease-mapping problem.

Parameter model: The joint distribution of $\boldsymbol{\theta}$ is

$$[\boldsymbol{\theta}] = [\boldsymbol{\beta}][\tau^2][\phi],$$

where $\boldsymbol{\beta} \sim U((-\infty, \infty)^p)$; $[\tau^2] \propto \exp(-b/\tau^2)$, for b a small positive number (e.g., $b = 0.01$); and $\phi \sim U(0, \phi_{\max})$, for $\phi_{\max}$ the largest parameter value (> 0) such that $(\mathbf{I} - \phi\mathbf{H})$ is positive-definite for $0 < \phi < \phi_{\max}$.

This particular parameter model is based on choosing noninformative, maximum-entropy prior distributions (e.g., Cressie, Richardson, and Jaussent, 2004). In problems where there is scientific theory to guide the behavior of parameters (e.g., the regression coefficients $\boldsymbol{\beta}$), one should choose more informative priors.

Recall the example of predicting the true rate at $\mathbf{s}_1$. The BHM's (squared-error loss) optimal predictor is $E(\exp\{Y(\mathbf{s}_1)\}|\mathbf{Z})$, where the parameters are integrated out (rather than estimated, as they were for the EHM). That is,

$$E(\exp\{Y(\mathbf{s}_1)\}|\mathbf{Z}) = \int [\exp\{Y(\mathbf{s}_1)\}|\mathbf{Z}, \boldsymbol{\beta}, \tau^2, \phi][\boldsymbol{\beta}, \tau^2, \phi|\mathbf{Z}] \, d\boldsymbol{\beta} d\tau^2 d\phi,$$

although the integration is generally analytically intractible. Once again, MCMC is overwhelmingly the method of choice to compute the optimal predictor, this time including uncertainty on $\boldsymbol{\theta}$ through the parameter model. Then $(\mathbf{Y}^{(1)}, \boldsymbol{\theta}^{(1)}), \ldots, (\mathbf{Y}^{(L)}, \boldsymbol{\theta}^{(L)})$ are samples from the posterior distribution $[\mathbf{Y}, \boldsymbol{\theta}|\mathbf{Z}]$, and the optimal spatial predictor of the true rate at $\mathbf{s}_1$ is approximated, as for the EHM, by

$$\frac{1}{L}\sum_{l=1}^{L} \exp\{Y(\mathbf{s}_1)^{(l)}\}.$$

Details of MCMC implementation for a BHM can be found in Banerjee, Carlin, and Gelfand (2004, Section A.7).

4.2.2 The Markov Random Field (MRF)

In this section, we define a class of spatial models known as Markov random fields, with the intention of using them as process models in an HM. For temporal data or data in $D_s \subset \mathbb{R}^1$, the Markov models discussed at the beginning of Section 4.2 have been a popular way of introducing statistical dependence. Such models assume a complete ordering of D_s; then the "present," conditioned on the "past," is assumed to depend only on the "immediate past." Financial time series, such as quarterly trade balances, are often modeled with a component that is Markov (superimposed on a seasonal component and other large-scale effects); for that component, only its immediate-past value influences the present value.

For spatial data, an analogous notion can be formulated that does not rely on a complete ordering of the spatial locations, but it is based on which locations are "neighbors" of any particular location (Besag, 1974; Cressie, 1993, Section 6.4). For most of this section, we assume that the process $Y(\cdot)$ is defined on the lattice $D_s \equiv \{s_1, \ldots, s_n\} \subset \mathbb{R}^d$. In general, $Y(\cdot)$ is characterized by its joint distribution,

$$[Y(s_1), \ldots, Y(s_n)],\tag{4.98}$$

from which the conditional probabilities, $[Y(s_i) \mid Y_{-i}]; \; i = 1, \ldots, n$, can be calculated, where we recall that $Y_{-i} \equiv (Y(s_1), \ldots, Y(s_{i-1}), Y(s_{i+1}), \ldots, Y(s_n))'$.

The *neighborhood* $N(s_i)$, of the ith location s_i, is formally defined to be the collection of all other locations $s_j (j \neq i)$ such that

$$[Y(s_i) \mid Y_{-i}] = [Y(s_i) \mid Y(N(s_i))], \qquad i = 1, \ldots, n,\tag{4.99}$$

where $Y(N(s_i)) \equiv (Y(u): u \in N(s_i))'$. For example, suppose that the right-hand side of (4.99) is a Poisson distribution,

$$Y(s_i) \mid Y(N(s_i)) \sim Poi\left(\exp\left\{\alpha_i + \sum_{j \in N(s_i)} \theta_{ij} Y(s_j)\right\}\right), \qquad i = 1, \ldots, n,$$

where $\theta_{ij} = \theta_{ji}$ (the reason for this symmetry in the parameters $\{\theta_{ij}\}$ will become clearer in Section 4.2.3). This is called the *auto Poisson model* (Besag, 1974).

In (4.99), if $s_j \in N(s_i)$ then s_j is said to be a *neighbor* of s_i, and it is straightforward to show that if s_j is a neighbor of s_i, then s_i is a neighbor of s_j. In words, (4.99) says that the conditional distribution of the Y at the ith location, conditioned on Y at all other locations, in fact depends only on its neighboring values $Y(N(s_i))$. In this sense, (4.99) is a spatial analogue of the temporal Markov property (4.90).

There is a way to represent the conditional dependencies in (4.99) using graph theory. An *undirected graph* is made up of vertices and (undirected) edges; we define an edge between vertices s_i and s_j to mean that $s_j \in N(s_i)$. Figure 4.10 shows the nodes and edges of an undirected graph for a simple example, where $n = 7$. Although a graphical representation shows the conditional *independencies* in a statistical model, it does not give the *type and strength of the dependencies*. Moreover, there are other ways to represent spatial dependence, through the covariance function or variogram (Section 4.1.1), or through a spatial moving average (Section 4.1.4). Further discussion of directed and undirected graphs can be found in Section 2.4.

Use of the spatial Markov property can be found in statistical image analysis (e.g., Geman and Geman, 1984) and small area estimation, particularly disease

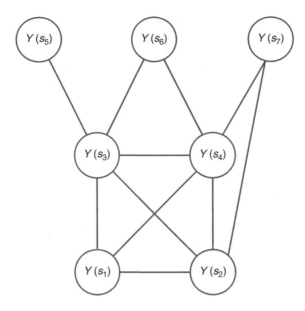

Figure 4.10 Undirected graph with seven vertices, showing the (undirected) edges between the vertices (this is the moral graph of Figure 4.14).

mapping (e.g., Besag, York, and Mollié, 1991). In image analysis, the spatial lattice D_s is typically a regular rectangular lattice of pixels; Geman and Geman (1984) proposed models based on (4.99) for the process model of (the hidden image) $\mathbf{Y}$ when the noisy image $\mathbf{Z}$ is observed. In small area estimation, the lattice is irregular and made up of location identifiers (e.g., centroids) of the small areas; for example, Besag, York, and Mollié (1991) used models based on (4.99) for the process model of (hidden) disease risks $\mathbf{Y}$ when (noisy) disease rates $\mathbf{Z}$ are observed in the Départements of France. More details on small area estimation are given in Section 4.2.6.

When the conditional probabilities on the right-hand side of (4.99) *define* the joint probability (4.98), the process $\{Y(\mathbf{s}) : \mathbf{s} \in D_s\}$ is called a *Markov random field* (*MRF*). This definition can be appropriately generalized for countable D_s; for example, see discussion of the Ising model in Section 4.2.4. A very attractive feature of working with an MRF is that modeling can be carried out at the *local* level by specifying the neighborhoods,

$$\{N(\mathbf{s}_i) : i = 1, \ldots, n\}, \tag{4.100}$$

and the conditional probabilities,

$$\{[Y(\mathbf{s}_i) \mid \mathbf{Y}(N(\mathbf{s}_i))] : i = 1, \ldots, n\}. \tag{4.101}$$

However, such specifications have to be made consistently, so that at a *global* level the joint distribution (4.98) is well defined.

Much of the material presented in this section follows closely the notation and development of Besag (1974, Section 3) and Cressie (1993, Chapter 6). Define the support of the probability distribution of $\mathbf{Y}$ to be $\Omega \equiv \{\mathbf{y} : \Pr(\mathbf{y}) > 0\}$, where $\Omega \subset D_s$ and $\mathbf{y} \equiv (y(\mathbf{s}_1), \ldots, y(\mathbf{s}_n))' \in \mathbb{R}^n$. Furthermore, define $\Omega_i \equiv \{y(\mathbf{s}_i) : \Pr(y(\mathbf{s}_i)) > 0\}$; $i = 1, \ldots, n$. Note that here we use $\Pr(\cdot)$ to denote either a probability density or a probability mass function.

The *positivity condition* is said to be satisfied if $\Omega = \Omega_1 \times \cdots \times \Omega_n$, which says that if each $y(\mathbf{s}_i)$ individually has positive probability, then $\mathbf{y}$ has positive probability. This allows results given below to be proved simply, although in Section 4.2.3 we shall assume a much weaker condition (the MRF support condition of Kaiser and Cressie, 2000) and obtain similar results.

A result in Besag (1974), which we call Besag's Lemma, relates joint probabilities to conditional probabilities:

$$\frac{\Pr(\mathbf{y})}{\Pr(\mathbf{w})} = \prod_{i=1}^{n} \frac{\Pr(y(\mathbf{s}_i) | y(\mathbf{s}_1), \ldots, y(\mathbf{s}_{i-1}), w(\mathbf{s}_{i+1}), \ldots, w(\mathbf{s}_n))}{\Pr(w(\mathbf{s}_i) | y(\mathbf{s}_1), \ldots, y(\mathbf{s}_{i-1}), w(\mathbf{s}_{i+1}), \ldots, w(\mathbf{s}_n))},$$

$$\mathbf{y}, \mathbf{w} \in \Omega. \qquad (4.102)$$

For example, if $n = 3$, the right-hand side of (4.102) is

$$\frac{\Pr(y(\mathbf{s}_1) | w(\mathbf{s}_2), w(\mathbf{s}_3))}{\Pr(w(\mathbf{s}_1) | w(\mathbf{s}_2), w(\mathbf{s}_3))} \cdot \frac{\Pr(y(\mathbf{s}_2) | y(\mathbf{s}_1), w(\mathbf{s}_3))}{\Pr(w(\mathbf{s}_2) | y(\mathbf{s}_1), w(\mathbf{s}_3))} \cdot \frac{\Pr(y(\mathbf{s}_3) | y(\mathbf{s}_1), y(\mathbf{s}_2))}{\Pr(w(\mathbf{s}_3) | y(\mathbf{s}_1), y(\mathbf{s}_2))}.$$

It is a simple matter to verify that this is equal to the left-hand side of (4.102).

The relation (4.102) has sometimes been called Brook's Lemma, where the article by Brook (1964) is cited. However, after close inspection of that article and that of Besag (1974), it would appear that the result should be properly credited to Besag. Notice that the right-hand side of (4.102) depends on the ordering of the locations, but the left hand side does not. Thus, specification of the conditional probabilities in (4.99) such that a joint distribution exists, is delicate. If it can be done coherently, then the joint probability is available from (4.102), up to a multiplicative normalizing constant.

In the rest of this section, we address how a Markov random field can be specified and discuss its properties. Recall from (4.99) the definition of neighbor and neighborhood. A *clique* is defined to be a set of locations in D_s that consists either of a single site or of a set of sites that are *all* neighbors of each other. For example, if $n = 3$, $\mathbf{s}_1 \in N(\mathbf{s}_2)$, $\mathbf{s}_1 \in N(\mathbf{s}_3)$, but $\mathbf{s}_2 \notin N(\mathbf{s}_3)$, then the cliques are $\{\mathbf{s}_1\}$, $\{\mathbf{s}_2\}$, $\{\mathbf{s}_3\}$, $\{\mathbf{s}_1, \mathbf{s}_2\}$, and $\{\mathbf{s}_1, \mathbf{s}_3\}$. Cliques are central to a particular representation of $[\mathbf{Y}]$ given by the Hammersley–Clifford Theorem, which is stated below.

In what follows, we assume that $\mathbf{0} \in \Omega$. This makes some of the algebra below easier, but Kaiser and Cressie (2000) show how the results based on a possibly *nonzero* reference value, $\mathbf{y}_0 \in \Omega$, follow in a similar manner.

Define

$$Q(\mathbf{y}) \equiv \log\{\Pr(\mathbf{y})/\Pr(\mathbf{0})\}, \qquad \mathbf{y} \in \Omega, \tag{4.103}$$

and call $Q(\cdot)$ the *negpotential function*. Note that (4.103) involves a *ratio* of probabilities. For example, if $\mathbf{Y} \sim Gau(\mathbf{0}, \boldsymbol{\Sigma})$, then $Q(\mathbf{y}) = -(1/2)\mathbf{y}'\boldsymbol{\Sigma}^{-1}\mathbf{y}$; $\mathbf{y} \in \mathbb{R}^n$. For discrete data, this yields

$$\Pr(\mathbf{y}) = \exp\{Q(\mathbf{y})\}/\sum_{\mathbf{x}\in\Omega} \exp\{Q(\mathbf{x})\}, \qquad \mathbf{y} \in \Omega, \tag{4.104}$$

where the sum exists and is finite because $\{\Pr(\mathbf{y}): \mathbf{y} \in \Omega\}$ is a probability mass function that sums to 1. For continuous data, the summation in the denominator of (4.104) is replaced with integration. Then, for the example above, it is a simple matter to use $Q(\mathbf{y}) = -(1/2)\mathbf{y}'\boldsymbol{\Sigma}^{-1}\mathbf{y}$, to recover the Gaussian density, $\Pr(\mathbf{y})$, with mean $\mathbf{0}$ and covariance matrix $\boldsymbol{\Sigma}$.

Let $\mathbf{j}_m \equiv (j(1), \ldots, j(m))'$ denote $1 \le m \le n$ distinct index values from $\{1, 2, \ldots, n\}$. Define the sets

$$T_m(p) \equiv \{\text{all distinct } p\text{-tuples formed from } \mathbf{j}_m\}, \qquad 1 \le p \le m.$$

Then for all $m = 1, \ldots, n$ and all $\mathbf{j}_m$, define the so-called *G-functions* through

$$y(\mathbf{s}_{j(1)}) \ldots y(\mathbf{s}_{j(m)}) G_{j(1),\ldots,j(m)}(y(\mathbf{s}_{j(1)}), \ldots, y(\mathbf{s}_{j(m)}))$$

$$\equiv \sum_{t=0}^{m-1} \sum_{\mathbf{j}_{m-t}\in T_m(m-t)} (-1)^t Q(\mathbf{y}: y(\mathbf{s}_h) = 0; h \notin \mathbf{j}_{m-t}), \tag{4.105}$$

where all arguments at which $Q(\cdot)$ is evaluated are assumed to be in the support Ω. For example, $y(\mathbf{s}_i)G_i(y(\mathbf{s}_i)) \equiv Q(0, \ldots, 0, y(\mathbf{s}_i), 0, \ldots, 0)$ and

$$y(\mathbf{s}_i)y(\mathbf{s}_j)G_{ij}(y(\mathbf{s}_i), y(\mathbf{s}_j)) \equiv Q(0, \ldots, 0, y(\mathbf{s}_i), 0, \ldots, 0, y(\mathbf{s}_j), 0, \ldots, 0)$$

$$- Q(0, \ldots, 0, y(\mathbf{s}_i), 0, \ldots, 0, 0, 0, \ldots, 0)$$

$$- Q(0, \ldots, 0, 0, 0, \ldots, 0, y(\mathbf{s}_j), 0, \ldots, 0). \tag{4.106}$$

Consequently, $Q(\cdot)$ can be expanded in terms of a subset of the *G*-functions (e.g., Cressie, 1993, Section 6.4.1). For any $\mathbf{y} \in \Omega$,

$$Q(\mathbf{y}) = \sum_{i=1}^{n} y(\mathbf{s}_i)G_i(y(\mathbf{s}_i)) + \sum_{1\le i<j\le n}\sum y(\mathbf{s}_i)y(\mathbf{s}_j)G_{ij}(y(\mathbf{s}_i), y(\mathbf{s}_j))$$

$$+ \cdots + y(\mathbf{s}_1)y(\mathbf{s}_2)\ldots y(\mathbf{s}_n)G_{12\ldots n}(y(\mathbf{s}_1), y(\mathbf{s}_2), \ldots, y(\mathbf{s}_n)). \tag{4.107}$$

Relations (4.105) and (4.107) are analogous to the Mobius inversion formulas (e.g., Lauritzen, 1996, p. 239). Observe that (4.105) defines G-functions, $G_{j(1),...,j(m)}(\cdot)$, for any $1 \leq m \leq n$ and any $j(1), \ldots, j(m) \in \{1, \ldots, n\}$, although only some of these functions appear in the expansion (4.107). For example, while (4.105) results in a valid definition for $G_{1,2,3}(\cdot)$, $G_{2,1,3}(\cdot)$, and so forth, only $G_{1,2,3}(\cdot)$ appears in (4.107). The joint probability $\{\Pr(\mathbf{y}): \mathbf{y} \in \Omega\}$, and hence $\{Q(\mathbf{y}): \mathbf{y} \in \Omega\}$, is *invariant to permutation of the indices*; consequently, the functions defined in (4.105) are invariant to permutation of the indices contained in each $\mathbf{j}_m$. It will be seen in Section 4.2.3 that this necessary condition, namely permutation invariance, is an important sufficient condition for construction of the joint probability from the conditional probabilities, via the G-functions.

The expression (4.107) is very general and, as yet, does not involve any neighborhood information. That appears in the Hammersley–Clifford Theorem, which says that, depending on the cliques (which depend on the neighborhoods $\{N(\mathbf{s}_i): i = 1, \ldots, n\}$) of the MRF, many of the G-functions are in fact *zero*.

Hammersley–Clifford Theorem (Hammersley and Clifford, 1971). Suppose that the random process on Ω is a Markov random field with neighborhood structure $\{N(\mathbf{s}_i): i = 1, \ldots, n\}$. Then the negpotential function Q given by (4.107) satisfies the following property:

If sites $i, j(2), \ldots, j(m)$ do not form a clique, then $G_{i,j(2),...,j(m)}(\cdot) \equiv 0$.

Another result is that the G-functions in the expansion (4.107) can be expressed in terms of conditional probabilities. Cressie (1993, Section 6.4.1), shows that for $i = 1, \ldots, n$,

$$y(\mathbf{s}_i)G_i(y(\mathbf{s}_i)) = \log\left[\frac{\Pr(y(\mathbf{s}_i) \mid \{0(\mathbf{s}_j): j \neq i\})}{\Pr(0(\mathbf{s}_i) \mid \{0(\mathbf{s}_j): j \neq i\})}\right], \tag{4.108}$$

where $0(\mathbf{s}_i)$ is shorthand to denote evaluation at $y(\mathbf{s}_i) = 0$; and

$$y(\mathbf{s}_i)y(\mathbf{s}_j)G_{ij}(y(\mathbf{s}_i), y(\mathbf{s}_j)) = \log\left[\frac{\Pr(y(\mathbf{s}_i) \mid y(\mathbf{s}_j), \{0(\mathbf{s}_k): k \neq i, j\})}{\Pr(0(\mathbf{s}_i) \mid y(\mathbf{s}_j), \{0(\mathbf{s}_k): k \neq i, j\})}\right]$$

$$- \log\left[\frac{\Pr(y(\mathbf{s}_i) \mid \{0(\mathbf{s}_k): k \neq i\})}{\Pr(0(\mathbf{s}_i) \mid \{0(\mathbf{s}_k): k \neq i\})}\right]. \tag{4.109}$$

The general expression for higher-order terms is given in Section 4.2.3.

There is a large class of models defined by truncating (4.107), after including the singleton and pairwise G-functions. This means only (4.108) and (4.109) are needed. Consider the *auto spatial models* of Besag (1974): For $i = 1, \ldots, n$,

$$[Y(\mathbf{s}_i)|\mathbf{Y}_{-i}] \equiv \exp\{A_i(\mathbf{Y}_{-i})B_i(Y(\mathbf{s}_i)) + C_i(Y(\mathbf{s}_i)) + D_i(\mathbf{Y}_{-i})\}, \qquad (4.110)$$

which are of exponential-family form. If

$$A_i(\mathbf{Y}_{-i}) = \alpha_i + \sum_{j=1}^{n} \theta_{ij}\{B_j(Y(\mathbf{s}_j)) - B_j(0)\}, \qquad i = 1, \ldots, n, \qquad (4.111)$$

where $\theta_{ii} = 0$ and $\theta_{ij} = \theta_{ji}$, we see from (4.107) that, up to an additive constant,

$$Q(\mathbf{y}) = \sum_{i=1}^{n}[\alpha_i\{B_i(y(\mathbf{s}_i)) - B_i(0)\} + C_i(y(\mathbf{s}_i))]$$
$$+ \sum\sum_{1 \leq i < j \leq n} \theta_{ij}\{B_i(y(\mathbf{s}_i)) - B_i(0)\}\{B_j(y(\mathbf{s}_j)) - B_j(0)\}. \qquad (4.112)$$

That is, the auto spatial models given by (4.110) imply that $Q(\cdot)$ is truncated. Furthermore, we can specify $N(\mathbf{s}_i)$ in (4.110) and (4.111) conveniently by

$$N(\mathbf{s}_i) = \{\mathbf{s}_j : \theta_{ij} \neq 0\}; \qquad (4.113)$$

hence $\{\theta_{ij}\}$ have a direct interpretation as spatial-dependence parameters.

For example, recall the *auto Poisson* model: For $i = 1, \ldots, n$, we have

$$[Y(\mathbf{s}_i)|\mathbf{Y}(N(\mathbf{s}_i))]$$
$$= \exp\{(\alpha_i + \sum_{j=1}^{n} \theta_{ij}Y(\mathbf{s}_j))Y(\mathbf{s}_i) - \log Y(\mathbf{s}_i)! - (\alpha_i + \sum_{j=1}^{n} \theta_{ij}Y(\mathbf{s}_j))\},$$
$$(4.114)$$

where $\theta_{ii} = 0$, $\theta_{ij} = \theta_{ji}$, and $\theta_{ik} = 0$ for $\mathbf{s}_k \notin N(\mathbf{s}_i)$. Then (4.112) becomes, up to an additive constant,

$$Q(\mathbf{y}) = \sum_{i=1}^{n}\{\alpha_i y(\mathbf{s}_i) - \log y(\mathbf{s}_i)!\} + \sum\sum_{1 \leq i < j \leq n} \theta_{ij}y(\mathbf{s}_i)y(\mathbf{s}_j). \qquad (4.115)$$

Recall that a necessary condition for (4.107) to define a joint probability distribution, is invariance of (4.105) to permutation of the indices. When $Q(\cdot)$ is truncated, this amounts to $y(\mathbf{s}_i)y(\mathbf{s}_j)G_{ij}(y(\mathbf{s}_i), y(\mathbf{s}_j)) = y(\mathbf{s}_j)y(\mathbf{s}_i)G_{ji}(y(\mathbf{s}_j), y(\mathbf{s}_i))$; for the auto spatial model (4.110), this amounts to

$$\theta_{ij}\{B_i(y(\mathbf{s}_i)) - B_i(0)\}\{B_j(y(\mathbf{s}_j)) - B_j(0)\}$$
$$= \theta_{ji}\{B_j(y(\mathbf{s}_j)) - B_j(0)\}\{B_i(y(\mathbf{s}_i)) - B_i(0)\},$$

which *is* satisfied because we assumed $\theta_{ij} = \theta_{ji}$.

Another necessary condition for (4.107) to define a joint probability distribution is that $\exp(Q(\cdot))$ integrates (or sums) to 1 over Ω; see (4.104). This may not always hold, as in the case of the auto Poisson given by (4.114): Clearly, if $\theta_{12} > 0$ (say) in (4.115), then $\exp(Q(\cdot))$ is not summable; that is, the auto Poisson model is defined only if all $\{\theta_{ij}\}$ are negative or zero (Besag, 1974).

The two necessary conditions of *permutation invariance* and *summability* turn out to be crucial for specification of a Markov random field from conditional probabilities. The full statement of this result is deferred to Section 4.2.3, where it is presented in its most general form.

In summary, the joint probability of **Y** yields $Q(\cdot)$, which yields the *G*-functions, which can be written in terms of the conditional probabilities. Since MRFs are defined locally (i.e., in terms of the conditional probabilities), our modeling strategy is based on having *checkable conditions* that allow us to go backwards through the sequence, from conditional probabilities, to *G*-functions, to $Q(\cdot)$, to the joint probability $\Pr(\cdot)$.

4.2.3 From the Conditional Probabilities to the Joint Probability

Notice that up to now we have *assumed* that a joint probability distribution (i.e., a MRF) for **Y** *exists* (e.g., in the Hammersley–Clifford Theorem), and we have derived properties of the MRF based on the conditional probabilities. We now consider the more difficult problem of finding the joint probability distribution (if it exists) from the conditional probability distributions used to define the MRF. Our approach is constructive and follows the presentation by Kaiser and Cressie (2000).

The derivation of the expression (4.109) involves an arbitrary choice of the ith site or the jth site to be featured in the (conditional) probability statement. Because the indices $1, 2, \ldots, n$ are only used as convenient labels, it is clear that the conditional-probability consistency conditions must include a permutation-invariance condition. We shall see that other conditions involve summability (integrability) and supports of probability distributions.

The positivity condition, $\Omega = \Omega_1 \times \cdots \times \Omega_n$, is sufficient to ensure that all of the arguments at which $Q(\cdot)$ is evaluated in (4.105) are contained in Ω. However, it is not necessary, as evidenced by examples given in Moussouris (1974). Let $\Omega_{j(1),\ldots,j(m)}$ be the support of the marginal probability, $\Pr(y(\mathbf{s}_{j(1)}), \ldots, y(\mathbf{s}_{j(m)}))$, and define $\Phi_i \equiv \Omega_{\{1,\ldots,n\}\setminus\{i\}}$ to be the support of the marginal probability, $\Pr(\mathbf{y}_{-i})$. Then the *MRF support condition* (Kaiser and Cressie, 2000) is defined as

$$\{0(\mathbf{s}_i)\} \times \Phi_i \subset \Omega, \qquad i = 1, \ldots, n, \tag{4.116}$$

where recall that $0(\mathbf{s}_i)$ denotes a value of zero at location $\mathbf{s}_i$. This condition is weaker than the positivity condition. A weaker condition yet is given by Besag (1994, Lemma 0.1). However, the MRF support condition is precisely what is needed to *construct* the joint probability from G-functions (which are defined in terms of the conditional probabilities).

Recall (4.108) and (4.109), expressions for the singleton and pairwise G-functions, respectively, in terms of the conditional probabilities. There is a general expression, which is established by Kaiser and Cressie (2000). Recall that $\mathbf{j}_m = (j(1), j(2), \ldots, j(m))'$ is an index of distinct integers, where $1 \leq m \leq n$. Without loss of generality, let $j(1) = i$ for some $i \in \{1, \ldots, n\}$. Also, define $\mathbf{j}_m^{(-i)} \equiv (j(2), \ldots, j(m))'$, and let $T_m^{(-i)}(p)$ be the set of all distinct p-tuples formed from $\mathbf{j}_m^{(-i)}$, $1 \leq p \leq m - 1$. For $1 \leq m \leq n$, define

$$y(\mathbf{s}_i) \ldots y(\mathbf{s}_{j(m)}) G_{i,\ldots,j(m)}(y(\mathbf{s}_i), \ldots, y(\mathbf{s}_{j(m)}))$$

$$\equiv \sum_{t=1}^{m-1} \sum_{\mathbf{j}_{m-t}^{(-i)} \in T_m^{(-i)}(m-t)}$$

$$(-1)^{t-1} \log \left[\frac{\Pr(y(\mathbf{s}_i)|\{y(\mathbf{s}_h): h \in \mathbf{j}_{m-t}^{(-i)}\}, \{0(\mathbf{s}_k): k \notin \mathbf{j}_{m-t}\})}{\Pr(0(\mathbf{s}_i)|\{y(\mathbf{s}_h): h \in \mathbf{j}_{m-t}^{(-i)}\}, \{0(\mathbf{s}_k): k \notin \mathbf{j}_{m-t}\})} \right]$$

$$+ (-1)^{m-1} \log \left[\frac{\Pr(y(\mathbf{s}_i)|\{0(\mathbf{s}_k): k \neq i\})}{\Pr(0(\mathbf{s}_i)|\{0(\mathbf{s}_k): k \neq i\})} \right], \tag{4.117}$$

if $m \geq 2$; and if $m = 1$, only the last term in (4.117) appears. This definition is valid for all $\mathbf{j}_m$, but we use it in $Q(\cdot)$ given by (4.107) for ordered indices, $i < j(2) < \cdots < j(m)$.

Kaiser and Cressie's construction gives conditions under which the relations (4.117), followed by (4.107), followed by (4.104), yield a joint probability whose conditional probabilities are the ones that are used to initiate the construction.

Theorem (Kaiser and Cressie, 2000). Assume that a set of conditional distributions, $\{[Y(\mathbf{s}_i)|\mathbf{Y}(N(\mathbf{s}_i))]: i = 1, \ldots, n\}$, have been specified and that the MRF support condition (4.116) holds. Then a joint probability, $[\mathbf{Y}]$, having those conditional distributions exists, and it may be specified up to a normalizing constant through the application of (4.117), (4.107), and (4.104), if and only if

(i) The G-functions constructed from the specified conditional probabilities using (4.117) are each invariant under permutation of their associated indices.

(ii) The negpotential function $Q(\cdot)$ constructed from the G-functions using (4.107) and (4.117), and defined on support $\Omega \equiv \{\mathbf{y}: \exp\{Q(\mathbf{y})\} > 0\}$, satisfies the summability (or more generally a Lebesgue–Stieltjes integrability) condition,

$$\sum_{\mathbf{t} \in \Omega} \exp\{Q(\mathbf{t})\} < \infty. \tag{4.118}$$

Several observations about this theorem will help in making model choices for specifying an MRF. The permutation-invariance condition of (i) is straightforward to check for any particular model specification. For example, the auto spatial models (Sections 4.2.2 and 4.2.4) defined through the one-parameter exponential family of conditional distributions, $[Y(\mathbf{s}_i)|\mathbf{Y}(N(\mathbf{s}_i))]$, given by (4.110) and (4.111), satisfy the permutation-invariance condition if $\theta_{ij} = \theta_{ji}$; $i, j = 1, \ldots, n$. More generally, Lee, Kaiser, and Cressie (2001) give a generalization of MRF auto spatial models that allows for nonzero G-functions for cliques of any size; those models satisfy (i). We have already seen that the auto Poisson requires all $\{\theta_{ij}\}$ to be negative or zero in order for (ii) to be satisfied.

4.2.4 Some Examples of Auto Spatial Models

We have already considered two examples of auto spatial models. The *auto Gaussian* model, more commonly called a conditional autoregressive (CAR) model, is given by (4.93) and (4.94); discussion of CAR models will be deferred to Section 4.2.5. The *auto Poisson* model for count data is given by (4.114).

When data are *binary* (taking values 0 and 1) and $G_A \equiv 0$ for $|A| \geq 3$, where A is an index set of ordered integers in $\{1, \ldots, n\}$, then Besag (1974) shows that for $i = 1, \ldots, n$,

$$[Y(\mathbf{s}_i)|\mathbf{Y}(N(\mathbf{s}_i))] = \frac{\exp\{\alpha_i y(\mathbf{s}_i) + \sum_{\mathbf{s}_j \in N(\mathbf{s}_i)} \theta_{ij} y(\mathbf{s}_i) y(\mathbf{s}_j)\}}{1 + \exp\{\alpha_i + \sum_{\mathbf{s}_j \in N(\mathbf{s}_i)} \theta_{ij} y(\mathbf{s}_j)\}}, \qquad y(\mathbf{s}_i) \in \{0, 1\},$$

$$\tag{4.119}$$

where $\theta_{ij} = \theta_{ji}$. This spatial model is often called an *auto logistic model*. Statistical independence in the model is achieved by putting $\theta_{ij} \equiv 0$. Furthermore, any large-scale inhomogeneities can be modeled via $\boldsymbol{\alpha} \equiv (\alpha_1, \ldots, \alpha_n)'$. For example, put $\boldsymbol{\alpha} = \mathbf{X}\boldsymbol{\beta}$, where $\mathbf{X}$ is an $n \times p$ matrix of known explanatory variables and $\boldsymbol{\beta}$ is a p-dimensional vector of unknown regression coefficients. When $\boldsymbol{\alpha} = (\alpha, \ldots, \alpha)'$, the model is homogeneous in large-scale effects, leaving the spatial-dependence parameters $\{\theta_{ij}\}$ to model any spatial inhomogeneities.

The *Ising model* is defined by (4.119) on a regular lattice with locations given by the countable set $D_s = \{(u, v): u, v = \ldots, -1, 0, 1, \ldots\} \subset \mathbb{R}^2$;

assume homogeneity of $\{\alpha(u, v)\}$ and assume a "nearest-neighbor" neighborhood structure, $N(u, v) = \{(u - 1, v), (u + 1, v), (u, v - 1), (u, v + 1)\}$. Thus, the numerator of (4.119) becomes

$$\exp[y(u, v)\{\alpha + \gamma_1(y(u - 1, v) + y(u + 1, v))$$

$$+ \gamma_2(y(u, v - 1) + y(u, v + 1))\}],$$

Where γ_1 and γ_2 represent a reparameterization. The model was originally presented by Ising (1925) under the added assumption that $\gamma_1 = \gamma_2$. Because the lattice D_s is countably infinite, a delicate mathematical question remains as to whether (4.119) yields a well defined probability measure for the countably infinite set, D_s. Indeed, there may be regions of the parameter space where two different probability measures give rise to the *same* conditional probabilities, (4.119) (physicists call this phenomenon *phase transition*). Furthermore, suppose that $\gamma_1 = \gamma_2 = \gamma$; then critical values of γ exist, below which the limiting nearest-neighbor correlation is zero, but above which the process exhibits long-range dependence. These issues are discussed by, for example, Pickard (1987).

Other MRFs based on (4.110) and (4.111) are the the *auto gamma model* and the *auto binomial model*. The *Winsorized auto Poisson model* (Kaiser and Cressie, 1997) is a modification of the auto Poisson that allows positive spatial dependence; see Møller and Rubak (2010) for a different lattice process that achieves the same result. The *auto beta model* (Kaiser and Cressie, 2000) comes from a bivariate exponential family of conditional distributions applied to the joint-distribution construction given in Section 4.2.3. Arguably, the most useful of all MRFs is the auto Gaussian model, or *CAR model*. [Cressie (1993), called it a conditionally specified Gaussian model, to contrast it with a simultaneously specified Gaussian model, but the terminology of CAR and SAR models, respectively, remains popular.]

4.2.5 The CAR Model

When data are continuous, a natural model to choose for the conditional distributions $\{[Y(\mathbf{s}_i)|\mathbf{Y}(N(\mathbf{s}_i))]: i = 1, \dots, n\}$ given by (4.110) and (4.111) is the Gaussian (or normal) distribution. For $i = 1, \dots, n$, we have

$$\Pr(y(\mathbf{s}_i) \mid \mathbf{y}(N(\mathbf{s}_i))) = (2\pi \tau_i^2)^{-1/2} \exp[-\{y(\mathbf{s}_i) - \theta_i\}^2 / 2\tau_i^2], \qquad (4.120)$$

where it is understood that θ_i is a function of $\mathbf{y}(N(\mathbf{s}_i))$ and that the left-hand side is the conditional density function of $Y(\mathbf{s}_i)$, given $\mathbf{Y}(N(\mathbf{s}_i)) = \mathbf{y}(N(\mathbf{s}_i))$. In (4.120),

$$\theta_i(\mathbf{y}(N(\mathbf{s}_i))) = E(Y(\mathbf{s}_i) \mid \mathbf{y}(N(\mathbf{s}_i)))$$

$$= \mu(\mathbf{s}_i) + \sum_{\mathbf{s}_j \in N(\mathbf{s}_i)} c_{ij}(y(\mathbf{s}_j) - \mu(\mathbf{s}_j)), \qquad (4.121)$$

and $\mu(\mathbf{s}_i) \equiv E(Y(\mathbf{s}_i))$. The general condition $\theta_{ij} = \theta_{ji}$ for auto spatial models (4.111), applied to (4.120) and (4.121), implies that $c_{ij}\tau_j^2 = c_{ji}\tau_i^2$. Furthermore, $c_{ii} = 0$, and $c_{ik} = 0$ for $\mathbf{s}_k \notin N(\mathbf{s}_i)$; $i, j = 1, \ldots, n$.

Let $\mathbf{C} = (c_{ij})$ and $\mathbf{M} = \mathrm{diag}(\tau_1^2, \ldots, \tau_n^2)$. Then Besag (1974) shows that, provided $(\mathbf{I} - \mathbf{C})^{-1}\mathbf{M}$ is symmetric and positive-definite, the Gaussian conditional distributions (4.120) define a joint Gaussian distribution given by

$$\mathbf{Y} \sim Gau(\boldsymbol{\mu}, (\mathbf{I} - \mathbf{C})^{-1}\mathbf{M}). \tag{4.122}$$

The MRF given by (4.120) is an auto Gaussian model, but it is known more commonly as a *conditional autoregressive (CAR) model*.

The CAR model in particular, and MRFs in general, are an attractive way to handle spatial statistical dependencies. For each location $\mathbf{s}_i$ in the lattice D_s, a univariate (*conditional*) distribution is posited for $Y(\mathbf{s}_i)$; $i = 1, \ldots, n$. Thus, potentially complicated joint statistical dependencies are modeled simply through a collection of conditional dependencies. Because the CAR model is a Gaussian MRF, it is particularly appropriate to discuss the relationship between the CAR model and the geostatistical models described in Section 4.1.

On the lattice $D_s = \{\mathbf{s}_1, \ldots, \mathbf{s}_n\}$, a geostatistical model specifies the mean and covariance matrix of $\mathbf{Y} \equiv (Y(\mathbf{s}_1), \ldots, Y(\mathbf{s}_n))'$:

$$E(\mathbf{Y}) = \boldsymbol{\mu}_Y \quad \text{and} \quad \mathrm{var}(\mathbf{Y}) = \boldsymbol{\Sigma}_Y. \tag{4.123}$$

Further specification of the geostatistical model often involves $E(Y(\mathbf{s}_i)) \equiv \mu_Y(\mathbf{s}_i) = \mathbf{x}(\mathbf{s}_i)'\boldsymbol{\beta}$ (linear model) and $\mathrm{cov}(Y(\mathbf{s}_i), Y(\mathbf{s}_j)) = (\boldsymbol{\Sigma}_Y)_{ij} = C_Y(\mathbf{s}_j - \mathbf{s}_i)$ (covariance stationarity). The intuitive notion of spatial dependence, that nearby values tend to be more alike than values far apart, is captured in the geostatistical model through

$$C_Y(\mathbf{s}_j - \mathbf{s}_i) \simeq 0 \ (\text{or} = 0), \qquad \text{for } \|\mathbf{s}_j - \mathbf{s}_i\| \text{ "large."} \tag{4.124}$$

The same intuitive notion is captured in the CAR model,

$$E(\mathbf{Y}) = \boldsymbol{\mu}_Y \text{ and } \mathrm{var}(\mathbf{Y}) = (\mathbf{I} - \mathbf{C})^{-1}\mathbf{M}, \tag{4.125}$$

through

$$c_{ij} \simeq 0 \ (\text{or} = 0), \qquad \text{for } \|\mathbf{s}_j - \mathbf{s}_i\| \text{ "large."} \tag{4.126}$$

That is, for geostatistical models, $\mathrm{var}(\mathbf{Y})$ is "sparse," and for CAR models, $(\mathrm{var}(\mathbf{Y}))^{-1}$ is "sparse."

Algebraically, there is a one-to-one relationship between a geostatistical model on D_s and a CAR model on D_s. Given a CAR model, $Gau(\boldsymbol{\mu}_Y, (\mathbf{I} - \mathbf{C})^{-1}\mathbf{M})$, the geostatistical model is $Gau(\boldsymbol{\mu}_Y, \boldsymbol{\Sigma}_Y)$, where $\boldsymbol{\Sigma}_Y \equiv (\mathbf{I} - \mathbf{C})^{-1}\mathbf{M}$. And, given a geostatistical model $Gau(\boldsymbol{\mu}_Y, \boldsymbol{\Sigma}_Y)$, define $(\boldsymbol{\Sigma}_Y)^{-1} \equiv (\sigma^{(ij)})$, $\mathbf{M} \equiv$

$\{\text{diag}(\sigma^{(11)}, \ldots, \sigma^{(nn)})\}^{-1}$, and $\mathbf{C} \equiv \mathbf{I} - \mathbf{M}\boldsymbol{\Sigma}_Y^{-1}$. Then $\mathbf{C}$ is an $n \times n$ matrix with zeros down its diagonal, $\mathbf{M}$ is a diagonal matrix with positive entries, and the CAR model is $Gau(\boldsymbol{\mu}_Y, (\mathbf{I} - \mathbf{C})^{-1}\mathbf{M})$. The two models really are different, because if the geostatistical model is sparse, the CAR model is typically not, and *vice versa*.

Because the CAR model possesses computational advantages (taking the inverse of the covariance matrix of $\mathbf{Y}$ is trivial), it is often of interest to approximate a geostatistical model with a sparse CAR model. This problem can be formulated as minimizing a "distance" between $\boldsymbol{\Sigma}_Y$ (given) and $(\mathbf{I} - \mathbf{C})^{-1}\mathbf{M}$, with respect to $\mathbf{M}$ and a sparse $\mathbf{C}$. Rue and Held (2005, Chapter 5) discuss this problem in considerable detail.

When scientific interest centers on the large-scale effects, the idea is to use a few extra small-scale (spatial-dependence) parameters so that the large-scale parameters are estimated more efficiently. Suppose that $\mathbf{Y}$ is modeled according to a CAR model and that the large-scale variation is modeled as $E(\mathbf{Y}) = \boldsymbol{\mu}_Y = \mathbf{X}\boldsymbol{\beta}$, where recall that $\mathbf{X}$ is an $n \times p$ matrix of covariates and $\boldsymbol{\beta}$ is a p-dimensional vector of fixed (but unknown) regression coefficients. The classical Gaussian linear model is $\mathbf{Y} \sim Gau(\mathbf{X}\boldsymbol{\beta}, \tau^2\mathbf{I})$. Compare this to (4.122) with $\boldsymbol{\mu} = \mathbf{X}\boldsymbol{\beta}$, which can be written equivalently as

$$\mathbf{Y} = \mathbf{X}\boldsymbol{\beta} + \boldsymbol{\delta}, \tag{4.127}$$

where the error $\boldsymbol{\delta}$ is an n-dimensional random vector with distribution,

$$\boldsymbol{\delta} \sim Gau(\mathbf{0}, (\mathbf{I} - \mathbf{C})^{-1}\mathbf{M}).$$

Notice that when $\mathbf{C} = \mathbf{0}$, an $n \times n$ matrix with all zero entries, and $\mathbf{M} = \tau^2\mathbf{I}$, the CAR (regression) model (4.127) reduces to the classical linear model with *iid* Gaussian errors.

When $\mathbf{M}$ and $\mathbf{C}$ are unknown, as is usually the case, they are often expressed in terms of a few (small-scale) parameters, at least one of which captures the spatial dependence; for example, we use $\mathbf{C} = \phi\mathbf{H}$ in Section 4.2.6. The parameter space of $\mathbf{C}$ is $\{\mathbf{C}: (\mathbf{I} - \mathbf{C})^{-1}\mathbf{M}$ is symmetric and positive-definite$\}$. When $\mathbf{C} = \phi\mathbf{H} \equiv \phi \cdot (h_{ij})$ and $\tau_i^2 h_{ji} = \tau_j^2 h_{ij}$, the parameter space becomes

$$\{\phi: \phi_{\min} < \phi < \phi_{\max}\}, \tag{4.128}$$

where $\phi_{\min} \equiv (\lambda_{(1)})^{-1} < 0$, $\phi_{\max} \equiv (\lambda_{(n)})^{-1} > 0$, and $\lambda_{(1)} \leq \cdots \leq \lambda_{(n)}$ are the ordered eigenvalues of $\mathbf{M}^{-1/2}\mathbf{H}\mathbf{M}^{1/2}$ (Cressie, 1993, p. 559). Other parameterizations of $\mathbf{C}$ and $\mathbf{M}$ are given below and in the Bibliographic Notes in Section 4.5.

The inhomogeneity in the conditional variances, $\{\tau_i^2\}$, can often be modeled through $\mathbf{M} = \tau^2\boldsymbol{\Delta}$, where the $n \times n$ diagonal matrix $\boldsymbol{\Delta}$ is known and has positive diagonal entries. In that case, a simple transformation yields a homogeneous CAR. Define $\widetilde{\mathbf{Y}} \equiv \mathbf{\Delta}^{-1/2}\mathbf{Y}$, $\widetilde{\mathbf{X}} \equiv \mathbf{\Delta}^{-1/2}\mathbf{X}$, $\widetilde{\boldsymbol{\delta}} \equiv \mathbf{\Delta}^{-1/2}\boldsymbol{\delta}$, and $\widetilde{\mathbf{H}} \equiv \mathbf{\Delta}^{-1/2}\mathbf{H}\mathbf{\Delta}^{1/2}$. Then (4.127) is equivalent to

$$\widetilde{\mathbf{Y}} = \widetilde{\mathbf{X}}\boldsymbol{\beta} + \widetilde{\boldsymbol{\delta}}, \qquad (4.129)$$

where $\widetilde{\boldsymbol{\delta}} \sim Gau(\mathbf{0}, \tau^2(\mathbf{I} - \phi\widetilde{\mathbf{H}}))$, and the full parameter space is $\{(\boldsymbol{\beta}', \tau^2, \phi):$ $\boldsymbol{\beta} \in \mathbb{R}^p$, $\tau^2 > 0$, and $\phi \in (\phi_{\min}, \phi_{\max})\}$. The likelihood, $\mathcal{L}(\boldsymbol{\beta}, \tau^2, \phi)$, is most conveniently written in terms of the joint distribution of $\mathbf{Y}$, and it can be maximized via a combination of analytical and numerical procedures. As we demonstrate in Section 4.2.6, there are alternative ways to do inference on a CAR model that is part of an HM.

On the *regular countable* spatial lattice $\{(u, v): u, v = \ldots, -1, 0, 1, \ldots\}$ in $\mathbb{R}^2$, spatial dependence in a constant-mean homogeneous CAR model is expressed through

$$E(Y(u, v) \mid \{y(k, l): (k, l) \neq (u, v)\})$$

$$= \mu + \sum_i \sum_j \gamma(i, j)(y(u - i, v - j) - \mu),$$

where $\gamma(i, j) = \gamma(-i, -j)$ and $\gamma(0, 0) = 0$. The first-order dependence model is the special case, $\gamma(1, 0) = \gamma(-1, 0) \equiv \gamma_1$, $\gamma(0, 1) = \gamma(0, -1) \equiv \gamma_2$, and all other $\gamma(i, j)$'s are zero, which is similar to the Ising model (for binary data) given in Section 4.2.4. For this first-order dependence model, it can be seen that the correlation between two observations decays rather slowly with increasing distance between their lattice sites (Besag and Kooperberg, 1995).

For an *irregular finite* spatial lattice, the $\{c_{ij}\}$ in (4.121) could be modeled as some function of distance, $d_{ij} \equiv \|\mathbf{s}_i - \mathbf{s}_j\|$, between the locations $\mathbf{s}_i$ and $\mathbf{s}_j$. Note that, although $\mathbf{C} \equiv (c_{ij})$ depends only on $\{d_{ij}: 1 \leq i < j \leq n\}$, the covariance, $(\mathbf{\Sigma}_Y)_{ij} \equiv \text{cov}(Y(\mathbf{s}_i), Y(\mathbf{s}_j))$, does *not* in general depend on $\|\mathbf{s}_i - \mathbf{s}_j\|$ or, for that matter, on $\mathbf{s}_i - \mathbf{s}_j$. Hence an MRF on a finite spatial lattice is generally *not stationary*, even when its conditional-probability specification is homogeneous.

Care must be taken with parameterizing the spatial-dependence matrix $\mathbf{C}$, as we now demonstrate. It is not difficult to show that $\{\text{corr}(Y(\mathbf{s}_i), Y(\mathbf{s}_j)) \mid \{y(\mathbf{s}_k): k \neq i, j\})\}^2 = c_{ij}c_{ji}$, which implies that $0 \leq c_{ij}c_{ji} \leq 1$. Recall the parameterization, $\mathbf{C} = \phi\mathbf{H}$, where $\mathbf{H} \equiv (h_{ij})$ is a given $n \times n$ matrix whose diagonal elements are all zero. Let $\mathbf{A} \equiv (a_{ij})$ denote the $n \times n$ spatial neighborhood matrix such that $a_{ij} = 1$ if $\mathbf{s}_j \in N(\mathbf{s}_i)$; otherwise, $a_{ij} = 0$. Then the number of neighbors of $\mathbf{s}_i$ is $|N(\mathbf{s}_i)| = \sum_{j=1}^n a_{ij}$. Also, write $\mathbf{M} = \tau^2\mathbf{\Delta}$, where $\mathbf{\Delta}$ is a diagonal matrix whose diagonal entries are known and positive. Cressie and Kapat (2008) give special cases of this class of CAR models. The simplest model to write down is the *homogeneous CAR (HCAR)* model with $\mathbf{\Delta} = \mathbf{I}$ and $\mathbf{H} = \mathbf{A}$.

The *weighted CAR (WCAR)* model with $\mathbf{\Delta} = \text{diag}(|N(\mathbf{s}_1)|^{-1}, \ldots, |N(\mathbf{s}_n)|^{-1})$ and $h_{ij} = a_{ij}|N(\mathbf{s}_i)|^{-1}$ was proposed by Besag, York, and Mollié (1991). The WCAR model has the property that the square of the partial correlation between $Y(\mathbf{s}_i)$ and $Y(\mathbf{s}_j)$ is $\phi^2 |N(\mathbf{s}_i)|^{-1} |N(\mathbf{s}_j)|^{-1}$, for $\mathbf{s}_j \in N(\mathbf{s}_i)$. Hence, $\phi^2 \in (0, |N(\mathbf{s}_i)| \, |N(\mathbf{s}_j)|)$, illustrating that the spatial-dependence parameter ϕ *cannot* be interpreted in the same manner as one would interpret a spatial correlation between 0 and 1.

The following model (called the *ACAR* model below),

$$\boldsymbol{\Delta} = \text{diag}(|N(\mathbf{s}_1)|^{-1}, \ldots, |N(\mathbf{s}_n)|^{-1}) \, ; \, h_{ij} = a_{ij} |N(\mathbf{s}_j)|^{1/2} |N(\mathbf{s}_i)|^{-1/2},$$
(4.130)

has partial correlation,

$$\text{corr}(Y(\mathbf{s}_i), Y(\mathbf{s}_j) | \{y(\mathbf{s}_k) : k \neq i, j\}) = \phi.$$

This, and a more general result for multivariate CAR models, was given in Sain and Cressie (2007). We call this model the *autocorrelated CAR (ACAR)* model. For further models, see the Bibliographic Notes in Section 4.5, which include a class of diagonally dominant CAR models due to Pettitt, Weir, and Hart (2002).

Finally, an attractive property of the CAR model is that there is an analytical expression for its joint distribution. In general, the normalizing constant of an MRF, $\sum_{\mathbf{t} \in \Omega} \exp(Q(\mathbf{t}))$ (or $\int_\Omega \exp(Q(\mathbf{t})) \, d\mathbf{t}$) given by the left-hand side of (4.118), is analytically intractable. The CAR model given by (4.120) is an exception. Its negpotential function given by (4.107) simplifies, and

$$\int_\Omega \exp(Q(\mathbf{t})) \, d\mathbf{t} = (2\pi)^{n/2} \left(\prod_{i=1}^n \tau_i^2 \right)^{1/2} |\mathbf{I} - \mathbf{C}|^{-1/2}.$$
(4.131)

However, for n large, computation of the determinant, $|\mathbf{I} - \mathbf{C}|$, in (4.131) can be problematic. Further discussion of this aspect of the CAR model can be found in Cressie, Perrin, and Thomas-Agnan (2005).

4.2.6 Hierarchical Modeling on a Spatial Lattice: Small Area Estimation

Thus far, the lattice process has been defined on a regular or irregular spatial lattice, $D_s = \{\mathbf{s}_1, \ldots, \mathbf{s}_n\}$ in $\mathbb{R}^d$. In fact, it is possible to define MRFs (and SAR models, SMA models, and so forth) without knowing exactly the coordinates $\{\mathbf{s}_1, \ldots, \mathbf{s}_n\}$ of the process $\{Y(\mathbf{s}_i) : i = 1, \ldots, n\}$; a crucial component of the spatial-dependence model is which elements of the matrix $\mathbf{H}$ in Section 4.2.5 (or $\mathbf{W}$ or $\mathbf{E}$ in Section 4.2.7 or 4.1.6, respectively) are zero. In the case of the CAR model (a MRF), nonzero elements of $\mathbf{H}$ determine the neighborhood sets, $\{N(\mathbf{s}_i) : i = 1, \ldots, n\}$, upon which the theory of joint-to-conditional (Section 4.2.2) and conditional-to-joint (Section 4.2.3) probabilities is based. Generally, for any MRF, the only spatial information one needs to specify is which subsets of D_s constitute the neighborhood sets.

Let $A_1, \ldots, A_n$ be disjoint sub-areas (henceforth called *small areas*) of $\mathbb{R}^d$ that are spatially proximate and $D_s = \cup_{i=1}^n A_i$; let $\mathbf{s}_1, \ldots, \mathbf{s}_n$ denote a well defined feature of the respective small areas, such as geometric centroid, political capital city, and so forth. Then $D_s \equiv \{s_1, \ldots, s_n\}$ defines a spatial lattice, and neighborhoods can be defined using geographical properties; for example, the neighborhood of the ith small area could be defined to be those small areas with which it shares a common border:

$$N(s_i) \equiv \{s_j : A_j \text{ borders } A_i\}. \tag{4.132}$$

That is, spatial relationships can be defined in ways other than the Euclidean distances between $\{s_i : i = 1, \ldots, n\}$. Indeed, Figure 4.10 shows a dependence relationship between nodes of a lattice that may or may not have a spatial context.

In this subsection, we shall use the problem of *small area estimation* to illustrate spatial modeling of data that have been aggregated up to small areas. Associated with each small area, A_i, is a datum $Z(s_i)$, but the datum itself is assumed to be an average (or a transformation of an average).

Example: Doctor-Prescription Amounts per Consultation

Cressie, Perrin, and Thomas-Agnan (2005) consider the average doctor-prescription amounts per consultation in cantons of the Midi-Pyrénées in southwest France; Kang, Liu, and Cressie (2009) take logs of the data and analyze them using an HM with a Gaussian data model and a Gaussian process model.

There were 268 cantons in the Midi-Pyrénées where average doctor-prescription amounts (per consultation) were reported for the period January 1, 1999–December 31, 1999. Let s_{ij} denote the location where the jth prescription was written within canton A_i; $j = 1, \ldots, M_i$, $i = 1, \ldots, 268$. Denote those prescription amounts by $\{P_{ij} : j = 1, \ldots, M_i; i = 1, \ldots, 268\}$. As is typical with health-related data, aggregation (here over cantons) is carried out to preserve doctor and patient confidentiality. That is, the individual-location and individual-prescription data $\{(s_{ij}, P_{ij})\}$ are unavailable. Instead, we only know that in canton A_i, there were M_i prescriptions written, and the average prescription amount was,

$$P_i \equiv \sum_{j=1}^{M_i} P_{ij}/M_i, \qquad i = 1, \ldots, 268.$$

Furthermore, we have geographic information, such as a shape file of the cantons' boundaries and the locations of their centroids, $\{s_i : i = 1, \ldots, 268\}$. Then we define the spatial lattice to be $D_s \equiv \{s_1, \ldots, s_{268}\}$, with concomitant spatial (attribute) data $\{P_1, \ldots, P_{268}\}$.

Kang, Liu, and Cressie (2009), *hereafter KLC*, find that a log transformation of the data gives an appropriate scale on which to fit CAR models (Section 4.2.5). They write $Z(s_i) = k \cdot \log(P_i)$, where k is an unspecified constant to preserve data confidentiality. They specify the data model as

$$Z(s_i)|Y(s_i), \sigma_\epsilon^2 \sim ind. Gau(Y(s_i), \sigma_\epsilon^2/M_i), \qquad i = 1, \ldots, 268.$$

and the process model as

$$Y|\boldsymbol{\beta}, \tau^2, \phi \sim Gau(\mathbf{X}\boldsymbol{\beta}, \tau^2(\mathbf{I} - \phi\mathbf{H})^{-1}\boldsymbol{\Delta}) ,$$

where $\mathbf{Y} \equiv (Y(\mathbf{s}_1), \ldots, Y(\mathbf{s}_{268}))'$; $\mathbf{X}$ is a 268×3 matrix made up of three covariates (1, percentage of patients ≥ 70 years, N-S coordinate of centroid) for each of the 268 cantons; $\boldsymbol{\beta}$ is a three-dimensional vector of regression coefficients; $\boldsymbol{\Delta} \equiv \text{diag}(M_1^{-1}, \ldots, M_{268}^{-1})$; $\mathbf{H}$ is a 268×268 matrix expressing the spatial dependence:

$$h_{ij} = \begin{cases} (M_j/M_i)^{1/2}, & \mathbf{s}_j \in N(\mathbf{s}_i), \\ 0, & \text{elsewhere};\end{cases}$$

$N(\mathbf{s}_i)$ is the (neighborhood) set of all cantons within 30 km of canton i; τ^2 is the process-variance parameter; and ϕ is the parameter expressing the amount of spatial dependence in the process, chosen so that the matrix inverse exists. This choice of CAR model has the same partial-correlation properties as the ACAR model given by (4.130); Cressie, Perrin, and Thomas-Agnan (2005) give a justification for it and call it the *spatial rates* model, which is discussed below, near (4.141).

The analysis of KLC involves fitting an EHM and a BHM and comparing them; for the EHM, σ_ε^2 is estimated via the method-of-moments, and $\boldsymbol{\beta}$, τ^2, and ϕ are estimated via maximum likelihood estimation. Figure 4.11 shows the 268 cantons and their centroids in the Midi-Pyrénées region, with a choropleth map of the data (the average prescription amounts $\{P_i\}$) superimposed. The centroids are the same as those shown in Figure 4.9. There is a good deal of variability in the data, which KLC conclude is mostly due to the measurement error in the data model: on the log scale, $\widehat{\sigma}_\varepsilon^2 = 292.9$, which is to be compared to $\widehat{\tau}^2 = 77.47$.

Figure 4.12 shows a choropleth map of the (estimated) posterior means:

$$E(g^{-1}(Y(\mathbf{s}_i))|\mathbf{Z}, \widehat{\boldsymbol{\beta}}, \widehat{\sigma}_\varepsilon^2, \widehat{\tau}^2, \widehat{\phi}) , \qquad i = 1, \ldots, 268 ,$$

where recall that $g(x) \propto \log x$, and $\mathbf{Z} \equiv (Z(\mathbf{s}_1), \ldots, Z(\mathbf{s}_{268}))'$ are the data on the log scale. The maps properly account for bias correction through log-Gaussian relationships (e.g., Cressie, 1993, p. 135). The degree of smoothing in these predicted doctor-prescription amounts (posterior means) is remarkable, and the smoothed map follows roughly the political boundaries of the eight Départements in the region, even though that information was *not* used in the HM.

Accompanying the map shown in Figure 4.12 is a map showing the variability (or uncertainty) associated with the predicted values. In Figure 4.13, we show a choropleth map of:

$$\{\text{var}(g^{-1}(Y(\mathbf{s}_i))|\mathbf{Z}, \widehat{\boldsymbol{\beta}}, \widehat{\sigma}_\varepsilon^2, \widehat{\tau}^2, \widehat{\phi})\}^{1/2} , \qquad i = 1, \ldots, 268 .$$

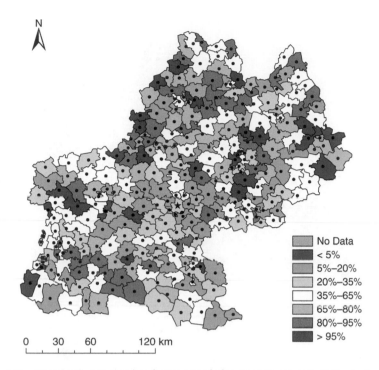

N

	No Data
■	< 5%
	5%–20%
	20%–35%
	35%–65%
	65%–80%
	80%–95%
■	> 95%

0   30   60   120 km

Figure 4.11 Choropleth map showing doctor-prescription amounts per consultation in the cantons of the Midi-Pyrénées (France). The "star" denotes the canton containing Toulouse. Percentiles used for shading are obtained from $\{P_i\}$.

On the original scale, predictions showing large average doctor-prescription amounts are accompanied by large variability (as expected). KLC also analyze the data using a BHM (with a prior on τ^2 and ϕ, and with $\widehat{\boldsymbol{\beta}}$ and $\widehat{\sigma}_\varepsilon^2$ fixed). A sensitivity study to compare results of the EHM and BHM is carried out using the parameter model:

$$\tau^2 \sim U(0, 380), \qquad \phi \sim U(0, \phi_{\max}),$$

where 380 is a value that is larger than the total estimated variation, and $\phi_{\max}$ is defined below equation (4.128). They find that the posterior means are largely unchanged, but the posterior standard deviations associated with the BHM are typically larger than those associated with the EHM (as expected). Consequently, the EHM can lead to inferences that are too liberal.

Disease Mapping

There is a literature closely related to small area estimation, known as *disease mapping*. Consider, as an example, the number of deaths caused by prostate cancer in the $n = 88$ counties of Ohio during the 10-year period, 1995–2004. Each individual (male) who died typically had a place of residence, which we denote as $\mathbf{s}_{ij}$ for the jth individual in A_i; $j = 1, \ldots, Z(\mathbf{s}_i)$, $i = 1, \ldots, n$,

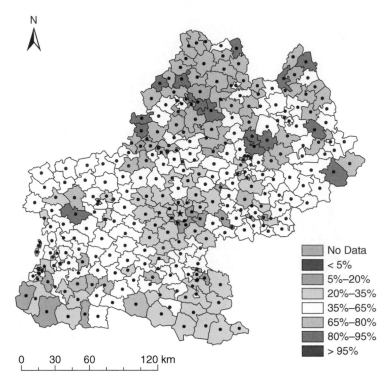

Figure 4.12 Choropleth map showing posterior mean of doctor-prescription amounts per consultation, in the cantons of the Midi-Pyrénées, based on the data in Figure 4.11. The "star" denotes the canton containing Toulouse. Percentiles used for shading are the same as in Figure 4.11.

where $\{Z(\mathbf{s}_i) : i = 1, \ldots, n\}$ are the *number* of deaths in the respective counties (small areas). A dominant question in disease mapping is whether the locations, $\{\mathbf{s}_{ij}\}$, exhibit spatial dependence, specifically clustering. The locations can be viewed as a realization of a spatial point process and could be tested for complete spatial randomness (Section 4.3.2). However, the data $\{\mathbf{s}_{ij}\}$ are typically unavailable, usually for confidentiality reasons, and they are aggregated to small areas and released to the public. Nevertheless, the question of clustering, now of small areas, is still relevant.

Assume for the moment that a given demographic group, males age $65-74$, are considered in the study of prostate-cancer deaths introduced above. (Combining several demographic groups will be considered later.) For reasons of confidentiality or even ease of analysis, often only the disease counts $\{Z(\mathbf{s}_i): i = 1, \ldots, n\}$ in the small areas $\{A_i : i = 1, \ldots, n\}$ are available. Further discussion of this aggregation to counts is given in Section 4.3.4. A concomitant variable $\{N_i : i = 1, \ldots, n\}$, the total numbers of *person* (males, age $65-74$) *years at risk*, should also be available (typically from census data). Then the disease *rate* in the ith small area is defined as

$$R(\mathbf{s}_i) \equiv Z(\mathbf{s}_i)/N_i . \tag{4.133}$$

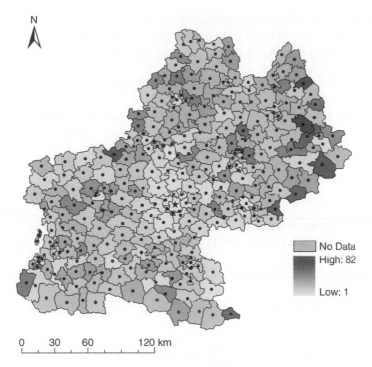

Figure 4.13 Choropleth map showing posterior standard error of doctor-prescription amounts per consultation, in the cantons of the Midi-Pyrénées, based on the data in Figure 4.11. The "star" denotes the canton containing Toulouse.

Under classical independence assumptions, one could model

$$Z(\mathbf{s}_i)|\{p(\mathbf{s}_j)\} \sim ind.\, Bin(N_i, p(\mathbf{s}_i)), \qquad i = 1, \ldots, n, \qquad (4.134)$$

where *Bin* denotes the binomial distribution, and $\{p(\mathbf{s}_j): j = 1, \ldots, n\}$ are the *disease risks* (i.e., the probabilities of getting the disease) in the small areas. Then, for $i = 1, \ldots, n$, we obtain

$$E(R(\mathbf{s}_i)|\{p(\mathbf{s}_j)\}) = p(\mathbf{s}_i) \qquad (4.135)$$

and

$$\mathrm{var}(R(\mathbf{s}_i)|\{p(\mathbf{s}_j)\}) = p(\mathbf{s}_i)(1 - p(\mathbf{s}_i))/N_i, \qquad i = 1, \ldots, n.$$

Consequently, small areas with smaller numbers of individuals at risk have observed rates that are more variable.

It is often the case that $\{p(\mathbf{s}_i)\}$ are all small and $\{N_i\}$ are all large, which is perfect for a Poisson approximation to the binomial distribution in (4.134). For a generic binomial random variable, $Bin(N, p)$, suppose $N \to \infty$ and $p \to 0$ such that $Np \to \mu$; then in distribution, $Bin(N, p) \to Poi(\mu)$.

The expected number of deaths in small area A_i is

$$N_i \, p(\mathbf{s}_i) = (N_i \overline{p})(p(\mathbf{s}_i)/\overline{p}) \equiv E_i \lambda(\mathbf{s}_i) \,,$$

where $\overline{p} \equiv \sum_{j=1}^{n} p(\mathbf{s}_j)/n$ is the average risk and $E_i \equiv N_i \overline{p}$ is a *baseline* expected number of deaths. Then we can interpret $\{\lambda(\mathbf{s}_i)\}$ as *relative risks*,

$$\lambda(\mathbf{s}_i) = \frac{p(\mathbf{s}_i)}{(E_i/N_i)} \,, \tag{4.136}$$

which is the risk divided by the "expected" risk for the ith small area; $i = 1, \ldots, n$. These calculations motivate replacing (4.133) with the assumption

$$Z(\mathbf{s}_i)|\{\lambda(\mathbf{s}_j)\} \sim ind. \, Poi(E_i \lambda(\mathbf{s}_i)), \qquad i = 1, \ldots, n \,. \tag{4.137}$$

Often, $\overline{p}$ and hence $\{E_i\}$ are unknown. A commonly used estimate of $\{E_i\}$ is

$$E_i \equiv N_i \left(\sum_{j=1}^{n} Z(\mathbf{s}_j) / \sum_{j=1}^{n} N_j \right), \qquad i = 1, \ldots, n \,. \tag{4.138}$$

A quantity often considered by epidemiologists is the *standardized mortality ratio (SMR)*, which is defined as

$$\mathrm{SMR}_i \equiv Z(\mathbf{s}_i)/E_i, \qquad i = 1, \ldots, n \,. \tag{4.139}$$

Consequently, if we assume (4.137), then

$$E(\mathrm{SMR}_i|\{\lambda(\mathbf{s}_j)\}) = \lambda(\mathbf{s}_i) \quad \text{and} \quad \mathrm{var}(\mathrm{SMR}_i|\{\lambda(\mathbf{s}_j)\}) = \lambda(\mathbf{s}_i)/E_i \,. \tag{4.140}$$

If $\{E_i\}$ have to be estimated [say using (4.138)], the equalities in (4.140) become approximations. Hence, up to these approximations, the SMR is an unbiased estimator of the relative risk with variability inversely proportional to the baseline expected number of deaths (equally, it is inversely proportional to the number of person years at risk). That is, for areas with a smaller E_i, the standardized mortality ratio, SMR_i, is a less precise estimator of its relative risk.

When the population in $D_s = \cup_{i=1}^{n} A_i$ is made up of several demographic groups or other obvious strata (e.g., age ranges, in the case of prostate cancer), then the calculation of the expected number of deaths E_i in the small area A_i is a little more involved: Define q_k to be the proportion of the at-risk population that are in group k; $k = 1, \ldots, K$, where K is the number of demographic groups. Then $\sum_{k=1}^{K} q_k = 1$. Consider the small area A_i. Because we have K

groups, the number of person-years-at-risk (N_i) for A_i can be decomposed into numbers of person-years-at-risk in each group ($\{N_{ik}\}$):

$$N_i = \sum_{k=1}^{K} N_{ik} .$$

Then the *baseline* expected number of deaths is defined by

$$E_i \equiv \sum_{k=1}^{K} N_{ik} q_k, \qquad i = 1, \ldots, n .$$

Often, $\{q_k : k = 1, \ldots, K\}$, and hence $\{E_i\}$, are unknown. A commonly used (internally standardized) estimate of q_k is

$$\widehat{q}_k = \sum_{j=1}^{n} Z(\mathbf{s}_j)_k / \sum_{j=1}^{n} N_{jk}, \qquad k = 1, \ldots, K,$$

where $Z(\mathbf{s}_j)_k$ is the observed number of deaths in small area A_j that occurred in the kth demographic group. Finally, the (internally standardized) estimate of the baseline expected number of deaths is defined by

$$E_i \equiv \sum_{k=1}^{K} N_{ik} \widehat{q}_k, \qquad i = 1, \ldots, n .$$

Much of the recent literature on disease mapping has involved fitting an HM to the data in order to "borrow strength" from the areas that are more precise (larger E_i); the approach is sometimes called *shrinkage*, or *super-population modeling*. For example, see Lawson and Cressie (2000) and the text by Lawson (2001) for a review of that literature.

The spatial dependence is typically incorporated into the process model through the logarithm of the true rates:

Data model: Conditional on $\{\lambda(\mathbf{s}_i)\}$ and for $i = 1, \ldots, n$,

$$Z(\mathbf{s}_i) | \lambda(\mathbf{s}_i) \sim Poi(E_i \lambda(\mathbf{s}_i)) .$$

Process model: Conditional on $\boldsymbol{\beta}_C$ and $\boldsymbol{\theta}$ and for $\mathbf{Y} \equiv (\log \lambda(\mathbf{s}_1), \ldots, \log \lambda(\mathbf{s}_n))'$,

$$\mathbf{Y} | \boldsymbol{\beta}, \boldsymbol{\theta}_C \sim Gau(\mathbf{X}\boldsymbol{\beta}, \boldsymbol{\Sigma}(\boldsymbol{\theta}_C)) ,$$

where

$$\boldsymbol{\Sigma}(\boldsymbol{\theta}_C) \equiv \sigma^2 \mathbf{D} + \tau^2 (\mathbf{I} - \phi \mathbf{H})^{-1} \boldsymbol{\Delta} ;$$

$\mathbf{D}$ and $\boldsymbol{\Delta}$ are known $n \times n$ diagonal matrices; $\mathbf{H}$ is a known $n \times n$ matrix with zeros down the diagonal; and the lattice-model covariance parameters are $\boldsymbol{\theta}_C \equiv (\sigma^2, \tau^2, \phi)'$, chosen so that the matrix inverse exists.

The first term in $\Sigma(\boldsymbol{\theta}_C)$ is a known (apart from the parameter, σ^2) diagonal matrix that accounts for inhomogeneities, such as extra-Poisson variation. The second term is the CAR model with spatial-dependence parameter ϕ and variance heterogeneity expressed through $\tau^2\Delta$, where Δ is a known diagonal matrix.

The model of Besag, York, and Mollié (1991) uses $\mathbf{D} = \mathbf{I}$ and $\phi = \phi_{\max}$, resulting in $\tau^2(\mathbf{I} - \phi\mathbf{H})^{-1}\Delta$ being only nonnegative-definite. That is, the lattice-model parameters are $\boldsymbol{\theta}_L = (\sigma^2, \tau^2)'$. Notice that, even when $\sigma^2 = 0$, it is still possible to obtain a proper posterior distribution through formal application of Bayes' Theorem. It reflects the often-seen, slowly decreasing spatial correlation as a function of distance between small areas. In contrast, the model of Cressie (1992) puts $\sigma^2 = 0$, and hence the lattice-model parameters are $\boldsymbol{\theta}_C = (\tau^2, \phi)'$; this latter model allows inference on the strength of the spatial-dependence parameter in the interval $(\phi_{\min}, \phi_{\max})$, the parameter space for ϕ in the model (4.128). Cressie and Hartfield (1996) use a similar model for regular two-dimensional plots in an agricultural field trial; they estimated a well defined, positive-definite CAR matrix $\mathbf{C}$. Wright, Stern, and Cressie (2003) leave all three parameters, σ^2, τ^2, and ϕ in the process model, although the preponderance of choice in the disease-mapping literature has been to specify $\phi = \phi_{\max}$.

Cressie and Chan (1989) and Cressie (1992) make the following choices of $\Delta \equiv \text{diag}(\Delta_1, \ldots, \Delta_n)$ and $\mathbf{H} \equiv (h_{ij})$, relating them to expected counts, $\{E_i\}$: For $i = 1, \ldots, n$,

$$\text{A1:} \quad \Delta_i = 1/E_i,$$

$$\text{A2:} \quad h_{ij} = \begin{cases} (E_j/E_i)^{1/2}, & \mathbf{s}_j \in N(\mathbf{s}_i) \\ 0, & \text{elsewhere}. \end{cases}$$

Importantly, the symmetry conditions, $\Delta_j h_{ij} = \Delta_i h_{ji}$, for all i, j, hold. This process model (like the data model given just above) results in smaller variances for areas with larger expected number of people at risk. Cressie, Perrin, and Thomas-Agnan (2005, Appendix A) give a justification of this choice of A1, A2 and called it the *spatial rates model*.

Besag, York, and Mollié (1991) made a different choice for Δ and $\mathbf{H}$. For $i = 1, \ldots, n$,

$$\text{B1:} \quad \Delta_i = 1/|N(\mathbf{s}_i)|,$$

$$\text{B2:} \quad h_{ij} = \begin{cases} 1/|N(\mathbf{s}_i)|, & \mathbf{s}_j \in N(\mathbf{s}_i) \\ 0, & \text{elsewhere}. \end{cases}$$

The symmetry conditions, $\Delta_j h_{ij} = \Delta_i h_{ji}$, for all i, j, hold. Recall that in Section 4.2.5, we called this a WCAR model.

One final way to compare the two models is to recall the result given in Section 4.2.5,

$$[\operatorname{corr}(Y(\mathbf{s}_i), Y(\mathbf{s}_j) | \{Y(\mathbf{s}_k) : k \neq i, j\})]^2 = \phi^2 h_{ij} h_{ji} \, . \tag{4.141}$$

In Section 4.2.5, we saw that for the WCAR (i.e., choose B1 and B2) model, the square of the partial correlation in (4.141) is $\phi^2 / |N(\mathbf{s}_i)||N(\mathbf{s}_j)|$, making ϕ difficult to interpret. For the spatial-rates model (i.e., choose A1 and A2), the square of the partial correlation in (4.141) is ϕ^2, which is invariant to the neighborhood structure. Consequently, ϕ is easily interpretable as a spatial-dependence parameter in $[-1, 1]$. The ACAR model defined in (4.130) has a similar structure to the spatial-rates model, where $N(\mathbf{s}_i)$ replaces E_i in the definition of Δ and $\mathbf{H}$. Both models have the property that ϕ can be interpreted as a partial correlation coefficient.

The HM just above becomes a BHM model by including a parameter model. We now give an example for a process model where $\mathbf{D} = \operatorname{diag}(1/E_1, \ldots, 1/E_n)$, and Δ and $\mathbf{H}$ are given in A1 and A2:

Parameter model: The joint distribution of the parameters is

$$[\boldsymbol{\beta}, \sigma^2, \tau^2, \phi] = [\boldsymbol{\beta}][\sigma^2][\tau^2][\phi] \, ,$$

where $\boldsymbol{\beta} \sim U((-\infty, \infty)^p)$; $[\sigma^2] \propto \exp(-b/\sigma^2)$, $[\tau^2] \propto \exp(-b/\tau^2)$, for b a small number (equal to 0.01); and $\phi \sim U(0, \phi_{\max})$.

Wright, Stern, and Cressie (2003) used this in a BHM for studying male lip cancer in Scotland. Implementation of the BHM is almost always through MCMC; see examples given in Gilks, Richardson, and Spiegelhalter (1996).

Change-of-Support in Small Areas: Ecological Bias

The *ecological fallacy* in its simplest form states that relationships seen at aggregated (here over space) levels could be very different from those seen at the individual level. Robinson (1950) coined the term and illustrated it with 1930s data on individuals in the United States, where part of the dataset contained the binary variables "foreign born" and "literate." At the individual level, these two variables showed a negative correclation of -0.11; however, at the state level (the lower 48 states in the United States), the percent foreign born and the percent literate had a correlation of $+0.53$. The Geography literature has referred to the way inferences vary according to the level of aggregation as the *modifiable areal unit problem (MAUP)*, and it is simply Simpson's Paradox in another guise (Chapter 1). In spatial statistics, the phenomenon is often called *change-of-support (COS)*; see Section 4.1.3. It is a difficult problem because typically one seeks explanation of an individual-level relationship, but all one has is aggregated-level data (due to data-collection methods or due to confidentiality requirements). Much has been written about the problem, and we refer the interested reader to the special issue of the *Journal of the Royal Statistical Society, Series A*, Vol. 164, Part 1 (2001).

The problem is inherently a statistical one; a perfect correlaton of ± 1 at the individual level implies a perfect correlation of ± 1, respectively, at all aggregated levels, but once the individual correlation lies *strictly between* -1 and 1, anything could happen to the correlation at the aggregated level. Our recommended approach to this vexing but fascinating problem is to use statistical modeling to resolve it; whenever possible, build statistical models at the individual level and look at their consequences under the operation of aggregation. Specifically, we recommend fitting the aggregated *individual-level model* to the *aggregated data*. While logically defensible, it hinges on the requirement that there is enough "knowledge" about the problem to build a good individual-level statistical model! But, if that knowledge is induced from aggregated data, there is a serious risk of being caught in the fallacy.

4.2.7 Simultaneously Specified Spatial Dependence

Whittle (1954) defined simultaneously specified spatial processes on the countable integer lattice in $\mathbb{R}^2$. Here we consider the finite irregular lattice; that is, $D_s \equiv \{s_1, \ldots, s_n\}$. Let $\boldsymbol{\nu} \equiv (\nu(s_1), \ldots, \nu(s_n))'$ denote a joint Gaussian distribution with zero mean and independent components. That is,

$$\boldsymbol{\nu} \sim Gau(\mathbf{0}, \boldsymbol{\Lambda}), \tag{4.142}$$

where $\boldsymbol{\Lambda} \equiv \text{diag}(\sigma_1^2, \ldots, \sigma_n^2)$. Analogous to (4.84), which recall is a first-order autoregressive model in $\mathbb{R}^1$, we define the *simultaneous autoregressive (SAR)* model in $\mathbb{R}^d$:

$$Y(s_i) = \mu(s_i) + \sum_{j=1}^{n} b_{ij}(Y(s_j) - \mu(s_j)) + \nu(s_i), \tag{4.143}$$

where $b_{ii} = 0$; $i = 1, \ldots, n$, and $(\mu(s_1), \ldots, \mu(s_n))' \equiv \boldsymbol{\mu}$ is an n-dimensional vector representing the mean of $\mathbf{Y}$. Notice that (4.143) requires no ordering of the locations $\{s_1, \ldots, s_n\}$. A special case of (4.143), for which the locations do have a type of ordering, is called a *unilateral process*. For example, D_s is a regular square lattice in $\mathbb{R}^2$ and b_{ij} is non-zero only if s_j is "southwest" of s_i (e.g., Tjostheim, 1983).

In terms of vectors and matrices, (4.143) can be written equivalently as

$$\mathbf{Y} - \boldsymbol{\mu} = \mathbf{B}(\mathbf{Y} - \boldsymbol{\mu}) + \boldsymbol{\nu};$$

that is,

$$\mathbf{Y} = \boldsymbol{\mu} + (\mathbf{I} - \mathbf{B})^{-1}\boldsymbol{\nu}, \tag{4.144}$$

where **B** has zeros down the diagonal, and it is assumed that the SAR coefficients, $\{b_{ij}\}$ are chosen such that $(\mathbf{I} - \mathbf{B})$ is invertible. Notice that **B** is not necessarily symmetric, and $(\mathbf{I} - \mathbf{B})$ is not necessarily positive-definite.

While **B** is typically sparse, $(\mathbf{I} - \mathbf{B})^{-1}$ is not. Nevertheless, the right-hand side of (4.144) expresses the spatial dependence in the SAR model as a spatial moving average of the elements of $\boldsymbol{v}$, which are *iid*.

If we write $\boldsymbol{\mu} = \mathbf{X}\boldsymbol{\beta}$, then (4.144) can be written as the general linear model,

$$\mathbf{Y} = \mathbf{X}\boldsymbol{\beta} + \boldsymbol{\delta}, \tag{4.145}$$

where now $\boldsymbol{\delta}$ is a spatial Gaussian process that satisfies $(\mathbf{I} - \mathbf{B})\boldsymbol{\delta} = \boldsymbol{v}$, and $\boldsymbol{v} \sim Gau(\mathbf{0}, \boldsymbol{\Lambda})$. Hence,

$$\boldsymbol{\delta} \sim Gau(\mathbf{0}, (\mathbf{I} - \mathbf{B})^{-1}\boldsymbol{\Lambda}(\mathbf{I} - \mathbf{B}')^{-1}). \tag{4.146}$$

This representation of a SAR model should be contrasted with the representation of a CAR model given by (4.127). From (4.146), the spatial dependence is captured by **B**. If $\mathbf{B} = \mathbf{0}$, the $n \times n$ matrix of zeros, then $\boldsymbol{\delta} \sim Gau(\mathbf{0}, \mathrm{diag}(\sigma_1^2, \ldots, \sigma_n^2))$, which is the joint distribution of independent components, $\boldsymbol{\delta}(\mathbf{s}_i) \sim Gau(0, \sigma_i^2)$, $i = 1, \ldots, n$. In the CAR given by (4.127), we obtain a similar result if $\mathbf{C} = \mathbf{0}$, but the interpretation of *nonzero* **C** in (4.127) is totally different to the interpretation of *nonzero* **B** in (4.145).

The area of research known as *spatial econometrics* (e.g., Paelinck and Klaassen, 1979; Anselin, 1988) views the matrix **B** as a type of spatial backward-shift operator; compare this with the temporal backward-shift operator found in (3.15). For $\boldsymbol{\mu} = \mathbf{0}$, the SAR model can be written as $\mathbf{Y} = \mathbf{B}\mathbf{Y} + \boldsymbol{v}$, which is analogous to the first-order autoregression in time series, namely $Y_t = BY_t + W_t$, where $BY_t \equiv Y_{t-1}$.

Every SAR model with a sparse **B** results in a CAR model with a sparse **C**. Define $\widetilde{\mathbf{Y}} \equiv \boldsymbol{\Lambda}^{-1/2}\mathbf{Y}$, where $\boldsymbol{\Lambda}$ is given in (4.142) and **Y** satisfies (4.144). Then

$$\mathrm{var}(\widetilde{\mathbf{Y}}) = (\mathbf{I} - \widetilde{\mathbf{B}})^{-1}(\mathbf{I} - \widetilde{\mathbf{B}}')^{-1}, \tag{4.147}$$

where $\widetilde{\mathbf{B}} \equiv \boldsymbol{\Lambda}^{-1/2}\mathbf{B}\boldsymbol{\Lambda}^{1/2}$. Because $\boldsymbol{\Lambda}$ is a diagonal matrix, **B** is sparse if and only if $\widetilde{\mathbf{B}}$ is sparse. From (4.147), we have

$$(\mathrm{var}(\widetilde{\mathbf{Y}}))^{-1} = (\mathbf{I} - \widetilde{\mathbf{B}}' - \widetilde{\mathbf{B}} + \widetilde{\mathbf{B}}'\widetilde{\mathbf{B}}) \equiv \mathbf{M}^{-1}(\mathbf{I} - \mathbf{C}),$$

where **M** is an $n \times n$ diagonal matrix, **C** is an $n \times n$ matrix with zeros down the diagonal, and the formulas for **M** and **C** can be derived straightforwardly. It is easy to see that if $\widetilde{\mathbf{B}}$ is sparse, so too is **C**, albeit less sparse than $\widetilde{\mathbf{B}}$. See Besag (1974) and Cressie (1993, Section 6.3), for comparisons between the SAR model and the CAR model.

There is one curiosity of the SAR model that illustrates once again the difficulty in generalizing from $s \in \mathbb{R}^1$ to $\mathbf{s} \in \mathbb{R}^d$. A simple calculation (e.g.,

Cressie, 1993, p. 409) shows that the autoregressive "errors" $\{\boldsymbol{\nu}(\mathbf{s}_i)\}$ in (4.143) are correlated with $\{Y(\mathbf{s}_i)\}$; specifically, $\text{cov}(\boldsymbol{\nu}, \mathbf{Y}) = \mathbf{\Lambda}(\mathbf{I} - \mathbf{B}')^{-1}$. That is, the SAR model has the property that the "noise" $\boldsymbol{\nu}$ correlates with the "signal" $\mathbf{Y}$, making the autoregression in (4.143) difficult to interpret.

A simple example of an HM involving the SAR model is given as follows. For illustrative purposes, suppose $\mathbf{B} = \rho\mathbf{W}$, where ρ is a real-valued parameter and $\mathbf{W}$ is known and has zeros down the diagonal. Furthermore, suppose that $\mathbf{\Lambda} = \sigma^2 \mathbf{I}$.

Data model: Conditional on σ_ε^2, and for $i = 1, \ldots, n$,

$$Z(\mathbf{s}_i)|Y(\mathbf{s}_i), \sigma_\varepsilon^2 \sim ind. \, Gau(Y(\mathbf{s}_i), \sigma_\varepsilon^2) \, .$$

Process model: Conditional on $\boldsymbol{\beta}$, σ^2, and ρ,

$$\mathbf{Y}|\boldsymbol{\beta}, \sigma^2, \rho \sim Gau(\mathbf{X}\boldsymbol{\beta}, \sigma^2[(\mathbf{I} - \rho\mathbf{W}')(\mathbf{I} - \rho\mathbf{W})]^{-1}) \, ,$$

where $\mathbf{W}$ is a known $n \times n$ matrix with zeros down the diagonal, and the parameter space of ρ ensures that the matrix inverse exists.

A BHM has a parameter (prior) model that specifies the distribution of $(\boldsymbol{\beta}', \sigma^2, \rho)$. Because of the Gaussian and additive structure of the HM, the model for the data $\mathbf{Z}$ could be represented additively in terms of the marginal distribution of $\mathbf{Z}$. That is,

$$\mathbf{Z} = \mathbf{X}\boldsymbol{\beta} + \boldsymbol{\delta} + \boldsymbol{\varepsilon} \, ,$$

where $\boldsymbol{\varepsilon} \equiv (\varepsilon(\mathbf{s}_1), \ldots, \varepsilon(\mathbf{s}_n))'$ are the measurement errors, often $\boldsymbol{\varepsilon} \sim Gau(\mathbf{0}, \sigma_\varepsilon^2 \mathbf{I})$, and $\boldsymbol{\delta}$ and $\boldsymbol{\varepsilon}$ are independent. Hence, the HM can be represented equivalently as a linear mixed model for "noisy" data $\mathbf{Z}$, with $E(\mathbf{Z}) = \mathbf{X}\boldsymbol{\beta}$ and $\text{var}(\mathbf{Z}) = \sigma^2[(\mathbf{I} - \rho\mathbf{W}')(\mathbf{I} - \rho\mathbf{W})]^{-1} + \sigma_\varepsilon^2 \mathbf{I}$. Inference is needed for $\boldsymbol{\beta}$, σ_ε^2, σ^2, ρ, $\boldsymbol{\delta}$, and hence the "signal" $\mathbf{Y}$. In an EHM, $\boldsymbol{\beta}$, σ_ε^2, σ^2, and ρ are estimated, whereas in a BHM, their uncertainty is captured by a parameter model. Obviously, analogous conclusions hold if a CAR model like (4.98) replaces the SAR model in the HM; see Section 4.2.6.

4.2.8   Other Topics

The SMA and SARMA Models

In Section 4.1, where we discussed geostatistical processes, we presented the spatial moving average (or process convolution) models (4.67). The discretized version could be viewed as a lattice model. By analogy to the (mean-zero) SAR model, $(\mathbf{I} - \rho\mathbf{W})\mathbf{Y} = \boldsymbol{\nu}$, we write the lattice *spatial moving average (SMA) model* as

$$\mathbf{Y} = (\mathbf{I} + \psi\mathbf{E})\boldsymbol{\nu} \, , \tag{4.148}$$

where $\mathbf{E}$ is an $n \times n$ matrix with zeros down the diagonal, and $\boldsymbol{\nu} \equiv (\nu(\mathbf{s}_1), \ldots, \nu(\mathbf{s}_n))'$ has mean zero and var$(\boldsymbol{\nu}) = \mathbf{\Lambda}$, a diagonal $n \times n$ matrix. Notice that when $\psi = 0$, $\mathbf{Y} = \boldsymbol{\nu}$, and hence the process $\mathbf{Y}$ exhibits no spatial dependence. From (4.148),

$$E(\mathbf{Y}) = \mathbf{0} \quad \text{and} \quad \text{var}(\mathbf{Y}) = (\mathbf{I} + \psi\mathbf{E})\mathbf{\Lambda}(\mathbf{I} + \psi\mathbf{E}')\,.$$

Haining (1978) gives a detailed discussion of this model.

A general linear model based on SMA dependence is obtained, if we write

$$\mathbf{Y} = \mathbf{X}\boldsymbol{\beta} + \boldsymbol{\delta}\,, \tag{4.149}$$

where now $\boldsymbol{\delta} = (\mathbf{I} + \psi\mathbf{E})\boldsymbol{\nu}$, and $\boldsymbol{\nu} \sim Gau(\mathbf{0}, \mathbf{\Lambda})$. Therefore,

$$\mathbf{Y} \sim Gau(\mathbf{X}\boldsymbol{\beta}, (\mathbf{I} + \psi\mathbf{E})\mathbf{\Lambda}(\mathbf{I} + \psi\mathbf{E}'))\,. \tag{4.150}$$

Notice that the spatial dependence is captured through (sparse) var$(\mathbf{Y})$, and hence (4.150) is closer in type to a (discretized) geostatistical model.

A *spatial autoregressive moving average (SARMA) model* for $\mathbf{Y}$ is defined as follows:

$$(\mathbf{I} - \rho\mathbf{W})\mathbf{Y} = (\mathbf{I} + \psi\mathbf{E})\boldsymbol{\nu}\,; \tag{4.151}$$

the spatial dependence in the SARMA model can be expressed through,

$$\mathbf{Y} = (\mathbf{I} - \rho\mathbf{W})^{-1}(\mathbf{I} + \psi\mathbf{E})\boldsymbol{\nu} \equiv \mathbf{F}\boldsymbol{\nu},$$

which, in fact, is a spatial moving average of the independent elements of $\boldsymbol{\nu}$. It is easy to see that $E(\mathbf{Y}) = \mathbf{0}$, and that

$$\text{var}(\mathbf{Y}) = \{(\mathbf{I} - \rho\mathbf{W})^{-1}(\mathbf{I} + \psi\mathbf{E})\}\mathbf{\Lambda}\{(\mathbf{I} - \rho\mathbf{W})^{-1}(\mathbf{I} + \psi\mathbf{E})\}'\,. \tag{4.152}$$

The general linear model based on SARMA dependence is sometimes called a *SARMAX model*. Define

$$\mathbf{Y} = \mathbf{X}\boldsymbol{\beta} + \boldsymbol{\delta}\,, \tag{4.153}$$

where the error term $\boldsymbol{\delta}$ follows the SARMA model. That is, $(\mathbf{I} - \rho\mathbf{W})\boldsymbol{\delta} = (\mathbf{I} + \psi\mathbf{E})\boldsymbol{\nu}$, where $\boldsymbol{\nu} \sim Gau(\mathbf{0}, \mathbf{\Lambda})$, and recall that $\mathbf{\Lambda} \equiv \text{diag}(\sigma_1^2, \ldots, \sigma_n^2)$. Hence,

$$\mathbf{Y} \sim Gau(\mathbf{X}\boldsymbol{\beta}, \mathbf{\Sigma}_Y)\,,$$

where $\mathbf{\Sigma}_Y$ is given by var$(\mathbf{Y})$ in (4.152). Spatio-temporal versions of these models can be found in Section 6.4.2.

Recall that our goal in this section is to present lattice models for $\mathbf{Y}$ that incorporate spatial dependence. When the SARMAX model (4.153) is used as a

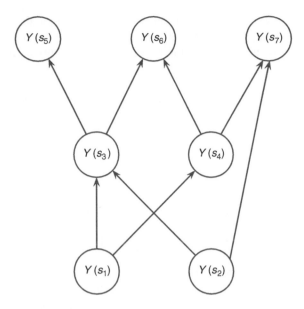

Figure 4.14 Directed graph with seven vertices, showing the (directed) edges between the vertices.

process model in an HM, which includes additive measurement error ε, data $\mathbf{Z}$ can be represented additively in terms of its marginal distribution,

$$\mathbf{Z} = \mathbf{Y} + \varepsilon = \mathbf{X}\boldsymbol{\beta} + \boldsymbol{\delta} + \varepsilon ,$$

where $\varepsilon \equiv (\varepsilon(\mathbf{s}_1), \ldots, \varepsilon(\mathbf{s}_n))'$, often $\varepsilon \sim Gau(\mathbf{0}, \sigma_\varepsilon^2 \mathbf{I})$, and $\boldsymbol{\delta}$ and ε are independent. To simplify discussion, assume that $\sigma_1^2 = \ldots = \sigma_n^2 = \sigma^2$. This gives a linear mixed model, as in Section 4.2.7, and inference is needed for $\boldsymbol{\beta}$, σ_ε^2, σ^2, ρ, ψ, $\boldsymbol{\delta}$, and hence the "signal" $\mathbf{Y}$. In an EHM, $\boldsymbol{\beta}$, σ_ε^2, σ^2, ρ, and ψ are estimated, whereas in a BHM, their uncertainty is captured by a parameter model.

The Partially Ordered Markov Model (POMM)
Another approach taken to modeling spatial dependence in lattice data has been to impose some sort of directionality or ordering on the integer lattice, and to define analogues to (4.84), (4.90), or (4.91) based on that ordering. Abend, Harley, and Kanal (1965) did this on an integer lattice with simple directional dependence that they called a *Markov mesh model*; Cressie and Liu (2001) developed this further in the case of a binary process. Goutsias (1989) started with processes that satisfy a spatial generalization of (4.91), and he showed that this is equivalent to a spatial generalization of (4.90).

Cressie and Davidson (1998) define *partially ordered Markov models (POMMs)* on an acyclic directed graph of spatial locations, $\{\mathbf{s}_i : i = 1, \ldots, n\}$, through conditional probabilities,

$$[Y(\mathbf{s}_i)|\mathbf{Y}(pa(\mathbf{s}_i))], \qquad i = 1, \ldots, n, \qquad (4.154)$$

where $pa(\mathbf{s}_i)$ is the set of "parents" of $\mathbf{s}_i$, defined by the directed graph. They note that this is precisely the class of processes that Whittle (1963) was looking for in his attempt to generalize the one-dimensional Markov property to higher dimensions.

A simple example of a directed graph is shown in Figure 4.14; the nodes are at $D_s = \{\mathbf{s}_1, \ldots, \mathbf{s}_7\}$. The set of parents, $pa(\mathbf{s}_i)$, is the set of all nodes $\mathbf{s}_j$ with a directed edge from $\mathbf{s}_j$ to $\mathbf{s}_i$. Further properties of such graphs are given by Lauritzen (1996).

Cressie and Davidson (1998) prove two main results. First, they prove

$$[\mathbf{Y}] = [\mathbf{Y}(D_0)] \prod_{\mathbf{s} \in D_s \backslash D_0} [Y(\mathbf{s})|\mathbf{Y}(pa(\mathbf{s}))], \qquad (4.155)$$

where $D_0 \subset D_s$ are all locations that have no parents (i.e., "minimum" elements in the partial ordering implied by the acyclic directed graph). From (4.155) we see that the joint distribution of POMMs can be written directly as a product of the conditional distributions (4.154), *without* the need to evaluate a normalizing constant. Of course, a (partial) ordering is needed on D_s in order to define (4.154), and so POMMs appear to be a rather restrictive class of spatial models for lattice data.

When taken out of its spatial context, we have seen in Section 2.4 that the acyclic directed graph represents precisely the type of relationships one sees in an HM. Suppose that the data model involves $[\mathbf{Z}|\mathbf{Y}, \boldsymbol{\theta}_D]$, the process model involves $[\mathbf{Y}|\boldsymbol{\theta}_P]$, and the parameter model involves $[\boldsymbol{\theta}]$, where $\boldsymbol{\theta} = \{\boldsymbol{\theta}_D, \boldsymbol{\theta}_P\}$. Then the directed graph that captures the dependence structure in the HM is given by Figure 2.2b. Consequently, the joint distribution $[\mathbf{Z}, \mathbf{Y}, \boldsymbol{\theta}_D, \boldsymbol{\theta}_P]$ can be obtained from (4.155), and it is

$$[\mathbf{Z}, \mathbf{Y}, \boldsymbol{\theta}_D, \boldsymbol{\theta}_P] = [\mathbf{Z}|\mathbf{Y}, \boldsymbol{\theta}_D][\mathbf{Y}|\boldsymbol{\theta}_P][\boldsymbol{\theta}_D, \boldsymbol{\theta}_P].$$

Cressie and Davidson's second result shows that POMMs are in fact MRFs, and hence they are not as restrictive as it might first seem. Define the *closure of the parents* of $\mathbf{s}_i$ as, $\overline{pa}(\mathbf{s}_i) \equiv pa(\mathbf{s}_i) \cup \{\mathbf{s}_i\}$. Then the *family* of $\mathbf{s}_i$ is defined as

$$fa(\mathbf{s}_i) \equiv \bigcup \{\overline{pa}(\mathbf{s}_j) : \mathbf{s}_j \in \overline{pa}(\mathbf{s}_i)\}; \qquad (4.156)$$

furthermore, remove $\mathbf{s}_i$ from the family and define $fa^*(\mathbf{s}_i) \equiv fa(\mathbf{s}_i)\backslash\{\mathbf{s}_i\}$. They show that a POMM's conditional probabilities are given by

$$[Y(\mathbf{s}_i)|\mathbf{Y}_{-i}] = [Y(\mathbf{s}_i)|\mathbf{Y}(fa^*(\mathbf{s}_i))], \qquad i = 1, \ldots, n. \qquad (4.157)$$

That is, $\mathbf{Y}$ is an MRF with $N(\mathbf{s}_i) = fa^*(\mathbf{s}_i)$; $i = 1, \ldots, n$.

Moreover, the conditional probabilities (4.157) that define the MRF can be calculated easily from (4.154). Define, for $i = 1, \ldots, n$,

$$R(Y(\mathbf{s}_i); \mathbf{Y}(fa^*(\mathbf{s}_i))) \equiv \prod [Y(\mathbf{s}_j)|\mathbf{Y}(pa(\mathbf{s}_j))], \qquad (4.158)$$

where the product in this expression is over $\{\mathbf{s}_j \in D_s : \mathbf{s}_i \in \overline{pa}(\mathbf{s}_j)\}$. Then, from Cressie and Davidson (1998), the conditional probabilities are

$$[Y(\mathbf{s}_i)|\mathbf{Y}_{-i}] = R(Y(\mathbf{s}_i); \mathbf{Y}(fa^*(\mathbf{s}_i))) \Big/ \sum_{t \in \Omega_i} R(t; \mathbf{Y}(fa^*(\mathbf{s}_i))),$$

where recall that Ω_i is the support of $Y(\mathbf{s}_i)$; $i = 1, \ldots, n$. In summary, POMMs are defined by the set of parents $\{pa(\mathbf{s}_i): i = 1, \ldots, n\}$, which then yield an MRF with neighborhoods and conditional probabilities defined by $\{fa^*(\mathbf{s}_i): i = 1, \ldots, n\}$. These neighborhoods are equivalently obtained by forming the moral graph from the acyclic directed graph (i.e., forming edges between all parents of each node and then making all directed edges undirected); see Lauritzen (1996, p. 47). In fact, the MRF defined by the (undirected) graph in Figure 4.10 is the moral graph obtained from the directed graph in Figure 4.14.

While the POMMs look like a curiosity from a purely spatial point of view, when the time dimension is added it becomes sensible to order spatio-temporal locations according to dynamic relations in a statistical model; see Figures 6.20 and 6.21 in Chapter 6.

4.3 SPATIAL POINT PROCESSES

A spatial point process is a stochastic process governing the location of events (equivalently, points) $\{\mathbf{s}_i\}$ in some set $D_s \subset \mathbb{R}^d$, where the number of such events in D_s is also random (e.g., Diggle, 2003). In the simplest case, the randomness is in the spatial locations and not in any attribute associated with the locations. For example, consider the locations of longleaf pines in 4 ha of a natural forest in Thomas county, Georgia, in 1979 (Platt, Evans, and Rathbun, 1988; Cressie, 1993; Rathbun and Cressie, 1994). Figure 4.15 shows the locations of adult and subadult trees. Trees develop for numerous reasons, due to seed dispersal, nutrients, water, light, competition, fire, animal foraging, and so forth. It is often reasonable to assume that their locations are the result of a superposition of many chance occurrences, and hence they can be modeled as a spatial point process. The proper definition of point processes requires some theoretical background, a brief description of which is given below.

Only *simple* spatial point processes in $\mathbb{R}^d$ (i.e., almost surely, either no event or a single event occurs at any point) will be considered. We characterize the spatial point process Z through subsets $A \subset D_s \subset \mathbb{R}^d$, which are Lebesgue measurable (i.e., subsets of D_s for which d-dimensional volume is defined).

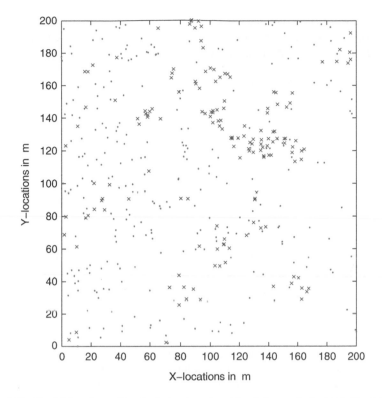

X–locations in m

Figure 4.15 Spatial locations of longleaf pine trees in a 4-ha study area in the Wade Tract, Thomas County, Georgia, USA; the $m_A = 271$ adult longleaf pine trees are shown as green dots, and the $m_S = 159$ subadult longleaf pine trees are shown as red crosses.

Let $Z(A)$ denote the number of events in $A \subset D_s$; then $Z(\cdot)$ is a stochastic (counting) process that is defined on the set of Lebesgue measurable subsets of D_s. Henceforth, assume that D_s is *bounded* and that $Z(A)$ is (almost surely) *finite* for all $A \subset D_s$. Then $\{Z(A): A \subset D_s\}$ characterizes the point process (e.g., Cressie, 1993, p. 619). We shall refer to the point process as $Z(\cdot)$ or Z, interchangeably.

An important, but simple, example is the *Poisson point process* Z, for which

$$Z(A)|\lambda^o \sim Poi(\lambda^o|A|), \qquad A \subset D_s, \tag{4.159}$$

where $\lambda^o > 0$ is a parameter of the Poisson point process, and recall that $|A|$ is the d-dimensional volume of A. More details on this spatial point process are given in Section 4.3.1.

One fundamental property of a spatial point process is the expected number of events in a given region A (i.e., $E(Z(A))$). This can be calculated in terms of an intensity function $\lambda(\mathbf{s})$ (with units of "per d-dimensional volume") that is a measure of the *potential* for an event to appear at any location $s \in D_s$. Let ds denote a small region located at s with volume $|ds|$. Then the *first-order intensity* function of the point process $Z(\cdot)$ is defined as

$$\lambda(s) \equiv \lim_{|ds| \to 0} E(Z(ds))/|ds|, \qquad s \in D_s, \qquad (4.160)$$

provided the limit exists. Hence,

$$E(Z(A)) = \int_A \lambda(s)\, ds, \qquad A \subset D_s. \qquad (4.161)$$

For the Poisson point process, characterized by (4.159), we obtain

$$\lambda(s) \equiv \lambda^o > 0, \qquad s \in D_s.$$

That is, the *potential* for an event to appear anywhere in D_s is *constant*.

An obvious nonparametric estimator of $\lambda(\cdot)$, based on $m = Z(D_s)$ event locations $\{s_1, s_2, \ldots, s_m\}$ in D_s, is (Diggle, 1985)

$$\widehat{\lambda}(s) \equiv \frac{1}{p_b(s)} \sum_{i=1}^{m} \kappa_b(s - s_i), \qquad s \in D_s, \qquad (4.162)$$

where $\kappa_b(\cdot)$ is a probability density (kernel) function symmetric about the origin, $b > 0$ is the *bandwidth* that determines the amount of smoothing, and $p_b(s) \equiv \int_{D_s} \kappa_b(s - x) dx$ is an edge correction. For example, in $\mathbb{R}^2$, consider the simple choice, $\kappa_b(x) = \rho_b(x_1)\rho_b(x_2)$, where $x = (x_1, x_2)'$ and $\rho_b(\cdot)$ is the Epanechnikov kernel,

$$\rho_b(x) = (3/4)b^{-1}\{1 - (x/b)^2\}I(|x| \le b). \qquad (4.163)$$

Choice of b in (4.162) is based on the usual trade-off between bias and variance. Diggle recommends using $b = 0.68m^{-1/5}$ in (4.162) and (4.163), for D_s a unit square, but this is only a guideline.

Based on the locations of the $m_A = 271$ adult pine trees in the 4-ha of forest, depicted in Figure 4.15, we obtain $\widehat{\lambda}(\cdot)$ using (4.162) and $b = 30$ m. The result is shown in Figure 4.16a, which indicates some inhomogeneity of intensity over D_s. In comparison, the $\widehat{\lambda}(\cdot)$ associated with the $m_S = 159$ subadults and the same $b = 30$ m, shown in Figure 4.16b, indicates an intensity surface that is even more inhomogeneous and with a localized peak.

Knowledge of $\lambda(\cdot)$ does not completely characterize the spatial behavior of a point process; there are higher-order moment measures that express complex spatial interactions (e.g., Cressie, 1993, p. 622). For example, spatial statistics based on the *second-order intensity* function (or second-order product density),

$$\lambda_2(s, x) \equiv \lim_{\substack{|ds| \to 0 \\ |dx| \to 0}} E(Z(ds)Z(dx))/(|ds|\,|dx|), \qquad s, x \in D_s, \qquad (4.164)$$

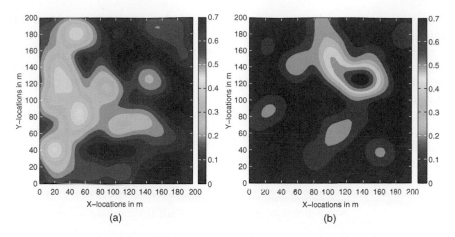

Figure 4.16 (a) Contour plot of estimated first-order intensity of $m_A = 271$ adult longleaf pine trees in the 4-ha study area in the Wade Tract; bandwidth $b = 30$ m. (b) Contour plot of estimated first-order intensity of $m_S = 159$ subadult longleaf pine trees in the same study area as (a); bandwidth $b = 30$ m.

are commonplace. Further discussion of $\lambda_2(\cdot, \cdot)$ is deferred until Section 4.3.2.

The study of spatial point processes has developed greatly in the last 15 years. It has been realized that many of the techniques in multivariate statistics have strong analogies in point processes. For example, the intensity function is like an unnormalized density function. Spatial dependence present in higher-order intensity functions is analogous to structure in multivariate density functions. Indeed, the theory for spatial point processes given in Section 4.3.3 shows that the spatial variability can be partitioned into $\Pr(Z(D_s) = m)$ and a conditional density function $f(\mathbf{s}_1, \dots, \mathbf{s}_m | m)$ that is proportional to the mth order intensity $\lambda_m(\mathbf{s}_1, \dots, \mathbf{s}_m)$. Therefore, many of the parametric models used in multivariate statistics have an analogue in spatial point processes (e.g., Møller and Waagepetersen, 2004; Illian et al., 2008).

4.3.1 The Poisson Point Process and the Cox Process

The canonical spatial point process that exhibits no spatial dependence (and is sometimes referred to as a *completely spatially random* process, or *CSR*) is the *homogeneous Poisson point process*. Here, $Z(A_1)$ and $Z(A_2)$ are independent whenever $A_1 \cap A_2 = \emptyset$, and $\lambda(\mathbf{s}) \equiv \lambda^o > 0$ in (4.160), for any $\mathbf{s} \in D_s$. As a consequence (e.g., Rogers, 1974, pp. 13–14), $Z(A) \sim Poi(\lambda^o | A|)$, which is the distributional result given in (4.159).

If we keep independence of $Z(\cdot)$ for non-overlapping sets, but choose a $\lambda(\cdot)$ in (4.160) that varies over D_s, the result is an *inhomogeneous Poisson point process*. Then,

$$Z(A) \sim Poi\left(\int_A \lambda(\mathbf{x})\, d\mathbf{x}\right), \qquad A \subset D_s. \tag{4.165}$$

The inhomogeneous Poisson point process is characterized by its first-order intensity $\lambda(\cdot)$; see, for example, Cressie (1993, Section 8.5.1).

If (4.165) is thought of as a data model in an HM, then an obvious process model is obtained by making $\lambda(\cdot)$ a spatial stochastic process. This is known as a Cox process (Cox, 1955); Møller and Waagepetersen (2004, Chapter 5) give a comprehensive discussion of the Cox process, which includes as special cases the Neyman–Scott process, the Thomas process, the Matérn Cluster process, the Shot-Noise Cox process, the Poisson-Gamma process, and the *Log-Gaussian Cox process* (LGCP). The latter process is often used in applications, and it is given below in the form of an HM.

Data model: Conditional on $\lambda(\cdot)$, the point process $Z(\cdot)$ is an inhomogeneous Poisson point process with intensity $\lambda(\cdot)$.

Process model: Conditional on β and $C_Y(\cdot, \cdot)$, $Y(\cdot) \equiv \log \lambda(\cdot)$ is a Gaussian process with the following properties:

$$E(Y(\mathbf{s})) = \mathbf{x}(\mathbf{s})'\beta \quad \text{and} \quad C_Y(\mathbf{s}, \mathbf{x}) \equiv \text{cov}(Y(\mathbf{s}), Y(\mathbf{x})).$$

Suppose the data model is written generically as $[Z|Y]$ and the process model as $[Y]$. The Cox process is actually defined via marginalization, namely $[Z] = \int [Z|Y][Y]dY$. It is only relatively recently (e.g., Møller, Syversveen, and Waagepetersen, 1998) that the full power of an HM approach has been realized through the *joint* distribution, $[Z, Y] = [Z|Y][Y]$.

An optimal spatial predictor of $\lambda(\mathbf{s}_0)$ is $\lambda^*(\mathbf{s}_0)$, the posterior expectation of $\lambda(\mathbf{s}_0)$ given the point-process data (i.e., given the point pattern). The data are the number of events $Z(D_s)$ in D_s *and* the locations $\mathbf{s}_1, \ldots, \mathbf{s}_{Z(D_s)}$ of those events. Hence, for the HM specified above, we have

$$\lambda^*(\mathbf{s}_0) = E(\exp(Y(\mathbf{s}_0))|Z(D_s), \{\mathbf{s}_1, \ldots, \mathbf{s}_{Z(D_s)}\}, \beta, C_Y(\cdot, \cdot)), \qquad (4.166)$$

which is obtained from Bayes' Theorem. Recall that

$$[Y(\cdot)|Z(D_s), \{\mathbf{s}_1, \ldots, \mathbf{s}_{Z(D_s)}\}, \beta, C_Y(\cdot, \cdot)]$$
$$\propto [Z(D_s), \{\mathbf{s}_1, \ldots, \mathbf{s}_{Z(D_s)}\}| \exp(Y(\cdot))][Y(\cdot)|\beta, C_Y(\cdot, \cdot)]. \qquad (4.167)$$

The second term in (4.167) is just the distribution of the Gaussian process Y. The first term is a distribution represented by the joint "density" function, $f((\mathbf{s}_1, \ldots, \mathbf{s}_m), m)$, of the inhomogeneous Poisson point process (e.g., Cressie, 1993, p. 660):

$$\exp\left(-\int_{D_s} \lambda(\mathbf{x})d\mathbf{x}\right) \times \begin{cases} 1, & m = 0, \\ \prod_{i=1}^m \lambda(\mathbf{s}_i)/m!, & m = 1, 2, \ldots, \end{cases} \qquad (4.168)$$

where $\lambda(\mathbf{s}) \equiv \exp(Y(\mathbf{s}))$; $\mathbf{s} \in D_s$. It will be seen in Section 4.3.3 that (4.168) can be used to simulate an inhomogeneous Poisson point process by first drawing $Z(D_s)(= m)$ from a $Poi(\int_{D_s} \lambda(\mathbf{x})d\mathbf{x})$ distribution and then drawing $\mathbf{s}_1, \ldots, \mathbf{s}_m$ iid from the density,

$$h(\mathbf{s}) \equiv \lambda(\mathbf{s})/(\int_{D_s} \lambda(\mathbf{x})\, d\mathbf{x})\,, \qquad \mathbf{s} \in D_s\,. \tag{4.169}$$

The homogeneous Poisson point process plays a role analogous to that of a white-noise geostatistical process in Section 4.1; that is, the intensity function of events is constant, there is independence between counts in nonoverlapping regions, and (hence) the relative locations of events show neither positive spatial dependence (clustering) nor negative spatial dependence (regularity). The inhomogeneous Poisson point process represents a small generalization; it is analogous to adding a spatially varying trend term to a zero-mean white-noise process in Section 4.1. Consequently, the Poisson point process cannot be used to model spatial statistical dependence, such as that found in higher-order moment (i.e., intensity) measures. For example in the next subsection, the pair-correlation function (4.170) is seen to capture departures from "Poissonness."

The next generalization introduces dependence through mixing of an independent process, namely the Cox process. On D_s, the density of the LGCP (with respect to a unit-intensity Poisson process) is proportional to the expected value of the expression (4.168), where recall that $\lambda(\cdot) = \exp(Y(\cdot))$ and the expectation is with respect to the Gaussian process Y. This is not generally known in closed form; however, it is not needed when taking an HM approach.

4.3.2 Spatial Statistical Dependence, Including the K Function

A spatial point process' second-order intensity function $\lambda_2(\cdot, \cdot)$, defined by (4.164), plays the analogous role to the covariance function for a geostatistical process (Section 4.1); we now consider some properties of λ_2. If $Z(d\mathbf{s})$ and $Z(d\mathbf{x})$ are statistically dependent, then $\lambda_2(\mathbf{s}, \mathbf{x})$ cannot be expressed simply as $\lambda(\mathbf{s})\lambda(\mathbf{x})$. Thus, $\lambda_2(\mathbf{s}, \mathbf{x})$ can be used as a summary measure of spatial dependence in a spatial point process, and *the pair-correlation function*,

$$g(\mathbf{s}, \mathbf{x}) \equiv \lambda_2(\mathbf{s}, \mathbf{x})/(\lambda(\mathbf{s})\lambda(\mathbf{x}))\,, \tag{4.170}$$

is often used (Stoyan and Stoyan, 1994, Section 14.4; Baddeley et al., 2000). For the inhomogeneous Poisson process, $\lambda_2(\mathbf{s}, \mathbf{x}) = \lambda(\mathbf{s})\lambda(\mathbf{x})$; hence, in this case, $g(\mathbf{s}, \mathbf{x}) = 1$.

Now suppose that (4.170) can be written as $g(\mathbf{s}, \mathbf{x}) = g^*(\mathbf{s} - \mathbf{x})$, which is a type of second-order stationarity *after weighting* by $\lambda(\cdot)$. We see below that g^* leads to a more general definition of the K function.

Suppose that $Z(\cdot)$ is stationary and isotropic (i.e., invariant under translation and rotation); then

$$\lambda(\mathbf{s}) \equiv \lambda^o \tag{4.171}$$

and

$$\lambda_2(\mathbf{s}, \mathbf{x}) \equiv \lambda_2^o(\|\mathbf{s} - \mathbf{x}\|), \qquad \mathbf{s}, \mathbf{x} \in D_s. \tag{4.172}$$

Furthermore, the pair-correlation function defined by (4.170) becomes,

$$g^o(h) \equiv \lambda_2^o(h)/(\lambda^o)^2, \qquad h > 0.$$

A plot of $g^o(h)$ versus h (e.g., Stoyan and Stoyan, 1994, Figure 94) shows ranges of h where $g^o(h) < 1$, $= 1$, or > 1. Small values of $g^o(h)$ occur if events at distance h-apart are rare; large values occur if events at distance h-apart appear frequently; a homogeneous Poisson point process has $g^o(h) \equiv 1$. In practice, $g^o(\cdot)$ is estimated by kernel-based methods (e.g., Illian et al., 2008, Section 4.3.3).

The K Function

For spatial point processes that are stationary and isotropic, there is another measure of spatial dependence, called the *K function* (Bartlett, 1964; Ripley, 1976). We now show a direct relationship between the second-order intensity function and the K function. Let $a(\mathbf{0}, dh)$ be an annulus of width dh on the sphere centered at $\mathbf{0}$ with radius h, and recall that $d\mathbf{0}$ is an infinitesimal region located at $\mathbf{0}$. Note that the surface area of a d-dimensional sphere of radius h is $d\pi^{d/2}h^{d-1}/\Gamma(1 + (d/2))$. Then, for $|d\mathbf{0}|$ and dh small, we obtain

$$
\begin{aligned}
E(Z(a(\mathbf{0}, dh))|Z(d\mathbf{0}) > 0) &= \frac{\Pr(Z(a(\mathbf{0}, dh)) > 0, Z(d\mathbf{0}) > 0)}{\Pr(Z(d\mathbf{0}) > 0)} \\
&= \frac{\lambda_2^o(h)\{d\pi^{d/2}h^{d-1}/\Gamma(1 + (d/2))\}dh}{\lambda^o}.
\end{aligned}
$$

Suppose $B(\mathbf{0}, h)$ is a d-dimensional sphere of radius h centered at $\mathbf{0}$. Then, consider

$$
\begin{aligned}
K(h) &\equiv (\lambda^o)^{-1}E(Z(B(\mathbf{0}, h))|Z(d\mathbf{0}) > 0) \\
&= (\lambda^o)^{-1}\int_0^h E(Z(a(\mathbf{0}, du))|Z(d\mathbf{0}) > 0) \\
&= (\lambda^o)^{-2}\{d\pi^{d/2}/\Gamma(1 + (d/2))\}\int_0^h u^{d-1}\lambda_2^o(u)\,du. \tag{4.173}
\end{aligned}
$$

Recall that the spatial point process is stationary and isotropic; hence, the quantity $E(Z(B(\mathbf{0}, h))|Z(d\mathbf{0}) > 0)$ is the expected number of extra events within distance h of an arbitary event. Finally, the definition of the *homogeneous K* function is (Ripley, 1976)

$$K(h) \equiv (\lambda^o)^{-1}E\left(\begin{matrix}\text{number of extra events within}\\\text{distance } h \text{ of an arbitrary event}\end{matrix}\right), \qquad h \geq 0. \tag{4.174}$$

Consequently, $K(\cdot)$ and $\lambda_2^o(\cdot)$ are related through the equation,

$$K(h) = (\lambda^o)^{-2}\{d\pi^{d/2}/\Gamma(1+(d/2))\} \int_0^h u^{d-1}\lambda_2^o(u)\,du, \qquad h \geq 0.$$

$$(4.175)$$

It is the K function that is famously used as a measure of spatial dependence in (stationary and isotropic) point processes. From (4.175), the second-order intensity is related directly to the K function by

$$\lambda_2^o(h) = \frac{(\lambda^o)^2\Gamma(1+(d/2))}{d\pi^{d/2}} \cdot \frac{K^{(\prime)}(h)}{h^{d-1}}, \qquad h \geq 0, \qquad (4.176)$$

where $K^{(\prime)}(h) \equiv dK(h)/dh$.

Also, from (4.175), the K function of the homogeneous Poisson point process in $\mathbb{R}^d$ is of the special form

$$K(h) = \pi^{d/2}h^d / \Gamma(1+(d/2)), \qquad h \geq 0. \qquad (4.177)$$

In $\mathbb{R}^2$, (4.177) is given by

$$K(h) = \pi h^2, \qquad h \geq 0. \qquad (4.178)$$

Because the homogeneous Poisson point process represents a spatial point process with no spatial dependence, clustering or regularity can be detected more easily by considering the function

$$L(h) \equiv \{K(h)\Gamma(1+(d/2))/\pi^{d/2}\}^{1/d} - h, \qquad h \geq 0. \qquad (4.179)$$

Ranges of h where the L function given by (4.179) is positive (negative) indicate clustering (regularity).

Estimation of the K function can be achieved by collecting and averaging pairs of events that are at distance h-apart or less from each other. Recall that D_s is a bounded region in $\mathbb{R}^d$. Then based on data $Z(D_s) = m$ and $\{s_1, \ldots, s_m\}$, an obvious (but biased) estimator of $K(h)$ is

$$(\widehat{\lambda}^o)^{-1} \sum_{\substack{i=1 \\ i \neq j}}^{m} \sum_{j=1}^{m} I(\|s_i - s_j\| \leq h)/m,$$

where $\widehat{\lambda}_0 \equiv m/|D_s|$.

The bias in this estimator is caused by the randomness in $m = Z(D_s)$ and by *edge effects*; when an event in D_s is near its edge, the sphere of radius h centered at the event will not be wholly within D_s for larger h. Hence, there may be events outside D_s that should contribute to the estimator above; they do not because they are unobserved. One way around this is to delete such events from the estimator.

Let d_j denote the distance from events $\mathbf{s}_j$ to the nearest edge of D_s; $j = 1, \ldots, m$. Then for $h > 0$, define the estimator

$$\widehat{K}(h) \equiv (|D_s|/m) \sum_{\substack{i=1 \\ i \neq j}}^{m} \sum_{j=1}^{m} I(\|\mathbf{s}_i - \mathbf{s}_j\| \leq h, d_j > h) / \sum_{j=1}^{m} I(d_j > h). \quad (4.180)$$

Other edge-corrected estimators are discussed by Cressie (1993, pp. 615–618). An estimator $\widehat{L}(\cdot)$ of the L function can be defined by substituting $\widehat{K}(\cdot)$ for $K(\cdot)$ in (4.179). In $\mathbb{R}^2$,

$$\widehat{L}(h) = (\widehat{K}(h)/\pi)^{1/2} - h, \qquad h > 0. \quad (4.181)$$

Figures 4.17a and 4.17b show $\widehat{K}(\cdot)$ and $\widehat{L}(\cdot)$, respectively, for the subadult trees shown in Figure 4.15. In Figure 4.17b, we have superimposed 95% pointwise confidence limits. These are obtained from $\{\widehat{L}^{(\ell)}(\cdot): \ell = 1, \ldots, 1000\}$, where each is estimated from 1000 simulations of CSR (Section 4.3.1) over the same region D_s and conditioned on there being 159 events. Clearly, from Figure 4.17, there is strong evidence of clustering at all scales.

From Figure 4.16a, we saw some heterogeneity in the first-order intensity function of adult trees. The K function also indicates mild clustering of adult trees at spatial scales less than 40 m; see Figure 4.18a, where the estimated L function is above the 95% confidence limits for $h < 40$ m. In order to calibrate this result, we show in Figure 4.18b the L function obtained from one simulated realization from CSR, conditioned on there being 271 events (the same as the number of adult trees). It appears that the adult trees are "settling down to a life of Poissonness"; contrast this to the subadult trees, which have yet to experience all the random attrition that an older tree would.

There is an *inhomogeneous* version of the K function based on $g^*(\mathbf{s} - \mathbf{x})$ defined just below (4.170) that might be more appropriate for the longleaf pine trees. From (4.175), $K(h)$ is related to $g^o(h) = \lambda_2^o(h)/(\lambda^o)^2$ through integration. This motivates the definition

$$K^*(h) \equiv \int_{B(\mathbf{0},h)} g^*(\mathbf{u}) \, d\mathbf{u}.$$

Since $g(\mathbf{s}, \mathbf{x}) = g^*(\mathbf{s} - \mathbf{x})$, it is true that for *any* set $A \subset \mathbb{R}^d$ we obtain

$$K^*(h) = \frac{1}{|A|} E \left\{ \sum_{\mathbf{s},\mathbf{x}}^* \frac{I(\|\mathbf{s} - \mathbf{x}\| \leq h)}{\lambda(\mathbf{s})\lambda(\mathbf{x})} \right\},$$

where $\sum_{\mathbf{s},\mathbf{x}}^*$ denotes summation over all events $\mathbf{s} \in Z \cap A$, $\mathbf{x} \in Z$, and such that $\mathbf{s} \neq \mathbf{x}$. Kernel estimation of $K^*(\cdot)$ is discussed by Illian et al. (2008, Section 4.3.3); Guan (2009) gives a nonparametric variance estimator for $K^*(\cdot)$;

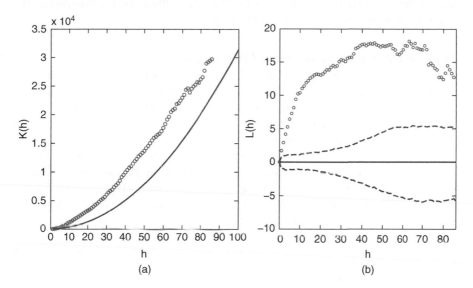

Figure 4.17 (a) Estimated K function for the $m_S = 159$ subadult longleaf pine trees (red circles) in the 4-ha study area in the Wade Tract; the theoretical K function for CSR (solid blue line) is superimposed. (b) Estimated L function for the $m_S = 159$ subadult longleaf pine trees (red circles) obtained from (a); the 95% pointwise confidence limits for L values based on 1000 CSR realizations (dashed blue lines) are superimposed.

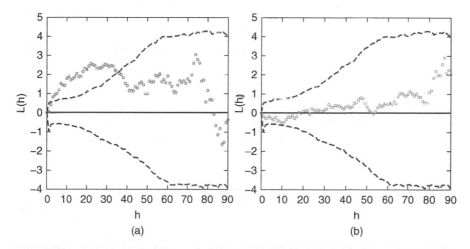

Figure 4.18 (a) Estimated L function for the $m_A = 271$ adult longleaf pine trees (green circles) in the 4-ha study area in the Wade Tract; the 95% confidence limits for L values based on 1000 CSR realizations (dashed blue lines) are superimposed. (b) Estimated L function for $m_A = 271$ locations generated from a single realization of a CSR process (black circles); the same 95% confidence limits for L values, as shown in (a) (dashed blue lines), are superimposed.

and Henrys and Brown (2009) present statistical inference for comparing two spatial point processes based on their respective $K^*(\cdot)$.

Dependence in the Log-Gaussian Cox Process

There are different ways that spatial statistical dependence can be modeled when the data are event locations in a spatial domain $D_s \subset \mathbb{R}^d$. Assuming an HM like that in Section 4.3.1 (e.g., with a LGCP), spatial dependence is present through a hidden geostatistical process that models the (log) intensity function. Then conditional on the intensity function $\lambda(\cdot)$, the events of $Z(\cdot)$ occur independently such that the number of events in non-overlapping subsets are independent Poisson. To emphasize further that the Poisson process has no spatial statistical dependence, it can be seen (e.g., Cressie, 1993, p. 651; Section 4.3.3) that conditional on $Z(D_s) = m$, the events $s_1, \ldots, s_m$ are *independent* and identically distributed according to the density,

$$h(\mathbf{s}) = \lambda(\mathbf{s}) I(\mathbf{s} \in D_s) / (\textstyle\int_{D_s} \lambda(\mathbf{x})\, d\mathbf{x}), \qquad \mathbf{s} \in \mathbb{R}^d.$$

We have already mentioned that, marginally, the point process $Z(\cdot)$ is known as a *Cox process*, which inherits spatial dependence from its so-called directing measure $\lambda(\cdot)$. We shall now calculate the second-order intensity function of the LGCP $Z(\cdot)$, where recall that $\lambda(\cdot)$ is a log Gaussian process.

$$
\begin{aligned}
E(Z(d\mathbf{s})Z(d\mathbf{x})) &= E\{E(Z(d\mathbf{s})Z(d\mathbf{x})|\lambda(\cdot))\} \\
&= E\{\lambda(d\mathbf{s})\lambda(d\mathbf{x})\} \\
&= E(e^{Y(\mathbf{s})} \cdot e^{Y(\mathbf{x})})|d\mathbf{s}|\,|d\mathbf{x}|,
\end{aligned}
\tag{4.182}
$$

where $\lambda(\cdot) \equiv \exp\{Y(\cdot)\}$. Since $Y(\cdot)$ is a Gaussian process, then using well known results for the lognormal distribution (e.g., Aitchison and Brown, 1957), we see that for the LGCP, the first-order intensity function defined by (4.151) is $E(e^{Y(\mathbf{s})}) = \exp\{\mu_Y(\mathbf{s}) + C_Y(\mathbf{s}, \mathbf{s})/2\}$, and the second-order intensity function defined by (4.164) is

$$\lambda_2(\mathbf{s}, \mathbf{x}) = \exp\{\mu_Y(\mathbf{s}) + \mu_Y(\mathbf{x}) + C_Y(\mathbf{s}, \mathbf{s})/2 + C_Y(\mathbf{x}, \mathbf{x})/2 + C_Y(\mathbf{s}, \mathbf{x})\}.$$
$$\tag{4.183}$$

Only when $C_Y(\mathbf{s}, \mathbf{x}) = 0$, can we write $\lambda_2(\mathbf{s}, \mathbf{x}) = \lambda(\mathbf{s})\lambda(\mathbf{x})$. Hence, *conditional* on $\lambda(\cdot)$, $Z(\cdot)$ has *no* spatial statistical dependence, but *marginally* $Z(\cdot)$ is an LGCP with spatial statistical dependence characterized by (4.183). Then $g(\mathbf{s}, \mathbf{x}) = \exp\{C_Y(\mathbf{s}, \mathbf{x})\}$, which is a function of $\mathbf{s} - \mathbf{x}$ if C_Y is stationary. More generally, spatial statistical dependence in the process model for $\lambda(\cdot)$ leads to spatial dependence in the Cox process $Z(\cdot)$.

4.3.3 Distribution Theory for Spatial Point Processes

Recall we assumed that $Z(\cdot)$ is simple (i.e., with probability 1, at any spatial location, only single events can occur). Then a spatial point process $Z(\cdot)$ can be characterized by a sequence of nonnegative, permutation-invariant intensity functions, $\{\lambda_m(\mathbf{s}_1, \ldots, \mathbf{s}_m): m = 1, 2, \ldots\}$, such that the conditional density function is expressed as

$$
\begin{aligned}
f(\mathbf{s}_1, &\ldots, \mathbf{s}_m | m) d\mathbf{s}_1 \ldots d\mathbf{s}_m \\
&\equiv \Pr(Z(d\mathbf{s}_1) = 1, \ldots, Z(d\mathbf{s}_m) = 1 | Z(D_s) = m) \qquad (4.184) \\
&= \frac{\lambda_m(\mathbf{s}_1, \ldots, \mathbf{s}_m) d\mathbf{s}_1 \ldots d\mathbf{s}_m}{\int_{D_s} \cdots \int_{D_s} \lambda_m(\mathbf{x}_1, \ldots, \mathbf{x}_m) d\mathbf{x}_1 \ldots d\mathbf{x}_m}, \quad m = 1, 2, \ldots,
\end{aligned}
$$

and the count distribution in D_s is given by

$$
\begin{aligned}
\Pr(Z(D_s) &= m) \equiv p_m \\
&\propto \begin{cases} e^{-|D_s|}, & m = 0, \\ (e^{-|D_s|}/m!) \int_{D_s} \cdots \int_{D_s} \lambda_m(\mathbf{x}_1, \ldots, \mathbf{x}_m) d\mathbf{x}_1 \cdots d\mathbf{x}_m, & m = 1, 2, \ldots, \end{cases}
\end{aligned}
$$

$$(4.185)$$

where $\sum_{m=0}^{\infty} p_m = 1$ (Daley and Vere-Jones, 1988, p. 129).

For example, because the (inhomogeneous) Poisson point process has independent counts in disjoint regions, for that model, (4.184) becomes

$$
f(\mathbf{s}_1, \ldots, \mathbf{s}_m | m) = \prod_{i=1}^{m} \{\lambda(\mathbf{s}_i) / \int_{D_s} \lambda(\mathbf{x}) \, d\mathbf{x}\},
$$

and from (4.185),

$$
p_m = \exp(-\int_{D_s} \lambda(\mathbf{x}) \, d\mathbf{x}) \{\int_{D_s} \lambda(\mathbf{x}) d\mathbf{x}\}^m / m!, \qquad m = 0, 1, \ldots,
$$

which is the probability mass function of a Poisson distribution. Consequently, the simulation of the Poisson point process is straightforward: Generate $Z(D_s) \sim Poi(\int_{D_s} \lambda(\mathbf{x}) \, d\mathbf{x})$ and, conditional on $Z(D_s) = m$, generate $\mathbf{s}_1, \ldots, \mathbf{s}_m$ *iid* according to the density, $\lambda(\cdot) / \int_{D_s} \lambda(\mathbf{x}) \, d\mathbf{x}$. In the special case of a homogeneous Poisson point process, this latter density is just the uniform density, $1/|D_s|$.

The likelihood for a simple spatial point process is the Radon–Nikodym derivative of the point-process measure with respect to the unit-intensity Poisson-process measure. That is,

$$
\ell(\boldsymbol{\theta}) = e^{-|D_s|} \lambda_m(\mathbf{s}_1, \ldots, \mathbf{s}_m; \boldsymbol{\theta}), \qquad (4.186)
$$

where λ_m is on the right-hand side of (4.184) and has been written to emphasize any unknown parameters $\boldsymbol{\theta}$. The simplicity of (4.186) belies its difficulty to use in practice. Typically, it is only known up to a normalizing constant (that is a function of $\boldsymbol{\theta}$). Geyer (1999) discusses optimization of (4.186). Alternatively, Jensen and Møller (1991) and Baddeley and Turner (2000) optimize a composite likelihood based on the Papangelou conditional intensity, while Guan (2006) bases his composite likelihoods on pairwise loglikelihoods.

In a classical Bayesian setting, there is a prior distribution on $\boldsymbol{\theta}$. Based on this prior and (4.186), the posterior distribution $[\boldsymbol{\theta}|Z]$ is available through an MCMC algorithm (Møller et al., 2006).

Now, the mth intensity function λ_m in (4.185) can be factored uniquely into its Gibbsian form (e.g., Daley and Vere-Jones, 1988, p. 129):

$$\lambda_m(\mathbf{s}_1, \ldots, \mathbf{s}_m) \propto \exp\{\sum_i g_i(\mathbf{s}_i) + \sum_{i<j} g_{ij}(\mathbf{s}_i, \mathbf{s}_j) + \cdots$$

$$+ g_{12\ldots m}(\mathbf{s}_1, \mathbf{s}_2, \ldots, \mathbf{s}_m)\}, \tag{4.187}$$

where it is important to remember that the proportionality constant here and in (4.184) is chosen so that $\sum_{m=0}^{\infty} p_m = 1$. For example, suppose $g_i(\mathbf{s}) \equiv \log \lambda^o$; $g_{ij}(\mathbf{s}, \mathbf{u}) \equiv (\log \gamma)I(\|\mathbf{s} - \mathbf{u}\| \leq \rho)$; and all higher-order g-functions are zero, where $\boldsymbol{\theta} \equiv (\lambda^o, \gamma, \rho)'$ are parameters. Then

$$\lambda_m(\mathbf{s}_1, \ldots \mathbf{s}_m) = (\lambda^o)^m \gamma^{Y_m(\rho)} / c(\lambda^o, \gamma, \rho), \tag{4.188}$$

where $Y_m(\rho)$ is the number of pairs of event locations in $\{\mathbf{s}_1, \ldots, \mathbf{s}_m\}$ whose distances are less than or equal to ρ, and $c(\lambda^o, \gamma, \rho)$ is a normalizing constant to guarantee that $\sum_{m=0}^{\infty} p_m = 1$. This spatial point process is known as the *Strauss process*; its parameter space is $\{(\lambda^o, \gamma, \rho): c(\lambda^o, \gamma, \rho) < \infty\} = (0, \infty) \times [0, 1] \times [0, \infty)$; see Kelly and Ripley (1976). For the Strauss process, the likelihood is

$$\ell(\lambda^o, \gamma, \rho) = e^{-|D_s|}(\lambda^o)^m \gamma^{Y_m(\rho)} / c(\lambda^o, \gamma, \rho).$$

An infinite-order interaction model is considered by Widom and Rowlinson (1970).

Notice that the decomposition (4.187) is obtained by direct analogy with the expression for the negpotential $Q(\cdot)$ in terms of the G-functions for lattice processes; see (4.107).

Markov Point Processes

A *Markov point process* is obtained when the representation (4.187) of λ_m is truncated at a fixed number of terms, for all $m = 1, 2, \ldots$. These have also been called *Gibbs processes*, because they were originally introduced into physics by Gibbs (1902); they have a long history in Statistical Mechanics.

An example of a Markov point process is when, for all i and j, $g_i(\mathbf{s})$ is $\xi(\mathbf{s}; \boldsymbol{\beta})$, $g_{i,j}(\mathbf{s}, \mathbf{u}) = \psi(\|\mathbf{s} - \mathbf{u}\|; \boldsymbol{\theta})$, and all the other g-functions are zero; here, $\boldsymbol{\beta}$ and $\boldsymbol{\theta}$ denote unknown parameters. Large-scale variation in Markov point processes can be captured through covariates $\mathbf{x}(\cdot)$, by putting $\xi(\cdot, \boldsymbol{\beta}) = \mathbf{x}(\cdot)'\boldsymbol{\beta}$. When $\xi(\cdot; \boldsymbol{\beta})$ is a constant, we obtain the *pair-potential Markov point process*, and a special case of this is the Strauss process given by (4.188), where $\xi(\mathbf{s}; \boldsymbol{\beta}) = \log(\lambda^o)$; $\mathbf{s} \in D_s$. In that case,

$$\psi(\|\mathbf{s} - \mathbf{u}\|; \boldsymbol{\theta}) = (\log \gamma) I(\|\mathbf{s} - \mathbf{u}\| \le \rho). \qquad (4.189)$$

Finally, a Markov point process with general $\xi(\mathbf{s}; \boldsymbol{\beta})$ and pair-potential given by (4.189) with $\rho = 0$, corresponds to no spatial dependence. This is an inhomogeneous Poisson point process with intensity function,

$$\lambda(\mathbf{s}) = \exp(\xi(\mathbf{s}; \boldsymbol{\beta})), \qquad \mathbf{s} \in D_s.$$

4.3.4 Disease Mapping from Event Locations

In Section 4.2.6 we saw examples of HMs on lattices, in particular a discussion of disease mapping. The data were small-area counts, and inference was on (hidden) relative risks. After introducing an HM for disease-event locations, we shall see that the HM in that section can be derived straightforwardly.

An HM for Disease-Event Locations
To keep it simple, we assume that individuals at risk come from a homogeneous population (e.g., a single sex-age stratum, like males, age 65–74 years). The spatial locations of these *individuals at risk* are modeled as "events" of an inhomogeneous Poisson point process $Z^0(\cdot)$, with first-order intensity function $\delta(\cdot)$. Generally, $\delta(\cdot)$ is known, obtained from independent demographic studies. From the random locations of individuals at risk, there are some who have the disease being studied. We model their locations randomly, via a "thinning function,"

$$T(\mathbf{s}) = \begin{cases} 1, & \text{if an individual at } \mathbf{s} \text{ has the disease,} \\ 0, & \text{otherwise.} \end{cases} \qquad (4.190)$$

For noninfectious diseases (e.g., cancer), we can assume that for $\mathbf{s}_1 \neq \mathbf{s}_2$, $T(\mathbf{s}_1)$ and $T(\mathbf{s}_2)$ are independent. The risk function, defined in terms of probability, is

$$p(\mathbf{s}) \equiv E(T(\mathbf{s})) = \Pr(\text{individual at } \mathbf{s} \text{ has the disease}), \qquad \mathbf{s} \in D_s. \quad (4.191)$$

This is a primary process of interest, and epidemiologists want to estimate it and map it.

Define a new spatial point process,

$$Z(ds) \equiv T(\mathbf{s})Z^0(ds), \qquad \mathbf{s} \in D_s, \tag{4.192}$$

where recall that ds is an infinitesimal region located at $\mathbf{s}$. Then by a well known result for thinned Poisson point processes (e.g., Cressie, 1993, p. 690), $Z(\cdot)$ is also a Poisson point process with (first-order) intensity function, $p(\cdot)\delta(\cdot)$. Since $\delta(\cdot)$ is assumed known from demographic studies, $p(\cdot)$ is the source of randomness in the process-model part of the following HM.

Data model: Conditional on $p(\cdot)$ (and $\delta(\cdot)$), the point process $Z(\cdot)$ is an inhomogeneous Poisson point process with intensity function $p(\cdot)\delta(\cdot)$.

Process model: Conditional on $\boldsymbol{\beta}$ and $C_\nu(\cdot, \cdot)$,

$$p(\cdot) \equiv \exp\{\mathbf{x}(\cdot)'\boldsymbol{\beta} + \nu(\cdot)\},$$

                              where $\nu(\cdot)$ is a zero-mean Gaussian process with covariance function $C_\nu(\cdot, \cdot)$, and $\mathbf{x}(\cdot)$ is a vector of covariates.

Data from the observed point pattern is $Z(D_s) = m$ and $\{\mathbf{s}_1, \ldots, \mathbf{s}_m\}$, from which we wish to make inference on $\boldsymbol{\beta}$ and $\nu(\cdot)$ (and hence on $p(\cdot)$). In particular, there may be interest in the null hypothesis that certain β_i are equal to zero. Furthermore, a *risk map*, $\{p(\mathbf{s}) : \mathbf{s} \in D_s\}$, could be inferred by computing the posterior distribution,

$$[p(\cdot)|Z(D_s), \{\mathbf{s}_1, \ldots, \mathbf{s}_{Z(D_s)}\}].$$

Of course, $\mathbf{x}(\cdot)'\boldsymbol{\beta} + \nu(\cdot)$ has to be negative to ensure $p(\cdot)$ is a probability. If this is problematic, a logistic transformation could be used in the process model instead.

Aggregation of Events to Small Areas

Now suppose that we have the region $D_s = \bigcup\limits_{j=1}^{J} A_j$, where $\{A_j : j = 1, \ldots, J\}$ are disjoint small areas. Then $\mathbf{Z} \equiv (Z(A_1), \ldots, Z(A_J))'$ represent the number of disease cases in the J small areas. Moreover, conditional on $p(\cdot)$, the data model above implies that

$$Z(A_j) \sim ind. Poi\left(\int_{A_j} p(\mathbf{u})\delta(\mathbf{u}) \, d\mathbf{u}\right), \qquad j = 1, \ldots, J. \tag{4.193}$$

The mean number of individuals at risk in the j-th small area is $N_j \equiv \int_{A_j} \delta(\mathbf{u}) \, d\mathbf{u}$, $j = 1, \ldots, J$. Now make the assumption that $p(\cdot)$ is (approximately) constant within each of the $\{A_j\}$. That is, for $\mathbf{s} \in A_j$, write $p(\mathbf{s}) \equiv p_j$; $j = 1, \ldots, J$. Consequently,

$$Z(A_j) \sim Poi(N_j p_j), \tag{4.194}$$

and an analogous development of (4.133) through (4.136) yields the relative risks,

$$\lambda_j \equiv \frac{p_j}{(E_j/N_j)}, \qquad (4.195)$$

where recall that $E_j \equiv N_j \overline{p}$ is the baseline expected number of disease incidences; $j = 1, \ldots, J$, and $\overline{p} \equiv \sum_{j=1}^{J} p_j/J$ is the average risk. That is, under aggregation of the data model and the process model into small areas, $\{A_j : j = 1, \ldots, J\}$, the previous HM has an aggregated form.

Data model: Conditional on $\{\lambda_j\}$ (and $\{E_j\}$), and for $j = 1, \ldots, J$,

$$Z(A_j)|\lambda_j \sim ind. \; Poi(E_j\lambda_j).$$

Process model: Conditional on $\boldsymbol{\beta}$, $\boldsymbol{\theta}_C$, and for $\mathbf{Y} \equiv (\log \lambda_1, \ldots, \log \lambda_J)'$,

$$\mathbf{Y}|\boldsymbol{\beta}_C, \boldsymbol{\theta} \sim Gau(\mathbf{X}\boldsymbol{\beta}, \boldsymbol{\Sigma}(\boldsymbol{\theta}_C)),$$

where $\boldsymbol{\Sigma}(\boldsymbol{\theta}_C)$ is a $J \times J$ positive-definite matrix that depends on covariance parameters $\boldsymbol{\theta}_C$.

For example, for the HM following (4.136)–(4.140) in Section 4.2.6, $\boldsymbol{\Sigma}(\boldsymbol{\theta}_C)$ was chosen to be a MRF plus a component representing extra, non-spatial variation. However, it is not generally known how to disaggregate such a model so that it corresponds to a well-defined spatial point process.

If the piecewise-constant assumption for $p(\cdot)$ is dropped, the data model is still

$$Z(A_j) \sim Poi(N_j p_j), \qquad (4.196)$$

but where now p_j is the weighted average,

$$p_j = \int_{A_j} p(\mathbf{u})\delta(\mathbf{u})\,d\mathbf{u} \Big/ \int_{A_j} \delta(\mathbf{x})\,d\mathbf{x}. \qquad (4.197)$$

Now this requires knowledge of $\delta(\cdot)$ at the point level; unfortunately, it may only be known at the small-area level, where it has been assumed that demographic studies yield $\{N_j = \int_{A_j} \delta(\mathbf{x})\,d\mathbf{x}: j = 1, \ldots, J\}$. Hence, keeping the piecewise-constant assumption for $p(\cdot)$ can be viewed as a simplifying assumption that allows the statistical analysis to move forward. A Bayesian way to deal with $\delta(\cdot)$ unknown would be to put a prior on it that respects the constraints, $N_j = \int_{A_j} \delta(\mathbf{x})\,d\mathbf{x}; \; j = 1, \ldots, J$.

Aggregation of the point-level process model given in this section requires careful calibration. Noting that $N_j p_j = E_j \lambda_j$, $j = 1, \ldots, J$, then making inference on the relative risks, $\{\lambda_j\}$, is equivalent to making inference on the risks, $\{p_j\}$. Intuitively, areas that have historically had more individuals at risk would have a risk value that is more certain because there would be a lot more past disease outcomes to assess. For this reason, Cressie (1992) proposed a heteroskedastic model for $\{\lambda_j\}$, such that $\mathrm{var}(\lambda_j)$ is inversely related to E_j, $j = 1, \ldots, J$. Define $Y_j \equiv \log \lambda_j$; $j = 1, \ldots, J$. Then, assuming a CAR model for $\mathbf{Y}$ (Section 4.2.5), the heteroskedasticity is captured through

$$\mathrm{var}(Y_j | \mathbf{Y}_{-j}) = \tau^2 / E_j, \tag{4.198}$$

and through the spatial-rates CAR model (Cressie, Perrin, and Thomas-Agnan, 2005),

$$\mathbf{\Sigma}(\boldsymbol{\theta}_C) = \tau^2 (\mathbf{I} - \phi \mathbf{H})^{-1} \mathbf{\Delta}, \tag{4.199}$$

where $\boldsymbol{\theta}_C = (\tau^2, \phi)'$,

$$\mathbf{\Delta} \equiv \mathrm{diag}(1/E_1, \ldots, 1/E_J), \quad \text{and}$$

$$(\mathbf{H})_{ij} = (E_j^{1/2} / E_i^{1/2}) I (A_j \text{ is a neighbor of } A_i).$$

There is a curious lacuna between the spatial point process models used in disease mapping from event locations, and the Markov random field models used for (aggregated) small area counts. Aggregation of a point-level log-Gaussian Cox process defined on D_s, does *not* yield an easily interpretable (i.e., "sparse") MRF defined on $\{A_j\}$ and, in general, aggregation of a "sparse" MRF does not yield a "sparse" aggregated MRF. Therefore, in spite of a tradition in the disease-mapping literature to use MRFs (particularly CAR models), perhaps the spatial process models of choice should be geostatistical-type models, which are able to maintain "sparseness" under aggregation?

4.3.5 Other Topics

Marked Point Processes
Recall the example shown in Figure 4.15 of longleaf pine tree locations in 4-ha of a natural forest. The trees have varying size, and if their *diameters at breast height (DBH)* are measured, along with their location, then a spatial statistical model should account for tree size through an additional process (e.g., Rathbun and Cressie, 1994). In fact, Figure 4.15 shows the trees stratified according to whether they are considered adults or subadults, a stratification that is defined by their DBH.

Any accompanying measurements associated with the events of the spatial point process are considered a sampling from a process that is called the *mark process*, and we denote it by $M(\cdot)$. A marked spatial point process on D_s consists of the initial spatial point process, $Z(\cdot)$. Then, conditional on the realization of $Z(\cdot)$, namely $Z(D_s)$, $\mathbf{s}_1, \ldots, \mathbf{s}_{Z(D_s)}$, there is a subsequent (geostatistical or lattice) model for the mark process, $M(\cdot)$:

$$[M(\mathbf{s}_1), \ldots, M(\mathbf{s}_{Z(D_s)}) | Z(\cdot)].$$

For example, see Rathbun and Cressie (1994) for a spatial statistical model (conditional on the initial point process) for DBHs of longleaf pine trees in a natural forest. For marked spatial point processes in an HM, the data model is partitioned into two levels, namely the top level for the spatial point process $Z(\cdot)$ and the next level for the mark process $M(\cdot)$, conditional on $Z(\cdot)$.

An example of an HM for a marked spatial point process can be easily developed, as follows.

Data model: Conditional on $\lambda(\cdot)$, the point process $Z(\cdot)$ is an inhomogeneous Poisson process with intensity $\lambda(\cdot)$.

Conditional on $Z(D_s) = m$, $\mathbf{s}_1, \ldots, \mathbf{s}_m$, and σ_ε^2,

$$M(\mathbf{s}_i)|L(\mathbf{s}_i), \sigma_\varepsilon^2 \sim ind. \; Gau(L(\mathbf{s}_i), \sigma_\varepsilon^2)$$

Process model: Conditional on $\boldsymbol{\beta}_Y$ and $C_Y(\cdot, \cdot)$, the log intensity function, $Y(\cdot) \equiv \log \lambda(\cdot)$, is a Gaussian process with the following properties:

$$E(Y(\mathbf{s})) = \mathbf{x}_Y(\mathbf{s})'\boldsymbol{\beta}_Y,$$

$$\mathrm{cov}(Y(\mathbf{s}), Y(\mathbf{x})) \equiv C_Y(\mathbf{s}, \mathbf{x}).$$

Conditional on $Y(\cdot)$, $L(\cdot)$, is a Gaussian process whose first moment depends on covariates $\mathbf{x}_L(\cdot)$ and possibly $Y(\cdot)$, and whose second moments exhibit spatial statistical dependence.

Further properties of marked spatial point processes can be found, for example, in Cressie (1993, Section 8.7), Baddeley and van Lieshout (1995), Schlather (2001), and Schlather, Ribeiro, and Diggle (2004).

Models for Location Error

In much of spatial statistics, it is assumed that spatial locations, $\mathbf{s}_1, \ldots, \mathbf{s}_m$, are known precisely. In reality, *both* attribute and location are subject to measurement errors. The locational information often comes from global positioning systems (GPSs), which are commonplace in modern society. Each comes with a declaration of its locational precision; generally, the greater the precision of the GPS, the higher its price!

Suppose that $Z^0(\cdot)$ is a point process on $D_s^0 \subset \mathbb{R}^d$, which is characterized by its number of events, $Z^0(D_s^0) = m$, and the event locations, $\{\mathbf{s}_1^0, \ldots, \mathbf{s}_m^0\}$. These might be locations of trees in a natural forest D_s, such as shown in Figure 4.15. If the trees in the forest are mapped using a GPS, then the resulting point pattern of trees is in D_s, where D_s is equal to D_s^0 *augmented* by a buffer zone to account for every tree's location in the forest. Consequently, if we model the point pattern as being generated by a point process $Z(\cdot)$, then $Z(D_s) = Z^0(D_s^0)$, in distribution. A reasonable model for the event locations of $Z(\cdot)$ is

$$\mathbf{s}_i = \mathbf{s}_i^0 + \boldsymbol{\varepsilon}_i, \qquad i = 1, \ldots, m, \tag{4.200}$$

for $\boldsymbol{\varepsilon}_1, \ldots, \boldsymbol{\varepsilon}_m$ *iid* random vectors in $\mathbb{R}^d$ that represent location error (e.g., the GPS's measurement error). The model (4.200) for location error was called the *feature-positioning model* by Cressie and Kornak (2003). Dobrushin (1963) showed that if the location-error variances tend to infinity, then under regularity conditions, $Z(\cdot)$ converges to a homogeneous Poisson point process no matter what the underlying point process $Z^0(\cdot)$ is.

The feature-positioning model can be expressed as an HM; an example is given below.

Data model: Conditional on $Z^0(\cdot)$ and R_ε, the point process $Z(\cdot)$ is given by $Z(D_s) = Z^0(D_s^0)$, and

$$\mathbf{s}_i = \mathbf{s}_i^0 + \boldsymbol{\varepsilon}_i, \qquad i = 1, \ldots, m,$$

where $\{\mathbf{s}_i^0\}$ are the event locations of Z^0 in D_s^0, $\{\boldsymbol{\varepsilon}_i\}$ are *iid* random d-dimensional locations uniform on the ball, $b(\mathbf{0}, R_\varepsilon) \equiv \{\mathbf{x} \colon \|\mathbf{x}\| \le R_\varepsilon\}$, and $D_s = \bigcup_{\mathbf{s} \in D_s^0} b(\mathbf{s}, R_\varepsilon)$.

Process model: Conditional on $\boldsymbol{\beta}$ and $\boldsymbol{\theta}$, $Z^0(\cdot)$ is a Markov point process with regression parameters $\boldsymbol{\beta}$ in $\xi(\mathbf{s}; \boldsymbol{\beta}) = \mathbf{x}(\mathbf{s})'\boldsymbol{\beta}$ and small-scale spatial dependence parameters $\boldsymbol{\theta}$ in (4.189).

At the level of the process model, we could alternatively express spatial dependence in the point process $Z^0(\cdot)$ as follows.

Process model 1: Conditional on $\lambda(\cdot)$, $Z^0(\cdot)$ is an inhomogeneous Poisson point process with intensity $\lambda(\cdot)$.

Process model 2: Conditional on $\boldsymbol{\beta}$ and $C_Y(\cdot, \cdot)$, $Y(\cdot) \equiv \log \lambda(\cdot)$ is a Gaussian process with the following properties:

$$E(Y(\mathbf{s})) = \mathbf{x}(\mathbf{s})'\boldsymbol{\beta} \quad \text{and} \quad C_Y(\mathbf{s}, \mathbf{x}) \equiv \text{cov}(Y(\mathbf{s}), Y(\mathbf{x})).$$

Diggle (1993, pp. 97–99) provides some results that relate to estimation of parameters of the hidden spatial point process $Z^0(\cdot)$, from data $Z(D_s^0) = m$ and $\mathbf{s}_1, \ldots, \mathbf{s}_m$. For a stationary, isotropic $Z^0(\cdot)$ and a radially symmetric distribution for the location errors $\{\boldsymbol{\varepsilon}_i\}$, the first-order intensity function for $Z(\cdot)$ is the same as that for $Z^0(\cdot)$. However, when $Z^0(\cdot)$ exhibits clustering, Diggle's general conclusion is that the K function for $Z(\cdot)$ is smaller than that for $Z^0(\cdot)$. That is, K-function estimators based on the data $Z(D_s^0) = m$ and $\mathbf{s}_1, \ldots, \mathbf{s}_m$, generally underestimate the K function for the hidden, location-error-free process $Z^0(\cdot)$.

Fanshawe and Diggle (2011) extend the feature-positioning model of Cressie and Kornak (2003) by adopting a BHM for a marked spatial point process that is based on (4.200). Their goal is optimal spatial prediction of the mark process.

Directed Markov Point Process (DMPP)

Recall from Section 4.2.8, the discussion of Partially Ordered Markov Models (POMMs), where a partial order (equivalently an acyclic directed graph) defines the spatial dependence in lattice data. This directional type of dependence in lattice processes has an analogue for spatial point processes. Intuitively, this is not surprising, if we view a point process as an ultra-fine-grid lattice process with pixel ds_j located at pixel center s_j; $j = 1, \ldots, J$, where $\bigcup_{j=1}^{J} ds_j = D_s$, and $Z(ds_j) = 1$ or 0, according to a spatially dependent binary process.

If a lattice process is a binary POMM on an ultra-fine grid, and hence it has a directed type of spatial dependence, we would expect it to approximate a spatial point process that also has a directed type of spatial dependence. Under regularity conditions, including $\max\{|ds_j|: j = 1, \ldots, J\} \to 0$ as $J \to \infty$, the binary POMM should converge to a spatial point process; Cressie et al. (2000b) show this to be the case. They define *Directed Markov Point Processes (DMPPs)* as limits of binary POMMs.

Define the coordinate-wise *partial order* (notated as $\prec$) between two locations in $\mathbb{R}^d$ as

$$\mathbf{s} \prec \mathbf{x} \text{ if } s_1 \le x_1 \text{ and } s_2 \le x_2 \ldots \text{and } s_d \le x_d \,,$$

where $\mathbf{s} \equiv (s_1, \ldots, s_d)'$ and $\mathbf{x} \equiv (x_1, \ldots, x_d)'$. Then the cone of $\mathbf{x} \in \mathbb{R}^d$ is defined as

$$\text{cone}(\mathbf{x}) \equiv \{\mathbf{s} \in D_s : \mathbf{s} \prec \mathbf{x} \text{ and } \mathbf{s} \ne \mathbf{x}\} \,.$$

Furthermore, let $\psi(\mathbf{s}, \mathbf{x})$ denote a spatial interaction function. Then Cressie et al. (2000b) show that a (homogeneous) DMPP can be written in terms of the joint "density" function as follows:

$$f((\mathbf{s}_1, \ldots, \mathbf{s}_m), m)$$

$$= \exp\{-|D_s|\} \exp\left\{-\lambda \int_{D_s} \prod_{\mathbf{s}_j \in \text{cone}(\mathbf{x})} \psi(\mathbf{x}, \mathbf{s}_j)\, d\mathbf{x}\right\} \lambda^m \prod_{i=1}^{m} \prod_{\mathbf{s}_j \in \text{cone}(\mathbf{s}_i)} \psi(\mathbf{s}_i, \mathbf{s}_j) \,.$$

$$(4.201)$$

In fact, DMPPs can be defined more generally, in terms of a directed conditional intensity function, which characterizes the spatial dependence in the DMPP. More details of the definition and the properties of this type of point process can be found in Baddeley, Nair, and Cressie (2002).

4.4 RANDOM SETS

Recall from Chapter 1 our discussion of the object view (versus the field view) of spatial (and dynamical) phenomena. This book is largely about the field view, but in this section we shall discuss the role of random objects in an HM framework. Consider the data to be a collection of objects whose variability we describe using the theory of random sets (Matheron, 1971, 1975). For example, Cressie and Hulting (1992) used random sets to describe the evolution of breast cancer cells growing in a nutrient medium on a glass plate. The datum at a given time was an image of breast cancer cells on the plate.

Analogous to the theory of random variables, where variability is modeled as a real-valued measurable mapping from a probability space to a measure space on the real numbers, a *random set* in $\mathbb{R}^d$ is a measurable mapping from a probability space into a particular measure space, which we now describe. Define $\mathcal{F}$ to be the set of all closed subsets of $\mathbb{R}^d$ (including the empty set $\emptyset$). Let $\mathcal{K}$ denote the set of all compact sets, and let $\mathcal{K}' \equiv \mathcal{K} \backslash \emptyset$ be the set of all nonempty compact sets. For any $A \subset \mathbb{R}^d$, define

$$\mathcal{F}_A \equiv \{F \in \mathcal{F}: F \cap A \neq \emptyset\} \quad \text{and} \quad \mathcal{F}^A \equiv \{F \in \mathcal{F}: F \cap A = \emptyset\}. \quad (4.202)$$

For K compact and $G_1, \ldots, G_n$ open, generate all sets of the form $\mathcal{F}^K \cap \mathcal{F}_{G_1} \cap \cdots \cap \mathcal{F}_{G_n}$. Matheron (1975) has shown that this class of subsets of $\mathcal{F}$ is a *base* of a topology on $\mathcal{F}$ (which he called the *hit-or-miss topology*) and that the topological space is compact, Hausdorff, and separable. Furthermore, Matheron (1975, p. 28) proved that only hit-or-miss information, either on the set of all compact sets or on the set of all open sets, is needed to specify a random set; we return to this point later. Equipped with a topology on $\mathcal{F}$, one can now be rigorous about convergence of a sequence of closed sets. Furthermore, by taking countable unions and intersections of the open sets of the topological space $\mathcal{F}$, a σ-algebra $\sigma_{\mathcal{F}}$ on $\mathcal{F}$ can be generated.

A *random closed set* or RACS (which is often just called a *random set*) is defined as a measurable mapping Y from a probability space $(\Omega, \mathcal{A}, Q)$ into the measure space $(\mathcal{F}, \sigma_{\mathcal{F}})$. This is a very general definition of a random quantity, which includes the definitions of familiar random quantities, such as random variables, random vectors, point processes, and so on. Let $\Pr(\cdot)$ be the law of Y, namely, the probability induced on $\sigma_{\mathcal{F}}$ by

$$\Pr(\nu) \equiv Q(Y^{-1}(\nu)), \qquad \nu \in \sigma_{\mathcal{F}}.$$

4.4.1 Hit-or-Miss Topology

The hit-or-miss topology is basic to the theory of random sets. It was chosen because it reflects the way image data in $\mathbb{R}^d$ are analyzed; that is, its roots are in practical applications. When studying an object Y (e.g., a work of art, whose authenticity is in question), some sort of systematic (nondestructive) probing is needed, which leads to the use of structuring elements B (chosen independently of Y) to check whether "B hits Y" ($B \cap Y \neq \emptyset$) or "B misses Y" ($B \cap Y = \emptyset$).

It can be shown that all the interesting set transformations (dilation, erosion, opening, closing, convexification, etc.) of a RACS Y are themselves RACS (Matheron, 1975, p. 28). The analogue to this for a random variable Y is that a transformation $g(Y)$ is also a random variable; this is true provided $g(\cdot)$ is measurable. Therefore, for a RACS to be useful in an HM approach to modeling random objects, the development of a collection of random-set models is essential. How can the models be specified? What are the important events that make two random sets different? For a partial answer, we return to the hit-or-miss topology. If we can specify $\Pr(Y \in \mathcal{F}^K \cap \mathcal{F}_{G_1} \cap \cdots \cap \mathcal{F}_{G_k})$ for all compact K, for all open $G_1, \ldots, G_k$, and for all integers k, in a consistent way, then Y is well defined. Fortunately, a great reduction of test sets *is* possible.

Definition: For any $K \in \mathcal{K}$, define *the hitting function T* as

$$T(K) \equiv \Pr(Y \in \mathcal{F}_K) = \Pr\{Y \cap K \neq \emptyset\}. \tag{4.203}$$

Henceforth, we refer to K in $\Pr\{Y \cap K \neq \emptyset\}$ as a *test set*.

The hitting function T defined in (4.203) has the following properties (Matheron, 1975, p. 29):

1. $T(\emptyset) = 0$ and $0 \leq T \leq 1$.
2. T is increasing.
3. T satisfies the following recurrence relations. For any $k \geq 0$, let $S_k(B_0; B_1, \ldots, B_k)$ denote the probability that Y misses B_0 but hits $B_1, \ldots, B_k$. Then

$$S_0(B_0) = 1 - T(B_0) \geq 0$$

$$S_1(B_0; B_1) = T(B_0 \cup B_1) - T(B_0) \geq 0$$

$$\vdots$$

$$S_k(B_0; B_1, \ldots, B_k) = S_{k-1}(B_0; B_1, \ldots, B_{k-1})$$
$$- S_{k-1}(B_0 \cup B_k; B_1, \ldots, B_{k-1}) \geq 0.$$

That is, T is a *Choquet capacity of infinite order* (Matheron, 1975, p. 30).

A powerful result, proved independently by Matheron (1971) and by Kendall (1974), is Choquet's Theorem in the context of random-set theory; it says that the converse of property 3. above is true. In other words, if a given T on $\mathcal{K}$ is a Choquet capacity of infinite order, there exists a *necessarily unique P_T* on $\sigma_{\mathcal{F}}$ such that

$$P_T(\mathcal{F}_K) = T(K), \qquad \text{for all } K \in \mathcal{K}. \tag{4.204}$$

An immediate example of its use is when the RACS Y is a simple spatial point process (i.e., no more than one event at any location) in $\mathbb{R}^d$. In Section 4.3, we denoted a point process as $Z(\cdot)$, and $Z(A)$ is the number of points in $A \subset D_s \subset \mathbb{R}^d$. Then Choquet's Theorem says the point process is completely specified from

$$T(K) = 1 - \Pr(Y \cap K = \emptyset)$$

$$= 1 - \Pr(Z(K) = 0), \qquad \text{for all } K \in \mathcal{K},$$

where recall that the RACS Y is the point process $Z(\cdot)$ in this example. This observation, that the point process is uniquely determined from $\{\Pr(Z(K) = 0) : K \in \mathcal{K}\}$, was made by Ripley (1976, p. 989). It is tempting to bracket Choquet's Theorem with the result that says that a random variable Y is well defined once the probabilities of events $\{Y \leq y\}$, for all $y \in (-\infty, \infty)$, are specified in a consistent way. But the two results, while being similar, are not exactly analogous. In fact, Choquet's Theorem for a random variable, where the RACS Y is a one-point set in $\mathbb{R}^1$, involves "test sets," $\{[a, b]: -\infty < a \leq b < \infty\}$; a little more work is needed to modify the necessary test sets down to $\{(-\infty, y]: -\infty < y < \infty\}$. It is in this domain where results (and hence random-set models) are scarce, namely finding ways to reduce the hitting-function test sets down from the full complement $\mathcal{K}$.

There are other ways to model uncertainty in objects and patterns. The theory of random patterns (i.e., Pattern Analysis) due to Grenander (1996) has proved amenable to incorporation into an HM (Grenander and Miller, 2007).

4.4.2 Hierarchical Models for Objects Based on Random Sets

There are a number of ways that random-set models of objects can be used in an HM. The *observed* RACS is denoted as Z, which we consider to be a "noisy" version of the hidden RACS Y. For the purpose of illustration, suppose that the true process Y is the union of compact sets. Then the *observed* boundaries of the individual compact sets could be modeled through independent Brownian Bridges superimposed on the respective boundary loci of the compact sets. [A Brownian Bridge with mean zero is a Gaussian process that has the property that it starts at 0 and always returns to 0 on a finite interval (e.g., Glasserman, 2004).] Then Z is the union of the sets defined by the *observed* boundaries.

Given the hierarchical nature of the model, it is straightforward to simulate from the joint distribution. Formally,

$$[Z, Y] = [Z|Y][Y];$$

first simulate Y from $[Y]$ and then Z from $[Z|Y]$. The posterior distribution is proportional to the joint distribution; that is,

$$[Y|Z] \propto [Z, Y] = [Z|Y][Y],$$

but the proportionality constant, which is $1/[Z]$, can be difficult to obtain.

In principle, a Metropolis or Metropolis–Hastings algorithm could be implemented to obtain a simulation from $[Y|Z]$; see Section 2.3.2. This approach to simulating from the posterior distribution is quite general and could be used for making inference on a hidden object Y, given an observed object Z.

Sets can also appear in spatial statistics as supports of density or intensity functions. Recall the inhomogeneous Poisson point process with intensity $\{\lambda(\mathbf{s}): \mathbf{s} \in D_s\}$. In the example of trees in a natural forest, there may be a region $B \subset D_s$ where soil conditions are conducive to growth, but not so outside B; that is, $\lambda(\mathbf{s}) \equiv 0$ for $\mathbf{s} \in D_s \backslash B$. Based on data, $Z(D_s) = m$ and $\{\mathbf{s}_1, \ldots, \mathbf{s}_m\}$ on the point process $Z(\cdot)$, we may wish to make inference on the support B. Define $Y(\mathbf{s}) \equiv I(\mathbf{s} \in B) = 1$ if $\mathbf{s} \in B$, and zero otherwise. Then the following HM is well defined for making inference on the indicator function $Y(\cdot)$ (equivalently, on B).

Data model: Conditional on $B_0 \subset D_s$ and $\mu_0(\cdot)$, the point process $Z_1(\cdot)$ is an inhomogeneous Poisson point process with intensity $\lambda_1(\mathbf{s}) \equiv \mu_0(\mathbf{s})I(\mathbf{s} \in B_0)$; $\mathbf{s} \in D_s$.

Process model 1:   Conditional on $\boldsymbol{\beta}$ and $C_Y(\cdot, \cdot)$, $Y_0(\cdot) \equiv \log \mu_0(\cdot)$ is a Gaussian process on B_0 with the following properties: $E(Y_0(\cdot)) = \mathbf{x}(\cdot)'\boldsymbol{\beta}$, and we write $C_Y(\mathbf{u}, \mathbf{v}) \equiv \mathrm{cov}(Y_0(\mathbf{u}), Y_0(\mathbf{v}))$.

Process model 2:   Conditional on random-set model parameters $\boldsymbol{\theta}_R$, B_0 is a RACS defined by its hitting function,

$$T(K; \boldsymbol{\theta}_R) \equiv \Pr(K \cap B_0 \neq \emptyset), \qquad K \in \mathcal{K}.$$

Figure 4.20a shows a simulation of the HM on the unit square: First, B_0 is a (discretized) Boolean model (Section 4.4.3); a realization is obtained by superimposing Figure 4.19a onto a fine spatial grid, resulting in the set of black pixels shown in Figure 4.19b. Second, a realization of $\mu_0(\cdot) \equiv \exp(Y_0(\cdot))$, a log-Gaussian process, is obtained (see Figure 4.19c). Third, $\lambda_1(\mathbf{s}) \equiv \mu_0(\mathbf{s})I(\mathbf{s} \in B_0)$ is shown in Figure 4.19d. Finally, a realization of the spatial point process $Z_1(\cdot)$ is shown in Figure 4.20a.

4.4.3 The Boolean Model

The random set simulated in Figure 4.19b is called a *Boolean model*, which is obtained by centering independent realizations of a compact random set S in $\mathbb{R}^d$ at each point of a realization $\{\mathbf{u}_i\}$ of a homogeneous Poisson point process Z_0 in $\mathbb{R}^d$, and taking the union of all the centered compact sets. That is,

$$B = \cup_i (S_i \oplus \mathbf{u}_i), \qquad (4.205)$$

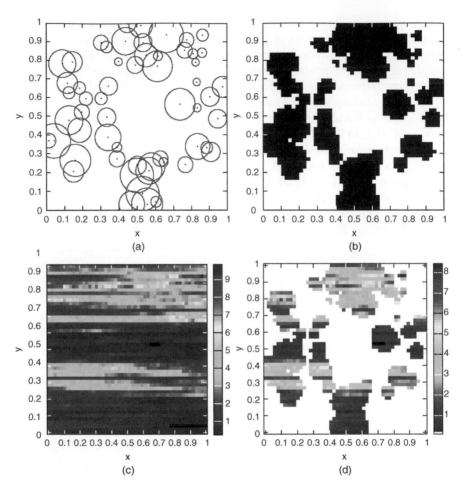

Figure 4.19 (a) Randomly generated disk centers and disk radii in the unit square D_s. A realization of the Boolean model is the union of the disks centered around the $Z_0(D_s) = 57$ foci locations shown. The 57 foci are from the CSR point process with intensity $\lambda^o = 50$, and the 57 radii are a random sample from the uniform distribution, $U[.02,.1]$. (b) Discretized Boolean model B_0 on a regular 50×50 grid of pixels on the unit square; its area $|B_0| = .3980$. A pixel is declared to be contained in the (discretized) Boolean model if the pixel center is contained in at least one of the disks shown in (a). (c) Log-Gaussian process discretized onto the 50×50 grid. The Gaussian process defining it is stationary and has mean 0, variance 1, and covariance function $C(\cdot)$ given by Figure 6.3, considered as a two-dimensional spatial covariance function. (d) Intensity function defined by the log-Gaussian process on the Boolean model, and defined to be zero elsewhere.

where $S \oplus \mathbf{u} \equiv \{\mathbf{s} + \mathbf{u} \colon \mathbf{s} \in S\}$; the random sets $\{S_i\}$ are independent RACS identically distributed as S; and $\{\mathbf{u}_i\}$ are the events of Z_0. Thus, there are two sources of randomness in the model, namely the homogeneous Poisson point process characterized by its intensity, λ^o, and the probability measure associated with the compact random set, S.

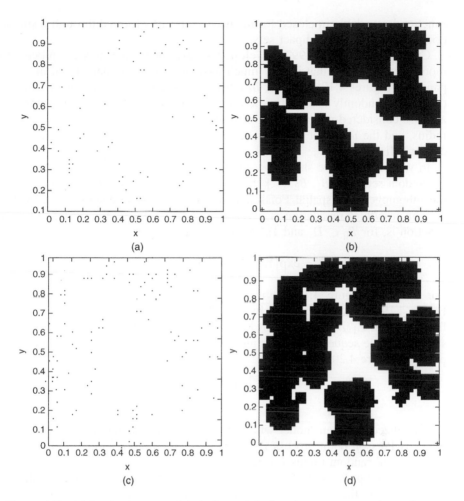

Figure 4.20 (a) Randomly generated foci of growth in the unit square, generated according to an inhomogeneous Poisson process with intensity function given by Figure 4.19d; there are $Z_1(D_s) = 70$ foci. (b) The (discretized) Boolean model B_1 is obtained the same way as in Figure 4.19b, using the same $U[.02,.1]$ distribution to generate the random radii; its area is $|B_1| = .5420$, indicating growth. (c) Using the same log-Gaussian process as in Figure 4.19c, the intensity function restricted like in Figure 4.19d yields randomly generated foci with $Z_2(D_s) = 114$. (d) The (discretized) Boolean model B_2 is obtained the same way as Figure 4.19b, using the same $U[.02,.1]$ distribution to generate the random radii; its area is $|B_2| = .6092$, indicating growth.

The hitting function of B given by (4.205) can be calculated. From the random set S, define $\check{S} \oplus K \equiv \{-\mathbf{s} + \mathbf{v} : \mathbf{s} \in S \text{ and } \mathbf{v} \in K\}$. Then the hitting function of B is (e.g., Cressie, 1993, p. 754)

$$T(K) = 1 - \exp\{-\lambda^o E(|\check{S} \oplus K|)\}, \qquad K \in \mathcal{K}, \qquad (4.206)$$

where recall that $|A|$ is the d-dimensional volume of a measurable set A. The Boolean model is a very useful model for random sets because its hitting function is available in closed form, and because it is formed through a simple operation (union) on compact sets.

Cressie and Hulting (1992) developed a set-valued autoregressive process to model tumor growth that is very much like the process model shown in select panels of Figures 4.19 and 4.20. *In vitro* breast-cancer cells on a glass slide at time 1 are randomly declared to be foci of growth with local growth rates that are also considered random. The local growth is modeled as a disk of random radius, and the *union* of all disks centered at the foci makes up the set of all cancer cells at time 2.

In what follows, we show how to simulate a process model for a sequence of random sets $\{B_0, B_1, B_2, \ldots\}$ that exhibit "random growth." Let Z_1 denote the inhomogeneous spatial Poisson point process whose events represent the foci of growth; a realization is given in Figure 4.20a. Its first-order intensity function is, for $B_0 \subset D_s$ and $Y_0(\cdot)$ a Gaussian process,

$$\lambda_1(\mathbf{s}) = \exp\{Y_0(\mathbf{s})\} I(\mathbf{s} \in B_0), \qquad \mathbf{s} \in D_s. \tag{4.207}$$

For example, Figure 4.19b shows B_0, Figure 4.19c shows $\exp\{Y_0(\cdot)\}$, and Figure 4.19d shows $\lambda_1(\cdot)$ given by (4.207). Then Figure 4.20a is a realization from Z_1 with $Z_1(D_s) = 70$ event locations, $\{\mathbf{u}_{1i} : i = 1, \ldots, 70\}$. Now we can start the whole sequence of steps again to generate a set-valued autoregressive process. Figure 4.20b shows

$$B_1 \equiv \bigcup_i (S_{1i} \oplus \mathbf{u}_{1i}), \tag{4.208}$$

a generalized Boolean model whose foci $\{\mathbf{u}_{1i}\}$ are generated by the *inhomogeneous* Poisson point process Z_1; in (4.208), $\{S_{1i}\}$ are *iid* random disks with center $\mathbf{0}$ and random radius $U[.02,.1]$.

By replacing B_0 with B_1, $Y_0(\cdot)$ with $Y_1(\cdot)$, and repeating, we obtain Z_2 and then B_2 in the same way B_1 was obtained in (4.208). Figure 4.20c shows Z_2 and Figure 4.20d shows B_2. The model that was simulated shows growth: $|B_0| = .3980$, $|B_1| = .5420$, and $|B_2| = .6092$. It is also possible to model a receding tumor through low intensities $\exp\{Y_0(\cdot)\}$, $\exp\{Y_1(\cdot)\}$, etc., and small disk radii of $\{S_{1i}\}$, $\{S_{2i}\}$, etc. Cressie and Hulting (1992) carry out statistical inference on intensities and local growth rates for *in vitro* breast cancer cells observed 72 hours apart. This discussion around Figures 4.19 and 4.20 opens up the possibility of building dynamical spatio-temporal set processes, something we refer to briefly in Section 6.5. There is a growing literature in growth processes using random sets (e.g., Jónsdóttir, Schmiegel, and Jensen, 2008).

The Boolean model's parameters can be estimated by discretizing its 0–1 values onto a fine grid and then using the method-of-moments on (4.206) for different test sets K (e.g., Cressie and Laslett, 1987). Writing down the Boolean model's likelihood has always been difficult to achieve, except for the simplest cases, because of the overlapping nature of the sets $\{S_i \oplus \mathbf{u}_i : i = 1, 2, \ldots\}$. The various combinations of possibilities of how an $\mathbf{s} \in D_s$ might be in or out of the Boolean model B has made the likelihood elusive. To deal with this, Møller and Helisova (2009) choose a model where there is dependence between the events $\{u_i\}$ and the sets $\{S_i\}$, they then define a conditional likelihood that is more conducive to MCMC analysis than the regular likelihood, and finally they use MCMC to (approximately) optimize the conditional likelihood.

Micheas and Wikle (2009) take a different approach and consider a random non-overlapping disk model to model objects from a hierarchical perspective. They model random disks and random foci in a multistage hierarchical Bayesian framework. The BHM approach facilitates inference without the need for tedious calculation of the hitting probabilities. Critically, their approach is based on modeling a point from the random set, instead of the set itself, which allows direct inference on the parameters of the model via MCMC. This also allows inference on *individual* random disks in the model. They also demonstrate how this methodology can be used for modeling the growth of objects.

4.5 BIBLIOGRAPHIC NOTES

A number of texts that cover spatial random processes have been mentioned in the introduction to this chapter. Review articles and other texts that give presentations of topics at various levels of difficulty include Yaglom (1957, 1962), Matérn (1960), Bartlett (1975), Cliff and Ord (1981), Ripley (1981), Upton and Fingleton (1985), Ripley (1988), Upton and Fingleton (1989), Cressie (1991, 1993), Possolo (1991), Bailey and Gatrell (1992), Hjort and Omre (1994), Gregoire et al. (1997), Griffith and Layne (1999), Moore (2001), Griffith (2003), Haining (2003), Møller (2003), Banerjee, Carlin, and Gelfand (2004), Waller and Gotway (2004), Longley et al. (2005), Schabenberger and Gotway (2005), Le and Zidek (2006), Bivand, Pebesma, and Gómez-Rubio (2008), Fortin and Dale (2009), LeSage and Pace (2009), Gaetan and Guyon (2010), and Gelfand et al. (2010, Part II).

This chapter has divided up naturally into four types of spatial processes. These are geostatistical processes, spatial lattice processes, spatial point processes, and random-set processes.

Geostatistical Processes
Matheron (1962, 1963) and Gandin (1963) wrote comprehensive accounts of statistics for spatial processes for audiences in mining and atmospheric sciences, respectively. Matheron coined the term "geostatistics," and a comprehensive account of mining geostatistics appears in the books by David (1977), Journel and Huijbregts (1978), Clark (1979), and Chilés and Delfiner (1999). Rivoirard (2005) summarizes the concept and methods in a review chapter. Various other accounts of geostatistical processes, for different purposes, can be found in Yaglom (1962), Yadrenko (1983), Bras and Rodriguez-Iturbe (1985), Isaaks and Srivastata (1989), Brooker (1991), Christakos (1992), Goovaerts (1997), Kitanidis (1997), Müller (1998), Hohn (1999), Stein (1999), Webster and Oliver (2001), and Lantuéjoul (2002).

Ripley (1981), Christensen (1991), and Cressie (1991, 1993) present a statistican's perspective of the subject and draw on examples beyond Mining, particularly in Crop Science, Hydrology, and the Environmental Sciences. These references do not use hierarchical models, by and large. Banerjee, Carlin, and Gelfand (2004) do, but they do not always distinguish clearly between the measurement error and the microscale variaton of the latent spatial process $Y(\cdot)$, occasionally resulting in spatial prediction of only the smooth component of $Y(\cdot)$. Le and Zidek (2006) and Diggle and Ribeiro (2007) also give a statistician's perspective, and their Bayesian presentations involve prediction of the hidden spatial process $Y(\cdot)$. Banerjee et al. (2008) and Finley et al. (2009) predict $Y(\cdot)$ through predictive processes defined on support points. Arab (2007) and Lindgren et al. (2011) use a spectral representation of $Y(\cdot)$ derived from a Galerkin expansion of a stochastic PDE.

Measures of Spatial Dependence
Fundamental to kriging and generally to calculating the predictive/posterior distribution is specification of the spatial covariance function. The variogram, along with the variance function, will often play the same role. Estimation of these important quantities in various scenarios has recently been considered by Stein, Chi, and Welty (2004), Zhang (2004), Stein (2005), Zhang and Zimmerman (2007), and Kaufman, Schervish, and Nychka (2008). An innovative approach to variogram estimation (and spatial prediction) based on block empirical likelihoods (which avoids specification of a joint likelihood from a parametric family) can be found in Nordman (2008a,b) and in Nordman and Caragea (2008).

Spatial dependence can also be summarized in the spectral domain, where estimation can likewise proceed (e.g., Fuentes, 2002, 2007; Im, Stein, and Zhu, 2007; Huang, Hsing, and Cressie, 2010). Other summaries of spatial dependence include the joint distribution and the spatial cumulative distribution function (Lahiri et al., 1999).

Covariance functions that are locally stationary have been considered by Silverman (1957) and by Sampson and Guttorp (1992). They transform spatial coordinates into a space where the covariance function is isotropic. Paciorek and Schervish (2006) consider process convolutions using inhomogeneous kernel functions. Global data have also fostered the need for nonstationary covariance models (Section 4.1.4; Cressie and Johannesson, 2008; Jun and Stein, 2008). The use of copulas to model spatial dependence is a more recent approach (e.g., Bárdossy and Li, 2008).

Proving that estimators of these measures of spatial dependence are consistent is complicated, requiring notions of a spatial domain that grows, along with samples that infill the domain. These issues are discussed by Ivanov and Leonenko (1989), Lahiri (1996), Lahiri et al. (1999), Stein (1999), and Park et al. (2009).

Spatial Prediction and Mapping
Kriging can be equated to spatial best linear unbiased prediction (Cressie, 1990). It is a special instance (i.e., it is linear) of optimal spatial prediction of

a hidden process $Y(\cdot)$ based on noisy, incomplete data $\mathbf{Z}$. This more general problem is solved by computing the posterior distribution $[g(Y(\cdot))|\mathbf{Z}, \widehat{\boldsymbol{\theta}}]$ for an EHM, or $[g(Y(\cdot))|\mathbf{Z}]$ for a BHM, where $g(Y(\cdot))$ is some functional of interest, like $Y(\mathbf{s}_0)$, $Y(B)$, $\nabla Y(\mathbf{s}_0)$ (Banerjee and Gelfand, 2006), or $\exp(Y(\mathbf{s}_0))$ (e.g., Cressie, 2006). A point predictor is obtained by summarizing the posterior distribution by its mean, or median, or mode, and so on.

The idea of using process models with parameters that are themselves processes was presented by Wikle, Berliner, and Cressie (1998) in the spatio-temporal context and was considered later by Gelfand et al. (2003) in the spatial-only context. Non-Gaussian HMs were considered in Section 4.1.2, to which contributions by Christensen and Waagepetersen (2002), Zhang (2002, 2003), Gelfand, Kottas, and MacEachern (2005), Cressie (2006), Monestiez et al. (2006), Zhu, Gu, and Peterson (2007), Crainiceanu, Diggle, and Rowlingson (2008), Musio, Augustin, and von Wilpert (2008), and Berliner et al. (2008) should be added.

Optimal spatial prediction of extremes of $Y(\cdot)$ is a nonlinear prediction problem, for which kriging is not well suited, since it "fills in the valleys" and "cuts off the hills." De Oliveira and Ecker (2002), Cooley, Nychka, and Naveau (2007), and Zhang, Craigmile, and Cressie (2008) use HMs for optimal spatial prediction of extremes.

Change-of-Support

In the climate and remote-sensing communities, the problem of change-of-support is usually referred to as *downscaling*, where inference is on $Y(\mathbf{s}_0)$ at the point or small-grid-cell level, based on data $Z(B_1), \ldots, Z(B_m)$. Upscaling is then concerned with inference on $Y(B)$ based on data $Z(\mathbf{s}_1), \ldots, Z(\mathbf{s}_m)$. It is the latter problem that mining engineers are particularly interested in, since ore is mined and sent to the mill in units made up of a block B. Also, environmental remediation or management of an ecological resource is typically made at the block level. Ecologists use the term *scale* instead of support, in the context of pattern and scale (e.g., Levin, 1992).

Change-of-support is commonplace in spatial statistics. Openshaw and Taylor (1979) show how hard the problem is in general to solve. The downscaling problem has been considered from a geostatistical viewpoint by Kyriakidis (2004). A comprehensive review of the statistical problem of change-of-support has been written by Gotway and Young (2002), and Section 4.1.3 features other approaches.

Spatial Moving Average (SMA) and Multiresolution Statistical Models

The SMA models are easy to define and easy to simulate from. They also offer a convenient way to model complicated spatial dependence with reduced rank models; see the review by Wikle (2010a). The temptation is to let the moving average weights (equivalently, process-convolution kernels) be as general as possible, but then they typically lack physical interpretation and lead to non-sparse covariance matrices. Choosing which reduced-rank model to use can be guided by the physical structure of the process. In the context of deterministic smoothing, Johannesson and Cressie (2004) give a method for choosing from among several families of spherical basis functions on the globe, based on a measure of *spatial coherence*. In the context of Fixed Rank Kriging, where the emphasis is on modeling a spatial covariance function, Shi and Cressie (2007) give a method for choosing among multiresolution wavelet basis functions. Beyond a general recommendation of multiresolutional structure, the question of basis-function choice is open. For the change-of-resolution models (Section 4.1.6), the random effects are "drawn upward" from fine resolution to coarse resolution through hierarchical representations (Kolaczyk, 1999; Huang and Cressie, 2001; Kolaczyk and Nowak, 2004; Huang, Cressie, and Gabrosek 2002; and Tzeng, Huang, and Cressie, 2005).

Multivariate Spatial Processes
There are classes of multivariate spatial models that assume symmetric dependence through $\text{cov}(Y_1(\mathbf{s}), Y_2(\mathbf{s} + \mathbf{h})) = \text{cov}(Y_2(\mathbf{s}), Y_1(\mathbf{s} + \mathbf{h}))$, most notably, the linear model of coregionalization, or LMC (e.g., Wackernagel, 1995; Webster, Atteia, and Dubois, 1994; Banerjee, Carlin, and Gelfand, 2004, Chapter 7). However, there is no *a priori* reason for this type of symmetry to hold. Ver Hoef and Cressie (1993) avoid making this assumption by defining and working with cross-variograms. Sain and Cressie (2007) and Sain, Furrer, and Cressie (2011) allow asymmetry parameters in their multivariate (lattice) spatial models and note an asymmetric multivariate spatial dependence in the data they analyze. Gneiting, Kleiber, and Schlather (2010) define Matérn cross-covariance functions that show considerable flexibility, including the possibility of asymmetry.

Generally, the goal is spatial prediction of the multivariate spatial process $\mathbf{Y}(\cdot)$, or of one component, say $Y_1(\cdot)$, based on multivariate (noisy) spatial data, $\{\mathbf{Z}(\mathbf{s}_1), \dots, \mathbf{Z}(\mathbf{s}_m)\}$. When the component $Y_1(\cdot)$ is predicted in an EHM setting, the associated methodology is called *cokriging*. References for multivariate spatial prediction include Myers (1982, 1992), Ver Hoef and Cressie (1993), Wackernagel (1995), Cressie and Wikle (1998b), and Huang et al. (2009). In a BHM setting, see the articles by Majumdar and Gelfand (2007) and by Finley et al. (2008).

Banerjee, Carlin, and Gelfand (2004) and Gelfand et al. (2004) make a comparison of the LMC defined in Section 4.1.5, with the conditional-probability approach in (4.83), which deserves revisiting, here for the bivariate case $K = 2$. Under the LMC, they report properties of the conditional-probability approach given by (4.83) that look unusual to them, which they interpret as casting doubt on the general applicability of (4.83). In fact, there are a couple of misconceptions that, once identified, clear up these unusual-looking properties. First, taking the conditional-probability approach requires modeling $[\mathbf{Y}_2|\mathbf{Y}_1] = [Y_2(\mathbf{s}_1), \dots, Y_2(\mathbf{s}_n)|\mathbf{Y}_1]$. Any consideration of the conditional behavior of a component of $\mathbf{Y}_2$, say $Y_2(\mathbf{s}_i)$, is always referred to the conditional distribution $[Y_2(\mathbf{s}_i)|\mathbf{Y}_1]$, *never* to $[Y_2(\mathbf{s}_i)|Y_1(\mathbf{s}_i)]$. Part of Gelfand et al.'s (2004) discussion refers to the behaviors of $[Y_2(\mathbf{s}_1)|Y_1(\mathbf{s}_1)], \ldots, [Y_2(\mathbf{s}_n)|Y_1(\mathbf{s}_n)]$. They point out, correctly, that trying to interpret these quantities in some joint manner makes no sense. However, (4.83) considers the joint behavior of $\{Y_2(\mathbf{s}_1), \ldots, Y_2(\mathbf{s}_n)\}$, conditional on the *vector* $\mathbf{Y}_1$. The reason for Gelfand et al.'s misconception appears to come from observing that, in the LMC,

$$\mathbf{Y}_2|\mathbf{Y}_1 \sim Gau\left(\frac{a_{21}}{a_{11}}\mathbf{Y}_1, a_{22}^2\mathbf{\Sigma}_{2|1}\right),$$

where the (i,j)th entry of $\mathbf{\Sigma}_{2|1}$ is $\rho_2(\mathbf{s}_i - \mathbf{s}_j)$. They then notice that in equation (4.82), $\mathbf{W}_2 \equiv (W_2(\mathbf{s}_1), \ldots, W_2(\mathbf{s}_n))' \sim Gau(\mathbf{0}, \mathbf{\Sigma}_{2|1})$. Finally, they put $\mathbf{W}_2(\mathbf{s})$ *equal to* the error in the regression equation; that is, they write

$$Y_2(\mathbf{s}_i) = \frac{a_{21}}{a_{11}}Y_1(\mathbf{s}_i) + a_{22}W_2(\mathbf{s}_i), \qquad i = 1, \ldots, n.$$

It is not clear to us, either algebraically or statistically, how this equation above is correct.

We conclude that the conditional-probability approach, when considered properly, has many modeling advantages. Even when $K \geq 3$, there are often nested relations that allow a decomposition of the joint probability (e.g., for $K = 3$, $[\mathbf{Y}_1, \mathbf{Y}_2, \mathbf{Y}_3] = [\mathbf{Y}_3|\mathbf{Y}_1, \mathbf{Y}_2][\mathbf{Y}_2|\mathbf{Y}_1][\mathbf{Y}_1]$).

Bayesian Hierarchical Geostatistical Model Computations

Computational issues in the Bayesian implementation of hierarchical spatial models are covered in the books by Banerjee, Carlin, and Gelfand (2004) and by Diggle and Ribeiro (2007), as well as in the review chapter by Wikle (2010b). The dominant method used is a Markov chain Monte Carlo (MCMC) approach. In cases where parameters are random, which we argue are more practical, extra care must often be taken to balance computational considerations (e.g., convergence, efficiency) with the choice of the prior distribution on the parameters. For example, Gaussian-process priors typically include parameters associated with the variance, spatial dependence, and smoothness. In many Bayesian analyses in the literature, the smoothness parameter is assumed to be known (as a percentage of total variance), and attention is focussed on the variance and spatial-dependence parameters. For example, inverse gamma or discrete uniform priors are often chosen for the spatial-dependence parameter. In certain cases, one can use more "objective" priors for spatial parameters (e.g., Berger, De Oliveira, and Sansó, 2001; Paulo, 2005), but typically the variance parameters are given a relatively noninformative conjugate prior (e.g., inverse gamma). However, the use of noninformative priors for variance components can be problematic (see Browne and Draper, 2006; Gelman, 2006). It is increasingly common to reparameterize the spatial dependence parameters (e.g., see Zhang, 2004, Christensen, Roberts, and Skold, 2006; Palacios and Steel, 2006; Diggle and Ribeiro, 2007; and Yan et al., 2007). Experience suggests that it can be difficult for certain datasets to be fitted to these models without a great deal of careful sensitivity analyses.

Information Content

In Section 2.2, a brief discussion was given of the notion of information content. This relates to the properties of statistical inference as the data size increases; as it tends to infinity, is the uncertainty in the inference removed? For standard, *iid* error assumptions, the answer is generally "yes." For the type of short-term temporal dependence typically seen in Chapter 3, the answer is again generally "yes." However, in cases of infill sampling in a fixed domain, the situation is delicate (Lahiri, 1996; Lahiri, Lee, and Cressie, 2002; Lee and Lahiri, 2002; Bhattacharjya, Eidsvik, and Mukerji, 2010).

Model Selection

This book is almost silent on model selection. However, there has been some innovative work in the area of geostatistical model selection; see Hoeting et al. (2006) and Huang and Chen (2007). Likewise, Zhu and Carlin (2000) and Zhu, Huang, and Reyes (2010) consider selection of models for spatial lattice data.

Spatial Lattice Processes

Such processes are distinguished from geostatistical processes by the finite (or countably infinite) size of the spatial index set D_s. However, there are methodologies that the two spatial statistical modeling approaches (lattice and geostatistical) can share, particularly because in practice geostatistical processes are evaluated on a fine (regular) grid $\{s_1, \ldots, s_n\}$. In Section 4.2, many of the lattice models are MRFs (Sections 4.2.2-4.2.5), which are based on a conditional-distribution specification of spatial dependence. This is different from the bivariate-moments specification of the geostatistical models in Section 4.1. Some comparison of the two will be given below in a separate set of bibliographic notes.

Not all lattice processes are MRFs, and in fact there is an area that has become known as Spatial Econometrics that is based around the simultaneous-spatial-dependence models such as SAR, SARMA, and SARMAX. These are specified in Sections 4.2.7 and 4.2.8. In that literature (e.g., Anselin, 1988; Arbia, 1989; Getis, Mur, and Zoller, 2004; LeSage and Pace, 2009), researchers have often written their models as

$$\mathbf{Y} = \mathbf{X}\boldsymbol{\beta} + \mathbf{B}\mathbf{Y} + \boldsymbol{\varepsilon},$$

by analogy to models in (temporal) econometrics. See Section 4.2.7 for definitions, and an explanation that $\mathbf{B}$ is now a "spatial-shift" operator in place of the usual time-series backward-shift operator. While the decomposition of variability above seems natural, it is not hard to see that $E(\mathbf{Y}) = (\mathbf{I} - \mathbf{B})^{-1}\mathbf{X}\boldsymbol{\beta}$, leading to a confounding of the covariates $\mathbf{X}$ and the spatial dependence in $(\mathbf{I} - \mathbf{B})^{-1}$. In general, for processes that include both CAR and SAR models with fixed effects (covariates), one must take care regarding potential confounding between fixed effects and random effects when making inference on the unknowns (Reich et al., 2006; Paciorek, 2010; Hodges and Reich, 2010).

An additive decomposition of variability does not generalize easily to non-Gaussian, nonlinear lattice models; a decomposition based on a sequence of conditional-probability models *does* generalize, which is a theme of this book.

Texts and monographs in the area of lattice processes include Cliff and Ord (1981), Ripley (1981, 1988), Anselin (1988), Griffith (1988), Haining (1990), Cressie (1991, 1993), Guyon (1995), Griffith and Layne (1999), Tiefelsdorf (2000), Fotheringham, Brunsdon, and Charlton (2002), Getis, Mur, and Zoller (2004), Rue and Held (2005), some chapters in Gamerman and Lopes (2006), Lloyd (2007), Le Sage and Pace (2009), and Gelfand et al. (2010, Part III). Those with an emphasis on epidemiology include Elliott et al. (2000), Lawson (2001), Waller and Gotway (2004), and Lawson (2009).

The Markov Random Field (MRF)

This is a very elegant way to incorporate dependence in *any* multivariate distribution, not just spatial dependence. The dependence is succinctly captured by an undirected graph (Sections 2.4 and 4.2.2), which actually shows the conditional *independencies* but does not show the type and strength of the dependencies.

There has been much written about the theoretical properties of MRFs, including their properties in the limit as the lattice extends to infinity (e.g., Spitzer, 1971; Prum and Fort, 1991; van den Berg, 1993; Guyon, 1995), and their properties as the lattice spacing tends to zero (e.g., Besag, Milne, and Zachary, 1982; Cressie et al., 2000b). However, the statistical-modeling implications of these properties were dispersed in hard-to-find places. The Hammersley–Clifford Theorem (Hammersley and Clifford, 1971) was in an unpublished Oxford University manuscript; Clifford (1990) gives some of the history surrounding the result, as well as the original proof. The articles by Brook (1964) and Moussouris (1974) are noteworthy, but the article that captured the past, the present (at the time the article was published), and in some sense the future (at the time of writing this), was Besag (1974). Its impact on spatial statistics has been enormous.

A downside to MRFs is that they do not aggregate. In other words, if $\{Y(\mathbf{s}_1), Y(\mathbf{s}_2), Y(\mathbf{s}_3), \ldots, Y(\mathbf{s}_n)\}$ forms a sparse MRF (i.e., local neighborhood structure), then $\{Y(\mathbf{s}_1) + Y(\mathbf{s}_2), Y(\mathbf{s}_3), \ldots, Y(\mathbf{s}_n)\}$ is typically *not* a sparse MRF. Furthermore, $\{Y(\mathbf{s}_2), Y(\mathbf{s}_3), \ldots, Y(\mathbf{s}_n)\}$ may not be a sparse MRF; that is, MRFs do not marginalize either. In applications of spatial statistics, aggregation and marginalization are commonplace. See Rue, Steinsland, and Erland (2004), Rue and Held (2005), and Rue, Martino, and Chopin (2009) for further discussion. Statistical image analysis often uses MRFs, and they are well suited to this application because the pixels are fixed and the data are usually complete. [For a generic review of statistical image analysis, see, for example, the encyclopedia entry by Cressie and Davidson (1998b).]

The fundamental problem for modelers using MRFs is to know when their conditional-probability models are specified coherently (i.e., give rise to a joint distribution). This is discussed at length in Section 4.2.3. The conditions are easy to check for CAR (i.e., Gaussian) models, but as spatial statistical models evolve toward nonlinear, non-Gaussian models to capture more real-world phenomena, conditions to ensure coherent MRF models will be essential (Kaiser and Cressie, 2000; Lee, Kaiser, and Cressie, 2001).

Finally, implementation of MRFs in HMs will almost always be done by numerical statistical approximations (e.g., rejection sampling, Laplace approximation, importance sampling, slice sampling, Markov chain Monte Carlo, etc., or some combination of these). The MRF generally has a normalizing constant that cannot be obtained analytically and, when found in an HM, the HM's normalizing constant is likewise unavailable. A review of the considerable literature on statistical computing for MRFs can be found in Rue and Held (2005), Martino and Rue (2009), and Rue, Martino, and Chopin (2009).

CAR Models

The conditionally autoregressive (CAR) models are more correctly called auto Gaussian models (in the terminology of Besag's auto spatial models). Cressie (1993) called them conditionally specified Gaussian (CG) models and contrasted them with simultaneously specified Gaussian (SG). The "CAR" terminology has remained, but it should be remembered that these models are specifically for *Gaussian* spatial data.

Besag (1974, 1981) had noticed that if one assumes a CAR model on a regular lattice in $\mathbb{R}^2$, where $\text{var}(\mathbf{Y}) = \tau^2(\mathbf{I} - \phi\mathbf{A})^{-1}$ and $\mathbf{A}$ is the nearest-neighbor adjacency matrix, then $\text{corr}(Y(s_1, s_2), Y(s_1 + 1, s_2))$ tends to 1 very slowly as $\phi \to \phi_{\max}$. That is, to obtain substantial spatial dependence, ϕ has to be *very close* to $\phi_{\max}$; Besag then recommended that $\phi = \phi_{\max}$, which results in a CAR model that is *not* defined in n-dimensional space, but it is defined on some lower-dimensional subspace. This has become known as the *intrinsic autoregressive* (IAR) model (e.g., Banerjee, Carlin, and Gelfand, 2004, Section 3.3). The time-series analogue to "CAR versus IAR" is a stationary autoregressive process versus a random walk, where it has long been recognized that the two processes' behaviors are fundamentally different (spawning a large literature on *unit-root tests*). The spatial-modeling literature has generally concentrated on the IAR model without any determination of whether a proper CAR or an IAR model is appropriate. Besag's concern seems to have its roots more in the choice of the *nearest-neighbor* adjacency matrix $\mathbf{A}$ than in finding $\hat{\phi}$ very close to $\phi_{\max}$. Hrafnkellsson and Cressie (2003) showed empirically that if a *range* parameter is introduced into the CAR model, ϕ may take reasonable values and still generate strong spatial correlation between neighbors.

A family of CAR models due to Pettitt, Weir, and Hart (2002), termed *diagonally dominant*, keeps $(\text{var}(\mathbf{Y}))^{-1}$ from being singular throughout the whole parameter space. In the notation of Section 4.2.5, we have

$$\text{var}(\mathbf{Y}) = (\mathbf{I} - \mathbf{C})^{-1}\mathbf{M},$$

where $\mathbf{C} = (c_{ij})$, $\mathbf{M} = \text{diag}(m_{11}, \ldots, m_{nn})$, $c_{ii} = 0$,

$$c_{ij} = \frac{\kappa g_{ij}}{1 + |\kappa| \sum_{s_k \in N(s_i)} g_{ik}}, \qquad i \neq j,$$

$$m_{ii} = \frac{1}{1 + |\kappa| \sum_{s_k \in N(s_i)} g_{ik}},$$

and $\mathbf{G} = (g_{ij})$ is a symmetric matrix whose diagonal entries are zero and whose nondiagonal entries are nonnegative. Notice the spatial-dependence parameter $\kappa \in (-\infty, \infty)$, and the CAR model is proper over the whole parameter space. Ferreira and De Oliveira (2007) modify this model slightly by specifying $\kappa \in [0, \infty)$.

Multivariate CAR Models

Mardia (1988) introduced a multivariate Markov random field (MRF) model for image processing. More recently, Billheimer et al. (1997), Kim, Sun, and Tsutakawa (2001), Pettitt, Weir, and Hart (2002), Carlin and Banerjee (2003), Gelfand and Vounatsou (2003), Jin, Carlin, and Banerjee (2005), Jin, Banerjee, and Carlin (2007), Sain and Cressie (2007), and Sain, Furrer, and Cressie (2011) have explored these multivariate MRF models and their role in Bayesian hierarchical modeling.

CAR Models versus Geostatistical Models

As we specified in Section 4.2.5, there is *always* a relationship between a geostatistical model and a CAR model defined on a finite number of small areas. It is their respective properties that we would like to exploit. For example, to take the inverse of a spatial-dependence matrix, we would like to model with a CAR model, but to derive properties of aggregated processes, we would like to model with a geostatistical model. An approach that has good success in limited settings (small to moderate n) is to approximate a geostatistical model with a CAR model, when needed (Rue and Tjelmeland, 2002; Rue, Steinsland, and Erland, 2004; Rue and Held, 2005, Chapter 5; Cressie and Verzelen, 2008; Rue, Martino, and Chopin, 2009). More direct comparisons between CAR models and geostatistical models can be found in Banerjee, Wall, and Carlin (2003), Hrafnkelsson and Cressie (2003), and Song, Fuentes, and Ghosh (2008).

Ecological Inference in a Spatial Setting

In spatial statistics, ecological inference is known as the change-of-support problem, and it is really a manifestation of Simpson's Paradox in a spatial setting where aggregation is commonplace. The book by King (1997) addresses the general problem; one would need to adapt these results to the spatial setting. In Section 4.2.6, the special issue of the *Journal of the Royal Statistical Society, Series A*, Vol. 164, Part 1 (2001) was mentioned as a resource for problems with ecological bias. The following articles in that special issue are particularly illuminating: Best et al. (2001), Darby, Deo, and Doll (2001), and Wakefield and Salway (2001). Using a powerful model of aggregation from spatial point processes (Section 4.3) to lattice processes (Section 4.2), Best, Ickstadt, and Wolpert (2000) give an analysis of public health and exposure to automobile emissions that allows data measured at disparate resolutions to be combined consistently. The review paper by Gotway and Young (2002) also covers statistical change-of-support for lattice data.

Spatial Point Processes

Matérn (1960) discussed spatial point processes as part of his landmark publication in spatial statistics. In the area of ecology, Pielou (1977) developed descriptive methods for spatial point patterns. Ripley's (1981) book and Diggle's (1983, 2003) editions put spatial point processes on a more mathematical footing, which continued with the monographs by Cressie (1991, 1993), Stoyan and Stoyan (1994), van Lieshout (2000), Møller and Waagepetersen (2004), Illian et al. (2008), and Gelfand et al. (2010, Part IV). The review by Møller and Waagepetersen (2007) takes a modern distributional point of view to modeling and estimation of spatial point processes. A part of that work involves Log-Gaussian Cox Processes; Møller, Syversveen, and Waagepetersen (1998) discussed their marginal properties and, importantly, saw their potential use in an HM.

Intensities for Spatial Point Processes

The first-order intensity function has played a prominent role in the modeling and analysis of spatial point patterns. There is an attractive alternative, namely the Papangelou conditional intensity, which is an intensity function of the spatial point process Z, *conditional* on there being an event of Z at $s \in \mathbb{R}^d$. Baddeley et al. (2005) use it to develop a residual analysis for spatial point processes.

First- and higher-order intensities are often estimated using kernel estimation, which emphasizes the strong connection between spatial point processes in $\mathbb{R}^d$ and multivariate analysis of random spatial locations. Inference for such nonparametric estimators has been more recently based on resampling/subsampling rather than on asymptotic Gaussian distribution theory (e.g., Guan, Sherman, and Calvin, 2004; Guan and Loh, 2007; Guan and Sherman, 2007).

The recent literature on spatial-point-process modeling and inference is statistically rich (e.g., Møller and Waagepetersen, 2007; Guan, 2008; Waagepetersen and Guan, 2009). Inference in the form of hypothesis testing can be handled through Monte Carlo testing, provided that the spatial point process is straightforward to simulate from. The idea was developed by Hope (1968), and it has proved effective in a number of applications (e.g., Kulldorf, 1997; Priebe, Olson, and Healy, 1997; Kornak, Irwin, and Cressie, 2006).

Marked Spatial Point Processes

This represents a very attractive generalization of the spatial point process, by combining a stochastic model for attributes (mark process), along with a stochastic model for event locations (point process). The mark process and the point process are typically dependent (e.g., Penttinen, Stoyan, and Henttonen, 1992; Henderson, Shimakura, and Gorst, 2002; Schlather, Ribeiro, and Diggle, 2004). Comas, Delicado, and Mateu (2010) consider marks that are modeled as random functions. One mark process that is a direct consequence of the spatial point process itself is the set of random Dirichlet (or Voronoi) tesselations associated with the random locations of the events. Let s_i be the ith event from among events, $\{s_1, s_2, \ldots\}$ of the point process. Then the Dirichlet cell associated with s_i is $C_i \equiv \{x : \|x - s_i\| = \min_j \|x - s_j\|\}$ (e.g., Cox and Isham, 1980, Chapter 6; Schoenberg, Barr, and Seo, 2008). For further connections to random sets, see Baddeley and Møller (1989).

Bayesian Inference for Spatial Point Processes

Much of the spatial-point-process literature is not concerned with hierarchical models. Rather, the spatial point process is characterized by $[Z|\theta]$ and a prior $[\theta]$ is put on θ (e.g., Heikkinen and Penttinen, 1999; Møller, 1999; Cressie and Lawson, 2000; Møller et al., 2006; Berthelsen and Møller, 2008). When the Cox process is viewed conditionally, a BHM approach to inference is natural (e.g., Kottas and Sansó, 2007; Møller and Waagepetersen, 2007). In principle, a BHM should allow change-of-support to be handled, provided that the process model is consistent through different levels of aggregation (e.g., Wolpert and Ickstadt, 1998).

Applications of Spatial Point Processes

Principal areas of application have been in forestry, earthquakes, rainfall modeling, astronomy, and epidemiology. See the review by Stoyan and Penttinen (2000) for spatial point process methods in forestry. Ogata et al. (1998) and Choi and Hall (2001) are two examples of articles that study earthquake point-process data. Point process models for rainfall were developed by Rodriguez-Iturbe and co-authors (e.g., Rodriguez-Iturbe, Cox, and Isham, 1988). In astronomy, there has been considerable development in astrostatistics, which includes spatial point processes (e.g., Babu and Feigelson, 1996). Epidemiology, particularly related to environmental factors, has a large spatial component; point process models are relevant when the disease locations are available (e.g., Diggle, 1993). Often epidemiologists are interested in testing for the presence of clusters; for example, see Wakefield, Kelsall, and Morris (2000) for a discussion of this methodology.

Random Set Processes

Matheron (1975) is a book that is path-breaking in the way one can take an object view of the world (Chapter 1) and model the uncertainty associated with that view with probability theory. Well known for his work in geostatistics, Matheron also established a group at the School of Mines in Fontainebleau, France, working on what he called Mathematical Morphology. Matheron (1975) contains the theory of random sets, interwoven with definitions of set transforms (e.g., set addition, opening, closing, etc.) that are useful in image analysis and that he showed defined other random sets. This was all done in $\mathbb{R}^d$, and stereology (i.e., the measurement of an object in lower-dimensional spaces that allow the object to be reconstructed—with some uncertainty—in $\mathbb{R}^d$) was also considered. Kendall (1974) published a very similar theory of random sets at about the same time, but it was the French group who took it further through one of Matheron's early students, who published a book (Serra, 1982) linking Mathematical Morphology directly with image analysis being done in their laboratory. Cressie (1979) presented a central limit theorem for sums of random sets, and Molchanov (1993) presented limit theorems for unions of random closed sets, which is a beginning to establishing a statistical theory for random sets. More recent developments in random-set theory can be found in Molchanov (2005) and Nguyen (2006).

In the related area of Pattern Analysis, a strong statistical component where uncertainties are expressed in an HM and patterns are quantified and compared statistically was developed by a U.S. group at Brown University (e.g., Grenander and Miller, 2007). There are a number of other related areas, and these approaches are left for the interested reader to pursue: Stochastic Geometry (e.g., Stoyan, Kendall, and Mecke, 1987; Stoyan and Stoyan, 1994), Geometric Probability (e.g., Solomon, 1978), and Shape Analysis (e.g., Dryden and Mardia, 1998). There is interesting cross-over work that relates the field view of the world with the object view (Adler, 1981).

Stereology has developed from a theory based on probability to a statistical theory based on sampling (of objects). Here the randomness is derived from random sampling with probes, something that is important in medical testing where biopsies are taken and imaged. Early work concentrated on the first moment of the estimator, but that changed when it was realized that sampling theory, albeit for more complicated populations, could be used to develop (estimates of) variances of the sample-based statistics (Baddeley and Jensen, 2005).

CHAPTER 5

Exploratory Methods
for Spatio-Temporal Data

Spatio-temporal processes typically involve dependencies across a large range of spatial and temporal scales. In order to understand such processes, scientific theories are developed and observations are taken. These spatio-temporal data are a window to the underlying process; our statistical goals are to visualize, summarize, and infer (including spatio-temporal prediction) the process' behavior within and between relevant scales of variability. Exploratory-data-analytic methods of visualization and summarization are considered in this chapter. The goal is to use these exploratory methods to suggest relationships that can be incorporated into spatio-temporal models for the purpose of inference (e.g., Section 9.1).

A key challenge in spatio-temporal data analysis is the extraction of information from potentially large spatio-temporal datasets generated by data-assimilation algorithms, deterministic models, observation networks, or remote-sensing platforms. There are a number of approaches that have proven to be helpful in exploratory data analysis and diagnostics for model building, when working with spatio-temporal data. In this chapter, we review them in some detail, occasionally extending them, and we provide applications for which they can be used. We note that some of these methods have been developed in subject-matter disciplines (primarily meteorology, climatology, and oceanography) where statisticians have not generally played a prominent role.

We realize that a static medium (e.g., pages in this book) can be limiting for data that are inherently dynamical, and we look forward to seeing e-books in the future with new media for exploratory methods (e.g., hyperlinks that allow presentation of animation). The development of exploratory and diagnostic methods for spatio-temporal data is an important research topic and will remain so in the future.

5.1   VISUALIZATION

As with any statistical data analysis, we should always try to visualize (summaries of) the data. There are particular challenges in visualizing spatio-temporal data, since there are typically a minimum of three dimensions (two-dimensional space × one-dimensional time) to consider simultaneously. Of course, there are as many visualization approaches as there are data analysts, so we must be selective. In this section, we describe several simple visualization tools that can be quite informative when applied in practice.

5.1.1   Animations

Perhaps the most useful visualization for spatio-temporal datasets with two or three spatial dimensions is to use the special nature of the temporal dimension to sequence the data's variability and show it as an animation, or "movie." In cases where the data are completely gridded in space and evenly spaced in time, the production of animations is relatively simple. In fact, some computational packages (e.g., Matlab®) have built-in tools to produce animations.

In cases where there are missing observations or where observation times are unequally spaced, a simple interpolation (in space and time) algorithm to fill in missing observations for the purposes of animation (in time) might be applied. Alternatively, for two-dimensional spatial data that are not on a regular lattice, animations can be created from scatterplots. For example, at any snapshot in time, observations can be represented by the size and/or color of circles at each spatial location (e.g., see Figure 5.5 below). By exploiting the unidirectionality of the time dimension, these types of maps can be sequenced into an animation. As mentioned in our introductory remarks, an e-book version would allow animations to be hyperlinked. Animations could also be made available at selected websites (e.g., Section 9.1 presents forecasts for sea surface temperature in the tropical Pacific Ocean that have been animated; see SSES, 2009).

5.1.2   Marginal and Conditional Plots

Space(1-D)/Time Plots

A common method of illustrating wave propagation in the geophysical sciences is by use of image plots showing one-dimensional (1-D) space (typically either latitude or longitude) on the x-axis and time on the y-axis, where time progresses as one looks from top to bottom of the plot. For example, if the x-axis represents longitude from west to east, then coherent patterns going down the plot and to the right suggest propagation eastward, and patterns slanting to the left down the page are indicative of propagation westward. These are called *Hovmöller diagrams* in the atmospheric-sciences literature (Hovmöller, 1949).

An illustration of a space/time plot is given in Figure 5.1, where monthly Pacific sea surface temperature (SST) anomalies (averaged from 1° South latitude to 1° North latitude) are plotted as a function of longitude (x-axis) for

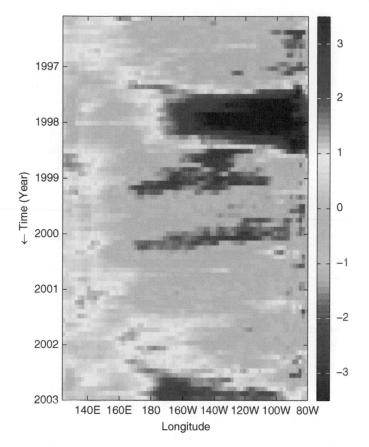

Figure 5.1   Sea surface temperature anomalies (°C) averaged between latitudes 1° S and 1° N. The
y axis refers to time in monthly increments (increasing down the page from 1996 to 2003), and the
x axis corresponds to longitude in 2° increments (throughout the equatorial Pacific region).

the period from January 1996 to December 2002. The dark-red anomalies correspond to a major El Niño event, and the dark-blue anomalies correspond to
La Niña events. Notice that there is evidence of propagation in this figure. For
example, both La Niña events show clear propagation from the eastern portion
of the domain into the western portion through time. There is also visual evidence to suggest that there is some precursor warming around 180° East (and
West) longitude, preceding the warm (El Niño) events.

Time-Series Plots
It is always helpful to plot time series associated with various spatial locations
or regions of space. For example, consider the tropical Pacific SST anomalies
discussed in the previous example. There are several regions in the tropical
Pacific that are deemed representative of the El Niño and La Niña phenomena.
One of these, the so-called "Niño 3" region, corresponds to an average of SSTs

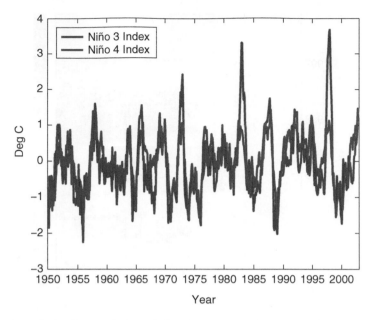

Figure 5.2 Monthly Niño 3 and Niño 4 indices from January 1950 to December 2002. The y axis shows anomalies in $°C$ and the x axis shows time in monthly increments.

over the region 5° N to 5° S and 150° W to 90° W. Another representative region, the "Niño 4" region, is an average of SSTs over 5° N to 5° S and 160° E to 150° W. Time series of these aggregates from January 1950 to December 2002 are shown in Figure 5.2. Clearly, these two time series are highly correlated, but they illustrate that the spatial regions they represent do not show identical warming and cooling.

It is often useful to consider aggregating over the entire spatial domain. Here we use as an illustrative example a study of the Eurasian Collared Dove (ECD, *Streptopelia decaocto*) in North America. The ECD was first observed in the USA in Florida during the mid-1980s (Romagosa and Labisky, 2000). Not only has its range increased as it has spread through the southeastern United States, but it has experienced growth in population as well (Section 9.3). Data from the North American Breeding Bird Survey (BBS; Robbins, Bystrak, and Geissler, 1986) are collected at many sampling routes; Figure 5.3 shows an aggregate of the BBS counts for the ECD from 1986 through 2003. One can see from this that the BBS counts have increased exponentially through time, as is characteristic for a recently introduced invasive species.

Spatial Maps

Just as it is useful to look at time series for individual spatial locations or for spatial regions, it is also useful to look at spatial maps for given times, sequences of times, or aggregates over time. Returning to the tropical Pacific

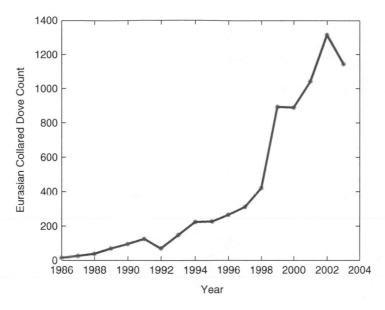

Figure 5.3   Yearly North American Breeding Bird Survey counts of Eurasian Collared Doves from 1986 to 2003. The y axis shows counts of the Eurasian Collared Dove and the x axis shows time in yearly increments.

SST example, Figure 5.4 shows monthly SST anomalies over the tropical Pacific region from February 1998 through January 1999. The observations are gridded at $2° \times 2°$ lat–lon resolution, and there are $m = 2261$ Pacific-Ocean $2° \times 2°$ pixels in the region of interest (from $30°$ South to $30°$ North latitude.) One can immediately see that the sequence of monthly maps shows the rapid transition from a warm event (El Niño) to a cold event (La Niña). This rapid transition from one extreme upper-ocean state to another is characteristic of the El Niño/Southern Oscillation (ENSO) phenomenon. It is also obvious from Figure 5.4 that the spatial pattern of the warm and cold events are not the same. This type of nonlinearity is another characteristic feature of the ENSO phenomenon. In Section 9.1, a BHM is fitted to these spatio-temporal data, and conclusions from this exploratory analysis are confirmed. Inference resulting from the fitted BHM is given by Berliner, Wikle, and Cressie (2000), and subsequent monthly updates can be found in SSES (2009).

The Pacific SST data in Figure 5.4 are on a regular grid. One can also look at a sequence of maps when the data are not on a regular grid, such as for the Eurasian Collared Dove (ECD) data. Figure 5.5 shows a 3-yearly sequence of yearly BBS sampling-route counts for the ECD from 1988 to 2003. In this figure, the ECD's relative abundance is represented by both the size and color of the circles. From this sequence of maps, it is immediately obvious that the range and abundance of the ECD has expanded substantially over the 15 years covered by these data.

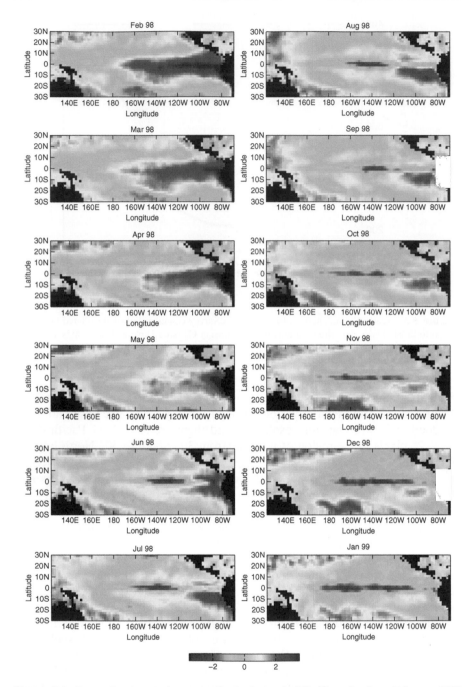

Figure 5.4 Sea surface temperature anomalies in the tropical Pacific region from Februrary 1998 to January 1999. The beginning of this period shows strong warming off the coast of South America (El Niño phenomenon). The end of this period shows the development of an area of cooling in the central Pacific (La Niña phenomenon).

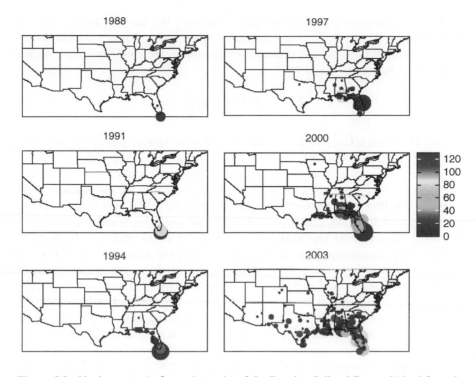

Figure 5.5 Yearly counts (at 3-year intervals) of the Eurasian Collared Dove, obtained from the North American Breeding Bird Survey. The color and radius of the circles are proportional to the counts.

5.1.3 Empirical Covariance/Correlation Functions

It can be quite informative to examine plots of empirical spatio-temporal covariance (or correlation) matrices. For example, assume we have observations $\mathbf{Z}_t \equiv (Z(\mathbf{s}_1; t), \ldots, Z(\mathbf{s}_m; t))'$, for $t = 1, \ldots, T$. An $m \times m$ *empirical* (averaged over time) *lag-τ spatial covariance matrix* is given by

$$\hat{\mathbf{C}}_Z^{(\tau)} \equiv \frac{1}{T - \tau} \sum_{t=\tau+1}^{T} (\mathbf{Z}_t - \hat{\boldsymbol{\mu}}_Z)(\mathbf{Z}_{t-\tau} - \hat{\boldsymbol{\mu}}_Z)', \qquad \tau = 0, 1, \ldots, T - 1, \quad (5.1)$$

where the *empirical spatial mean*, $\hat{\boldsymbol{\mu}}_Z$, is given by

$$\hat{\boldsymbol{\mu}}_Z \equiv \frac{1}{T} \sum_{t=1}^{T} \mathbf{Z}_t. \qquad (5.2)$$

Notice that in (5.1) we choose to divide by $(T - \tau)$ rather than T. If we divide by T, the sequence of empirical lag-τ ($\tau = 0, 1, \ldots, T - 1$) covariance matrices is guaranteed to be nonnegative definite. We use the divisor $(T - \tau)$ here because it more effectively mitigates against bias when a presumed stationary covariance is being estimated. Furthermore, the *empirical lag-τ spatial correlation matrix* is given by

$$\hat{\mathbf{R}}_Z^{(\tau)} \equiv \hat{\mathbf{D}}_Z^{-1/2} \hat{\mathbf{C}}_Z^{(\tau)} \hat{\mathbf{D}}_Z^{-1/2}, \tag{5.3}$$

where $\hat{\mathbf{D}}_Z \equiv \text{diag}(\hat{\mathbf{C}}_Z^{(0)})$ is a diagonal matrix with spatially indexed empirical variances (defined by averaging over time) on the main diagonal.

As an example, consider the empirical lag-0 covariance and correlation matrices for SST anomalies for locations in a domain *along the equator* in the western Pacific Ocean. A useful way to present these matrices is as an image plot. Figure 5.6 shows image plots for the empirical lag-0 covariance (given by (5.1) with $\tau = 0$) and correlation (given by (5.3) with $\tau = 0$) matrices for the SST anomalies. The covariance plot (Figure 5.6a) shows clearly that the variability is greater in the eastern portion of the domain and that there is a fairly strong spatial dependence throughout the domain. The associated correlation plot (Figure 5.6b) shows that there is negative dependence between the extreme western portion of the domain and the eastern portion of the domain. It is also informative to check for spatio-temporal dependence at lags $\tau = 1, 2, \ldots$. Since ocean dynamics operate on relatively slow time scales, it is reasonable to expect dependence over quite large time lags. Consider the empirical lag-6 (month) covariance and correlation matrices for the equatorial SST anomalies, shown in Figure 5.7. They demonstrate very strong positive 6-month-lag dependence in the western portion of the domain. Note that, based on the definition of the cross-covariance and cross-correlation functions, these lag matrices are not symmetric, but $\hat{\mathbf{C}}_Z^{(\tau)} = (\hat{\mathbf{C}}_Z^{(-\tau)})'$. A similar relation holds for lag-correlation matrices.

It is also of interest to compute the empirical cross-covariances or cross-correlations between different spatio-temporal variables. For example, consider two data sets, $\mathbf{Z}_t \equiv (Z(\mathbf{s}_1; t), \ldots, Z(\mathbf{s}_m; t))'$ and $\mathbf{X}_t \equiv (X(\mathbf{x}_1; t), \ldots, X(\mathbf{x}_\ell; t))'$, for $t = 1, \ldots, T$, where the locations in $\mathbf{Z}_t$ and $\mathbf{X}_t$ need not coincide, and these vectors need not be of the same dimension. An *empirical lag-τ cross-covariance matrix* is given by

$$\hat{\mathbf{C}}_{Z,X}^{(\tau)} \equiv \frac{1}{T - \tau} \sum_{t=\tau+1}^{T} (\mathbf{Z}_t - \hat{\boldsymbol{\mu}}_Z)(\mathbf{X}_{t-\tau} - \hat{\boldsymbol{\mu}}_X)', \tag{5.4}$$

where recall that the empirical spatial mean, $\hat{\boldsymbol{\mu}}_Z$, is given by (5.2), and likewise

$$\hat{\boldsymbol{\mu}}_X \equiv \frac{1}{T} \sum_{t=1}^{T} \mathbf{X}_t. \tag{5.5}$$

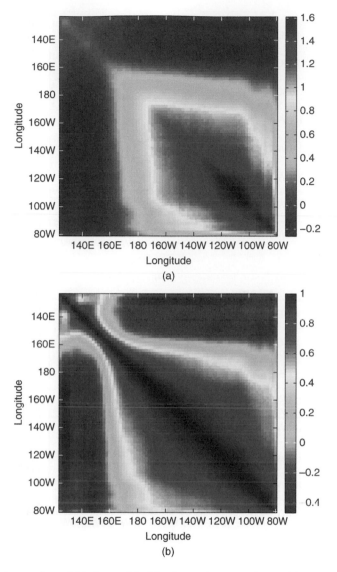

Figure 5.6 Image plots of (**a**) the empirical lag-0 covariance matrix and (**b**) the empirical lag-0 correlation matrix for the sea surface temperature anomalies along the equator in the Pacific region.

Note that the empirical lag-τ cross-covariance matrix (5.4) is an $m \times \ell$ matrix, as is the empirical *lag-τ spatial cross-correlation matrix* given by

$$\hat{\mathbf{R}}_{Z,X}^{(\tau)} \equiv \hat{\mathbf{D}}_Z^{-1/2} \hat{\mathbf{C}}_{Z,X}^{(\tau)} \hat{\mathbf{D}}_X^{-1/2}, \tag{5.6}$$

where $\hat{\mathbf{D}}_Z \equiv \mathrm{diag}(\hat{\mathbf{C}}_Z^{(0)})$ and $\hat{\mathbf{D}}_X \equiv \mathrm{diag}(\hat{\mathbf{C}}_X^{(0)})$.

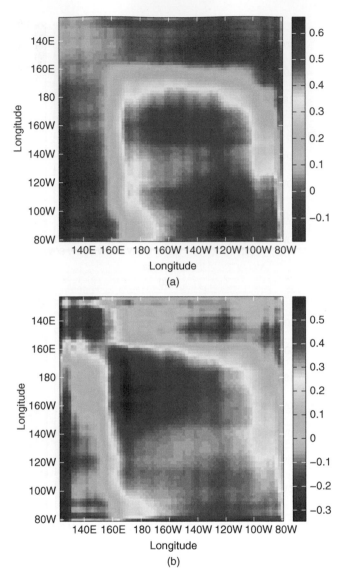

Figure 5.7 Image plot of **(a)** the empirical lag-6 covariance matrix and **(b)** the empirical lag-6 correlation matrix for the sea surface temperature anomalies along the equator in the Pacific region.

For example, Figure 5.8 shows the lag-6 cross-correlation for the special case of $\ell = 1$, where the X-variable is the near-surface zonal (i.e., east–west) wind component at (155° E, 5° N) and the Z-variable is the monthly SST anomaly for each of the $m = 2,261$ 2° × 2° pixels in the tropical Pacific region. The time index t increases in one-month increments from January 1970 through December 2000. In this case, since we are computing the lag-6 cross-correlation

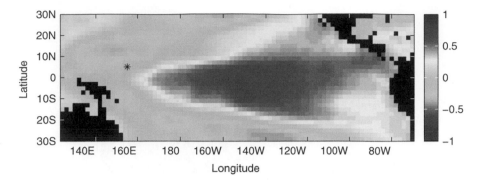

Figure 5.8 Image plot of the lag-6 cross-correlation between the near-surface zonal wind component at 155° E, 5° N (shown with an asterisk) and the monthly sea surface temperature anomalies from January 1970 to December 2000. In this case, the time series of the near-surface zonal wind component lags the sea surface temperature anomalies by 6 months.

for a spatio-temporal field relative to a time series for one spatial location (i.e., $\ell = 1$), we can plot the results as a spatial map. Note that the plot shows a very high correlation between the zonal wind component at this location and the Pacific SST anomalies at spatially coherent locations. In particular, we note a clear El Niño-type pattern in the lag-correlations, suggesting that the zonal wind component at (155° E, 5° N) could be a useful 6-month-ahead predictor of a future El Niño event (e.g., see Berliner, Wikle, and Cressie, 2000). This is incorporated into a BHM presented in Section 9.1.

As we shall see in Section 6.2, the characterization of the joint spatio-temporal covariance structure of a spatio-temporal process is important for optimal prediction. Thus, it is important to examine the empirical covariance function at various space and time lags. Making the (implicit) assumption that the first moment depends on space but not on time, and the second moment depends only on spatial and temporal *lag differences*, then the estimated spatio-temporal covariance at spatial lag $\mathbf{h}$ and time lag τ is given by

$$\hat{C}_Z(\mathbf{h}; \tau) \equiv \frac{1}{|N_s(\mathbf{h})|} \frac{1}{|N_t(\tau)|}$$

$$\sum_{\mathbf{s}_i, \mathbf{s}_j \in N_s(\mathbf{h})} \sum_{t, r \in N_t(\tau)} (Z(\mathbf{s}_i; t) - \hat{\mu}_Z(\mathbf{s}_i))(Z(\mathbf{s}_j; r) - \hat{\mu}_Z(\mathbf{s}_j)), \quad (5.7)$$

where recall from (5.2) that $\hat{\mu}_Z(\mathbf{s}_i) \equiv (1/T) \sum_{t=1}^{T} Z(\mathbf{s}_i; t)$, $N_s(\mathbf{h})$ refers to the pairs of spatial locations with spatial lag within some tolerance of $\mathbf{h}$, $N_t(\tau)$ refers to the pairs of time points with time lag within some tolerance of τ, and $|N(\cdot)|$ refers to the cardinality (i.e., number of elements) of the set $N(\cdot)$. Note that, as with purely spatial covariogram and variogram estimation (Section 4.1.1), potentially anisotropic spatio-temporal dependence can be investigated by allowing spatial lags $\mathbf{h}$ to have various directions. From (5.7), we can construct the lag-τ empirical covariance matrices $\hat{\mathbf{C}}^{(\tau)}$; $\tau = 0, 1, 2, \ldots$.

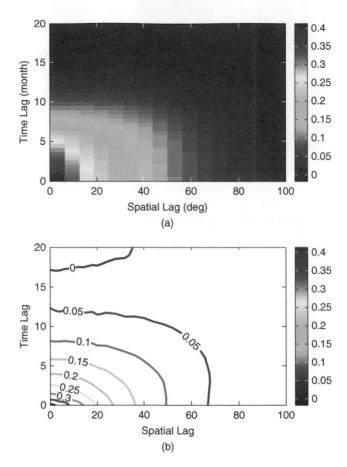

Figure 5.9 Empirical spatio-temporal covariance plots for the sea surface temperature anomalies in the tropical Pacific region (January 1970 to December 2002). The *y* axis shows temporal lag in months and the *x* axis shows spatial lag in degrees. (**a**) An image plot. (**b**) A contour plot.

Figure 5.9 shows the empirical spatio-temporal covariance function for temporal lag τ in months and the modulus of the spatial lag $h \equiv \|\mathbf{h}\|$ in degrees, for the tropical Pacific SST anomaly dataset from January 1970 through December 2002. Of course, we are free to visualize this information in different ways with our favorite types of plots. For example, we show both an image plot and a contour plot for illustration. See Sections 6.1 and 6.2 for more discussion about how spatio-temporal covariance plots can be used to characterize spatio-temporal dependence.

5.1.4   Spatio-Temporal LISAs

Local Indicators of Spatial Association (LISAs) decompose global statistics into components where each component is associated with a spatial coordinate

(Anselin, 1995) or, in our case, with a spatio-temporal coordinate. The important property of a LISA is that an "average" (in the very general sense of the word) of the local components yields the global component. In a purely spatial setting, a LISA applied to an empirical covariance function can show unusual components at various locations, thereby allowing a visualization of spatial outliers or departures from stationarity. Cressie and Collins (2001) study LISAs for empirical pair correlation functions of spatial point patterns.

Examples of LISAs: In a spatio-temporal setting, consider the yearly empirical covariance matrix $\hat{\mathbf{C}}_Z^{(0)}$ for SST anomalies, which is a 12-monthly average of cross-products; each of these local (in time) averages is taken over January through December in any given year from 1970 through 2002. A plot of the leading eigenvalues of these *spatial* covariance matrices versus year would investigate a type of local (yearly) temporal variability that is ignored in a typical principal components analysis. As we saw in Section 4.1.1 and will see in much more detail in Section 5.3, a principal components analysis (i.e., an eigenvector/eigenvalue decomposition) of a spatial covariance matrix is often termed an EOF analysis in the geophysics literature. In this case, the eigenvectors correspond to patterns of maximal variability, with the largest eigenvalue corresponding to the "dominant pattern" of variability over the time period used to calculate the spatial covariance matrix. We now visualize the leading eigenvalue and its associated eigenvector as a function of year, from 1970 to 2002. Each yearly value and map could be considered as a LISA because they approximate the empirical spatial covariance matrix from that year, and the overall empirical spatial covariance matrix is linearly related to the yearly empirical covariance matrices.

A LISA plot of the leading eigenvalue for the SST data for consecutive 12-month periods is shown in Figure 5.10. One can see clearly from this plot that the leading EOF varies greatly across the 33-year period. In addition, the years in which the leading eigenvalue is greatest typically corresponds to years in which the El Niño and La Niña phenomena are most active. To illustrate this, Figure 5.11 shows the corresponding leading eigenvector (EOF) maps for 1981 and 1982. Note that the 1981 EOF does not show the clear ENSO structure that is apparent in 1982. The abrupt transition into an ENSO state is evidence of the likely lack of temporal stationarity in these data.

As another example, consider the *temporal* empirical covariance function for the *monthly* SST anomaly data from January 1970 to December 2002, for each $2° \times 2°$ pixel. Figure 5.12 shows a spatial plot of the temporal empirical autocovariances at lag $\tau = 1$ (month). Again, there is noticeably higher temporal autocovariance in the ENSO region of the eastern Pacific, suggesting a lack of spatial stationarity in the lag-1 temporal autocovariances. These visualizations show that a geostatistical analysis of SST that assumes stationarity in space and/or time (Section 6.1.2) would be inappropriate.

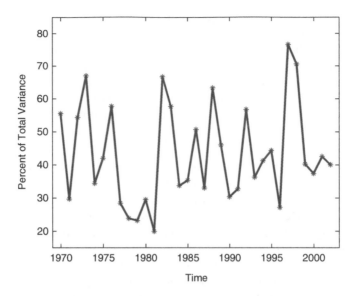

Figure 5.10 LISA plot showing the eigenvalue of the leading EOF for the monthly sea surface temperature anomaly data for consecutive 12-month periods starting in January 1970. For presentation purposes, the leading EOF eigenvalue is normalized by the total variance to show the percent variance accounted for by the leading EOF for each year.

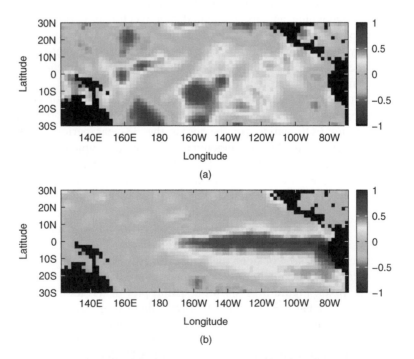

Figure 5.11 The spatial map of the leading EOF of the monthly sea surface temperature anomaly data associated with the LISA analysis in Figure 5.10. (a) 1981. (b) 1982.

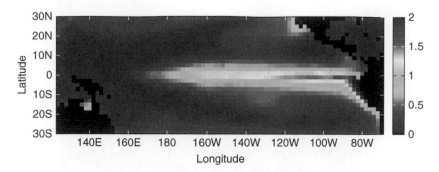

Figure 5.12 LISA plot showing the lag-1-month temporal autocovariance at each spatial location for the monthly sea surface temperature anomaly data.

5.1.5 Spatio-Temporal Parallel Coordinates Plot

The *Parallel Coordinates* (PC) plot is a way of visualizing multivariate data (Inselberg, 1985; Wegman, 1990). Visually, the vertical axes are placed in parallel in some predetermined order. Each component of a given multivariate observation is plotted on its respective axis. Then a piecewise straight line is drawn between corresponding values on each axis. For many multivariate observations, the PC plot shows an array of piecewise straight lines that may be difficult to interpret. An enhancement is to compare multivariate dependence between different classes by coloring their respective arrays with different colors.

Now consider spatio-temporal multivariate data $\{Z_t(\mathbf{s}_i) : \mathbf{s}_i \in D_s, t = 1, 2, \ldots\}$. The obvious use of PC plots for such data is to treat the observations as multivariate (spatial) vectors in time. For example, say there are observations at $i = 1, \ldots, m$ spatial locations for each time t. Recall that we denoted these as vectors $\mathbf{Z}_t$. In this case, varying the index t generates a "sample," $\mathbf{Z}_1, \ldots, \mathbf{Z}_T$, of m-variate vectors. Hence, each vertical axis of the PC plot represents a spatial location, and the corresponding T values associated with a location are plotted on the vertical axis. Consequently, this spatio-temporal PC plot shows T lines, each one representing $m - 1$ connected line segments. A potential difficulty with such a representation is that with large m and T, it may be difficult to extract much information from these plots due to the "visual clutter" inherent with greater line density (e.g., Edsall, 2003). One approach to reduce this clutter is to collapse the m spatial locations into fewer components, and a natural way to do this in the spatio-temporal context is to project the data onto the first p_α EOFs (e.g., see Section 5.3.2). The associated principal component (p_α-variate) time series associated with these projections becomes the new dataset. In this case, the data are represented in terms of p_α-variate vectors, which suggests that a vertical axis now represents a particular EOF rather than a location in physical space, and the ordering of the axes is naturally from the first EOF to the p_αth.

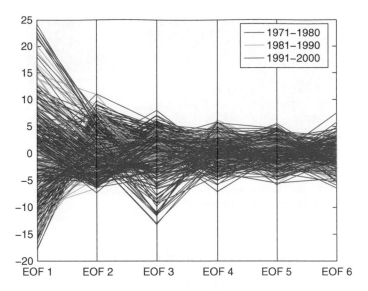

Figure 5.13 Parallel coordinates (PC) plot for the monthly sea surface temperature anomalies in the tropical Pacific region. The data were projected onto the first six EOFs and the associated principal components represent the x axis coordinates. Each connected line represents the values of these EOF variables for a given month (over the 30-year period from January 1971 to December 2000). Lines associated with the decades are indicated by different colors (blue: 1971–1980; green: 1981–1990; red: 1991–2000).

Example: Figure 5.13 shows a PC plot for the monthly SST anomaly dataset for the 30-year period from January 1971 to December 2000. Specifically, this plot shows the PC plot based on the projection of the data onto the first six EOFs, and there are $T = 12 \times 30 = 360$ piecewise straight lines superimposed. The use of color to differentiate the decades (1971–1980: blue; 1981–1990: green; 1991–2000: red) shows that the loadings on the EOFs are quite different between the first (blue) and last (red) ten-year periods, especially for the first four EOFs. This matches with the example in Section 5.3.4, which illustrates that the first four EOFs are associated with the El Niño/La Niña phenomena, and these are known to vary substantially across decades.

There are other ways that one could use PC plots to analyze spatio-temporal data. Of course, the approach described above could be used, but with T-dimensional vectors $\mathbf{Z}(\mathbf{s}_i)$; $i = 1, \ldots, m$, so that the vertical axes now represent successive time points. This is a useful way to examine multivariate time series in general but suffers from the same "visual clutter" problem described when m is large. However, projecting onto the p_α leading (spatial) EOFs would reduce the number of lines from m to p_α (e.g., $m = 2{,}261$ and $p_\alpha = 6$).

For spatio-temporal data, we have had success with a linked PC plot, where the PC plot is based on T-variate vectors $\{\mathbf{Z}(\mathbf{s}_i): i = 1, \ldots, m\}$, and it is linked dynamically to a map showing spatial coordinates $\{\mathbf{s}_i : i = 1, \ldots, m\}$.

By highlighting (brushing) either in the PC-plot view or in the spatial view, there is linked highlighting in the other view; see Ahlqvist et al. (2010).

5.2   SPECTRAL ANALYSIS

Building on the univariate and bivariate spectral-analysis methods discussed in Sections 3.5.3 and 3.5.4, one can use spectral analysis to gain insight into spatio-temporal data as well. This can be accomplished by several exploratory methods. Here, we focus on the use of cross-spectral analysis between several data locations separated in space (Section 5.2.1), as well as so-called *spatio-temporal spectral analysis* (Section 5.2.2).

5.2.1   Cross-Spectral Analysis

Careful application of the basic cross-spectral-analysis methods outlined in Section 3.5.4 can be used to explore spatio-temporal data. In particular, such methods can be used to discover properties of spatio-temporal features such as propagating waves. Wikle, Madden, and Chen (1997) provide a cross-spectral analysis of upper atmospheric winds in a study of tropical waves in the atmosphere. Of particular interest to these authors was a type of equatorial wave in the lower stratosphere known as a *mixed Rossby-gravity wave* (MRGW). These waves have a westward phase propagation and a period of about 3–5 days.

Recall that in Section 3.5.4 we considered the cross-spectral analysis between the u- and v-components of the wind in the lower stratosphere for a station (on Chuuk Island) in the tropical Pacific (see Figure 3.22). Recall also that the u-component is the east/west (or zonal) component and that the v-component is the north/south (or meridional) component. Figure 3.22 shows a squared coherence peak in the frequency range corresponding to the MRGW and, more importantly, showed that the v-component of the wind leads the u-component by a quarter of a cycle, in remarkable agreement with equatorial wave theory (e.g., Matsuno, 1966). However, the cross-spectral analysis at a single station does not provide information from which to infer the movement of these waves. For that, one must consider time series from multiple spatial locations.

To illustrate our point, we use once-daily upper air weather balloon (i.e., rawinsonde) observations during the period, 1 January 1962–31 December 2007 (a different dataset than the one used in Wikle, Madden, and Chen, 1997). We focus on the observations from the 70-hPa level of constant pressure (in the lower stratosphere, approximately 18.5 km above the surface). We considered the daily data at the four tropical Pacific stations (Koror, Chuuk—formerly Truk, Ponape, and Majuro) shown in Figure 5.14; all of these stations are in a fairly narrow latitude band.

To study the average propagation properties of wavelike disturbances in this dataset, consider the cross-spectral magnitude squared coherence (MSC)

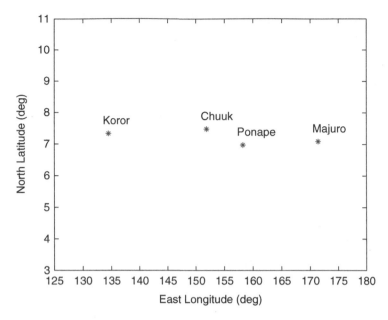

Figure 5.14   Locations of tropical stations for the Western Pacific equatorial wave cross-spectral analysis. The *y* axis and *x* axis show °N latitude and °E longitude, respectively.

and the phase spectrum (see Section 3.5.4 for their definitions) between the *v*-components at each of the six possible combinations of the four stations (Koror, Chuuk, Ponape, and Majuro). A portion of the MSC (top panel) and phase spectrum (bottom panel) plots are shown in Figure 5.15.

The figure shows that the MSC between the various pairs of stations are relatively large throughout this portion of the frequency domain, although it is generally smaller as station separation increases. The associated phase spectra are quite different, but suggest propagation. For instance, at 0.25 cycles per day (cpd), the Chuuk–Majuro phase is negative, implying that the Majuro *v*-component leads that at Chuuk. Similarly, the Chuuk–Koror phase at the same frequency is positive, implying that the Chuuk *v*-component leads that at Koror. Since Koror is west of Chuuk, and Chuuk is west of Majuro, the average phase propagation must be toward the west. Furthermore, the magnitudes of these phase differences are indicative of the horizontal scale of the wave. Wikle, Madden, and Chen (1997) show that one can use this information to perform more formal inference concerning wave properties.

5.2.2   Spatio-Temporal Spectral Analysis

Spectral analysis of time series is discussed in Section 3.5. In the spatial setting, two-dimensional spectral analysis has been used to explore both the structure and patterns of spatial datasets (e.g., Renshaw and Ford, 1983). It is natural to

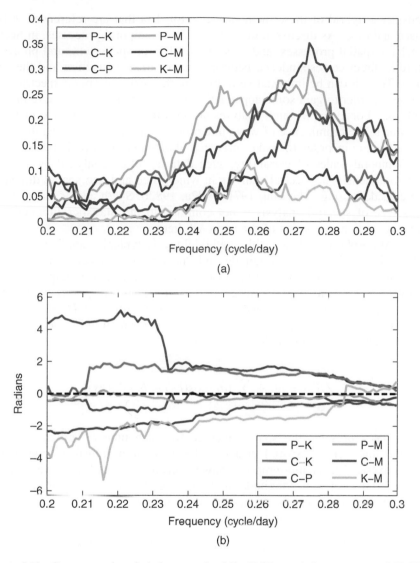

Figure 5.15 Cross-spectral analysis between the daily 70-hPa v-wind component at 0:00 UTC (midnight Greenwich Mean Time) at pairs of tropical Pacific stations for the period from 1 January 1962 through 31 December 2007. Results were obtained using a smoothed periodogram with smoothing bandwidth of 0.04 cycles per day. **(a)** The magnitude squared coherence (MSC) (see Section 3.5.4) for the pairs of stations. **(b)** The corresponding phase spectrum (in radians). Note that only a portion of the frequency domain is shown. Station labels are given by the first letter of the station name as shown in Figure 5.14. For example, "P-K" represents the MSC or phase spectrum between v-wind components at Ponape and Koror.

consider a hybrid of these methodologies for data that are referenced in both space and time. As discussed in Section 3.5 for temporal processes, in Section 4.1.1 for spatial processes, and in Section 6.1.5 for spatio-temporal processes, there is direct correspondence between the covariance function and the spectrum. Thus, it can be informative to explore the spatio-temporal spectrum of a dataset in order to gain some appreciation for its dependence structure in space and time. For example, such analyses are useful in climatology and meteorology due to the prominence of wave-like processes in their governing dynamics. In particular, in order to make inference about relationships between spatial and temporal scales of variability, such data are often analyzed by a variant of two-dimensional spectral analysis in which time and one spatial dimension are considered (e.g., Hayashi, 1971, 1982a, 1982b; Speth and Madden, 1983). This type of spectral analysis is not common in the Statistics literature, and thus we outline the basics of the approach here.

In Atmospheric Science, this methodology is typically applied to data in which the spatial axis is longitude and "positive (negative)" corresponds to eastward (westward) propagation. Assume that a given spatio-temporal process is cyclic in one-dimensional space $s \in D_s$ (e.g., s corresponds to longitude and s is positive to the east) and limited to discrete time $t \in D_t = \{1, \ldots, T\}$. Denote the data by $\{Z_t(s): s \in D_s, t \in D_t\}$, and expand it in Fourier harmonics in the spatial dimension with *wavenumber* k:

$$Z_t(s) = m_t + \sum_{k=1}^{\infty} \{a_{t,k}\cos(ks) + b_{t,k}\sin(ks)\}, \tag{5.8}$$

where m_t represents the spatial average for each time t, and $a_{t,k}$ and $b_{t,k}$ are the time-varying spatial cosine and sine Fourier transform coefficients, respectively. The spatio-temporal power spectrum, P, of positive traveling (eastward if s refers to longitude) and negative traveling (westward if s refers to longitude) waves can be computed according to

$$P(k, \pm \omega) = \frac{1}{4}[f_a(k, \omega) + f_b(k, \omega) \pm 2q_{a,b}(k, \omega)], \tag{5.9}$$

where the $+$ and $-$ refer to positive and negative traveling waves, respectively, ω is the time frequency, $f_a(k, \omega)$ and $f_b(k, \omega)$ are the temporal power spectra for $\{a_{k,t} : t = 1, \ldots, T\}$ and $\{b_{k,t} : t = 1, \ldots, T\}$, respectively, and $q_{a,b}(k, \omega)$ is the quadrature spectrum of the time series $\{a_{t,k}\}$ and $\{b_{t,k}\}$ (see Section 3.5.4 for the definition of the quadrature spectrum). This formula is a generalization of Deland's (1964, 1972) observation that since the cosine and sine coefficients of traveling waves are $90°$ out of phase, the quadrature spectrum indicates the squared amplitude of traveling waves, and its sign indicates the direction of phase propagation. The spatio-temporal power spectrum of the standing oscillation, ST, for the kth spatial wavenumber and time-frequency ω, can then be expressed as

$$ST(k, |\omega|) = \{\frac{1}{4}[f_a(k, \omega) - f_b(k, \omega)]^2 + c_{a,b}^2(k, \omega)\}^{1/2}, \tag{5.10}$$

where $c_{a,b}(k, \omega)$ is the co-spectrum (see Section 3.5.4 for more details) of the time series $\{a_{t,k}\}$ and $\{b_{t,k}\}$. It is then possible to isolate the corresponding "pure" eastward and westward propagating components, PU, as

$$PU(k, \pm\omega) = P(k, \pm\omega) - \frac{1}{2}ST(k, |\omega|). \tag{5.11}$$

As outlined by Hayashi (1982a), this method of partitioning space-time power spectra into standing and traveling parts is based on the following definitions and assumptions:

- Standing waves are defined as consisting of eastward and westward moving components that are of equal amplitude and have high coherence (see Section 3.5.4 for the definition of the coherence measure).
- Traveling waves are defined as consisting of eastward and westward moving components that have low coherence with each other.
- Standing and traveling waves are of a different origin and have low coherence with each other.

The validity and applicability of these assumptions are often called into question; for a discussion, see von Storch and Zwiers (1999, pp. 242–244). In addition to considering the validity of these assumptions, in practice one must consider all of the usual concerns of one-dimensional spectral analysis (e.g., stationarity, end effects, aliasing, statistical consistency, window length, etc., as discussed in Section 3.5).

Empirical Spatio-Temporal Spectrum

Calculation of the spatio-temporal spectrum proceeds using the basic approaches for classical univariate and bivariate spectral analysis described in Section 3.5. Specifically, consider spatio-temporal data from a lattice in one-dimensional space and discrete, equally spaced time points, $\{Z_t(\mathbf{s}_i): i = 1, \ldots, m, t = 1, \ldots, T\}$, where for simplicity of presentation, we assume that m and T are both even numbers. One algorithm proceeds as follows:

1. Take the *spatial* discrete Fourier transform (DFT) of the elements in the m-dimensional vector, $\mathbf{Z}_t \equiv (Z_t(\mathbf{s}_1), \ldots, Z_t(\mathbf{s}_m))'$, for each time, t. Denote the cosine and sine coefficients from these DFTs as $\hat{a}_{t,k}$ and $\hat{b}_{t,k}$, respectively, where k refers to the spatial wave number; $k = 0, 1, \ldots, m/2$.

2. Calculate the power spectra and cross-spectra for the time series from the calculations given in step 1.

   (a) Calculate the temporal power spectra for each of the sine and cosine wavenumber time series from step 1 using the smoothed periodogram approach (e.g., see Section 3.5.3). Denote these as $\hat{f}_a(k, \omega_j)$ and $\hat{f}_b(k, \omega_j)$, for wavenumber $k = 0, \ldots, m/2$ and temporal frequency $\omega_j = 2\pi j/T$; $j = 1, \ldots, T$.

   (b) Calculate the temporal cross-spectrum between the sine and cosine wavenumber time series using the smoothed cross-periodogram approach (e.g., see Section 3.5.4). Denote this by $\hat{f}_{a,b}(k, \omega_j)$, where the real and imaginary components give the associated co-spectra and quadrature spectra, respectively: $\hat{f}_{a,b}(k, \omega_j) = \hat{c}_{a,b}(k, \omega) - i\hat{q}_{a,b}(k, \omega)$, where $i \equiv \sqrt{-1}$.

3. Calculate the spatio-temporal power-spectrum components from the calculations given in step 2.

   (a) Calculate the spatio-temporal power-spectrum components (5.9) for eastward (positive) and westward (negative) traveling waves, respectively:

   $$\hat{P}(k, +\omega) = \frac{1}{4}[\hat{f}_a(k, \omega) + \hat{f}_b(k, \omega) + 2\hat{q}_{a,b}(k, \omega)], \quad (5.12)$$

   $$\hat{P}(k, -\omega) = \frac{1}{4}[\hat{f}_a(k, \omega) + \hat{f}_b(k, \omega) - 2\hat{q}_{a,b}(k, \omega)]. \quad (5.13)$$

   (b) Calculate the spatio-temporal power-spectrum of the standing oscillation component (5.10):

   $$\hat{ST}(k, |\omega|) = \{\frac{1}{4}[\hat{f}_a(k, \omega) - \hat{f}_b(k, \omega)]^2 + \hat{c}_{a,b}^2(k, \omega)\}^{1/2}. \quad (5.14)$$

   (c) Calculate the spatio-temporal power-spectrum components (5.11) for the "pure" eastward and westward propagating components, respectively:

   $$\hat{PU}(k, +\omega) = \hat{P}(k, +\omega) - \frac{1}{2}\hat{ST}(k, |\omega|), \quad (5.15)$$

   $$\hat{PU}(k, -\omega) = \hat{P}(k, -\omega) - \frac{1}{2}\hat{ST}(k, |\omega|). \quad (5.16)$$

Example: Once again, consider the tropical Pacific SST data discussed in Section 5.1. In particular, consider the monthly SST anomalies averaged over the region from $1°$ South to $1°$ North for the equatorial Pacific region (see Figure 5.1). We now consider the spatio-temporal spectral analysis of these data over the 33-year period from January 1970 to December 2002; the empirical spectral density for these data are shown by the contour plots in Figure 5.16. The top panel in this plot shows the total power spectrum, $\hat{P}(k, \pm\omega)$, for

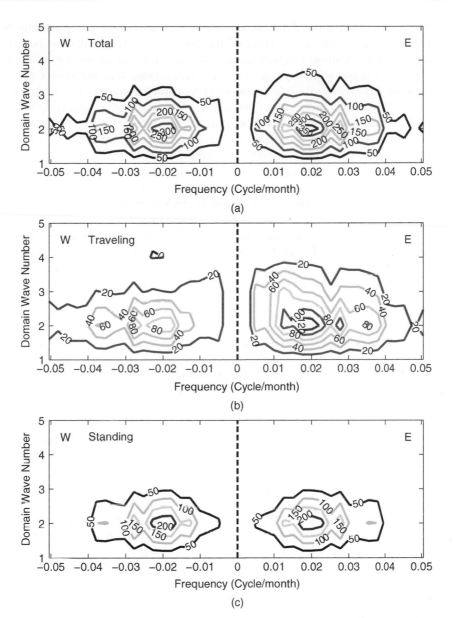

Figure 5.16 Spatio-temporal spectral analysis for SST anomalies at the equator (averaged from 1°
N to 1° S, across the Pacific region). **(a)** Total power spectral density ($\hat{P}$). **(b)** Pure traveling power
spectral density ($\hat{PU}$). **(c)** Standing power spectral density ($\hat{ST}$).

a portion of the temporal frequency domain (x axis) and the wave-number domain (y axis). The left portion of the plot shows the results for negative (westward propagating) frequencies and the right portion shows the results for the positive (eastward propagating) frequencies. Note that the power associated with the westward- and eastward-propagating waves is not symmetric; specifically, there is more power associated with westward-propagating waves.

As discussed above, the power-spectral density can be decomposed into pure travelling waves and pure standing waves. These components, $\hat{PU}(k, \pm\omega)$ and $\hat{ST}(k, \omega)$, are shown in the middle and bottom panels of Figure 5.16, respectively. Clearly, most of the power is associated with the traveling waves; within these, the most power is associated with oscillations at frequencies of about ± 0.026 cycles per month (i.e., a period of 38.5 months or 3.2 years), which is essentially the average frequency of the ENSO phenomena. In addition, we see that the power is centered around the (domain) wavenumber of about 2 to 3. That is, we would see between 2 to 3 waves (in space) over the equatorial Pacific region, since spatial "wavenumber" is defined relative to the longitudinal spatial extent of the domain D_s.

5.3 EMPIRICAL ORTHOGONAL FUNCTION (EOF) ANALYSIS

Empirical orthogonal functions (EOFs) are the geophysicist's terminology for the eigenvectors in the classical eigenvalue/eigenvector decomposition of a covariance (or a correlation) matrix. In its discrete formulation, EOF analysis is simply Principal Component Analysis or PCA (e.g., Hotelling, 1933; Jolliffe, 2002), while in its spatially continuous fomulation, it is a Karhunen–Loève (K–L) expansion (e.g., Loève, 1963) as described in Section 4.1.4. Depending on the application, EOFs are usually used (1) in a diagnostic mode to find principal (in terms of explanation of variance) spatial structures, along with the corresponding time variation of those structures, and (2) to reduce the dimension (spatially or temporally) in large spatio-temporal datasets, while simultaneously reducing noise. An extensive review of EOFs, their theory, and their application to meteorology and oceanography is contained in Preisendorfer (1988). In addition, von Storch and Zwiers (1999), Jolliffe (2002), and Wilks (2006) give quite complete overviews of EOF analysis.

5.3.1 Spatially Continuous Formulation

We first consider data $\{Z_t(\mathbf{s}) : \mathbf{s} \in D_s, t = 1, 2, \dots\}$ from a continuous spatial process measured at discrete time intervals. Our goal is to find an optimal and separable orthogonal decomposition of this process; that is, we wish to write

$$Z_t(\mathbf{s}) = \sum_{k=1}^{\infty} \alpha_t(k)\phi_k(\mathbf{s}), \qquad (5.17)$$

such that $\text{var}(\alpha_t(1)) > \text{var}(\alpha_t(2)) > \ldots$, and $\text{cov}(\alpha_t(i), \alpha_t(k)) = 0$, for all $i \neq k$. As described in Section 4.1.4, a well known solution to this problem is obtained through a Karhunen–Loève (K–L) expansion (e.g., see Papoulis, 1965, p. 457–461). Suppose that $E(Z_t(\mathbf{s})) = 0$, and define the spatial covariance function as $E(Z_t(\mathbf{s})Z_t(\mathbf{r})) \equiv C_Z^{(0)}(\mathbf{s}, \mathbf{r})$, which need not be stationary in space but is assumed invariant in time. Then the K–L expansion allows the covariance function to be decomposed as follows:

$$C_Z^{(0)}(\mathbf{s}, \mathbf{r}) = \sum_{k=1}^{\infty} \lambda_k \phi_k(\mathbf{s})\phi_k(\mathbf{r}), \qquad (5.18)$$

where $\{\phi_k(\cdot) : k = 1, 2, \ldots\}$ are the eigenfunctions and $\{\lambda_k : k = 1, 2, \ldots\}$ are the associated eigenvalues of the Fredholm integral equation,

$$\int_{D_s} C_Z^{(0)}(\mathbf{s}, \mathbf{r})\phi_k(\mathbf{s})\, d\mathbf{s} = \lambda_k \phi_k(\mathbf{r}), \qquad (5.19)$$

where

$$\int_{D_s} \phi_k(\mathbf{s})\phi_l(\mathbf{s})\, d\mathbf{s} = \begin{cases} 1 & \text{for } k = l, \\ 0 & \text{otherwise.} \end{cases} \qquad (5.20)$$

Assuming completeness of the eigenfunctions (see Section 3.5.1), we can then expand $Z_t(\mathbf{s})$ according to

$$Z_t(\mathbf{s}) = \sum_{k=1}^{\infty} \alpha_t(k)\phi_k(\mathbf{s}), \qquad (5.21)$$

where we call $\{\phi_k(\mathbf{s}) : \mathbf{s} \in D_s\}$ the k-th EOF, and we often refer to the associated time series $\{\alpha_t(k) : t = 1, 2, \ldots\}$ as the kth principal-component time series, or kth "amplitude" time series. This time series is stochastic and is derived from the projection of the process $\{Z_t(\mathbf{s})\}$ onto the EOF basis; specifically,

$$\alpha_t(k) = \int_{D_s} Z_t(\mathbf{s})\phi_k(\mathbf{s})\, d\mathbf{s}, \qquad t = 1, 2, \ldots. \qquad (5.22)$$

It is easy to verify that each of these time series is uncorrelated, with variances equal to the corresponding eigenvalues; that is, $E(\alpha_t(i)\alpha_t(k)) = \lambda_k \delta_{ik}$, where δ_{ik} is the Kronecker delta function (equal to one when $i = k$, and equal to zero otherwise).

If we truncate the expansion (5.17) at p_α, yielding

$$Z_{p_\alpha, t}(\mathbf{s}) \equiv \sum_{k=1}^{p_\alpha} \alpha_t(k)\phi_k(\mathbf{s}), \qquad (5.23)$$

then it can be shown (e.g., Freiberger and Grenander, 1965) that the finite EOF decomposition minimizes the variance of the truncation error, $E(Z_t(\mathbf{s}) - Z_{p_\alpha,t}(\mathbf{s}))^2$, and is thus optimal in this regard when compared to all other bases.

Since data are always discrete, in practice we must solve the Fredholm integral equation (5.19) numerically to obtain the EOF basis functions. Cohen and Jones (1969) and Buell (1972, 1975) give numerical-quadrature solutions to this problem. The numerical-quadrature approaches for discretizing the Fredholm integral equation give estimates for the eigenfunctions and eigenvalues that are weighted according to the spatial distribution of the data locations, but only for the eigenfunctions at the locations $\{\mathbf{s}_1, \ldots, \mathbf{s}_n\}$ for which there are data. Obled and Creutin (1986) have presented an elegant spline-based method for discretizing the K–L integral equation and for interpolating the eigenfunctions to locations where data are not available.

5.3.2 Spatially Discrete Formulation

Although the continuous K–L representation of EOFs is often the most realistic from the point of view of modeling a geophysical process, it is rarely considered in applications. This is due simply to the discrete nature of where and when data are observed, and to the difficulty of solving the K–L integral equation. In cases where there are repeat observations (e.g., over time) or some additional information (e.g., deterministic model output or "historical" observations), one can calculate an empirical covariance matrix and perform a PCA analysis. For example, consider a spatially discrete formulation of EOF analysis by using the PCA formulation as given in standard multivariate statistics books (e.g., Johnson and Wichern, 1992), modified according to the spatio-temporal notation we have introduced.

In that case, let $\mathbf{Z}_t \equiv (Z_t(\mathbf{s}_1), \ldots, Z_t(\mathbf{s}_m))'$ and define the kth discrete EOF to be $\boldsymbol{\psi}_k \equiv (\psi_k(\mathbf{s}_1), \ldots, \psi_k(\mathbf{s}_m))'$, where $\boldsymbol{\psi}_k$ is the vector in the linear combination $a_t(k) = \boldsymbol{\psi}_k' \mathbf{Z}_t$; $k = 1, \ldots, m$. (Notice that for discrete EOFs, we deliberately use $\psi_k(\mathbf{s}_i)$ to refer to the i-th element of the eigenvector to distinguish it notationally from the continuous eigenfunction element $\phi_k(\mathbf{s}_i)$ evaluated at $\mathbf{s}_i$; see Section 5.3.1.) Recall we are assuming that var$(\mathbf{Z}_t)$ does not depend on time t. Then, $\boldsymbol{\psi}_1$ is the vector that allows var$(a_t(1))$ to be maximized subject to the constraint $\boldsymbol{\psi}_1' \boldsymbol{\psi}_1 = 1$, and $\boldsymbol{\psi}_2$ is the vector that maximizes var$(a_t(2))$ subject to the constraints $\boldsymbol{\psi}_2' \boldsymbol{\psi}_2 = 1$ and cov$(a_t(1), a_t(2)) = 0$. In general, $\boldsymbol{\psi}_k$ is the vector that maximizes var$(a_t(k))$ subject to the constraints $\boldsymbol{\psi}_k' \boldsymbol{\psi}_k = 1$ and cov$(a_t(k), a_t(j)) = 0$ for all $j \neq k$. This is equivalent to solving the eigensystem,

$$\mathbf{C}_Z^{(0)} \boldsymbol{\Psi} = \boldsymbol{\Psi} \boldsymbol{\Lambda},$$

where $\mathbf{C}_Z^{(0)} \equiv$ var$(\mathbf{Z}_t)$ is the lag-0 spatial covariance matrix; $\boldsymbol{\Psi} \equiv (\boldsymbol{\psi}_1, \ldots, \boldsymbol{\psi}_m)$ is the $m \times m$ orthonormal matrix of eigenvectors ($\boldsymbol{\Psi}' \boldsymbol{\Psi} = \mathbf{I}$); $\boldsymbol{\Lambda} \equiv$ diag$(\lambda_1, \ldots, \lambda_m)$ is the $m \times m$ diagonal matrix of eigenvalues decreasing down the diagonal, $\mathrm{var}(a_t(k)) = \lambda_k$, $k = 1, \ldots, m$; and the mean of $\mathbf{Z}_t$ is assumed to be $\mathbf{0}$ without loss of generality. The solution is obtained by a symmetric decomposition of $\mathbf{C}_Z^{(0)}$, given by $\mathbf{C}_Z^{(0)} = \mathbf{\Psi}\mathbf{\Lambda}\mathbf{\Psi}'$, which is a PCA formulation.

It is straightforward to show (e.g., Cohen and Jones, 1969; Buell, 1972) that if a discretization of the spatially continuous Fredholm integral equation (5.19) assumes equal areas of influence for each observation location, then such a discretization is equivalent to the spatially discrete PCA formulation of EOFs. Conversely, a PCA decomposition of irregularly spaced data (i.e., without consideration of the relative area associated with each observation location) leads to improper weighting of the significance of each element of the covariance matrix $\mathbf{C}_Z^{(0)}$ in the discretization of the spatially continuous equation (5.19). This improper weighting can give erroneous results (see Jolliffe, 2002, p. 297) and is the source of many incorrect EOF analyses in the literature. For a discussion of the effects of ignoring this distinction between the continuous and the discrete formulation, see Karl, Koscielny, and Diaz (1982).

5.3.3 Temporal Formulation

Although the most common formulation of EOFs in the literature is the spatial formulation discussed above, it is also perfectly reasonable to consider a temporal formulation of EOFs (e.g., see Preisendorfer, 1988). In this case, define the T-dimensional vectors $\mathbf{Z}(\mathbf{s}_i) \equiv (Z_1(\mathbf{s}_i), \ldots, Z_T(\mathbf{s}_i))'$, for $i = 1, \ldots, m$. Let the $T \times T$ covariance matrix be given by $\mathbf{\Gamma}_Z \equiv \mathrm{var}(\mathbf{Z}(\mathbf{s}_i))$, for all $\mathbf{s}_i \in D_s$. Then, the development of the EOF decomposition is completely analogous to the spatial formulation, and we can write the spectral decomposition as $\mathbf{\Gamma}_Z = \mathbf{\Psi}^{(s)}\mathbf{\Lambda}^{(s)}\mathbf{\Psi}^{(s)'}$, where the superscript is used to remind us that we are decomposing a (T-dimensional) vector spatial process, $\mathbf{\Psi}^{(s)} \equiv (\boldsymbol{\psi}_1^{(s)}, \ldots, \boldsymbol{\psi}_T^{(s)})'$, and $\mathbf{\Lambda}^{(s)} \equiv \mathrm{diag}(\lambda_1^{(s)}, \ldots, \lambda_T^{(s)})$. In this case, the EOFs $\{\boldsymbol{\psi}_k^{(s)} : k = 1, \ldots, T\}$ are T-dimensional temporal patterns. Associated with the kth EOF is a spatial field given by $a_k(\mathbf{s}_i) = (\boldsymbol{\psi}_k^{(s)})'\mathbf{Z}(\mathbf{s}_i)$, for $i = 1, \ldots, m$. Typically, one considers such an analysis when T, the number of time points, is much less than m, the number of spatial locations, and interest is in considering the variability associated with common temporal patterns at various spatial locations.

5.3.4 Calculation of EOFs

In this section, we focus on the calculation of the *spatial* EOFs. Analogous calculations can be performed to obtain temporal EOFs. Since EOF analysis depends on the (weighted) decomposition of a covariance matrix, $\mathbf{C}_Z^{(0)}$, in practice, we must obtain this matrix empirically. Assume that our spatio-temporal observations are given by the vectors $\mathbf{Z}_t = (Z_t(\mathbf{s}_1), \ldots, Z_t(\mathbf{s}_m))'$; $t = 1, \ldots, T$. Let $\hat{\mathbf{C}}_Z^{(0)}$ be the empirical temporal lag-0 covariance matrix obtained from (5.1).

Given that $\hat{\mathbf{C}}_Z^{(0)}$ is symmetric and nonnegative definite (so that all eigenvalues are greater than or equal to zero), the spectral decomposition, $\hat{\mathbf{C}}_Z^{(0)} = \hat{\mathbf{\Psi}}\hat{\mathbf{\Lambda}}\hat{\mathbf{\Psi}}'$, yields the empirical eigenvectors and eigenvalues. Note that Lawley (1956) derived approximate formulas for the bias and variance of empirical eigenvalues and eigenvectors. Subsequently, von Storch and Hannoschöck (1985) extended Lawley's results by allowing for possible temporal dependence in $\{\mathbf{Z}_t : t = 1, \ldots, T\}$. Based on theory and Monte Carlo simulation, they found that the empirical eigenvalue $\hat{\lambda}_k$ is biased relative to λ_k. This bias is positive for the larger λ_k's and negative for the smaller λ_k's. Furthermore, it has been shown that the sampling error associated with the covariance matrix $\hat{\mathbf{C}}_Z^{(0)}$ leads to numerical instability in the EOFs, $\hat{\mathbf{\Psi}}$ (e.g., Gray, 1981; North et al., 1982). This has led to sampling-based selection strategies for the level of truncation, p_α. Many of these strategies are described in Preisendorfer (1988).

We note that in the presence of white-noise measurement error, the EOFs corresponding to the true, non-noisy process (say, Y) are the same as for the data (say, $Z = Y+$ noise), but the eigenvalues are different. In addition, the "amplitude" time series for both the data (Z) and true process (Y) have the same mean (zero), but the variance of the true process' "amplitude" time series is less. Thus, if white-noise measurement error is present, and EOFs are calculated based on the data, then the EOF spatial patterns are not affected; however, the variance accounted for by each pattern must be adjusted accordingly, by subtracting the estimated white-noise variance from each estimated eigenvalue.

Calculation When $m > T$

Consider the situation in which the number of spatial locations m is larger than the number of time periods T, and we would like to calculate the EOFs associated with the spatial covariance matrix $\widehat{\mathbf{C}}_Z^{(0)}$ given by (5.1). In this case, the $m \times m$ covariance matrix is not positive-definite, since it only has $T - 1$ nonzero eigenvalues. Thus, there are a maximum of $T - 1$ unique EOFs available for consideration. In many cases, $m >> T$, and it is computationally inefficient to perform the spectral decomposition on $\widehat{\mathbf{C}}_Z^{(0)}$. However, we can make use of a convenient matrix-algebra result (e.g., von Storch and Hannoschöck, 1984). Consider an $m \times T$ matrix $\mathbf{W}$. It can be shown that the nonzero eigenvalues of the $m \times m$ matrix $\mathbf{WW}'$ are the same as the nonzero eigenvalues of the $T \times T$ matrix $\mathbf{W}'\mathbf{W}$. Furthermore, it can be shown that if $\mathbf{\xi}_i$ is an eigenvector of $\mathbf{W}'\mathbf{W}$ corresponding to nonzero eigenvalue λ_i, then $\mathbf{\psi}_i \equiv \mathbf{W}\mathbf{\xi}_i/\sqrt{\mathbf{\xi}_i'\mathbf{W}'\mathbf{W}\mathbf{\xi}_i}$ is the eigenvector of $\mathbf{WW}'$ associated with λ_i.

For a spatio-temporal dataset that does not have missing values, we can define the $m \times T$ matrix of data, $\tilde{\mathbf{Z}} \equiv (\tilde{\mathbf{Z}}_1, \ldots, \tilde{\mathbf{Z}}_T)$, where $\tilde{\mathbf{Z}}_t \equiv \mathbf{Z}_t - \hat{\mathbf{\mu}}_Z$ and $\hat{\mathbf{\mu}}_Z$ is given by (5.2). Now, define the $T \times T$ matrix, $\mathbf{A} \equiv \tilde{\mathbf{Z}}'\tilde{\mathbf{Z}}$; then there are a maximum of $T - 1$ nonzero eigenvalues associated with $\mathbf{A}$. Next, calculate the spectral decomposition, $\mathbf{A} = \hat{\mathbf{\Xi}}\hat{\mathbf{\Lambda}}\hat{\mathbf{\Xi}}'$, where $\hat{\mathbf{\Xi}} \equiv (\hat{\mathbf{\xi}}_1, \ldots, \hat{\mathbf{\xi}}_T)$. Then, for each nonzero $\hat{\lambda}_i$, one obtains the associated EOF of $\hat{\mathbf{C}}_Z^{(0)}$ by using the matrix-algebra result above: $\hat{\boldsymbol{\psi}}_i \equiv \tilde{\mathbf{Z}}\hat{\boldsymbol{\xi}}_i / \sqrt{\hat{\boldsymbol{\xi}}_i'\tilde{\mathbf{Z}}'\tilde{\mathbf{Z}}\hat{\boldsymbol{\xi}}_i}$; $i = 1, \ldots, T - 1$.

Example: Consider the monthly SST anomaly dataset $\{\mathbf{Z}_t : t = 1, \ldots, 396\}$ for the 33-year period from January 1970 to December 2002, discussed in Section 5.1. Figure 5.17 shows the first and second EOFs and the associated "amplitude" time series for the 33-year period. Now, EOF 1 and EOF 2 account for 38.8% and 9.3% of the variation in the dataset, respectively. Note that the spatial pattern for the first EOF looks very much like the El Niño pattern shown in Figure 5.4. Indeed, the associated "amplitude" time series shows peaks corresponding to the peaks in the two El Niño time series shown in Figure 5.2. The first EOF accounts for a remarkably large percentage of the variation over the 30-plus years of data, illustrating just how important the El Niño phenomenon is in the tropical Pacific. The second EOF also shows an El Niño-like "signature," but it is much more constrained to the eastern portion of the tropical Pacific region. In contrast, Figure 5.18 shows the third and fourth EOFs and associated "amplitude" time series; these account for 8.5% and 4.2% of the variation, respectively.

Although La Niña signatures appear in the central portion of the equatorial Pacific, there are other spatial regions showing large (in magnitude) EOF coefficients (sometimes called loadings) as well. This illustrates an important point about EOF analysis, namely the constraint of orthogonality limits the physical interpretability of all but the first EOF. However, this example also illustrates the incredible dimension-reduction capability of EOF analysis, something we use when fitting a BHM to the SST anomaly dataset in Section 9.1. In this case, the first four EOFs account for over 60% of the variation of a spatial vector that has $m = 2,261$ elements (i.e., the number of ocean pixels in the domain of interest). Figure 5.19 shows the cumulative percentage of variation accounted for by the first 100 EOFs; the first 100 EOFs account for over 97% of the SST-anomaly variation.

5.4 EXTENSIONS OF EOF ANALYSIS

The eigenvalue/eigenvector decomposition underlying EOF analysis can be applied to a variety of other situations involving spatio-temporal data. In most cases, these can be thought of as summarizing in some manner an augmented data matrix. We briefly discuss three of these cases below. For the interested reader, the Bibliographic Notes in Section 5.8 contain references that give considerably more detail.

5.4.1 Complex (Hilbert) EOFs

One advantage of the EOF approach described in Section 5.3 is that the complicated variability of spatio-temporal data can be compressed into a relatively

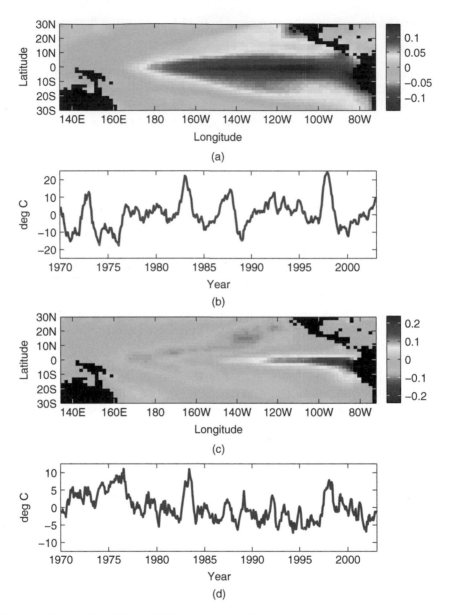

Figure 5.17 (a) First EOF for SST anomaly data. (b) Associated amplitude time series for the first EOF, which accounts for 38.8% of the variation in the monthly anomalies from January 1970 through December 2002. (c) Second EOF for SST anomaly data. (d) Associated amplitude time series for the second EOF, which accounts for 9.3% of the variation in these data. Note that the EOFs are unitless in these plots, and the amplitude time series are in the same units as the data, °C.

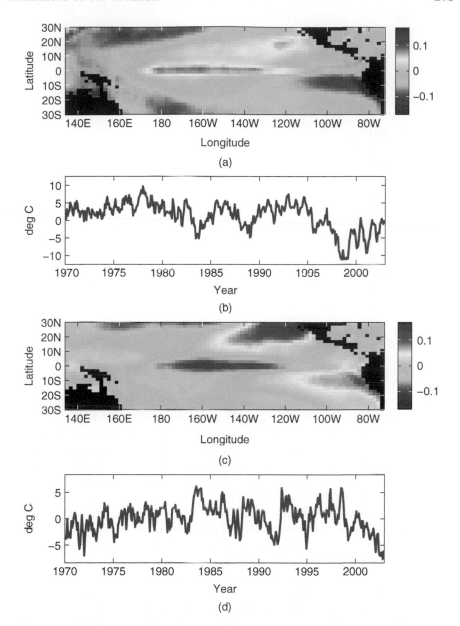

Figure 5.18 (a) Third EOF for SST anomaly data. (b) Associated amplitude time series for the third EOF, which accounts for 8.5% of the variation in the monthly anomalies from January 1970 through December 2002. (c) Fourth EOF for SST anomaly data. (d) Associated amplitude time series for the fourth EOF, which accounts for 4.2% of the variation in these data. Units are the same as in Figure 5.17.

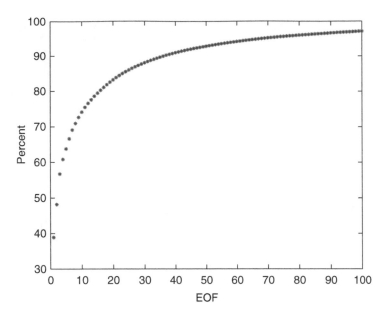

Figure 5.19 Cumulative variance, expressed as a percent of total variance, accounted for by the first 100 EOFs for the monthly Pacific SST anomaly data from January 1970 through December 2002. The y axis shows cumulative variance (percent) and the x axis shows EOF index.

small set of eigenvectors. However, such an EOF analysis only detects spatial structures that do not propagate in time. To extend the EOF analysis to the study of spatial structures that can propagate in time, Wallace and Dickinson (1972) developed *complex principal component* analysis in the frequency domain. The technique involves the computation of complex eigenvectors from cross-spectral matrices. The limitation of this technique is that it only gives the decomposition for individual (i.e., very narrow) frequency bands. Consequently, if the power of a phenomenon is spread over a wide frequency band (as is generally the case with environmental phenomena), then several EOF spatial maps (one for each spectral estimate) are needed to evaluate the phenomenon, and this can complicate the interpretation.

Complex empirical orthogonal function (CEOF) analysis, or *Hilbert EOF (HEOF)* analysis, in the time domain, was developed as an alternative to the frequency-domain approach described above (Rasmusson, Arkin, and Chen, 1981). This method differs from the frequency-domain approach in that Hilbert transforms are used to shift the time series of the data at each location by a quarter of a cycle. That is, for a data vector $\mathbf{Z}_t = (Z_t(\mathbf{s}_1), \ldots, Z_t(\mathbf{s}_m))'$, let

$$\tilde{\mathbf{Z}}_t \equiv \mathbf{Z}_t + i\mathbf{Z}_t^H, \tag{5.24}$$

where $i = \sqrt{-1}$ and $\mathbf{Z}_t^H$ is the *Hilbert transformed* vector defined by (e.g., von Storch and Zwiers, 1999, Section 16.2.2):

$$\mathbf{Z}_t^H \equiv \sum_{j=0}^{\infty} \frac{2}{(2j+1)\pi}(\mathbf{Z}_{t+2j+1} - \mathbf{Z}_{t-2j+1}), \tag{5.25}$$

for $t = \ldots, -1, 0, 1, \ldots$.

The original data and its Hilbert transform allow the examination of propagating disturbances. Specifically, one simply performs the EOF analysis (described in Section 5.3) on the empirical covariance matrix of the complex augmented data, $\{\tilde{\mathbf{Z}}_t : t = 1, \ldots, T\}$. Since this covariance matrix is Hermitian, it has complex eigenvectors and real, nonnegative eigenvalues (e.g., von Storch and Zwiers, 1999, p. 359). Barnett (1983) and Horel (1984) give excellent discussions of some of the theoretical and practical issues related to such analyses.

If one can compute the Hilbert transform (5.25), then the EOF analysis of $\{\tilde{\mathbf{Z}}_t\}$ proceeds directly after calculating its empirical covariance matrix and performing the eigenvector/eigenvalue decomposition, exactly as in the usual EOF analysis. One should be sure to take the complex conjugate of $(\mathbf{Z}_{t-\tau} - \hat{\mu}_Z)$ in (5.1) when calculating the (lagged) empirical covariance matrix. In practice, finite-sample Hilbert transforms can be computed fairly easily, as discussed in Barnett (1983) and von Storch and Zwiers (1999, Section 16.2.4). Of course, the eigenvectors (EOFs) and the principal component ("amplitude") time series are both complex-valued. Thus, one typically has to develop some intuition regarding the interpretation of results. The following example is provided to illustrate a basic HEOF analysis.

Example: Consider the monthly SST anomaly dataset $\{\mathbf{Z}_t : t = 1, \ldots, 396\}$ for the 33-year period from January 1970 to December 2002, discussed in Section 5.1. Then, $\{\tilde{\mathbf{Z}}_t\}$ is constructed as in (5.24), where $\{\mathbf{Z}_t^H\}$ defined by (5.25) is calculated in the manner suggested by von Storch and Zwiers (1999, Section 16.2.4). The first complex EOF accounts for 42.4% of the variation in this dataset. (Since the augmented covariance matrix is Hermitian, recall that the eigenvalues are real and thus this percentage is calculated by simply dividing the largest eigenvalue by the sum of all eigenvalues.) Image plots of the real and imaginary part of the first complex EOF are shown in the top and bottom panels of Figure 5.20, respectively. Figure 5.21 shows the corresponding real and imaginary "amplitude" time series for the first complex EOF in the top panel. The bottom panel shows the associated *phase* through time, given by $\arctan\{Im[a_t(1)]/Re[a_t(1)]\}$, where $a_t(1)$ is the complex-valued "amplitude" time series associated with the first complex EOF, and $Im[\cdot]$ and $Re[\cdot]$ correspond to the imaginary and real components, respectively. Note that the real part of the first complex EOF resembles the spatial pattern of the El

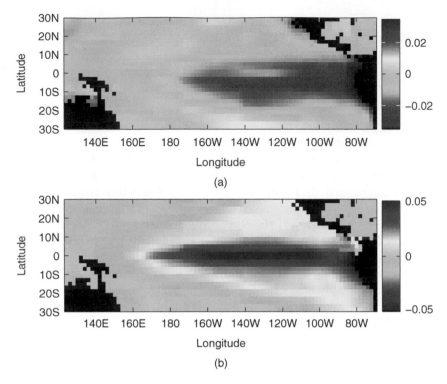

Figure 5.20 The first complex (Hilbert) EOF from the monthly Pacific SST anomaly data from January 1970 to December 2002. **(a)** The real part of the first complex EOF. **(b)** The imaginary part of the first complex EOF. This complex EOF accounts for approximately 42.4% of the total variability of the Hilbert transform-augmented Pacific SST anomalies [see (5.24)] over this time period, as derived from the largest eigenvalue of the associated covariance matrix. The EOFs are unitless.

Niño signal when the real part of $a_t(1)$ is negative, and somewhat resembles spatial pattern of the La Niña signal when the real part of $a_t(1)$ is positive. Similarly, the pattern of the corresponding imaginary part of the first complex EOF resembles a narrower (in a latitudinal sense) El Niño pattern when the imaginary part of $a_t(1)$ is positive, and it resembles a La Niña pattern when the imaginary part of $a_t(1)$ is negative. In essence, these patterns, and the associated time series, show an idealized and filtered view of the ENSO phenomena.

Let ψ_1 be the first complex EOF; then our CEOF analysis suggests that one cycle of ENSO follows roughly the sequence: $Re\{\psi_1\}$, $-Im\{\psi_1\}$, $-Re\{\psi_1\}$, $Im\{\psi_1\}$. Graphically, this corresponds to the top panel in Figure 5.20, followed 1/4 cycle later by the negative of the bottom panel of Figure 5.20, followed by the negative of the top panel, followed by the bottom panel.

The real and imaginary parts of the time series shown in Figure 5.21 are roughly a quarter cycle out of phase, as expected, since the imaginary part is the Hilbert transform of the real part (von Storch and Zwiers, 1999, Sec. 16.3.14).

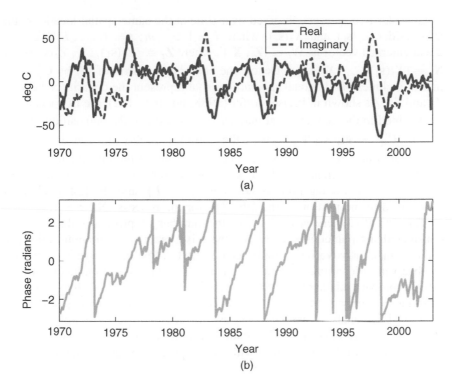

Figure 5.21 The first complex (Hilbert) EOF amplitude time series corresponding to the CEOFs shown in Figure 5.20. (a) The real (blue) and imaginary (red) portions of the amplitude time series. (b) The phase (green) associated with the real and imaginary portions (i.e., the arctan of the imaginary part divided by the real part of the complex-valued time series).

More importantly, the bottom panel of Figure 5.21 shows the associated phase in radians of the ENSO cycle discussed above. Each "sawtooth" in the phase plot represents a filtered ENSO oscillation. Clearly, the period of these cycles varies considerably throughout the data record.

As discussed in von Storch and Zwiers (1999, Sec. 16.3.12), the interpretation of complex EOF analysis can be difficult and is based on some tenuous assumptions. They wisely state: "Prudence is clearly advisable" (von Storch and Zwiers, 1999, p. 363).

5.4.2 Multivariate EOF Analysis

There is often interest in the simultaneous analysis of two or more spatio-temporal datasets. Kutzbach (1967) used a form of EOF analysis that simultaneously considered several meteorological variables at many spatial locations and times, and Preisendorfer (1988) discussed this approach at length. A brief description of the basic idea behind the multivariate EOF analysis follows.

Consider two datasets observed over time at the same spatial locations; that is, consider $Z_t(\mathbf{s}_i)$ and $X_t(\mathbf{s}_i)$, where $i = 1, \ldots, m$; $t = 1, \ldots, T$. We write the augmented vector as $\mathbf{W}_t \equiv (\mathbf{Z}'_t, \mathbf{X}'_t)'$, where $\mathbf{Z}_t \equiv (Z_t(\mathbf{s}_1), \ldots, Z_t(\mathbf{s}_m))'$ and $\mathbf{X}_t \equiv (X_t(\mathbf{s}_1), \ldots, X_t(\mathbf{s}_m))'$. Denote the covariance matrix of $\mathbf{W}_t$ by $\mathbf{C}_W^{(0)}$. This matrix includes off-diagonal submatrices that represent the covariance between $\mathbf{Z}_t$ and $\mathbf{X}_t$. As shown in Preisendorfer (1988, pp. 161–162), the EOFs can then be obtained in the conventional manner from the eigen-decomposition of $\mathbf{C}_W^{(0)}$; that is, $\mathbf{C}_W^{(0)} = \mathbf{\Psi}_W \mathbf{\Lambda}_W \mathbf{\Psi}'_W$, where the columns of $\mathbf{\Psi}_W$ are the eigenvectors (i.e., EOFs) and $\mathbf{\Lambda}_W$ is a diagonal matrix containing the eigenvalues of $\mathbf{C}_W^{(0)}$. Then, the first m elements of the kth eigenvector correspond to the portion of the kth EOF for the process $\{\mathbf{Z}_t : t = 1, \ldots, T\}$, and the last m elements correspond to the portion of the kth EOF for the process $\{\mathbf{X}_t : t = 1, \ldots, T\}$.

Theoretically, there is no limit to the number of processes that could be considered simultaneously. However, there is a practical limitation to this procedure, since the covariance matrix can easily become very large if the number of observation locations or variables increases. Bretherton, Smith, and Wallace (1992) compare this approach to other multivariate methods such as Canonical Correlation Analysis (see Section 5.6) and find that, in some cases, the multivariate EOF analysis has large biases and does not perform well when the signal-to-noise ratio is small. Calculation of multivariate EOFs proceeds as with single-process EOFs, by starting with the empirical covariance matrix $\hat{\mathbf{C}}_W^{(0)}$.

5.4.3 Extended EOF Analysis

Extended EOFs (e.g., Weare and Nasstrom, 1982) are simply multivariate EOFs in which the additional variables are lagged versions of the same process. For example, we could let the augmented data vector be $\mathbf{W}_t = (\mathbf{Z}'_t, \mathbf{Z}'_{t-\tau})'$, for $\tau = 1, 2, \ldots$. In this case, if temporal invariance is assumed, then the diagonal submatrices of $\mathbf{C}_W^{(0)}$ are equivalent, and the off-diagonal submatrices are just the lag-τ covariance matrices $\mathbf{C}_Z^{(\tau)}$. In this way, we can examine the propagation of EOF spatial patterns in time by noting that the first m coefficients of a particular eigenvector correspond to the lag-zero representation of that EOF, and the next m coefficients correspond to the lag-τ representation of the same EOF. This approach is closely linked with time-lagged Canonical Correlation Analysis discussed below in Section 5.6.

Example: Consider the monthly SST anomaly dataset $\{\mathbf{Z}_t : t = 1, \ldots, 396\}$ for the 33-year period from January 1970 through December 2002, discussed in Section 5.1. In this case, we form the augmented data vector with the SST anomaly data at time t and at time $t - 6$ (i.e., $\tau = 6$ months) throughout the data record. The extended EOF patterns for the first eigenvector are shown in Figure 5.22. The top panel shows the portion of the first eigenvector corresponding to the SST anomalies at time t, while the lower panel shows the portion of the same eigenvector corresponding to the anomalies at time $t - 6$.

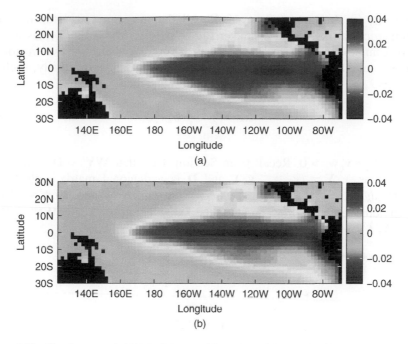

Figure 5.22 The first extended EOF of the monthly Pacific SST anomaly data from January 1970 to December 2002. **(a)** The portion of the eigenvector associated with the current time t and **(b)** the portion of the eigenvector associated with time-lagged $t - 6$. This extended EOF accounts for 31% of the variation in the augmented data vector. Note that these eigenvectors are unitless.

This first extended EOF accounts for 31% of the variation in the augmented data vector. The ENSO pattern is evident in both plots in Figure 5.22, suggesting that there is substantial persistence across 6 months. Nonetheless, there are differences in the spatial pattern of these EOFs, indicating that there is variability in the spatial pattern throughout the ENSO cycle.

5.5 PRINCIPAL OSCILLATION PATTERNS (POPs)

Recall from Section 3.2.1 that a spectral decomposition of the *propagator matrix* for a first-order dynamical system elucidates many features of its underlying dynamics. In essence, Principal Oscillation Pattern (POP) analysis is just the spectral decomposition of the operator for a spatio-temporal process expressed as a first-order dynamical system.

To gain insight into the interpretation of the POPs in space and time, we consider an idealized first-order discrete linear system, as discussed in Section 3.2.1:

$$\mathbf{Z}_t = \mathbf{M}\mathbf{Z}_{t-1}, \tag{5.26}$$

where $\mathbf{Z}_t \equiv (Z_t(\mathbf{s}_1), \ldots, Z_t(\mathbf{s}_m))'$. Recall that for an $m \times m$ full-rank non-symmetric matrix $\mathbf{M}$, the characteristic equation, $|\mathbf{M} - \lambda \mathbf{I}| = 0$, has m (possibly complex) roots. Corresponding to a root λ_k, there are two vectors $\mathbf{w}_k$ and $\mathbf{v}_k$, called the "right" and "left" *singular vectors*, respectively, such that $\mathbf{M}\mathbf{w}_k = \lambda_k \mathbf{w}_k$ and $\mathbf{M}'\mathbf{v}_k = \lambda_k \mathbf{v}_k$; $k = 1, \ldots, m$. Then,

$$\mathbf{M} = \sum_{k=1}^{m} \frac{\lambda_k}{d_k} \mathbf{w}_k \mathbf{v}_k', \tag{5.27}$$

where $d_k \equiv \mathbf{v}_k' \mathbf{w}_k > 0$. Recall from Section 3.2.1 that $\mathbf{W}\mathbf{V}' = \mathbf{D}$, where $\mathbf{W} \equiv (\mathbf{w}_1, \ldots, \mathbf{w}_m)$, $\mathbf{V} \equiv (\mathbf{v}_1, \ldots, \mathbf{v}_m)$, and $\mathbf{D}$ is a diagonal matrix with the elements $\{d_k : k = 1, \ldots, m\}$ on the main diagonal. Now normalize $\mathbf{w}_k$ and $\mathbf{v}_k$ by dividing each by $d_k^{1/2}$ and use the same notation. Then, $\mathbf{W}\mathbf{V}' = \mathbf{I}$, and $\mathbf{M} = \mathbf{W}\boldsymbol{\Lambda}\mathbf{V}' = \sum_{k=1}^{m} \lambda_k \mathbf{w}_k \mathbf{v}_k'$. Consequently, we can write

$$\mathbf{Z}_t = \mathbf{W}\mathbf{V}'\mathbf{Z}_t = \mathbf{W}\mathbf{a}_t = \sum_{k=1}^{m} a_t(k)\mathbf{w}_k, \tag{5.28}$$

where

$$\mathbf{a}_t \equiv \mathbf{V}'\mathbf{Z}_t \tag{5.29}$$

and $\mathbf{a}_t \equiv (a_t(1), \ldots, a_t(m))'$. The essence of POP analysis is the decomposition represented by (5.27) and (5.29). The right singular vectors $\{\mathbf{w}_k : k = 1, \ldots, m\}$ are called *principal oscillation patterns* and, although they constitute a linear basis, they are not orthonormal. Each of these vectors does represent a spatial field, as each component of the vector is spatially referenced. The elements of the time series $\{a_t(k) : t = 1, 2, \ldots\}$ are known as POP coefficients. The left singular vectors $\{\mathbf{v}_k : k = 1, \ldots, m\}$ are called *adjoint bases*. We note that, although the basis vectors $\{\mathbf{w}_k\}$ are not orthogonal with themselves, any $\mathbf{w}_k$ is orthogonal to $\mathbf{v}_j$; $j \neq k$.

The right singular vectors $\{\mathbf{w}_k : k = 1, \ldots, m\}$ of the matrix $\mathbf{M}$ are sometimes referred to as the *normal modes* of the first-order dynamical system. Because $\mathbf{M}$ is not in general symmetric, some or all of its eigenvalues and eigenvectors are complex, as discussed in Section 3.2.1. Furthermore, because $\mathbf{M}$ is real, the complex conjugates, $\bar{\lambda}_k$ and $\bar{\mathbf{w}}_k$, also satisfy the singular-vector equation, $\mathbf{M}\bar{\mathbf{w}}_k = \bar{\lambda}_k \bar{\mathbf{w}}_k$.

Now, writing (5.26) in terms of its decompositions (5.27) and (5.28) and pre-multiplying by $\mathbf{V}'$, we obtain from (5.29)

$$\mathbf{a}_t = \mathbf{V}'\mathbf{W}\boldsymbol{\Lambda}\mathbf{V}'\mathbf{Z}_{t-1} = \boldsymbol{\Lambda}\mathbf{a}_{t-1}, \tag{5.30}$$

or

$$a_t(k) = \lambda_k a_{t-1}(k), \qquad k = 1, \ldots, m, \tag{5.31}$$

which is a collection of m first-order homogeneous difference equations, each with solution $a_t(k) = (\lambda_k)^t$ (assuming $a_0(k) = 1$), as described in Section 3.2.

If λ_k is complex, then $\lambda_k \equiv \lambda_k^R + i\lambda_k^I$ (recall $i \equiv \sqrt{-1}$), which can be written in polar form as $\lambda_k^R = \gamma_k \cos(\phi_k)$ and $\lambda_k^I = \gamma_k \sin(\phi_k)$. Then, $\lambda_k = \gamma_k e^{i\phi_k}$, where $\gamma_k = |\lambda_k| = \{(\lambda_k^R)^2 + (\lambda_k^I)^2\}^{1/2}$ and $\phi_k = \arctan(\lambda_k^I/\lambda_k^R)$. Thus, the coefficients evolve according to, $a_t(k) = \gamma_k^t e^{i\phi_k t}$. Under the conditions, $|\lambda_k| \leq 1$; $k = 1, \ldots, m$, $a_t(k)$ evolves as a damped spiral in the complex plane with a characteristic damping rate γ_k and frequency ϕ_k, for $k = 1, \ldots, m$. Notice that here ϕ_k is an *angle* in the complex plane and should not be confused with the basis functions and their associated vectors that we use in EOF representations of spatio-temporal processes (e.g., Section 5.3).

We now decompose the right singular vector (i.e., normal mode) $\mathbf{w}_k$ as the sum of a real and an imaginary term: $\mathbf{w}_k = \mathbf{w}_k^R + i\mathbf{w}_k^I$. Note that for $\mathbf{M}$ real, the normal modes occur in complex conjugate pairs if they are complex. Hence, the general evolution of a damped normal mode (i.e., $\gamma_k \leq 1$) can be described in a two-dimensional subspace spanned by $\mathbf{w}_k^R$ and $\mathbf{w}_k^I$ [see, e.g., von Storch et al. (1995)]; it occurs in the succession,

$$\ldots \to \mathbf{w}_k^R \to -\mathbf{w}_k^I \to -\mathbf{w}_k^R \to \mathbf{w}_k^I \to \mathbf{w}_k^R \to \ldots, \tag{5.32}$$

with a period of $2\pi/\phi_k$; and each stage in (5.32) occurs a quarter of a cycle apart. Note the similarity of this to the complex (Hilbert) EOF example shown in Section 5.4.1. In the case of POPs, the time τ_k needed to reduce an initial *amplitude* $a_0(k)$ to $a_0(k)/e$ is referred to as the *e-folding time* and is given by $\tau_k \equiv -1/\ln(\gamma_k)$.

5.5.1 Calculation of POPs

The previous section emphasized the physical motivation and interpretation behind a POP analysis. If the system were *deterministic*, then the normal-mode approach leading to (5.32) would be directly interpretable. However, data come with uncertainty, and we need to account for it. Thus, we assume that the data follow a first-order vector autoregressive process (i.e., VAR(1), as discussed in Section 3.4.7):

$$\mathbf{Z}_t = \mathbf{M}\mathbf{Z}_{t-1} + \boldsymbol{\eta}_t, \tag{5.33}$$

where $\boldsymbol{\eta}_t$ is an m-dimensional additive error vector such that $E(\boldsymbol{\eta}_t) = \mathbf{0}$, $E(\boldsymbol{\eta}_t \mathbf{Z}'_{t-1}) = \mathbf{0}$, and $E(\boldsymbol{\eta}_t \boldsymbol{\eta}'_r) = \mathbf{C}_\eta^{(0)}$ when $t = r$, and $\mathbf{0}$ otherwise. As discussed in Section 3.4.7, under second-order stationarity, $\mathbf{M} = \mathbf{C}_Z^{(1)} (\mathbf{C}_Z^{(0)})^{-1}$, where $\mathbf{C}_Z^{(\tau)}$ is the lag-τ cross-covariance matrix for $\{\mathbf{Z}_t\}$.

In order to perform a POP analysis in practice, the propagator matrix $\mathbf{M}$ in (5.33) must be estimated. As discussed in Section 3.4.7, a method-of-moments estimator for $\mathbf{M}$ is $\hat{\mathbf{M}} = \hat{\mathbf{C}}_Z^{(1)} (\hat{\mathbf{C}}_Z^{(0)})^{-1}$, where $\hat{\mathbf{C}}_Z^{(\tau)}$; $\tau = 0, 1$, are given by (5.1). An eigenvector/eigenvalue decomposition of $\hat{\mathbf{M}}$ then gives estimated right singular vectors $\{\hat{\mathbf{w}}_k: k = 1, \ldots, m\}$ and estimated eigenvalues $\{\hat{\lambda}_k: k = 1, \ldots, m\}$. The adjoint-vector (left-singular-vector) estimates can be obtained from $\hat{\mathbf{V}}' = \hat{\mathbf{W}}^{-1}$, and the POP-coefficient estimates can then be obtained from $\hat{\mathbf{a}}_t = \hat{\mathbf{V}}'\mathbf{Z}_t$; see (5.29). Similarly, estimates of $\{\gamma_k\}$ and $\{\phi_k\}$ can be obtained from the estimates $\{\hat{\lambda}_k\}$.

The estimated eigenvectors $\hat{\mathbf{W}}$ are sometimes referred to as *empirical* normal modes, analogous to the deterministic decomposition. It is then *assumed* that these empirical normal modes behave as one would expect the deterministic normal modes to behave. For example, for damped empirical modes (i.e., $\hat{\gamma}_k \leq 1$, where $\hat{\gamma}_k \equiv |\hat{\lambda}_k|$) one might expect the succession (5.32). However, in the presence of noise, this relationship may not hold. To check if this relationship is valid in practice, a cross-spectral analysis is often performed between the estimates of the real component $\hat{a}_t^R(k)$ and the imaginary component $\hat{a}_t^I(k)$ of $\hat{a}_t(k)$ which, according to the deterministic analysis, should vary coherently with a frequency ϕ_j and phase lag $\pi/2$, with $\hat{a}_t^R(k)$ lagging $\hat{a}_t^I(k)$. If this is not observed, then the interpretation based on (5.32) is not valid.

Although POPs can be used for both prognostic and diagnostic purposes, from a statistical perspective they are probably best considered as diagnostic, exploratory tools. As diagnostics, POPs are used to examine the oscillation properties and spatial structure of spatio-temporal dynamical processes. In this case, one looks at the estimated frequencies $\{\hat{\phi}_k\}$, amplitudes $\{\hat{\gamma}_k\}$, and e-folding times $\{\hat{\tau}_k\}$, as well as the right singular vectors (POPs) $\{\hat{\mathbf{w}}_k\}$ and amplitude time series $\{\hat{a}_t(k)\}$. These quantities give insight into the interpretation of the empirical normal modes. Often, the data are initially filtered (usually in time) to focus on a particular phenomenon of interest, assuming the appropriate frequency band in which to filter is known *a priori*. In some cases, the data are projected onto a reduced set of basis functions (e.g., EOFs) and the POP analysis is performed in the reduced-dimensional space. This is in the spirit of dimension reduction presented in Section 7.2.6, and we demonstrate the idea in the following example.

Example: Consider the monthly SST anomaly dataset $\{\mathbf{Z}_t\}$ from January 1970 to December 2002, discussed in Section 5.1. For diagnostic purposes, assume a VAR(1) structure,

$$\mathbf{Z}_t = \mathbf{M}\mathbf{Z}_{t-1} + \boldsymbol{\eta}_t, \tag{5.34}$$

with the same assumptions as given below (5.33). A POP analysis considers the decomposition of the estimated propagator matrix $\hat{\mathbf{M}}$, however there are $T = 33 \times 12 = 396$ time points (months) and $m = 2{,}261$ ocean pixels (spatial locations) in the dataset. Thus, the method-of-moments estimate, $\hat{\mathbf{M}} \equiv \hat{\mathbf{C}}_Z^{(1)}(\hat{\mathbf{C}}_Z^{(0)})^{-1}$, whose components are given by (5.1), is not well defined (the $2{,}261 \times 2{,}261$ matrix, $\hat{\mathbf{C}}_Z^{(0)}$, has rank $T - 1 = 395$). Yet, as we have seen, most of the variability in the monthly SST anomalies can be accounted for by a relatively small number of EOFs. Thus, let us assume we can approximate the SST anomaly data by projecting onto the first p_α EOFs, given by the $m \times p_\alpha$ matrix $\boldsymbol{\Psi}$: From Section 5.3.2, $\mathbf{Z}_t \simeq \boldsymbol{\Psi} \cdot (a_t(1), \ldots, a_t(p_\alpha))'$, where

'·' is used here to emphasize matrix–vector multiplication. Hence, *define* the (dimension-reduced) p_α-variate vector,

$$\boldsymbol{\alpha}_t \equiv \boldsymbol{\Psi}'\mathbf{Z}_t.$$

Then, ignoring the truncation error and using orthogonality of the EOFs, we can rewrite (5.34) as

$$\boldsymbol{\alpha}_t = \boldsymbol{\Psi}'\mathbf{M}\boldsymbol{\Psi}\boldsymbol{\alpha}_{t-1} + \boldsymbol{\Psi}'\boldsymbol{\eta}_t \equiv \mathbf{M}_\alpha\boldsymbol{\alpha}_{t-1} + \boldsymbol{\eta}_{\alpha,t}, \qquad (5.35)$$

where $\mathbf{M}_\alpha \equiv \boldsymbol{\Psi}'\mathbf{M}\boldsymbol{\Psi}$ and $\boldsymbol{\eta}_{\alpha,t} \equiv \boldsymbol{\Psi}'\boldsymbol{\eta}_t$. Now, the POP analysis can be performed on the p_α-dimensional vectors, $\{\boldsymbol{\alpha}_t : t = 1, \ldots, T\}$, leading to the estimates $\hat{\mathbf{C}}_\alpha^{(\tau)}$ and hence to $\hat{\mathbf{M}}_\alpha \equiv \hat{\mathbf{C}}_\alpha^{(1)}(\hat{\mathbf{C}}_\alpha^{(0)})^{-1}$. Notice that there is no concern about the singularity of the lag-0 covariance matrix when $p_\alpha < T$. Furthermore, interpretations of the POPs can still be considered in physical space. To see this, note that the POP analysis yields the singular value decomposition, $\hat{\mathbf{M}}_\alpha = \hat{\mathbf{W}}_\alpha\hat{\boldsymbol{\Lambda}}_\alpha\hat{\mathbf{V}}_\alpha'$, and thus we can define $\hat{\mathbf{M}} \equiv \boldsymbol{\Psi}\hat{\mathbf{M}}_\alpha\boldsymbol{\Psi}' = \boldsymbol{\Psi}\hat{\mathbf{W}}_\alpha\hat{\boldsymbol{\Lambda}}_\alpha\hat{\mathbf{V}}_\alpha'\boldsymbol{\Psi}'$. We can then consider the kth POP in physical space by making image plots of the back-transformed right singular vectors, $\boldsymbol{\Psi}\hat{\mathbf{w}}_{\alpha,k}$, for each $k = 1, \ldots, p_\alpha$, and where $\hat{\mathbf{W}}_\alpha \equiv (\hat{\mathbf{w}}_{\alpha,1}, \ldots, \hat{\mathbf{w}}_{\alpha,p_\alpha})$.

For the monthly tropical Pacific SST anomaly data, consider the $p_\alpha = 20$ leading EOFs (which correspond to about 83% of the variation as shown in Figure 5.19). In this case, the decomposition of $\hat{\mathbf{M}}_\alpha$ is summarized in Table 5.1.

Table 5.1 Eigenvalue Spectrum of $\hat{\mathbf{M}}_\alpha$

$\hat{\lambda}_{\alpha,k}$	$\hat{\gamma}_{\alpha,k}$	$2\pi/\hat{\phi}_{\alpha,k}$
0.4529 + 0.0938i	0.4625	30.8
0.4529 − 0.0938i	0.4625	−30.8
0.6010 + 0.2146i	0.6381	18.3
0.6010 − 0.2146i	0.6381	−18.3
0.4703	0.4703	—
0.5027	0.5027	—
0.7246 + 0.2155i	0.7559	21.7
0.7246 − 0.2155i	0.7559	−21.7
0.9060	0.9060	—
0.8677 + 0.0798i	0.8713	68.5
0.8677 − 0.0798i	0.8713	−68.5
0.7223 + 0.1409i	0.7359	32.6
0.7223 − 0.1409i	0.7359	−32.6
0.8645	0.8645	—
0.7644 + 0.0600i	0.7668	80.2
0.7644 − 0.0600i	0.7668	−80.2
0.6583 + 0.0533i	0.6604	77.7
0.6583 − 0.0533i	0.6604	−77.7
0.7765	0.7765	—
0.6967	0.6967	—

We note from this table that all of the damping rates $\{\hat{\gamma}_{\alpha,k}: k = 1, \ldots, 20\}$ are less than one, implying that there is no explosive growth potential in these data. We also note that there are many different oscillatory and non-oscillatory patterns present in the dataset. The oscillation frequencies vary quite a bit, with the estimated values of the associated periods, $2\pi/\hat{\phi}_{\alpha,k}$, falling between 18.3 to 80.2 months. As an example, consider the POP with estimated period of 68.5 months. The POP patterns associated with this oscillatory component are shown in Figure 5.23. The four panels in this figure show the POP evolution as indicated in (5.32). The associated POP-coefficient time series (real and imaginary components) are shown in Figure 5.24. We interpret Figures 5.23 and 5.24 as follows. The POPs show some similarity with the El Niño and La Niña patterns, and the time series in Figure 5.24 show increased amplitude during the major ENSO events. However, we note that the period of 68.5 months seems long for the average ENSO oscillation. Yet, there is nothing in the POP analysis to prevent a physical signal such as ENSO from being "distributed" among multiple normal modes. Examination of the other normal modes (not shown here) suggest that there are ENSO features found in multiple normal modes.

5.6 SPATIO-TEMPORAL CANONICAL CORRELATION ANALYSIS (CCA)

Canonical Correlation Analysis (CCA) is a long-standing multivariate statistical technique (Hotelling, 1936) that obtains linear combinations of two sets of random variables whose correlations are maximal. This approach has sometimes been used when the two random variables of interest are indexed by space and time. In this regard, it is related to multivariate EOFs, which are discussed in Section 5.4.2.

5.6.1 Two-Field Spatio-Temporal CCA

We assume that, in addition to the dataset $\{\mathbf{Z}_t \equiv (Z_t(\mathbf{s}_1), \ldots, Z_t(\mathbf{s}_m))' : t = 1, \ldots, T\}$, we are interested in another, related dataset $\{\mathbf{X}_t \equiv (X_t(\mathbf{x}_1), \ldots, X_t(\mathbf{x}_\ell))' : t = 1, \ldots, T\}$, with a possibly different spatial domain, but the same temporal domain. As before, we denote the covariance matrices by $\mathbf{C}_Z^{(0)} = \text{var}(\mathbf{Z}_t)$, $\mathbf{C}_X^{(0)} = \text{var}(\mathbf{X}_t)$, and $\mathbf{C}_{Z,X}^{(0)} = \text{cov}(\mathbf{Z}_t, \mathbf{X}_t)$, which have dimensions $m \times m$, $\ell \times \ell$, and $m \times \ell$, respectively. We then seek certain linear combinations of each of the data vectors, $a_t(k) = \boldsymbol{\xi}_k' \mathbf{Z}_t$ and $b_t(k) = \boldsymbol{\psi}_k' \mathbf{X}_t$, where $\boldsymbol{\xi}_k \equiv (\xi_k(1), \ldots, \xi_k(m))'$ and $\boldsymbol{\psi}_k \equiv (\psi_k(1), \ldots, \psi_k(\ell))'$. For $k = 1, 2, \ldots, \min\{m, \ell\}$, define the kth *canonical correlation* as

$$r_k \equiv \text{corr}(\boldsymbol{\xi}_k' \mathbf{Z}_t, \boldsymbol{\psi}_k' \mathbf{X}_t) = \frac{\boldsymbol{\xi}_k' \mathbf{C}_{Z,X}^{(0)} \boldsymbol{\psi}_k}{(\boldsymbol{\xi}_k' \mathbf{C}_Z^{(0)} \boldsymbol{\xi}_k)^{1/2} (\boldsymbol{\psi}_k' \mathbf{C}_X^{(0)} \boldsymbol{\psi}_k)^{1/2}}. \tag{5.36}$$

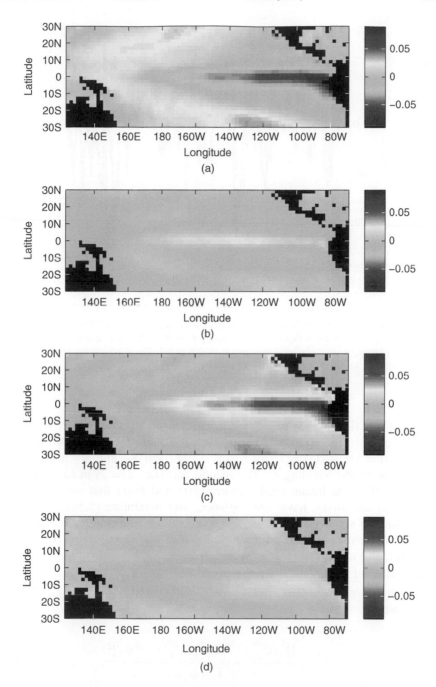

Figure 5.23 Image plots of the POP for the tropical monthly Pacific SST anomalies from January 1970 to December 2002. The POP corresponds to the 10th eigenvalue $\lambda_{\alpha,10} = 0.8677 + 0.0798i$, with damping rate 0.8713 and oscillation period 68.5 months, as shown in Table 5.1. (a) Real part $(\Psi \hat{\mathbf{w}}^R_{\alpha,10})$. (b) Negative imaginary part $(-\Psi \hat{\mathbf{w}}^I_{\alpha,10})$. (c) Negative real part $(-\Psi \hat{\mathbf{w}}^R_{\alpha,10})$. (d) Imaginary part $(\Psi \hat{\mathbf{w}}^I_{\alpha,10})$.

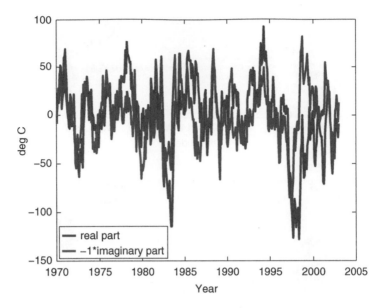

Figure 5.24 Monthly tropical Pacific SST anomaly data. Shown are the POP coefficient time series corresponding to the POPs in Figure 5.23. The real part of the POP coefficient time series is shown in blue and the negative of the imaginary part is shown in red. The y axis shows amplitude in units of $°C$, and the x axis shows time in units of months.

The first pair (i.e., $k = 1$) of canonical variables associated with r_1 are defined as the set of linear combinations, $a_t(1) = \boldsymbol{\xi}_1' \mathbf{Z}_t$ and $b_t(1) = \boldsymbol{\psi}_1' \mathbf{X}_t$, such that $\mathrm{var}(a_t(1)) = \mathrm{var}(b_t(1)) = 1$, for $t = 1, \ldots, T$, and $\boldsymbol{\xi}_1$, and $\boldsymbol{\psi}_1$ maximize the correlation (5.36), yielding r_1. The second pair (i.e., $k = 2$) of canonical variables are then the linear combinations $a_2(t)$ and $b_2(t)$ that are uncorrelated with $a_1(t)$ and $b_1(t)$, have unit variance, and maximize (5.36), yielding r_2. Then, the kth set of canonical variables are the linear combinations $a_t(k)$ and $b_t(k)$ that are uncorrelated with the previous $k - 1$ canonical pairs, have unit variance, and maximize (5.36), yielding r_k.

Initially, let $k = 1$ and note that since $\mathbf{C}_Z^{(0)}$ and $\mathbf{C}_X^{(0)}$ are positive-definite, they can be written as $\mathbf{C}_Z^{(0)} = (\mathbf{C}_Z^{(0)})^{1/2}(\mathbf{C}_Z^{(0)})^{1/2}$ and $\mathbf{C}_X^{(0)} = (\mathbf{C}_X^{(0)})^{1/2}(\mathbf{C}_X^{(0)})^{1/2}$. Then, we can write

$$r_1^2 = \frac{[\tilde{\boldsymbol{\xi}}_1'(\mathbf{C}_Z^{(0)})^{-1/2}\mathbf{C}_{Z,X}^{(0)}(\mathbf{C}_X^{(0)})^{-1/2}\tilde{\boldsymbol{\psi}}_1]^2}{(\tilde{\boldsymbol{\xi}}_1'\tilde{\boldsymbol{\xi}}_1)(\tilde{\boldsymbol{\psi}}_1'\tilde{\boldsymbol{\psi}}_1)}, \tag{5.37}$$

where $\tilde{\boldsymbol{\xi}}_1 \equiv (\mathbf{C}_Z^{(0)})^{1/2}\boldsymbol{\xi}_1$ and $\tilde{\boldsymbol{\psi}}_1 \equiv (\mathbf{C}_X^{(0)})^{1/2}\boldsymbol{\psi}_1$. The problem is now reduced to finding $\tilde{\boldsymbol{\xi}}_1$ and $\tilde{\boldsymbol{\psi}}_1$ that maximize (5.37). It can be shown (e.g., Johnson and Wichern, 1992, p. 463) that r_1^2 is the largest singular value of the singular value decomposition of the cross-correlation matrix,

$$(\mathbf{C}_Z^{(0)})^{-1/2}\mathbf{C}_{Z,X}^{(0)}(\mathbf{C}_X^{(0)})^{-1/2}, \tag{5.38}$$

where $\tilde{\boldsymbol{\xi}}_1$ and $\tilde{\boldsymbol{\psi}}_1$ are the left and right singular vectors corresponding to r_1^2, respectively. Consequently, we can obtain $\boldsymbol{\xi}_1$ and $\boldsymbol{\psi}_1$ through $\boldsymbol{\xi}_1 \equiv (\mathbf{C}_Z^{(0)})^{-1/2}\tilde{\boldsymbol{\xi}}_1$ and $\boldsymbol{\psi}_1 \equiv (\mathbf{C}_X^{(0)})^{-1/2}\tilde{\boldsymbol{\psi}}_1$, respectively. These are called the first CCA patterns, and they can be mapped on their respective regions. We can also obtain the time series of canonical variables, $a_t(1) \equiv \boldsymbol{\xi}_1'\mathbf{Z}_t$ and $b_t(1) \equiv \boldsymbol{\psi}_1'\mathbf{X}_t$, for $t = 1, \ldots, T$.

In general, $\tilde{\boldsymbol{\xi}}_k$ and $\tilde{\boldsymbol{\psi}}_k$ are the left and right singular vectors, respectively, associated with the kth singular value r_k^2 from the singular value decomposition of (5.38). Then, for $k > 1$, $\boldsymbol{\xi}_k$, $\boldsymbol{\psi}_k$, $\{a_t(k)\}$, and $\{b_t(k)\}$ can be obtained analogously to the $k = 1$ case.

To calculate the singular value decomposition in (5.38), empirical covariance matrices, $\hat{\mathbf{C}}_Z^{(0)}$, $\hat{\mathbf{C}}_X^{(0)}$, and $\hat{\mathbf{C}}_{Z,X}^{(0)}$, are needed. These are given by (5.1) and (5.4), as discussed in Section 5.1.3. Then, the empirical singular values and singular vectors are obtained from the singular value decomposition of $(\hat{\mathbf{C}}_Z^{(0)})^{-1/2}\hat{\mathbf{C}}_{Z,X}^{(0)}(\hat{\mathbf{C}}_X^{(0)})^{-1/2}$. The CCA from these matrices is often unsatisfactory because the empirical covariance matrices are noisy (or singular) when calculated with sample sizes common in many spatio-temporal applications. To compensate for this, the data are often projected onto a truncated set of EOFs, just as in Section 5.5.1, before applying the singular value decomposition (e.g., von Storch and Zwiers, 1999, Chapter 4). As in Section 5.5.1 for POPs, we get a benefit from the reduction of spatial dimension; this is necessary for computational stability or if $\min\{m, \ell\} > T$ (otherwise, the method-of-moments estimate of (5.38) is undefined).

Example: To illustrate the exploratory application of CCA to spatio-temporal datasets, consider the tropical Pacific SST anomalies (Section 5.1), averaged over January through March (JFM) for each year from 1970 through 1999, as well as a dataset from the U.S. Fish and Wildlife Service Breeding Population Survey (BPS). Different from the BBS, the BPS is based on yearly aerial surveys that seek to assess the breeding population of waterfowl in North America. This survey has been conducted each year (since 1955) and consists of 18-mile linear segments (1/4 mile wide) over which the aircraft pilot and an observer count and speciate the waterfowl population. For this example, we consider "raw indicated pair count" data for Mallards from 1970 through 1999. The "indicated pair counts" consist of pairs (male and female) and "lone drakes" (individual males). Although there is clearly detection error in these counts, we ignore such error for this exploratory spatio-temporal data analysis. In addition, for simplicity of illustration, we only consider the ℓ BPS sampling locations for which there were no missing data for each of the 30 years from 1970 through 1999.

Figure 5.25 shows a spatial map of the empirical means and standard deviations of these counts at each of these sampling locations over the period of interest. We note that the largest average counts (and variability) occur in the center portion of the flyway. From a biological standpoint, one expects to see persistence in waterfowl breeding location as individuals tend to return to their natal landscape for breeding (i.e., "site philopatry"). However, there is inherent spatial variability in indicated pair counts since wetland and upland habitat

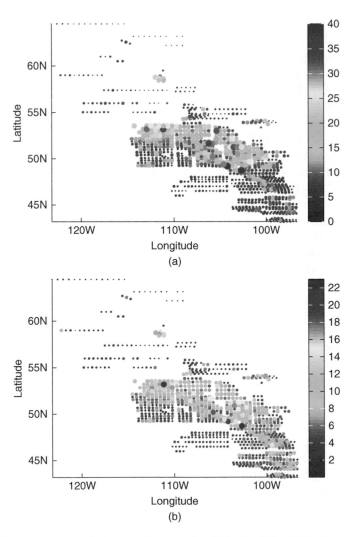

(a)

(b)

Figure 5.25 Summaries of indicated pair counts for Mallards, 1970–1999, obtained from the Breeding Population Survey; the region shown is the Prairie Pothole region of North America, and the color and radius of the circles are proportional to the size of each quantity plotted. (**a**) Averages taken over years. (**b**) Standard deviations taken over years.

conditions vary across the landscape. In addition, the waterfowl may fly over their natal landscape if the conditions are poor in any given year (e.g., in a drought), imposing temporal variability in breeding counts. Thus, one might hypothesize that since there is a strong connection between tropical Pacific SST conditions and the weather over North America (i.e., there is a *teleconnection* over large distances), there might be some evidence of a relationship between tropical Pacific SST anomalies and BPS counts. Therefore, we compare the average of the JFM SST anomalies from 1970 to 1999, to the BPS counts for the same period. The JFM period was chosen for the SST data, since the habitat conditions encountered by the migrating waterfowl would be determined from weather conditions in the late winter to early spring.

Figure 5.26 shows the first CCA patterns for both tropical Pacific SST anomalies and BPS counts. Figure 5.27 shows the time series associated with these patterns. These figures suggest that the relatively cooler ocean anomalies extending from the western Pacific up to the northern tropical Pacific (as well as cooler than normal SSTs off the coast of South America) are correlated with increased Mallard pair counts in the area centered on 110° W and between 50° and 55° N, as well as decreased counts in the area between 100° and 110° W and around 50° N. The two time series of canonical variables shown

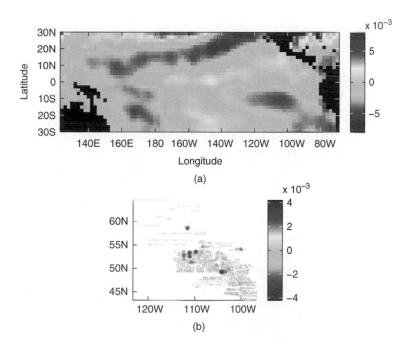

Figure 5.26 Yearly tropical Pacific SST anomaly data based on January–March averages, and yearly indicated pair counts for Mallards from the Breeding Population Survey. (a) First CCA pattern for SST anomalies. (b) First CCA pattern for the Mallard indicated pair counts. The CCA patterns are unitless.

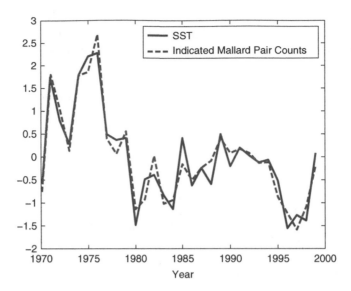

Figure 5.27 Time series of first canonical variables for yearly SST anomalies (blue solid line) and for yearly indicated pair counts for Mallards (red dashed line), associated with Figure 5.26. The x axis shows time in yearly increments. The time series are unitless (since CCA is based on correlations).

in Figure 5.27 show a very strong relationship (the canonical correlation is 0.96) and they both show decade-scale oscillations with their associated CCA patterns.

5.6.2 Time-Lagged CCA

When only one dataset (say $\{\mathbf{Z}_t : t = 1, \ldots, T\}$) is considered, the CCA technique can be used to find the canonical correlation patterns between $\mathbf{Z}_t$ and $\mathbf{Z}_{t-\tau}$, for some time lag τ. In this case, we obtain the vectors $\boldsymbol{\xi}_k$ and $\boldsymbol{\psi}_k$ such that the marginal correlation between $a_t(k) \equiv \boldsymbol{\xi}_k' \mathbf{Z}_t$ and $b_{t-\tau}(k) \equiv \boldsymbol{\psi}_k' \mathbf{Z}_{t-\tau}$ is maximized. To do this, we obtain the kth left and right singular vectors from the singular value decomposition applied to $(\mathbf{C}_Z^{(0)})^{-1/2} \mathbf{C}_Z^{(\tau)} (\mathbf{C}_Z^{(0)})^{-1/2}$, where $\mathbf{C}_Z^{(\tau)}$ is the lag-τ cross-covariance matrix of $\{\mathbf{Z}_t\}$, which is assumed to be temporally stationary. Analogous to the two-field CCA previously described, to obtain $\boldsymbol{\xi}_k$ and $\boldsymbol{\psi}_k$ we have to weight the singular vectors obtained from this singular value decomposition by premultiplying them with $(\mathbf{C}_Z^{(0)})^{-1/2}$.

The time-lagged CCA outlined here is similar to the POP analysis discussed in Section 5.5. When considering POPs and time-lagged CCA (for $\tau = 1$), recall that the singular value decomposition must be performed on certain matrices, which we specify below.

$$\text{POP:} \quad \mathbf{C}_Z^{(1)}(\mathbf{C}_Z^{(0)})^{-1}, \tag{5.39}$$

$$\text{CCA:} \quad (\mathbf{C}_Z^{(0)})^{-1/2}\mathbf{C}_Z^{(1)}(\mathbf{C}_Z^{(0)})^{-1/2}. \tag{5.40}$$

Clearly, these two matrices are similar in that they include some form of the lag-one covariance matrix and the inverse of the lag-zero covariance matrix. It is straightforward to show that the singular values are the same for the decomposition of (5.39) and (5.40) and that the singular vectors from the CCA decomposition (5.40) are equivalent to those from the POP decomposition (5.39) scaled by the matrix $(\mathbf{C}_Z^{(0)})^{-1/2}$.

5.7 SPATIO-TEMPORAL FIELD COMPARISONS

There are numerous instances in spatio-temporal statistical analysis where there is strong interest in comparing two spatio-temporal "fields." This might occur when comparing the output from two models (deterministic or statistical), comparing a historical forecast to the actual observations (or some smooth representation of them), or comparing model output/data for two or more time periods. For the purposes of this exposition, consider two spatio-temporal datasets represented by the $m \times T$ matrices, $\mathbf{Z} \equiv (\mathbf{Z}_1, \ldots, \mathbf{Z}_T)$ and $\mathbf{X} \equiv (\mathbf{X}_1, \ldots, \mathbf{X}_T)$.

There is a substantial literature on field comparison in the context of forecast verification in the atmospheric sciences (e.g., see the overview in Wilks, 2006, Chapter 7). Given that weather forecasters are often judged by the accuracy of their forecasts, there is a definite need for objective and quantitative forecast-verification methodologies to compare a forecasted field to the field that was subsequently observed. One such measure, commonly used by statisticians as well, is the *root mean squared error* (RMSE), which can be defined as (e.g., Briggs and Levine, 1997),

$$\text{RMSE} \equiv \frac{\| \mathbf{Z} - \mathbf{X} \|_F}{\sqrt{mT}},$$

where $\| \cdot \|_F$ is the Frobenius (i.e., Euclidean) norm. (The matrix $\mathbf{B} \equiv (b_{ij})$ has Frobenius norm, $\|\mathbf{B}\|_F \equiv \{\sum_i \sum_j b_{ij}^2\}^{1/2}$.)

Another commonly used measure is the *anomaly correlation coefficient* (ACC), which is the average gridpoint correlation between the anomalies from the two fields [where the anomalies are relative to some common underlying field, $\mathbf{C}$ (e.g., climatology)]. For example, Briggs and Levine (1997) write it as

$$\text{ACC} \equiv \frac{tr\{(\mathbf{Z} - \mathbf{C})'(\mathbf{X} - \mathbf{C})\}}{\| \mathbf{Z} - \mathbf{C} \|_F \| \mathbf{X} - \mathbf{C} \|_F}.$$

Such simple univariate summaries are not typically sufficient to describe the differences between fields. For example, the ACC measures the average linear association between the fields but does not account for the bias, whereas the RMSE does not take into account the linear association but is a good measure of average accuracy (Murphy, 1995; Briggs and Levine, 1997).

There are different approaches to obtaining more information about the fields. A classic analysis in this regard is the paper by Preisendorfer and Barnett (1983). In this case, they also consider the Frobenius norm between the two matrices but, more importantly, they show that this norm can be decomposed as the sum of three terms (i.e., "trinity statistics") that relate to the difference in the centroids of the two spatio-temporal fields, their variability, and their evolution patterns. Significance tests can then be developed for these measures using a permutation procedure. One can also examine these measures across different spatial or temporal scales. For example, Branstator, Mai, and Baumhefner (1993) consider EOF-based diagnostics to compare fields by spatial scale. Similarly, Briggs and Levine (1997) use discrete wavelet transforms to decompose field verification measures. Direct comparison of *thresholded* fields through summary measures were given by Zhang, Craigmile, and Cressie (2008).

The methods described above provide overall summary statistics of the "difference" between two fields, but they are often unsatisfactory when comparing "spatially coherent" aspects. A spatial comparison of two fields was given by Shen, Huang, and Cressie (2002), who used the notion of false discovery rate in wavelet space to declare wavelet coefficients present or absent in the differenced field. In situations where a *feature* of one map (say a region of precipitation) is compared to another, traditional pixelwise comparisons may yield a poor match if the features are not aligned. It may be that just being able to capture the correct scale or orientation of the feature is suggestive of a "good" forecast, even if the spatial phase is not correct. That is, a forecast may have value even if a traditional field comparison suggests that the fields do not agree. For example, there may be a small location error causing the forecast and "truth" fields to barely overlap. In fact, the forecast might represent the size, shape, and intensity of the feature quite well, and a forecaster with expert knowledge could adjust the forecast to account for the uncertainty in location. Ebert and McBride (2000) describe a field-comparison procedure that differentiated location error from other sources of error. Micheas et al. (2007) extended methodology in morphometrics to field comparisons by using a Procrustes measure to decompose the "difference" in terms of location, scale, rotation angle, and intensity.

5.8 BIBLIOGRAPHIC NOTES

Visualization
The suggestions for data visualization presented in this section are quite simple, but they can be very useful. For example, the Hovmöller diagrams are quite helpful for visualizing propagating features. A more recent perspective on such diagrams can be found in Martius, Schwierz, and Davies (2006). In general, the visualization of statistical data is a topic that is constantly moving forward in response to new computational tools, software, exploratory techniques, and ever-more-complicated models. Chen, Hardle, and Unwin (2008)

and Carr and Pickle (2010) contain comprehensive and recent overviews of many of these methods. An older, but still quite useful, reference is Wegman and Carr (1993). The application and modification of these methods to the case of spatio-temporal data will be an exciting research topic in coming years.

Notice that the estimation of covariance matrices discussed in this section is covered in detail in almost any text that describes multivariate time series (e.g., Lütkepohl, 2005). In addition, estimation in the spatio-temporal geophysical context is discussed in von Storch and Zwiers (1999, Chapter 12).

Anselin (1995) defined the concept of local indicators of spatial association. A recent overview can be found in Lloyd (2007, Section 4.2.1). The foundations of visualizing multivariate data with parallel coordinates (PC) plots can be found in Inselberg (1985) and Wegman (1990). A recent example that considers spatio-temporal data can be found in Edsall (2003). A relatively recent overview of PC plots for spatial data can be found in Longley et al. (2005, Chapter 15).

Spectral Analysis

Cross-spectral analysis of time series is described in most advanced books on time-series analysis (e.g., Shumway and Stoffer, 2006; see also the Bibliographic Notes in Section 3.7). The data analysis by Wikle, Madden, and Chen (1997) illustrates how one can use a combination of cross-spectral analyses to make inference on propagating features in spatio-temporal datasets. Spatiotemporal spectral analysis (or *frequency–wavenumber analysis*) is summarized in von Storch and Zwiers (1999, Section 11.5).

EOFs

The definitive reference to EOFs is the monograph by Preisendorfer (1988). Additional general discussion from the geophysical perspective can be found in von Storch and Zwiers (1999) and Wilks (2006). The definitive monograph in Statistics that considers EOFs is Jolliffe (2002). In addition, any book on multivariate statistics (e.g., Johnson and Wichern, 1992) considers the closely related topic of principle components analysis.

In the meteorological literature, one finds extensive use of EOFs since their introduction by Lorenz (1956). For example, they have been used for describing climate (e.g., Kutzbach, 1967; Barnett, 1977), for comparing simulations of general circulation models (e.g., Preisendorfer and Barnett, 1983), for developing regression forecast techniques (e.g., Peagle and Haslam, 1982), in weather classification (e.g., Christensen and Bryson, 1966), in map typing (e.g., Richman, 1981), in the interpretation of geophysical fields (Obled and Creutin, 1986), and in the simulation of random fields, particularly nonhomogeneous processes (Braud and Obled, 1991). In addition, as in the psychometric literature for PCAs and as advocated by Richman (1981, 1986) and others, orthogonal and oblique rotation of EOFs often aids in the interpretation of spatio-temporal data (e.g., see Wilks, 2006, Section 11.5; Jolliffe, 2002, Chapter 11).

Because EOFs have difficulty resolving traveling-wave disturbances, complex EOF analysis was introduced by Wallace and Dickinson (1972) and was shown to be very useful in applications to certain meteorological problems (e.g., Wallace, 1972; Barnett, 1983; Horel, 1984). For an overview from the geophysical perspective, see von Storch and Zwiers (1999, Chapter 16). From a statistical perspective, Brillinger (2001, Chapter 9) derives principal components in the frequency domain. We note that the notion of *extended EOF analysis* is related to so-called *singular spectrum analysis (SSA)*, which considers principal components of an augmented data vector made up of lagged values from a univariate time series (e.g., Elsner and Tsonis, 1996; Jolliffe, 2002, Section 12.2.1). Indeed, in the case where one considers augmented vectors made up of lagged values from a multivariate dataset, then so-called *multichannel SSA (MSSA)* is equivalent to extended EOF analysis.

Although calculation of EOFs were obtained through the empirical covariance matrix, we note that it is equivalent to calculate EOFs through a singular value decomposition of the (centered) data matrix (e.g., von Storch and Zwiers, 1999, Section 13.2.9). In some software implementations, it may be more efficient to calculate them by this approach.

In cases where there is missing information or basis functions are needed for locations that are not observed, one can "shrink" the empirical covariance estimates to some parametric-based covariance matrix (e.g., Nott and Dunsmuir, 2002), or do likewise in the spectral domain (Daniels and Cressie, 2001). Alternatively, one can implement a preliminary smoothing procedure and then estimate the covariance matrix (e.g., Wikle and Cressie, 1999).

POPs

Principal Oscillation Patterns (POPs) were originally formulated as a specific case of Principal Interaction Patterns (PIPs) developed by Hasselmann (1988). POPs were reformulated by von Storch et al. (1988). Subsequently, there was a substantial increase in the number of POP applications in the literature and a comprehensive overview of POPs can be found in von Storch et al. (1995) and von Storch and Zwiers (1999). A recent example of the use of POPs in an ecological context to study the growth dynamics of shortleaf pine trees is given in Hooten and Wikle (2007).

The notion of complex POP (CPOP) analysis was introduced by Bürger (1993) as an extension of conventional POP analysis. Bürger notes that while POP analysis is able to model *traveling oscillations*, it is unable to model *standing oscillations*. In fact, he shows the inherent impossibility of modeling standing oscillations in first-order linear dynamical systems. Thus, CPOP analysis is a natural extension to POP analysis, in some ways analogous to the relationship between EOFs and CEOFs. That is, CEOFs are able to detect traveling disturbances, which cannot be detected by EOFs; and CPOPs can detect standing oscillations, which cannot be detected by POPs.

Traditional time-series-analysis techniques (including the vector-autoregression case that is analogous to POPs) require an assumption of second-order temporal stationarity (i.e., constant mean with autocorrelation depending only on time lag). This assumption clearly breaks down when the physical process under consideration has known cycles (e.g., solar-influenced annual and semiannual cycles in atmospheric processes). In that case, the mean and variance (at least) are also periodic. Traditionally, these cycles are removed, and then it is hoped that the stationarity assumption is satisfied. Often, there is still evidence of nonstationarity, at least with regard to the variance. However, from a statistical perspective, it makes sense to use the redundant information contained in the periodically correlated statistics (i.e., cyclostationarity) optimally, rather than to remove it. An excellent discussion of the analysis of periodically correlated atmospheric time series can be found in Lund et al. (1995). Blumenthal (1991) first published the idea of using periodically correlated statistics in the POP framework; the approach is summarized in von Storch et al. (1995).

A more general decomposition that accounts for the variation in the data (EOFs) as well as the dynamics (POPs) is the *predictive oscillation pattern* methodology of Kooperberg and O'Sullivan (1996).

CCA

Canonical correlation analysis is described in detail in almost any text that covers multivariate statistics (e.g., Johnson and Wichern, 1992; Jolliffe, 2002). In the geophysical context, excellent overviews are contained in von Storch and Zwiers (1999) and Wilks (2006).

We note that Bretherton, Smith, and Wallace (1992) performed a comparison of methods for finding coupled patterns in climate data (including CCA and multivariate EOFs) and were supportive of a variant of CCA known (unfortunately) as Singular Value Decomposition (SVD). This is related to, but not the same as, the well known matrix-algebra technique of the same name. In this regard, von Storch and Zwiers (1999, Section 14.1.7) suggest that since this "SVD" approach effectively finds patterns that maximize the *covariance* between spatio-temporal fields, it is more appropriate to call this *maximum covariance analysis*. Some authors (e.g., Cherry, 1997) have pointed out that there are difficulties with the interpretation of CCA and "SVD" results, particularly the tendency for the methods to produce spurious spatial patterns. Nevertheless, the approach can be a useful exploratory tool with multivariate spatio-temporal data. In the atmospheric sciences, CCA has been used in diagnostic climatological studies (e.g., Glahn, 1968; Nicholls, 1987; Barnett and Preisendorfer, 1987), in the forecast of El Niño (Graham and Michaelsen, 1987; Barnston and Ropelewski, 1992), and in the forecast of long-range temperature and precipitation (Barnston, 1994).

The time-lagged CCA approach outlined here is similar to the POP analysis and to the minimum/maximum autocorrelation factor (MAF) analysis (Shapiro and Switzer, 1989; Cressie and Helterbrand, 1994; Solow, 1994). In the MAF case, one is interested in the eigenvectors proportional to those obtained from the singular value decomposition of $(\mathbf{C}_Z^{(0)})^{-1}\mathbf{V}$, where the matrix $\mathbf{V}$ is the first-difference covariance matrix given by $\mathbf{V} \equiv E[(\mathbf{Z}_t - \mathbf{Z}_{t-1})(\mathbf{Z}_t - \mathbf{Z}_{t-1})']$.

Field Comparisons

Spatio-temporal field comparison can borrow techniques and motivation from the forecast-verification literature (e.g., see von Storch and Zwiers, 1999, Chapter 18; Wilks, 2006, Chapter 7, and the references therein). Although a significant portion of that literature is related to categorical and probabilistic forecast *skill measures*, there is also a substantial component of the literature devoted to continuous-variable field comparisons. The methods of Preisendorfer and Barnett (1983) are particularly useful for spatio-temporal datasets. In addition, the review by Wigley and Santer (1990) contains many univariate and multivariate measures that are useful across a broad range of applications. We note that, given the statistical dependence usually found in spatio-temporal datasets, most of the methods of comparison rely on resampling or Monte Carlo tests (e.g., Stanford and Ziemke, 1994). Field comparisons based on "objects" have seen substantial development in the last few years (e.g., Hoffman et al., 1995; Ebert and McBride, 2000; Micheas et al., 2007). In addition, measures that explicitly account for distributional forecasts (or ensembles) are the subject of much interest (see Wilks, 2006, Section 7.7.1; Micheas et al., 2007).

A closely related area to field comparisons has developed out of what is known as "optimal fingerprint" analysis in the study of climate change (e.g., Hasselmann, 1979, 1993). It was developed for "distinguishing between the anticipated externally generated time-dependent climate-change signal and the natural internal variability of the climate system" (Hasselmann, 1993, p. 1957). This methodology has been extended into a Bayesian framework by Leroy (1998) and by Berliner, Levine, and Shea (2000).

CHAPTER 6

Spatio-Temporal Statistical Models

Nearby values tend to be more alike than those far apart; this chapter explores this notion, where "nearby" refers to being proximal in both space and time. Let $\{Y(\mathbf{s}; t) \colon \mathbf{s} \in D_s, t \in D_t\}$ denote a spatio-temporal random process that is a statistical model for a phenomenon evolving through the spatio-temporal index set $D_s \times D_t$. For example, $Y(\mathbf{s}; t)$ might be the air pressure at time t and at geographical coordinates $\mathbf{s} = (\text{latitude, longitude, height})'$; conceptually, $D_s = $ sphere $\times \mathbb{R}$ and $D_t = \mathbb{R}$. Or, $Y(\mathbf{s}; t)$ might be the yearly breast-cancer incidence rate in each of the 88 counties of Ohio; conceptually, $D_s = \{\mathbf{s}_1, \ldots, \mathbf{s}_{88}\}$, the set of centroids of each county, and D_t is a subset of the positive integers (denoting years). There may also be instances where the spatio-temporal index set should be written more generally as $D_{s,t}$, to account for temporally evolving spatial index sets or curved reference frames (see Einsteinian physics in Chapter 1).

In this book, we emphasize *dynamical* spatio-temporal statistical models, because we believe that the holy grail of Science, namely the discovery of causation, is within our grasp when we model how current process values have evolved from past process values. In cases where scientific understanding is not available to develop a dynamical spatial statistical model, a *descriptive* statistical model based on first- and second-order moments (means, variances, and covariances) can be developed. Because the dynamical models typically yield first- and second-order moments, the descriptive models are mathematically more general but are scientifically less interpretable.

The dynamical statistical approach is built from *conditional* probability distributions, modeling how the current value $Y(\mathbf{s}; t)$ behaves given the behavior of "nearby" current and past values taken from the set $\{Y(\mathbf{x}; r) \colon \mathbf{x} \in D_s, r < t\} \cup \{Y(\mathbf{x}; t) \colon \mathbf{x} \neq \mathbf{s}\}$. These conditional-probability specifications come from scientific knowledge. In the absence of adequate knowledge, the data can still provide information about the spatio-temporal variability, and this is typically achieved through *descriptive* models based on *marginal* probability distributions. An example of this difference in approach to statistical modeling occurs in linear mixed models, where one chooses to either (a) make explicit the random components through conditional probability distributions or (b) make explicit the mean vector and covariance matrix through marginal probability distributions.

Since marginal probabilities can be obtained from weighted integrals of conditional probabilities, models based on conditional probabilities are closer to the etiology of the phenomenon under study. Indeed, different physical processes could imply the same marginal probabilities; see the example given at the beginning of Section 4.2, where a symmetric spatial process is matched to a unilateral spatial process. That is, the etiology of the phenomenon under study can be masked by using a first- and second-order-moment description. Nevertheless, descriptive spatio-temporal statistical models based on marginal probability distributions do have a place when the modeler's knowledge is limited. Otherwise, our preference is to build dynamical spatio-temporal models based on conditional probability distributions.

Physical Statistical Models

When there is scientific knowledge about a process Y, it can often be described in terms of a partial differential equation (PDE), sometimes in time, sometimes in space, and sometimes in both. Heine (1955) considers such equations in two dimensions—in particular, the general second-order, linear, nonstochastic PDE:

$$\left\{ a \frac{\partial^2}{\partial u^2} + 2h \frac{\partial^2}{\partial u \partial v} + b \frac{\partial^2}{\partial v^2} + 2g \frac{\partial}{\partial u} + 2f \frac{\partial}{\partial v} + c \right\} Y(u, v) = 0.$$

He shows that by simple changes of variables, this PDE reduces to several special cases.

Parabolic: $\quad \left\{ \left(\frac{\partial}{\partial u} + \alpha \right)^2 - \gamma^2 \left(\frac{\partial}{\partial v} \pm \beta \right) \right\} Y(u, v) = 0,$

Elliptic: $\quad \left\{ \left(\frac{\partial}{\partial u} - \alpha \right)^2 + \frac{\partial^2}{\partial v^2} \pm \gamma^2 \right\} Y(u, v) = 0,$

Hyperbolic: $\quad \left\{ \left(\frac{\partial}{\partial u} + \alpha \right) \left(\frac{\partial}{\partial y} + \beta \right) \pm \gamma^2 \right\} Y(u, v) = 0,$

Degenerate: $\quad \left\{ \gamma \frac{\partial^2}{\partial v^2} + \alpha \frac{\partial}{\partial v} \pm \beta \right\} Y(u, v) = 0,$

where α, β, and γ are generic, nonnegative parameters.

A nonstochastic (or deterministic) PDE can be converted into a *stochastic* PDE by replacing 0 on the PDE's right-hand side with a (mean-zero) stochastic term. In a remarkable early contribution to the Statistics literature, Hotelling (1927) investigated a number of one-dimensional (in time) stochastic PDEs.

Heine (1955) did the same thing in two dimensions, based on the equations given above; here, we write the stochastic term in the PDE as $\delta(u, v)$, where $\delta(\cdot, \cdot)$ is a mean-zero, two-dimensional stochastic process that models either (a) random impulses from smaller-order contributions or (b) uncertainty in the scientific relationship expressed through the PDE. The resulting equation is an example of a *physical statistical model* (Berliner, 2003). Clearly, the process $Y(\cdot, \cdot)$ is now a stochastic process, and its moments are of interest. Because $E(\delta(u, v)) \equiv 0$, linearity of the PDE implies that $E(Y(u, v)) \equiv 0$. What is $\text{cov}(Y(u, v), Y(p, q))$?

The two-dimensional co-ordinates (u, v) could be purely spatial or they could be spatio-temporal. We consider the case of a spatial u and a temporal v, and we define the spatio-temporal process $\{Y(s; t): s \subset D_s \subset \mathbb{R}, t \in D_t \subset \mathbb{R}\}$ according to a stochastic PDE that is, for illustration, parabolic. In particular, we consider the spatio-temporal process presented by Heine (1955) and Jones and Zhang (1997), which is governed by the following *stochastic* PDE:

$$\frac{\partial Y(s; t)}{\partial t} - \beta \frac{\partial^2 Y(s; t)}{\partial s^2} + \alpha Y(s; t) = \delta(s; t), \tag{6.1}$$

where $\alpha > 0$, $\beta > 0$, and $\delta(\cdot; \cdot)$ is an *error process* that is random and has mean zero. Clearly, a $Y(\cdot; \cdot)$ that satisfies (6.1) is an example of a dynamical spatio-temporal statistical model.

Whittle (1963) considers the same class, but where **s** is more generally a spatial location in $\mathbb{R}^d$ (see also Section 6.3.1). These models were called *diffusion-injection models* by Whittle (1986, p. 431), and we shall adopt that terminology here ("injection" here refers to injection of variability from the random component δ). In all that follows in this chapter, $\delta(\cdot; \cdot)$ is assumed to be a spatio-temporal process with mean zero, independent in time, and potentially dependent in space (at any fixed time). The special case of independence in space corresponds to the covariance structure, $\text{cov}(\delta(s; t), \delta(x; r)) = \sigma_\delta^2 I(s = x, t = r)$, which is white noise in $\mathbb{R}^1$.

The *deterministic* PDE associated with (6.1) is, using obvious shorthand,

$$\frac{\partial Y}{\partial t} = \beta \frac{\partial^2 Y}{\partial s^2} - \alpha Y, \tag{6.2}$$

which is a homogeneous reaction-diffusion model (homogeneous because every term contains the dependent variable, Y, or its derivatives). In (6.2), it is understood that the partial derivatives are evaluated at s and t. The equation specifies that the rate of change in Y is equal to the "spread" of Y in space (diffusion) offset by the "loss" of a certain multiple of Y (reaction). From a given initial condition, $Y(s; 0)$, the process $Y(\cdot; \cdot)$ governed by the deterministic PDE (6.2) dampens to zero as time t increases, which is not a very realistic behavior for many dynamical processes seen in nature (e.g., meteorological processes). Figure 6.1 shows several plots of $Y(s; t)$ defined by (6.2), as a function of space s and time t, for different choices of α and β. (The solutions shown in Figure 6.1 are obtained numerically.)

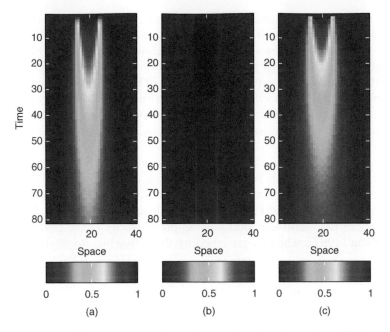

Figure 6.1 Several plots of $Y(s; t)$ defined by the deterministic reaction-diffusion equation described in (6.2), as a function of space s and time t for different choices of α and β: **(a)** $\alpha = 1$, $\beta = 20$; **(b)** $\alpha = 0.05$, $\beta = 0.05$; **(c)** $\alpha = 1$, $\beta = 50$. The starting values are $Y(s; 0) = 1$ for $15 \leq s \leq 24$, and 0 otherwise. (The solutions are obtained numerically for $s \in D_s \equiv \{\Delta_s, 2\Delta_s, \ldots, 40\Delta_s\}$, where $\Delta_s = 1$, and $t \in D_t \equiv \{\Delta_t, 2\Delta_t, \ldots, 80\Delta_t\}$, where $\Delta_t = 0.1$.)

By including the random process $\delta(\cdot; \cdot)$ in (6.1), a statistical balance is reached between (a) the "disturbance" caused by $\delta(\cdot; \cdot)$ and (b) the smoothing effect of both the diffusion component and the loss component. That is, from a given initial condition, the stochastic PDE results in a process that eventually achieves both spatial and temporal stationarity. Figure 6.2 shows several simulations of $Y(s; t)$ defined by the stochastic PDE (6.1), for $\alpha = 1$, $\beta = 20$, δ is white noise, and different choices of its variance σ_δ^2; these should be compared to Figure 6.1a, the (numerical) solution of the corresponding deterministic PDE.

Typically, stochastic PDEs like those considered by Heine (1955) are difficult to deal with analytically. In the case of the stochastic PDE (6.1), Heine (1955) shows that $Y(\cdot; \cdot)$ has a stationary covariance function $C_Y(\cdot; \cdot)$, and he derives an analytical expression for the corresponding spatio-temporal correlation function: For $h \in \mathbb{R}$ and $\tau \in \mathbb{R}$, we obtain

$$C_Y(h; \tau)/C_Y(0; 0) \equiv \rho_Y(h; \tau)$$

$$= (1/2) \left\{ e^{-h(\alpha/\beta)^{1/2}} Erfc \left(\frac{2\tau(\alpha/\beta)^{1/2} - h/\beta}{2(\tau/\beta)^{1/2}} \right) \right.$$

$$\left. + e^{h(\alpha/\beta)^{1/2}} Erfc \left(\frac{2\tau(\alpha/\beta)^{1/2} + h/\beta}{2(\tau/\beta)^{1/2}} \right) \right\}, \qquad (6.3)$$

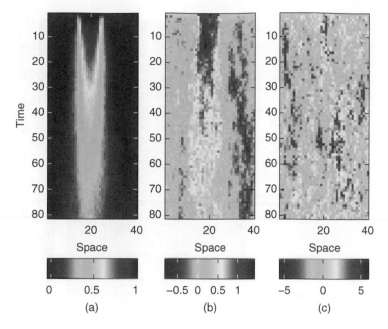

Figure 6.2 Simulations of $Y(s;t)$ defined by the stochastic PDE (6.1) as a function of space $s \in D_s$ and time $t \in D_t$, and δ is mean-zero white noise with variance σ_δ^2. The same $\alpha = 1$, $\beta = 20$, and starting values, $Y(s;0)$, as in Figure 6.1a are used: **(a)** $\sigma_\delta = 0.01$, **(b)** $\sigma_\delta = 0.1$, and **(c)** $\sigma_\delta = 1$.

where $Erfc(z)$ is the "complementary error function,"

$$Erfc(z) \equiv (2/\pi^{1/2}) \int_z^\infty e^{-v^2} dv, \qquad z \geq 0,$$

and for $z < 0$, $Erfc(z) = 2 - Erfc(-z)$. Figure 6.3 shows a contour plot of $\rho_Y(h;\tau)$ given by (6.3) as a function of spatial lag h and temporal lag τ, for $\alpha = 1$ and $\beta = 20$ (the same parameter values used in Figure 6.1a and Figure 6.2).

Special cases include the spatial correlation function at a given time:

$$\rho_Y(h;0) = e^{-h(\alpha/\beta)^{1/2}}, \qquad h > 0, \tag{6.4}$$

and the temporal correlation function at a given spatial location:

$$\rho_Y(0;\tau) = Erfc(\tau^{1/2}\alpha^{1/2}), \qquad \tau > 0. \tag{6.5}$$

Figure 6.4a shows a plot of $\rho_Y(h;0)$ given by (6.4) as a function of spatial lag h, and Figure 6.4b shows a plot of $\rho_Y(0;\tau)$ given by (6.5) as a function of temporal lag τ; both figures are for $\alpha = 1$ and $\beta = 20$, as in Figure 6.2.

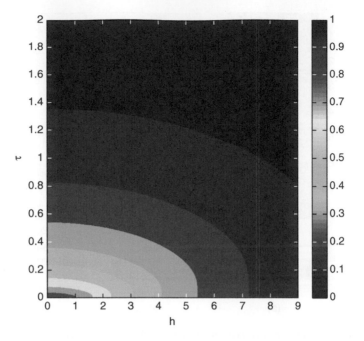

Figure 6.3 Contour plot of $\rho_Y(h; \tau)$ defined in (6.3) as a function of spatial lag h and temporal lag τ; $\alpha = 1$ and $\beta = 20$.

The stochastic PDEs considered above are second-order linear. Whittle (1963) discussed the more general case of

$$\mathcal{L}Y(\mathbf{s}; t) = \delta(\mathbf{s}; t),$$

where $\mathcal{L}$ is a linear operator. The spatial version of this is $\mathcal{L}Y(\mathbf{s}) = \delta(\mathbf{s})$; $\mathbf{s} \in D_s \subset \mathbb{R}^d$. He gives the example

$$\left\{ \frac{\partial^2}{\partial s_1^2} + \cdots + \frac{\partial^2}{\partial s_d^2} - \alpha^2 \right\}^p Y(\mathbf{s}) = \delta(\mathbf{s}), \qquad (6.6)$$

where $\mathbf{s} = (s_1, \ldots, s_d)'$, $\delta(\cdot)$ is a mean-zero, white-noise process in $\mathbb{R}^d$ (i.e., $\mathrm{cov}(\delta(\mathbf{s}), \delta(\mathbf{x})) = \sigma_\delta^2 I(\mathbf{s} = \mathbf{x}))$, and the linear operator on the left-hand side is a fractional Laplacian (of fraction p) defined through its Fourier representation (e.g., Fuentes, Chen, and Davis, 2008). Upon reparameterizing, $\theta_1 = 1/\alpha > 0$, $\theta_2 = 2p - d/2 > 0$ (i.e., restrict $p > d/4$), Whittle (1963) shows that the (spatial, stationary, isotropic) covariance function of $Y(\cdot)$ defined by (6.6) is given by

$$C_Y(\mathbf{h}) \propto \{\|\mathbf{h}\|/\theta_1\}^{\theta_2} K_{\theta_2}(\|\mathbf{h}\|/\theta_1), \qquad (6.7)$$

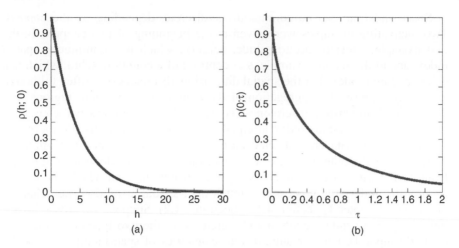

Figure 6.4 (a) Plot of marginal spatial correlation $\rho_Y(h; 0)$, given in (6.4), as a function of spatial lag h; $\alpha = 1$ and $\beta = 20$. (b) Plot of marginal temporal correlation $\rho_Y(0; \tau)$, given in (6.5), as a function of temporal lag τ; $\alpha = 1$ and $\beta = 20$.

where K_{θ_2} is a modified Bessel function of the second kind of order θ_2 (e.g., Abramowitz and Stegun, 1964, pp. 374–379). The covariance function (6.7) is known as the *Matérn covariance function*; see (4.6).

We now discuss some initial data analysis that addresses the question of whether there is spatio-temporal dependence in the dataset under study. Griffith (1988) considered the Space–Time Index (STI) as a type of Moran's I statistic for the spatio-temporal setting. Suppose that there are m spatial locations $\mathbf{s}_1, \ldots, \mathbf{s}_m$, at each of which there are T mean-corrected observations, $\{Z(\mathbf{s}_i; t) : i = 1, \ldots, m; t = 1, \ldots, T\}$. Henebry (1995) discussed the properties of

$$
\mathrm{STI} \equiv \frac{m(T-1) \sum_{t=2}^{T} \sum_{j=1}^{m} \sum_{i=1}^{m} w_{ij,t-1} Z(\mathbf{s}_i; t) Z(\mathbf{s}_j; t-1)}{(\sum_{t=2}^{T} \sum_{j=1}^{m} \sum_{i=1}^{m} w_{ij,t-1})(\sum_{t=1}^{T} \sum_{i=1}^{m} Z(\mathbf{s}_i; t)^2)},
$$

where $\{w_{ij,t}\}$ are spatio-temporal weights indicating spatial "neighborliness" at each snapshot of time.

The permutation distribution of STI (i.e., permute the locations $\{\mathbf{s}_i : i = 1, \ldots, m\}$ and the time points $\{1, 2, \ldots, T\}$, and recompute STI for each permutation) serves as a baseline for the variability of STI under the null hypothesis (H_0) of *no* spatio-temporal dependence. An initial check to see whether it is worthwhile fitting a spatio-temporal model to data could be carried out as follows: Generate the permutation distribution of STI, which is very computationally intensive. Observe where the actual *observed* STI falls in the distribution generated. If it is below the $100(\alpha/2)$th percentile or above the $100(1 - \alpha/2)$th percentile, then reject H_0 at the $100(1 - \alpha)\%$ significance level. Practically speaking, a rejection of H_0 means that the spatio-temporal dependence is present and a spatio-temporal model is needed.

Space and time can be continuous or discrete, depending on the context. Two motivating examples were given at the beginning of this chapter: In the first example, $\mathbf{s}$ =(latitude, longitude, height)$'$, which is a continuous spatial index; and in the second example, $\mathbf{s}$ = centroid of a county in Ohio, which is a discrete spatial index. For the spatial dimension, discreteness is often (although not always) caused by aggregation of the continuous index into regions. For the temporal dimension, discreteness is often (although not always) caused by sampling the continuous index at equally spaced time intervals. Furthermore, it could be that data are collected based on one type of index but inference is desired for the other type. For example, the problem of downscaling comes from having data for a given, coarse spatial resolution, from which one wishes to infer the underlying process at a much finer spatial resolution (i.e., change-of-support; Chapter 1, Section 4.1.3, Section 7.1.2). Suppose we cross-classify the two types of index (continuous/discrete) with the two types of dimension (spatial/temporal), which results in four categories of spatio-temporal models. Where appropriate, we shall mention the category to which a given model belongs. For the temporal index, we use a notational prop: When time is continuous, an element of the spatio-temporal process is written as $Y(\mathbf{s}; t)$, and when time is discrete, an element of the spatio-temporal process is written as $Y_t(\mathbf{s})$.

Spatio-temporal covariance functions offer a succinct but informative summary of random processes on $D_s \times D_t$. Indeed, it is very common to consider the covariance function as a characterization of the spatio-temporal process $Y(\cdot; \cdot)$. An example given in Chapter 1 for Gaussian processes shows that modeling based purely on the covariance function is ambiguous with respect to the model's dynamics. In this chapter, we discuss spatio-temporal covariance modeling (based on marginal probabilities), along with dynamical modeling (based on conditional probabilities). It is worth reemphasizing that, when possible, we prefer to work with dynamical models directly, where the etiology of the phenomenon is at its most apparent and causative effects can be incorporated. In that sense, this chapter is a bridge between the exploratory methods presented in Chapter 5 and the dynamical spatio-temporal HMs presented in Chapter 7.

6.1 SPATIO-TEMPORAL COVARIANCE FUNCTIONS

To motivate spatio-temporal covariance functions in cases where the dynamical structure is unknown, write the spatio-temporal process $Y(\cdot; \cdot)$ as

$$Y(\mathbf{s}; t) \equiv \mu(\mathbf{s}; t) + \beta(\mathbf{s}) + \gamma(t) + \kappa(\mathbf{s}; t) + \delta(\mathbf{s}; t), \qquad \mathbf{s} \in D_s, \quad t \in D_t, \tag{6.8}$$

which is similar to the mixed-effects model discussed by Wikle (2003a). In (6.8), $\mu(\mathbf{s}; t)$ is a *deterministic* mean; $\beta(\mathbf{s})$ is a mean-zero *random* effect representing location-specific variability common to all times; $\gamma(t)$ is a mean-zero *random* effect representing time-specific variability common to all locations; $\kappa(\mathbf{s}; t)$ is a mean-zero *random* effect capturing the spatio-temporal interaction not found in the larger-scale deterministic $\mu(\mathbf{s}; t)$; $\delta(\mathbf{s}; t)$ is a mean-zero *random* effect representing the microscale spatio-temporal variability that is modeled by white noise in $D_s \times D_t$; and all random effects are mutually statistically independent. To make the exposition simple, we present (6.8) as a continuous-space, continuous-time model. Further, the second-order moments are written as

$$\text{cov}(\beta(\mathbf{s}), \beta(\mathbf{x})) \equiv C_\beta(\mathbf{s}, \mathbf{x}) \tag{6.9}$$

$$\text{cov}(\gamma(t), \gamma(r)) = C_\gamma(t, r) \tag{6.10}$$

$$\text{cov}(\kappa(\mathbf{s}; t), \kappa(\mathbf{x}; r)) \equiv C_\kappa(\mathbf{s}, \mathbf{x}; t, r) \tag{6.11}$$

$$\text{var}(\delta(\mathbf{s}; t)) \equiv \sigma_\delta^2. \tag{6.12}$$

Covariance models for (6.9) can be found in Chapter 4, covariance models for (6.10) can be found in Chapter 3, and covariance models for (6.11) are discussed at length in this section.

We now present some examples of (6.8), where, for simplicity, we assume that the deterministic mean $\mu(\mathbf{s}; t) \equiv 0$. Using marginal probabilities, we calculate the resulting spatio-temporal covariance functions, although we note that there is a conditional-probability interpretation of (6.8); see Section 6.6.

Regional-Effects Model (Reinsel et al., 1981; Bloomfield et al., 1983)
Suppose that $Y(\cdot; \cdot)$ can be written as

$$Y(\mathbf{s}; t) = \gamma(t) + \kappa_k(t) + \delta(\mathbf{s}; t), \qquad \mathbf{s} \in D_s^{(k)}, \tag{6.13}$$

where D_s is made up of mutually exclusive regions $\{D_s^{(k)} : k = 1, \ldots, K\}$. The random effect, $\kappa_k(t)$, is a "regional" component of variation *common* to all locations $\mathbf{s}$ in the kth region $D_s^{(k)}$; they are independent for $k = 1, \ldots, K$. Suppose that all random effects are white noise:

$$\text{var}(\gamma(t)) \equiv \sigma_\gamma^2, \qquad \text{var}(\kappa_k(t)) \equiv \sigma_\kappa^2, \qquad \text{var}(\delta(\mathbf{s}; t)) = \sigma_\delta^2. \tag{6.14}$$

This model results in temporal independence but induces "block" spatial covariances. For all t, we have

$$\text{cov}(Y(\mathbf{s}; t), Y(\mathbf{x}; t)) = \begin{cases} \sigma_\gamma^2 + \sigma_\kappa^2 + \sigma_\delta^2, & \text{if } \mathbf{s} = \mathbf{x} \\ \sigma_\gamma^2 + \sigma_\kappa^2, & \text{if } \mathbf{s}, \mathbf{x} \in D_s^{(k)}, \ \mathbf{s} \neq \mathbf{x}; \\ & k = 1, \ldots, K \\ \sigma_\gamma^2, & \text{otherwise.} \end{cases} \tag{6.15}$$

The contribution of Bloomfield et al. (1983) was to augment the spatio-temporal random effect, $\kappa_k(t)$ in (6.13), with another spatio-temporal random effect $\eta(\cdot; \cdot)$ that exhibits temporal correlation. Suppose that

$$Y(\mathbf{s}; t) \equiv \gamma(t) + \kappa_k(t) + \eta(\mathbf{s}; t) + \delta(\mathbf{s}; t), \qquad (6.16)$$

where for *all* t, r:

$$\operatorname{cov}(\eta(\mathbf{s}; t), \eta(\mathbf{x}; r)) = \begin{cases} \sigma_\eta^2, & \text{if } \mathbf{s} = \mathbf{x}, \\ C_\eta(\mathbf{s}, \mathbf{x}), & \text{if } \mathbf{s} \neq \mathbf{x}. \end{cases} \qquad (6.17)$$

Then (6.15) is generalized to become

$$\operatorname{cov}(Y(\mathbf{s}; t), Y(\mathbf{x}; r)) = \begin{cases} \sigma_\gamma^2 + \sigma_\kappa^2 + \sigma_\eta^2 + \sigma_\delta^2, & \text{if } \mathbf{s} = \mathbf{x}, \\ \sigma_\gamma^2 + \sigma_\kappa^2 + C_\eta(\mathbf{s}, \mathbf{x}), & \text{if } \mathbf{s}, \mathbf{x} \in D_s^{(k)}, \mathbf{s} \neq \mathbf{x}; \\ & k = 1, \dots, K, \\ \sigma_\gamma^2 + C_\eta(\mathbf{s}, \mathbf{x}), & \text{otherwise.} \end{cases}$$
$$(6.18)$$

Mixture Model (Oehlert, 1993)

Consider the expression (6.8), with (6.9) given by $C_\beta(\mathbf{s}, \mathbf{x}) = \sigma_\beta^2 I(\mathbf{s} = \mathbf{x})$, and (6.11) given by a separable covariance, $C_\kappa(\mathbf{s}, \mathbf{x}; t, r) = C_\kappa^{(s)}(\mathbf{s}, \mathbf{x}) \cdot C_\kappa^{(t)}(t, r)$. Then

$$\operatorname{cov}(Y(\mathbf{s}; t), Y(\mathbf{x}; r))$$
$$= \begin{cases} \sigma_\beta^2 + C_\gamma(t, t) + C_\kappa^{(s)}(\mathbf{s}, \mathbf{s}) \cdot C_\kappa^{(t)}(t, t) + \sigma_\delta^2, & \text{if } \mathbf{s} = \mathbf{x}, t = r, \\ C_\gamma(t, r) + C_\kappa^{(s)}(\mathbf{s}, \mathbf{x}) \cdot C_\kappa^{(t)}(t, r), & \text{otherwise.} \end{cases} \qquad (6.19)$$

When C_γ, $C_\kappa^{(s)}$, and $C_\kappa^{(t)}$ in (6.19) are stationary (in space or time), we obtain the type of mixture models proposed by De Iaco, Myers, and Posa (2001); see (6.30) below.

Invariant-Temporal-Covariance Model (Stein, 1986)

Consider (6.8) with $\gamma(t) \equiv 0$, and (6.11) given by the temporally invariant covariance function, $C_\kappa(\mathbf{s}, \mathbf{x}; t, r) \equiv C_\kappa^{(s)}(\mathbf{s}, \mathbf{x})$, which is exactly the same model form as (6.17). Then

$$\operatorname{cov}(Y(\mathbf{s}; t), Y(\mathbf{x}; r)) = \begin{cases} C_\beta(\mathbf{s}, \mathbf{s}) + C_\kappa^{(s)}(\mathbf{s}, \mathbf{s}) + \sigma_\delta^2, & \text{if } \mathbf{s} = \mathbf{x}, t = r, \\ C_\beta(\mathbf{s}, \mathbf{x}) + C_\kappa^{(s)}(\mathbf{s}, \mathbf{x}), & \text{otherwise.} \end{cases}$$
$$(6.20)$$

The two spatial covariance functions, C_β and $C_\kappa^{(s)}$, are not identifiable in this model; to deal with this, Stein (1986) assumes that they are individually specified.

The spatio-temporal covariance functions above are representative of models in the early spatio-temporal statistics literature. More recently, there has been considerable development of large classes of spatio-temporal covariance functions; the rest of this section presents an overview.

6.1.1　Theoretical Properties

A covariance function is a *nonnegative-definite function*, and vice versa. Therefore, investigating nonnegative-definite functions in space and time has been an important endeavor in spatio-temporal statistics.

Definition 6.1. A function $\{f(\mathbf{u}, \mathbf{v}) : \mathbf{u}, \mathbf{v} \in D\}$ defined on $D \times D$ is said to be *nonnegative-definite*, if for any complex numbers $\{a_i : i = 1, \ldots, m\}$, any $\{\mathbf{u}_i : i = 1, \ldots, m\}$ in D, and any integer m, we have

$$\sum_{i=1}^{m} \sum_{j=1}^{m} a_i \overline{a}_j f(\mathbf{u}_i, \mathbf{u}_j) \geq 0, \tag{6.21}$$

where recall that $\overline{a}$ denotes the complex conjugate of a.

Positive-definiteness of $f(\cdot, \cdot)$ involves the inequality above being strictly positive whenever $\mathbf{a} \equiv (a_1, \ldots, a_m)'$ is a nonzero vector. In this book, we shall be considering, almost exclusively, covariance functions that are positive-definite. We now give some examples of D.

If D is a subset of the integers $\mathbb{Z}$, f is a (temporal) covariance function for a discrete-index time series (Chapter 3), and if $D \subset \mathbb{R}^d$, then f is a (spatial) covariance function for a continuous-index spatial process (Chapter 4). In the spatio-temporal setting, D could be a subset of $\mathbb{R}^d \times \{\ldots, -1, 0, 1, \ldots\}$ or of $\mathbb{R}^d \times \mathbb{R}$. Hence, a spatial covariance function in $\mathbb{R}^{d+1}$ (see Chapter 4) could serve as a spatio-temporal covariance function in $\mathbb{R}^d \times \mathbb{R}$. In (6.21), we write $\mathbf{u} = (\mathbf{s}; t)$ and $f(\mathbf{u}_i, \mathbf{u}_j) \equiv f((\mathbf{s}_i; t_i), (\mathbf{s}_j; t_j))$, to obtain a spatio-temporal covariance function.

6.1.2　Stationarity in Space or Time

Definition 6.2. We say that f is a *stationary spatio-temporal covariance function* on $\mathbb{R}^d \times \mathbb{R}$, if it satisfies Definition 6.1 and can be written as

$$f((\mathbf{s}; t), (\mathbf{x}; r)) = C(\mathbf{s} - \mathbf{x}; t - r), \qquad \mathbf{s}, \mathbf{x} \in \mathbb{R}^d, \ t, r \in \mathbb{R}.$$

If a random process $Y(\cdot; \cdot)$ has a constant expectation and a stationary covariance function, $C_Y(\mathbf{h}; \tau)$, then it is said to be *second-order (or weakly) stationary*. Strong stationarity of $Y(\cdot; \cdot)$ corresponds to the equivalence of the two probability measures defining the random processes $Y(\cdot; \cdot)$ and $Y(\cdot + \mathbf{h}; \cdot + \tau)$, respectively, for all $\mathbf{h} \in \mathbb{R}^d$ and all $\tau \in \mathbb{R}$.

When there is no ambiguity, we drop dependence on Y and write simply, $C(\mathbf{h}; \tau)$, unless clarity demands otherwise. Upon rewriting (6.21) in terms of $C(\cdot; \cdot)$, we see that the defining property of a stationary spatio-temporal covariance function $C(\cdot; \cdot)$ on $\mathbb{R}^d \times \mathbb{R}$ becomes

$$\sum_{i=1}^{m} \sum_{j=1}^{m} a_i \bar{a}_j C(\mathbf{s}_i - \mathbf{s}_j; t_i - t_j) \geq 0,\qquad (6.22)$$

for any $\{a_i\}$, any $\{(\mathbf{s}_i; t_i)\}$, and any m. Notice that $C(\mathbf{h}; 0)$, $\mathbf{h} \in \mathbb{R}^d$, corresponds to a stationary spatial covariance function and that $C(\mathbf{0}; \tau)$, $\tau \in \mathbb{R}$, corresponds to a stationary temporal covariance function.

The *stationary spatio-temporal correlation function* associated with $C(\cdot; \cdot)$ is

$$\rho(\mathbf{h}; \tau) \equiv C(\mathbf{h}; \tau)/C(\mathbf{0}; 0), \qquad \mathbf{h} \in \mathbb{R}^d, \ \tau \in \mathbb{R},\qquad (6.23)$$

an example of which is given by (6.3). The correlation function (6.23) represents spatio-temporal dependence in a continuous-space ($\mathbb{R}^d$), continuous-time ($\mathbb{R}$) model.

The intuitive notion that values tend to be weakly correlated when they are "far apart" can be captured by using covariance functions that tend to zero as their spatio-temporal coordinates move farther apart. Covariance models are often used that are identically zero when separated by more than a fixed distance in space or in time; these are sometimes referred to as *compactly supported* covariances.

It is possible that stationarity of the covariance function be considered separately for space and time. *Spatial stationarity* of the covariance function corresponds to

$$\text{cov}(Y(\mathbf{s}; t), Y(\mathbf{x}; r)) \equiv C(\mathbf{s} - \mathbf{x}; t, r),$$

and *temporal stationarity* of the covariance function corresponds to

$$\text{cov}(Y(\mathbf{s}; t), Y(\mathbf{x}; r)) \equiv C(\mathbf{s}, \mathbf{x}; t - r).$$

Recall that *spatio-temporal stationarity* of the covariance function corresponds to

$$\text{cov}(Y(\mathbf{s}; t), Y(\mathbf{x}; r)) \equiv C(\mathbf{s} - \mathbf{x}; t - r).$$

Now we turn our attention to isotropy. Similar to spatial stationarity, *spatial isotropy* corresponds to

$$\text{cov}(Y(\mathbf{s}; t), Y(\mathbf{x}; r)) \equiv C(\|\mathbf{s} - \mathbf{x}\|; t, r).$$

Geometric spatial anisotropy corresponds to

$$\text{cov}(Y(\mathbf{s}; t), Y(\mathbf{x}; r)) \equiv C(\{p_1(s_1 - x_1)^2 + \cdots + p_d(s_d - x_d)^2\}^{1/2}; t, r),$$

where $p_1 > 0, \ldots, p_d > 0$. Finally, *geometric spatio-temporal anisotropy* corresponds to

$$\text{cov}(Y(\mathbf{s}; t), Y(\mathbf{x}; r)) = C(\{p_1(s_1 - x_1)^2 + \cdots + p_d(s_d - x_d)^2 + q(t - r)^2\}^{1/2}),$$

where $p_1 > 0, \ldots, p_d > 0,\ q > 0$.

6.1.3 Separability and Full Symmetry

Definition 6.3. A random process $Y(\cdot; \cdot)$ is said to have a *separable spatio-temporal covariance function* if, for all $\mathbf{s}, \mathbf{x} \in \mathbb{R}^d$, $t, r \in \mathbb{R}$, we obtain

$$\text{cov}(Y(\mathbf{s}; t), Y(\mathbf{x}; r)) = C^{(s)}(\mathbf{s}, \mathbf{x}) \cdot C^{(t)}(t, r), \qquad (6.24)$$

where $C^{(s)}$ and $C^{(t)}$ are spatial and temporal covariance functions, respectively.

As a consequence of (6.24), a simple class of spatio-temporal covariance functions is given by the *product* of individual spatial and temporal covariance functions. When $C^{(s)}$ and $C^{(t)}$ are, respectively, spatially and temporally stationary, (6.24) becomes

$$C(\mathbf{h}; \tau) = C^{(s)}(\mathbf{h}) \cdot C^{(t)}(\tau), \qquad \mathbf{h} \in \mathbb{R}^d,\ \tau \in \mathbb{R}. \qquad (6.25)$$

Also, separability implies that the spatio-temporal correlation function $\rho(\cdot; \cdot)$ given by (6.23) satisfies

$$\rho(\mathbf{h}; \tau) = \rho(\mathbf{h}; 0) \cdot \rho(0; \tau), \qquad \mathbf{h} \in \mathbb{R}^d,\ \tau \in \mathbb{R}. \qquad (6.26)$$

Clearly the converse is true, and hence (6.26) is a characterization of separability in second-order stationary processes. This is a nice result that allows one to make a visual inspection of whether separability holds, by *comparing* the contours of $C(\mathbf{h}; \tau)$ with those of $C(\mathbf{h}; 0) \cdot C(0; \tau)$. Figure 6.5a is an example of (6.26), where we chose the same parameter values, $\alpha = 1$ and $\beta = 20$, that were used in Figure 6.2. In the figure, $\rho(h; 0)$ is given by (6.4), and $\rho(0; \tau)$ is given by (6.5). By contrast, Figure 6.5b shows the corresponding spatio-temporal correlation function (6.3) derived from (6.1); this is the same correlation function shown in Figure 6.3. A comparison of the contours in Figure 6.5b with those in Figure 6.5a shows that the diffusion-injection model given by (6.1) does *not* yield a separable covariance function. This is usually the case; spatio-temporal models constructed dynamically (i.e., causally) often have important components of spatio-temporal interaction, for which a separable covariance function is inadequate.

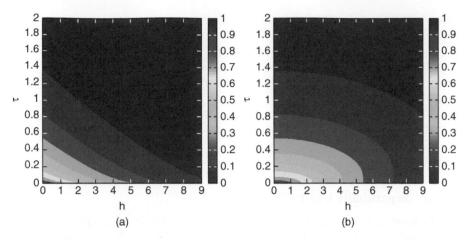

Figure 6.5 **(a)** Contour plot of separable correlation function, given by (6.26), as a function of spatial lag h and temporal lag τ; $\alpha = 1$ and $\beta = 20$. **(b)** Contour plot of nonseparable correlation function (6.3); $\alpha = 1$, $\beta = 20$. (This is for comparison to **(a)**, and it is the same plot as given in Figure 6.3.)

Because of their ease of definition, and because (matrix) computations in spatial statistical analysis can be much simpler, separable covariance models dominated the literature up until the beginning of the twenty-first century. But, they have very particular properties that are rarely seen in empirical studies of spatio-temporal dependence. For example, separability implies that $C(\mathbf{h}_1; \tau) \propto C(\mathbf{h}_2; \tau)$; $\tau \in \mathbb{R}$, which means that each time series has *identical* cross-correlational properties with any other time series at *any* displaced location, both near and far! Likewise, $C(\mathbf{h}; \tau_1) \propto C(\mathbf{h}; \tau_2)$; $\mathbf{h} \in \mathbb{R}^d$. The resulting contour lines for a separable $\{C(\mathbf{h}; \tau): \mathbf{h} \in \mathbb{R}^d, \tau \in \mathbb{R}\}$ show a remarkably regular structure.

To illustrate this, Figure 6.6 shows spatial and temporal profiles of the plots in Figure 6.5. That is, plots of $\rho(\cdot; \tau_i)$ for *separable* $\rho(\cdot; \cdot)$ given by (6.26) and different values of τ_i are shown in Figure 6.6a. Similar plots of $\rho(h_i; \cdot)$ for *separable* $\rho(\cdot; \cdot)$ given by (6.26) and different values of h_i are shown in Figure 6.6b. The corresponding profile plots for *nonseparable* $\rho(\cdot; \cdot)$ given by (6.3) are shown in Figures 6.6c and 6.6d, respectively. Upon comparing Figure 6.6a with Figure 6.6c, and Figure 6.6b with Figure 6.6d, we see the rather regular structure that separability imposes on the profile plots.

Another property of spatio-temporal covariance functions that is sometimes assumed, but which is usually not appropriate, particularly when modeling flow processes, is *full symmetry*.

Definition 6.4. A random process $Y(\cdot; \cdot)$ is said to have a *fully symmetric spatio-temporal covariance function* if, for all $\mathbf{s}, \mathbf{x} \in \mathbb{R}^d$, $t, r \in \mathbb{R}$,

$$\text{cov}(Y(\mathbf{s}; t), Y(\mathbf{x}; r)) = \text{cov}(Y(\mathbf{s}; r), Y(\mathbf{x}; t)). \qquad (6.27)$$

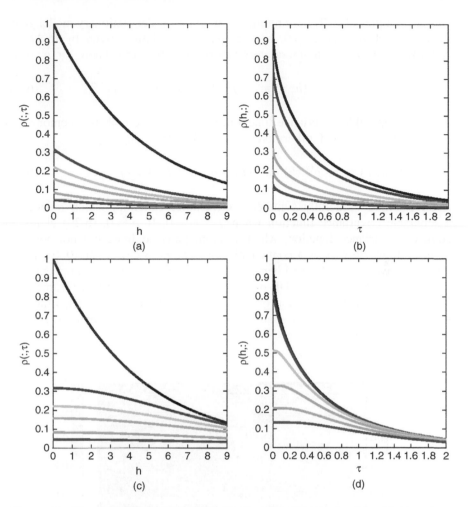

Figure 6.6 Top panels (**a**) and (**b**) show a *separable* correlation function: (**a**) Plot of sep arable correlation function described in (6.26), versus spatial lag h, for temporal lags $\{\tau_i\} = \{0, 0.5, 0.75, 1.0, 1.5, 2.0\}$; $\alpha = 1$, $\beta = 20$. (**b**) Plot of separable correlation function described in (6.26), versus temporal lag τ, for spatial lag $\{h_i\} = \{0, 1, 3, 5, 7, 9\}$; $\alpha = 1$, $\beta = 20$. Bottom panels (**c**) and (**d**) show a *nonseparable* correlation functon: (**c**) Plot of nonseparable correlation function described in (6.3), versus spatial lag h, for the same temporal lags as in (**a**); $\alpha = 1$, $\beta = 20$. (**d**) Plot of nonseparable correlation function described in (6.3), versus temporal lag τ, for the same spatial lags as in (**b**); $\alpha = 1$, $\beta = 20$.

If Y is a variable like (the average maximum and minimum) daily temperature, (6.27) would say that the covariance between yesterday's temperature in St. Louis, MO, and today's temperature in Columbus, OH, is identical to that between yesterday's temperature in Columbus, and today's temperature in St. Louis. Because St. Louis is west of Columbus, this would be an unlikely spatio-temporal covariance model for daily local temperatures.

For examples of (6.27), we return to the second-order-stationary model given by (6.3). Let $\rho^{(s)}(h)$; $h \geq 0$, be the spatial correlation given by (6.4) and $\rho^{(t)}(\tau)$; $\tau \geq 0$, be the temporal correlation given by (6.5). Then, for $p > 0$,

$$C(h; \tau) \equiv p \cdot \rho^{(s)}(h) \cdot \rho^{(t)}(\tau), \tag{6.28}$$

defines a separable covariance function. Indeed, Figure 6.4b is a contour plot of (6.28) with $p = 1$. Furthermore, for $p > 0$, $q \geq 0$, and $r \geq 0$,

$$C(h; \tau) \equiv p \cdot \rho^{(s)}(h) \cdot \rho^{(t)}(\tau) + q \cdot \rho^{(s)}(h) + r \cdot \rho^{(t)}(\tau) \tag{6.29}$$

is an example of a fully symmetric covariance function, which reduces to a separable covariance function when $q = r = 0$. If $p = 0$, (6.29) yields an additive covariance function, which is nonnegative-definite but not positive-definite. Figure 6.7 gives a contour plot of $\rho(h; \tau) \equiv C(h; \tau)/C(0; 0)$, where $C(\cdot; \cdot)$ is given by (6.29) and hence is fully symmetric; chosen parameters are $p = q = r = 1/3$, and the PDE parameters are $\alpha = 1$ and $\beta = 20$ (same as in Figure 6.2). Further discussion of covariance functions like (6.29), which are sums and products of purely spatial or temporal covariance functions, is given below in Section 6.1.4.

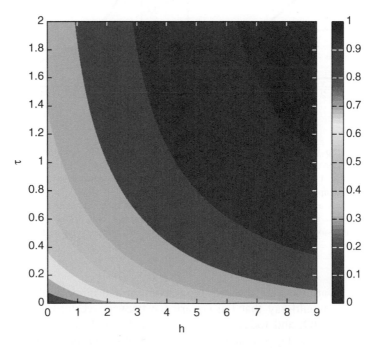

Figure 6.7 Contour plot of fully symmetric correlation function derived from (6.29); $\alpha = 1$, $\beta = 20$, and $p = q = r = \frac{1}{3}$.

Notice that, in general, the class of processes whose covariances are separable, are contained within the class of processes whose covariances are fully symmetric. Figure 6.8 shows several simulations from a mean-zero, stationary, Gaussian, spatio-temporal process with nonseparable covariance function proportional to (6.3); Figure 6.9 shows several simulations corresponding to the fully symmetric covariance function given by (6.29) with $p = q = r = 1/3$; and Figure 6.10 shows several simulations corresponding to the separable covariance function given by (6.28) with $p = 1$. All figures use the same PDE parameters, $\alpha = 1$ and $\beta = 20$ (as in Figure 6.2), the same respective random number seeds, and they are calibrated to correspond to covariances with the same variance, $C(0; 0)$. Notice how difficult it is to distinguish between processes with nonseparable, fully symmetric, and separable covariance functions simply by inspecting their *realizations*. Yet, the difference between the spatio-temporal *covariance functions* shown in Figure 6.3 (nonseparable), Figure 6.7 (fully symmetric), and Figure 6.5a (separable), is apparent.

Because separability implies full symmetry, rejection of the hypothesis of full symmetry implies rejection of the hypothesis of separability. Statistical testing procedures, where the null hypothesis is either separability or is full symmetry, have been considered by Mitchell, Genton, and Gumpertz (2005), Scaccia and Martin (2005), Fuentes (2006), Li, Genton, and Sherman (2007), and Crujeiras, Fernandez-Casal, and González-Manteiga (2010).

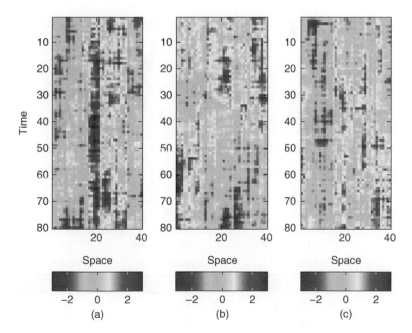

(a)   (b)   (c)

Figure 6.8 The three independent simulations shown in (**a**), (**b**), and (**c**) are from a stationary Gaussian process with mean zero and nonseparable covariance function proportional to (6.3). Here, $s \in D_s \equiv \{\Delta_s, \ldots, 40\Delta_s\}$ with $\Delta_s = 1$, and $t \in D_t \equiv \{\Delta_t, \ldots, 80\Delta_t\}$ with $\Delta_t = .01$.

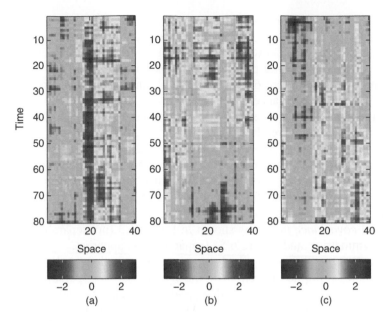

Figure 6.9 The three independent simulations shown in (**a**), (**b**), and (**c**) are from a stationary Gaussian process with mean zero and fully symmetric covariance function given by (6.29); D_s and D_t are the same as in Figure 6.8.

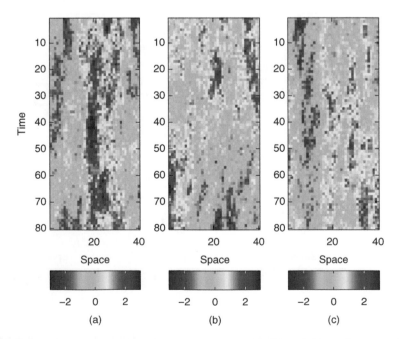

Figure 6.10 The three independent simulations shown in (**a**), (**b**), and (**c**) are from a stationary Gaussian process with mean zero and separable covariance function given by (6.28); D_s and D_t are the same as in Figure 6.8.

6.1.4 Sums and Products of Covariance Functions

Because the sum of two nonnegative-definite functions is nonnegative-definite, the following function is a valid spatio-temporal covariance function:

$$C(\mathbf{h}; \tau) \equiv pC^{(s_1)}(\mathbf{h}) \cdot C^{(t_1)}(\tau) + qC^{(s_2)}(\mathbf{h}) + rC^{(t_2)}(\tau), \qquad (6.30)$$

where $p > 0$, $q > 0$, and $r > 0$, $C^{(s_1)}$ and $C^{(s_2)}$ are spatial covariance functions, and $C^{(t_1)}$ and $C^{(t_2)}$ are temporal covariance functions. A special case of this covariance function has already been considered in (6.29). The class of covariance functions given by (6.30) was considered by De Iaco, Myers, and Posa (2001), and it can be derived from a general result given by Gneiting, Genton, and Guttorp (2007):

Theorem 6.1. Let μ be a finite, nonnegative measure on a non-empty set Θ. Suppose that for each $\theta \in \Theta$, $C^{(s_\theta)}$ and $C^{(t_\theta)}$ are stationary covariance functions on $\mathbb{R}^d$ and $\mathbb{R}$, respectively, and suppose that $\int_\Theta |C^{(s_\theta)}(\mathbf{0}) \cdot C^{(t_\theta)}(0)| d\mu(\theta) < \infty$. Then,

$$C(\mathbf{h}; \tau) \equiv \int_\Theta C^{(s_\theta)}(\mathbf{h}) \cdot C^{(t_\theta)}(\tau) \, d\mu(\theta), \qquad \mathbf{h} \in \mathbb{R}^d, \ \tau \in \mathbb{R}, \qquad (6.31)$$

is a stationary spatio-temporal covariance function.

We have seen in Section 6.1.3 that separability implies full symmetry; Theorem 6.1 shows that the converse is not true. While each component of the mixture on the right-hand side of (6.31) is separable, and hence fully symmetric, $C(\cdot; \cdot)$ given by (6.31) is not separable; however, it *is* fully symmetric. Finally, (6.30) is a special case of (6.31), since $C^{(s)}(\cdot) = 1$ or $C^{(t)}(\cdot) = 1$ are covariance functions of a random process trivially equal to a single random variable (with unit variance) for all $s \subset D_s$ or all $t \in D_t$, respectively.

6.1.5 Spatio-Temporal Variogram

There is another way to express dependence, related to the covariance function. The *spatio-temporal variogram* of the process $Y(\cdot; \cdot)$ is defined to be

$$\text{var}(Y(\mathbf{s}; t) - Y(\mathbf{x}; r)) \equiv 2\gamma(\mathbf{s}, \mathbf{x}; t, r), \qquad (6.32)$$

along with its stationary version, $2\gamma(\mathbf{h}; \tau)$; $\mathbf{h} \in \mathbb{R}^d$, $\tau \in \mathbb{R}$. The quantity γ is called the *semivariogram*. The process $Y(\cdot; \cdot)$ is said to be *intrinsically stationary*, if it has constant expectation and its variogram is stationary. If $Y(\cdot; \cdot)$ is second-order stationary with (stationary) covariance function $C(\mathbf{h}; \tau)$, then, as in the purely spatial setting (Section 4.1.1), $Y(\cdot; \cdot)$ is intrinsically stationary with semivariogram,

$$\gamma(\mathbf{h}; \tau) = C(\mathbf{0}; 0) - C(\mathbf{h}; \tau), \qquad \mathbf{h} \in \mathbb{R}^d, \ \tau \in \mathbb{R}. \qquad (6.33)$$

Similarly to Section 6.1.2, we can define separately the notions of spatial or temporal intrinsic stationarity, and so on, of the variogram. In general, there is no reason why the space dimension and the time dimension should behave alike.

6.1.6   Spectral Representation

Stationary spatio-temporal covariance functions have a spectral representation, in an analogous manner to the purely spatial (Chapter 4) and purely temporal (Chapter 3) stationary covariance functions. In fact, the spectral representation can be viewed simply as Theorem 4.1 (Bochner's Theorem) in $\mathbb{R}^{d+1}$. Written to emphasize space and time separately, it is

$$C(\mathbf{h}; \tau) = \int \int e^{i\mathbf{h}'\omega + i\tau\xi} \, dF(\omega; \xi), \qquad \mathbf{h} \in \mathbb{R}^d, \ \tau \in \mathbb{R}, \qquad (6.34)$$

where F is a finite, nonnegative, symmetric measure on $\mathbb{R}^d \times \mathbb{R}$, called the *spectral measure*. If the spectral measure can be written as $dF(\omega; \xi) = f(\omega; \xi) \, d\omega d\xi$, then $f(\cdot; \cdot)$ is called the *spectral density*, and $\int f(\omega; \tau) \, d\omega d\tau = C(\mathbf{0}; 0)$. This happens if C is integrable (i.e., $\int \int |C(\mathbf{h}; \tau)| \, d\mathbf{h} d\tau < \infty$), and then the inverse result holds:

$$f(\omega; \xi) = (2\pi)^{-(d+1)} \int \int e^{-i\mathbf{h}'\omega - i\tau\xi} C(\mathbf{h}; \tau) \, d\mathbf{h} d\tau. \qquad (6.35)$$

That is, f is the Fourier transform of C (and C is the inverse Fourier transform of f). Furthermore, nonnegativity of f corresponds to nonnegative-definiteness of C, and the two functions are equivalent ways to represent (second-order stationary) spatio-temporal dependence.

   The spectral representation (6.34) offers a convenient way to construct valid stationary spatio-temporal covariance functions. The essential property of nonnegative-definiteness is difficult to establish directly from its definition but, through Bochner's Theorem, we only have to establish nonnegativity of $f(\cdot; \cdot)$. A related strategy is to start with a family of nonnegative f and take each member's inverse Fourier transform to obtain a family of nonnegative-definite functions C. In the spatio-temporal context, Cressie and Huang (1999) proved the following theorem:

   Theorem 6.2. Suppose that C is a symmetric, continuous, bounded, integrable function on $\mathbb{R}^d \times \mathbb{R}$. Then C is a stationary spatio-temporal covariance function if and only if,

$$\alpha(\boldsymbol{\omega}; \tau) \equiv (2\pi)^{-d} \int e^{-i\mathbf{h}'\boldsymbol{\omega}} C(\mathbf{h}; \tau) \, d\mathbf{h}, \qquad \tau \in \mathbb{R}, \qquad (6.36)$$

is nonnegative-definite in τ, for almost all $\boldsymbol{\omega} \in \mathbb{R}^d$. (Here, "almost all $\boldsymbol{\omega}$" means that nonnegative-definiteness of (6.36) may fail for some $\boldsymbol{\omega} \in \mathbb{R}^d$, but the Lebesgue measure of the set of all such $\boldsymbol{\omega}$ is equal to zero.)

The idea here is that α is only a *one-dimensional* function of τ, for which there are many results for guaranteeing nonnegative-definiteness (e.g., Cressie, 1993, p. 86). One first establishes a suitable family for $\alpha(\boldsymbol{\omega}; \tau)$, where members need only be nonnegative-definite in τ, and $\int |\alpha(\boldsymbol{\omega}; \tau)| \, d\boldsymbol{\omega} < \infty$. Then, for given τ, the inverse Fourier transform of $\alpha(\cdot; \tau)$,

$$C(\mathbf{h}; \tau) \equiv \int e^{i\mathbf{h}'\boldsymbol{\omega}} \alpha(\boldsymbol{\omega}; \tau) \, d\boldsymbol{\omega}, \qquad \mathbf{h} \in \mathbb{R}^d, \tau \in \mathbb{R}, \qquad (6.37)$$

yields a spatio-temporal covariance function. Generally, families constructed in this way will not be separable. (Separability occurs when $\alpha(\boldsymbol{\omega}; \tau) \equiv k(\boldsymbol{\omega}) \cdot \rho(\tau)$.)

Example(Cressie and Huang, 1999): Let

$$\alpha(\boldsymbol{\omega}; \tau) \equiv \exp\{-\|\boldsymbol{\omega}\|^2 |\tau|/4\} \exp\{-\delta\tau^2\} \exp\{-c_0\|\boldsymbol{\omega}\|^2/4\},$$

where $\delta > 0$ and $c_0 > 0$. This satisfies the conditions of Theorem 6.2 and results in the following nonseparable family:

$$C(\mathbf{h}; \tau) = \sigma^2 \exp\{-b^2\|\mathbf{h}\|^2/(a^2\tau^2 + 1)\}/(a^2\tau^2 + 1)^{d/2}, \qquad \mathbf{h} \in \mathbb{R}^d, \tau \in \mathbb{R}, \qquad (6.38)$$

where $\sigma^2 = C(\mathbf{0}; 0)$, and $a \geq 0$ and $b \geq 0$ are scaling parameters for time and space, respectively. Figure 6.11a shows a contour plot of the spatio-temporal covariance function (6.38) in one-dimensional space (i.e., $d = 1$, $a = 2$, $b = 0.2$, and $\sigma^2 = 1$). Figure 6.11b shows a realization from a Gaussian process with mean zero and spatio-temporal covariance function given by (6.38). The smoothness of the realization in space is remarkable, and it is due to the behavior of (6.38) for small $\|\mathbf{h}\|$; notice that it is differentiable in $\|\mathbf{h}\|$ at $\|\mathbf{h}\| = 0$, resulting in smooth sample paths (e.g., Cressie, 1993, p. 60).

Consider the separable spatio-temporal covariance function, $C(\mathbf{h}; 0) \cdot C(\mathbf{0}; \tau)$, where $C(\cdot; \cdot)$ is given by (6.38). (From the discussion in Section 6.1.3, the product is separable and positive-definite.) Figure 6.12a shows a contour plot of this covariance function, and Figure 6.12b shows a realization from the corresponding mean-zero Gaussian process (using the same random number seed as that used in Figure 6.11b). Once again, we see

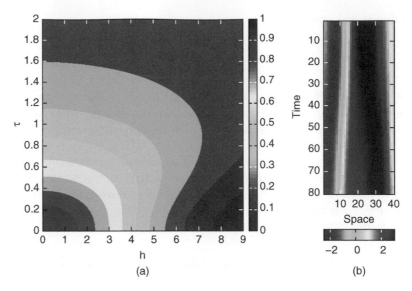

Figure 6.11 (a) Contour plot of the nonseparable covariance function given by (6.38); $d = 1$, $a = 2$, $b = 0.2$, and $\sigma = 1$. (b) Simulation from a stationary Gaussian process with mean zero and the nonseparable covariance function shown in (a). Here, D_s and D_t are the same as in Figure 6.8.

that nonseparability is hard to detect by comparing directly the realizations shown in Figure 6.11b and Figure 6.12b, but their difference is obvious when comparing their covariance functions in Figure 6.11a and Figure 6.12a.

Another construction of $C(\mathbf{h}; \tau)$ based on Theorem 6.2 is due to Gneiting (2002), and his construction does not require integrability of C. He shows that

$$C(\mathbf{h}; \tau) \equiv \sigma^2 \phi(\|\mathbf{h}\|^2/\psi(|\tau|^2))/\{\psi(|\tau|^2)\}^{d/2}, \qquad \mathbf{h} \in \mathbb{R}^d, \ \tau \in \mathbb{R}, \quad (6.39)$$

is a valid spatio-temporal covariance function, provided $\{\phi(x): x \geq 0\}$ is a completely monotone function and $\{\psi(x): x \geq 0\}$ is a positive function with a completely monotone derivative.

Example(Gneiting, 2002): Choose

$$\phi(x) = \exp\{-px^\gamma\}, \qquad x \geq 0, \ p > 0, \ 0 < \gamma \leq 1,$$
$$\psi(x) = (qx^\alpha + 1)^\beta, \qquad x \geq 0, \ q > 0, \ 0 < \alpha \leq 1, \ 0 \leq \beta \leq 1.$$

This results in

$$C(\mathbf{h}; \tau) = \sigma^2 \exp\{-p\|\mathbf{h}\|^{2\gamma}/(q|\tau|^{2\alpha} + 1)^{\beta\gamma}\}/(q|\tau|^{2\alpha} + 1)^{\beta d/2}. \quad (6.40)$$

Suppose we put $\gamma = 1$, $\alpha = 1$, and $\beta = 1$ in (6.40) as a special case; then we obtain the same covariance function given by (6.38) by putting $p = b^2$ and $q = a^2$.

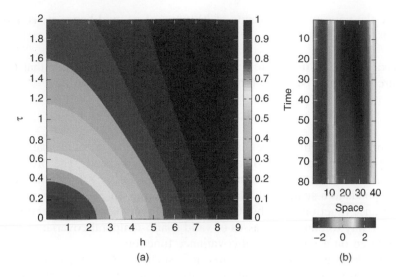

Figure 6.12 (a) Contour plot of the separable covariance function derived from (6.38) as the product of its marginal correlation functions; $d = 1$, $a = 2$, $b = 0.2$, and $\sigma = 1$. (b) Simulation from a stationary Gaussian process with mean zero and the separable covariance function shown in (a). Here, D_s and D_t are the same as in Figure 6.8.

Other examples of $\phi(\cdot)$ and $\psi(\cdot)$ are given by Gneiting (2002) and include, for $x \geq 0$,

$$\phi(x) = (1 + px^\gamma)^{-\nu}; \quad p > 0, \, 0 < \gamma \leq 1, \, \nu > 0,$$

$$\phi(x) = 2^\nu \{\exp(px^{1/2}) + \exp(-px^{1/2})\}^{-\nu}, \qquad p > 0, \, \nu > 0,$$

$$\phi(x) = (2^{\nu-1}\Gamma(\nu))^{-1}(px^{1/2})^\nu K_\nu(px^{1/2}), \qquad p > 0, \, \nu > 0,$$

where $K_\nu(\cdot)$ is a modified Bessel function of the second kind of order ν (e.g., Abramowitz and Stegun, 1964, pp. 374–379), and

$$\psi(x) = (qx^\alpha + r)/(r(qx^\alpha + 1)), \qquad q > 0, \, 0 < r \leq 1, \, 0 < \alpha \leq 1,$$

$$\psi(x) = \log(qx^\alpha + r)/\log(r), \qquad q > 0, \, r > 1, \, 0 < \alpha \leq 1.$$

6.1.7 Taylor's Hypothesis

Sometimes a curious relationship is observed between dependence in space and dependence in time, a relationship that was originally hypothesized for certain processes in fluid dynamics (Taylor, 1938, p. 478).

Definition 6.5. A stationary spatio-temporal covariance function, $C(\mathbf{h}; \tau)$; $\mathbf{h} \in \mathbb{R}^d$, $\tau \in \mathbb{R}$, satisfies *Taylor's hypothesis* if there exists a vector $\mathbf{u}_0 \in \mathbb{R}^d$ such that

$$C(\mathbf{0}; \tau) = C(\mathbf{u}_0\tau; 0), \qquad \tau \in \mathbb{R}, \tag{6.41}$$

where the units of $\mathbf{u}_0$ are (units of $\mathbf{h}$)/(units of τ), and hence $\mathbf{u}_0$ is a velocity vector.

Example: Let $\mathbf{u}_0$ denote a given velocity vector and assume that $C^{(s)}(\cdot)$ is a purely spatial covariance function. Then, it is easy to see that

$$C(\mathbf{h}; \tau) \equiv C^{(s)}(\mathbf{h} - \mathbf{u}_0\tau), \tag{6.42}$$

is nonnegative-definite (Definition 6.1) and hence is a valid spatio-temporal covariance function. It also satisfies Taylor's hypothesis. The process corresponding to (6.42) is sometimes referred to as *Taylor's frozen field*, since it corresponds to a spatial field that moves with constant velocity. Notice that the covariance function given by (6.42) is generally not separable, and it represents another way to construct classes of valid spatio-temporal covariance functions, here based on a purely spatial covariance function.

If $C^o(h)$ is a covariance function in $\mathbb{R}$ such that $C^o(\|\mathbf{h}\|)$ is a valid covariance function in $\mathbb{R}^d$, then the geometrically anisotropic covariance function (Section 6.1.2),

$$C(\mathbf{h}; \tau) \equiv C^o(\{p\|\mathbf{h}\|^2 + q|\tau|^2\}^{1/2}), \qquad \mathbf{h} \in \mathbb{R}^d, \ \tau \in \mathbb{R},$$

where $p > 0$, $q > 0$, is a spatio-temporal covariance function that satisfies Taylor's hypothesis with $\mathbf{u}_0 = (q^{1/2}/p^{1/2}, 0, \ldots, 0)'$. Finally, separable models can satisfy Taylor's hypothesis. Again, let $C^o(\cdot)$ be a covariance function in $\mathbb{R}$ such that $C^o(\|\mathbf{h}\|)$ is a valid covariance function in $\mathbb{R}^d$. Then,

$$C(\mathbf{h}; \tau) \equiv C^o(\|\mathbf{h}\|)C^o(|\tau|), \qquad h \in \mathbb{R}^d, \ \tau \in \mathbb{R},$$

satisfies Taylor's hypothesis with any velocity vector $\mathbf{u}_0$ such that $\|\mathbf{u}_0\| = 1$.

6.1.8 Spatio-Temporal Dynamical Models

While the classes of spatio-temporal covariance functions given in this section are quite flexible and can exhibit interaction between space and time, they are derived from moments of bivariate probability distributions, and hence they play a *descriptive* role in representing the spatio-temporal dependence in the process $Y(\cdot; \cdot)$. That is, it is very difficult to look at a covariance function and determine the etiology of the spatio-temporal process under study. We prefer a dynamical specification of the spatio-temporal process, where the dependence is motivated by the evolution of the physical, chemical, biological, economic, and so on, processes through time and in space; see the examples given in Chapter 9. When the model is built mechanistically, any spatio-temporal covariance function derived from the model will automatically be nonnegative-definite. For example, the stochastic diffusion-injection model (6.1) results in a spatio-temporal covariance function given by the stationary (in space and time) positive-definite function (6.3). This same approach can be taken whether the temporal index t is discrete or continuous; further discussion is given in Section 6.3.1.

6.2 SPATIO-TEMPORAL KRIGING

Apart from characterizing statistical dependencies in space and time, what can spatio-temporal covariance functions be used for? We have already seen in Chapter 4 how optimal linear spatial prediction (kriging) can be formulated based on the processes' spatial statistical dependencies. These are typically quantified through a spatial variogram or a spatial covariance function. In the spatio-temporal context, recall from Section 6.1.5 that the variogram is defined as

$$2\gamma(\mathbf{s}, \mathbf{x}; t, r) \equiv \mathrm{var}(Y(\mathbf{s}; t) - Y(\mathbf{x}; r)), \qquad \mathbf{s}, \mathbf{x} \in \mathbb{R}^d, \ t, r \in \mathbb{R}. \qquad (6.43)$$

The goal of kriging is to predict $Y(\mathbf{s}_0; t_0)$ from incomplete and noisy data. Any unbiased linear predictor, $Y^@(\mathbf{s}_0; t_0)$, of $Y(\mathbf{s}_0; t_0)$, has the property that its mean squared prediction error, $E(Y^@(\mathbf{s}_0; t_0) - Y(\mathbf{s}_0; t_0))^2$, can be expressed in terms of the variogram. It can also obviously be expressed in terms of the covariance function, which we shall do below.

Recall the spatio-temporal *covariance function*,

$$C(\mathbf{s}, \mathbf{x}; t, r) \equiv \mathrm{cov}(Y(\mathbf{s}; t), Y(\mathbf{x}; r)), \qquad (6.44)$$

and notice that the the semivariogram is easily obtained from the formula,

$$\gamma(\mathbf{s}, \mathbf{x}; t, r) = (1/2)\{C(\mathbf{s}, \mathbf{s}; t, t) + C(\mathbf{x}, \mathbf{x}; r, r)\} - C(\mathbf{s}, \mathbf{x}; t, r).$$

Section 6.1 gives valid (i.e., nonnegative-definite) stationary models for (6.44). Essentially, stationarity is an assumption of convenience for parameter estimation and sometimes for computing; however, it may be too strong an assumption over large spatio-temporal domains.

In fact, kriging does *not* require a stationarity assumption, as we illustrate in the rest of Section 6.2. In what follows, we shall develop spatio-temporal kriging based on the general descriptive specification of dependence given by the covariance function, (6.44). We do it for the continuous-time case, although it is equally appropriate for discrete time. Suppose that the data are

$$Z(\mathbf{s}_i; t_{ij}) = Y(\mathbf{s}_i; t_{ij}) + \varepsilon(\mathbf{s}_i; t_{ij}), \qquad j = 1, \ldots, T_i, \ i = 1, \ldots, m, \quad (6.45)$$

where $\{\varepsilon(\mathbf{s}_i; t_{ij})\}$ is independent of $Y(\cdot; \cdot)$ and represents the measurement error that is henceforth assumed to be *iid* with mean zero and variance σ_ε^2. Write $\mathbf{Z}^{(i)} \equiv (Z(\mathbf{s}_i; t_{ij}): j = 1, \ldots, T_i)'; \ i = 1, \ldots, m$. Then we wish to predict the hidden value $Y(\mathbf{s}_0; t_0)$, based on all the data defined by (6.45). This would be appropriate for a retrospective analysis (called a *re-analysis* in the climate sciences). That is, we are not concerned with filtering (Section 8.1) in this discussion of spatio-temporal kriging.

6.2.1 Simple Kriging

The *simple-kriging* (*sk*) predictor, $Y^*(\mathbf{s}_0; t_0)$, takes the form of a linear combination of the data:

$$Y^*(\mathbf{s}_0; t_0) \equiv \sum_{i=1}^{m} \sum_{j=1}^{T_i} \ell_{ij} Z(\mathbf{s}_i; t_{ij}) + c$$

$$\equiv \boldsymbol{\ell}'\mathbf{Z} + c, \tag{6.46}$$

where $\mathbf{Z} \equiv (\mathbf{Z}^{(1)\prime}, \ldots, \mathbf{Z}^{(m)\prime})'$, and $\boldsymbol{\ell}$ and c are optimized (i.e., the mean squared prediction error is minimized); see below.

Assume for the moment that the mean function,

$$\mu(\mathbf{s}; t) \equiv E(Y(\mathbf{s}; t)), \qquad \mathbf{s} \in D_s, \ t \in D_t,$$

is *known*. Should the mean function be unknown, different versions of kriging can be developed: If the mean function is assumed constant over space and time, then we can derive the *ordinary-kriging* predictor (Section 6.2.2); if the mean function is a linear combination of covariates, then we can derive the *universal-kriging* predictor (Cressie, 1993, Section 3.4).

From the point of view of kriging, time is simply another dimension, and Section 4.1.2 can be consulted for carrying out kriging in Euclidean spaces. Clearly, any spatio-temporal covariance function (or variogram) would have to respect that distances in time would be treated differently from distances in space. We shall now illustrate this important point with simple kriging, but there are analogous ordinary-kriging and universal-kriging equations that are straightforward to derive in the spatio-temporal setting (Section 6.2.2). Write $\mathbf{C}_Z \equiv \text{var}(\mathbf{Z})$, $\mathbf{c}_0' \equiv \text{cov}(Y(\mathbf{s}_0; t_0), \mathbf{Z})$, and $C_{0,0} \equiv \text{var}(Y(\mathbf{s}_0; t_0))$. If both the hidden process $Y(\cdot; \cdot)$ and the measurement-error process $\varepsilon(\cdot; \cdot)$ are assumed to be Gaussian processes and we write $\mathbf{Z} = \mathbf{Y} + \boldsymbol{\varepsilon}$, then $\mathbf{Y}$ and $\boldsymbol{\varepsilon}$ follow Gaussian distributions with covariance matrices, $\boldsymbol{\Sigma}_Y$ and $\boldsymbol{\Sigma}_\varepsilon$, respectively. From (6.45) and Section 4.1.2, we have

$$\begin{bmatrix} Y(\mathbf{s}_0; t_0) \\ \mathbf{Z} \end{bmatrix} \sim Gau\left(\begin{bmatrix} \mu(\mathbf{s}_0; t_0) \\ \boldsymbol{\mu} \end{bmatrix}, \begin{bmatrix} C_{0,0} & \mathbf{c}_0' \\ \mathbf{c}_0 & \mathbf{C}_Z \end{bmatrix} \right), \tag{6.47}$$

where $\boldsymbol{\mu} \equiv (\mu(\mathbf{s}_i; t_{ij}): j = 1, \ldots, T_i, \ i = 1, \ldots, m)'$, and $\mathbf{C}_Z = \boldsymbol{\Sigma}_Y + \boldsymbol{\Sigma}_\varepsilon$. Thus, the posterior distribution is (e.g., Rencher, 2002, p. 88),

$$Y(\mathbf{s}_0; t_0)|\mathbf{Z} \sim Gau(\mu(\mathbf{s}_0; t_0) + \mathbf{c}_0'\mathbf{C}_Z^{-1}(\mathbf{Z} - \boldsymbol{\mu}), C_{0,0} - \mathbf{c}_0'\mathbf{C}_Z^{-1}\mathbf{c}_0). \tag{6.48}$$

Recall that the *simple-kriging predictor* of $Y(\mathbf{s}_0; t_0)$ takes the form $Y^*(\mathbf{s}_0; t_0) = \boldsymbol{\ell}'\mathbf{Z} + c$, where $\boldsymbol{\ell}$ and c are chosen to minimize the mean squared prediction error, $E(Y(\mathbf{s}_0; t_0) - \boldsymbol{\ell}'\mathbf{Z} - c)^2$. Under the joint-Gaussian assumption (6.47), it is easy to see that the simple-kriging predictor is just the posterior mean of (6.48). That is,

$$Y^*(\mathbf{s}_0; t_0) = E(Y(\mathbf{s}_0; t_0)|\mathbf{Z}) = \mu(\mathbf{s}_0; t_0) + \mathbf{c}_0'\mathbf{C}_Z^{-1}(\mathbf{Z} - \boldsymbol{\mu}). \qquad (6.49)$$

The simple kriging variance is the minimized mean squared prediction error; under the joint-Gaussian assumption (6.47), this is just the posterior variance. That is,

$$\sigma_{sk}^2(\mathbf{s}_0; t_0) \equiv E(Y(\mathbf{s}_0; t_0) - Y^*(\mathbf{s}_0; t_0))^2 = C_{0,0} - \mathbf{c}_0'\mathbf{C}_Z^{-1}\mathbf{c}_0. \qquad (6.50)$$

Now drop the joint Gaussian assumption; it is easy to see that (6.49) and (6.50) are still appropriate formulas for the simple-kriging predictor and its mean squared prediction error (Section 4.1.2).

Notice that the kriging equations involve taking the inverse of the $T_+ \times T_+$ positive-definite matrix $\mathbf{C}_Z = \text{var}(\mathbf{Z})$, where $T_\parallel = \sum_{i=1}^m T_i$, but this is often impossible for the sizes of spatio-temporal datasets one sees in geophysical and environmental applications. If $\mathbf{C}_Z$ could be simplified, then the impossible might become possible. This practical limitation to spatio-temporal kriging is one reason why separable covariance functions (Section 6.1.3) have been chosen to represent covariances between the data; then $\mathbf{C}_Z$ has block structure that makes computation of $\mathbf{C}_Z^{-1}$ much easier (see Section 6.2.2). However, separability is not necessary for fast computations; Cressie, Shi, and Kang (2010) use a spatio-temporal random effects model that is nonseparable (and nonstationary), for which kriging is possible, even for massive spatio-temporal datasets.

In the spatio-temporal setting, there are two different ways of writing the data vector $\mathbf{Z}$. In (6.46), we have written it as a multivariate spatial process, where $\mathbf{Z}^{(i)}$ is the T_i-dimensional vector of temporal data at the ith site; $i = 1, \ldots, m$. Alternatively, we could collect all the data at time point t and call it $\mathbf{Z}_t$. The concatenation of such $\{\mathbf{Z}_t : t = 1, \ldots, T\}$ amounts to a reordering of the data vector $\mathbf{Z}$ in (6.46).

For illustrative purposes, suppose that one datum is observed at each location $\{\mathbf{s}_i : i = 1, \ldots, m\}$ and at each time $t = 1, \ldots, T$. Then writing $\mathbf{Z} = (\mathbf{Z}^{(1)\prime}, \ldots, \mathbf{Z}^{(m)\prime})'$ is motivated by a model that assumes a *multivariate* (in time) *spatial* process. There is a large literature on multivariate spatial prediction and cokriging (e.g., Myers, 1982; Ver Hoef and Cressie, 1993; Wackernagel, 1995). The optimal prediction itself is quite straightforward. Since cokriging takes an EHM approach, there remains the problem of building and fitting valid cross-variograms, for substitution into the cokriging equations. Section 4.1.5 discusses how difficult it can be to find flexible classes of valid multivariate spatial models, except when the cross-dependence is modeled conditionally.

The data could also be written as $(\mathbf{Z}_1', \ldots, \mathbf{Z}_T')'$, which is motivated by a model that assumes a *multivariate* (in space) *time series* (e.g., the VAR(1) model presented in Section 3.4.7). Which of the two orderings of data in $\mathbf{Z}$ to use will generally be determined by how the physical process is believed to behave, and by the parsimony of parameterization that is achievable.

6.2.2   Ordinary Kriging

We now consider kriging for the case where $Y(\cdot;\cdot)$ has *constant* unknown mean μ; this is called *ordinary kriging* (*ok*). Then $\boldsymbol{\mu} = \mu\mathbf{1}$, where $\mathbf{1}$ is a T_+-dimensional vector of ones. From Section 4.1.2, substituting the generalized-least-squares estimator,

$$\widehat{\mu}_{gls} \equiv (\mathbf{1}'\mathbf{C}_Z^{-1}\mathbf{1})^{-1}\mathbf{1}'\mathbf{C}_Z^{-1}\mathbf{Z}, \tag{6.51}$$

for $\mu(\cdot;\cdot) \equiv \mu$ into (6.49) yields the ordinary-kriging predictor,

$$\widehat{Y}(\mathbf{s}_0; t_0) \equiv \widehat{\mu}_{gls} + \mathbf{c}_0'\mathbf{C}_Z^{-1}(\mathbf{Z} - \widehat{\mu}_{gls}\mathbf{1})$$
$$\equiv \boldsymbol{\lambda}'\mathbf{Z}, \tag{6.52}$$

where $\boldsymbol{\lambda}' \equiv \{\mathbf{c}_0 + \mathbf{1}(1 - \mathbf{1}'\mathbf{C}_Z^{-1}\mathbf{c}_0)/(\mathbf{1}'\mathbf{C}_Z^{-1}\mathbf{1})\}'\mathbf{C}_Z^{-1}$. Formula (6.52) gives the predictor that minimizes the mean squared prediction error over all linear unbiased predictors. Clearly, it takes the same form as ordinary kriging in the purely spatial setting; see (4.51). The minimized mean squared prediction error is the ordinary kriging variance,

$$\sigma_{ok}^2(\mathbf{s}_0; t_0) \equiv C_{0,0} - \mathbf{c}_0'\mathbf{C}_Z^{-1}\mathbf{c}_0 + (1 - \mathbf{1}'\mathbf{C}_Z^{-1}\mathbf{c}_0)^2/(\mathbf{1}'\mathbf{C}_Z^{-1}\mathbf{1}). \tag{6.53}$$

There are also versions of (6.52) and (6.53) that could be derived for universal kriging (uk) in the spatio-temporal setting, but we omit them here.

We apply ordinary kriging to several spatio-temporal datasets obtained by subsampling the realization shown in Figure 6.9a, which recall was generated from a mean-zero Gaussian process with covariance function (6.3). Figures 6.13, 6.14, and 6.15 show the effect of different sampling locations and different sample sizes. Figure 6.13a shows the true surface, $\{Y(\mathbf{s}_0; t_0): \mathbf{s}_0 \in D_s, t_0 \in D_t\}$, and Figure 6.13b shows the kriged surface, $\{\widehat{Y}(\mathbf{s}_0; t_0): \mathbf{s}_0 \in D_s, t_0 \in D_t\}$, based on a subsampling of the true surface. Notice that we use the true spatio-temporal covariance function (6.3) when calculating $\widehat{Y}(\mathbf{s}_0; t)$ in (6.52). Since there is no measurement error in this example, $\mathbf{Z} = \mathbf{Y}$, and $\widehat{Y}(\mathbf{s}_i; t_{ij}) \equiv Z(s_i; t_{ij})$ is an exact interpolator through the data. Comparison of Figure 6.13b (kriged surface) with Figure 6.13a (true surface) shows how much smoother the kriged surface is. Figure 6.13c shows the kriging-standard-error surface $\{\sigma_{ok}(\mathbf{s}_0; t_0): \mathbf{s}_0 \in D_s, t_0 \in D_t\}$ obtained from (6.53); the farther $(\mathbf{s}_0; t_0)$ is from data locations, the larger the kriging standard error. Figures 6.14 and 6.15 are similarly interpreted.

Notice the ubiquitousness of $\mathbf{C}_Z^{-1}$ in all the kriging formulas. Pragmatic assumptions are sometimes made to compute the inverse of $\mathbf{C}_Z$. For example,

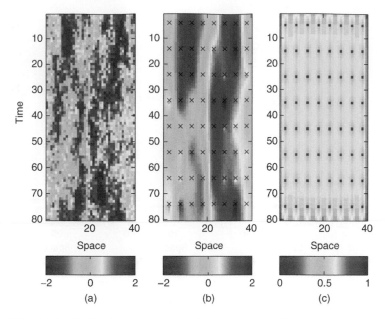

Figure 6.13 (a) Realization from a stationary Gaussian process with mean zero and covariance function derived from (6.3); $\alpha = 1$ and $\beta = 20$. (b) Kriged surface based on $n = 64$ observations; the black crosses denote the locations of the $n = 64$ regularly spaced observations subsampled from the realization in (a). (c) Kriging-standard-error surface; smaller standard errors occur near the observation locations. Here, D_s and D_t are the same as in Figure 6.8.

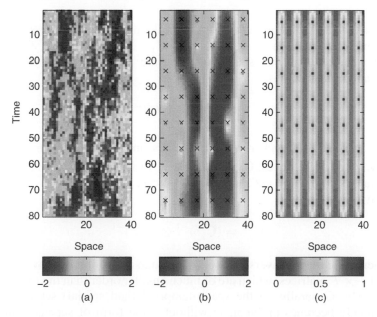

Figure 6.14 (a) Same realization as given in Figure 6.13a. (b) Kriged surface based on $n = 48$ observations; the black crosses denote the locations of the $n = 48$ regularly spaced observations subsampled from the realization in (a). (c) Kriging-standard-error surface; smaller standard errors occur near the observation locations. Here, D_s and D_t are the same as in Figure 6.8.

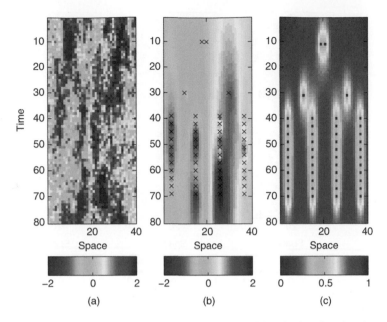

Figure 6.15 (a) Same realization as given in Figure 6.13a. (b) Kriged surface based on $n = 48$ observations; the black crosses denote the locations of the $n = 48$ irregularly spaced observations subsampled from the realization in (a). (c) Kriging-standard-error surface; smaller standard errors occur near the observation locations. Here, D_s and D_t are the same as in Figure 6.8.

consider a spatio-temporal dataset where a datum, $Z(\mathbf{s}_i; t)$, is observed at each location $\mathbf{s}_i$ and at each time point t; $i = 1, \ldots, m$, $t = 1, \ldots, T$. One pragmatic assumption is that space and time are separable when modeling the covariation of Z; that is,

$$\mathbf{C}_Z = \mathbf{C}_Z^{(s)} \otimes \mathbf{C}_Z^{(t)}, \tag{6.54}$$

where $\otimes$ is the Kronecker product, $\mathbf{C}_Z^{(s)}$ is an $m \times m$ covariance matrix of purely spatial covariances, $\mathbf{C}_Z^{(t)}$ is a $T \times T$ covariance matrix of purely temporal covariances, and $T_+ = mT$. In this special case, where $\mathbf{C}_Z$ is given by (6.54), we have

$$\mathbf{C}_Z^{-1} = (\mathbf{C}_Z^{(s)})^{-1} \otimes (\mathbf{C}_Z^{(t)})^{-1}, \tag{6.55}$$

and hence the matrix inverses in (6.49) through (6.53) involve inverses of $m \times m$ and $T \times T$ matrices, which are of much smaller order than the $(mT) \times (mT)$ matrix $\mathbf{C}_Z$. Generally, in the spatio-temporal (and spatial) setting, inverting $\mathbf{C}_Z$ quickly becomes problematic without some form of separable model, or dimension reduction, or approximation of $\mathbf{C}_Z^{-1}$ [Cressie, Shi, and Kang (2010, Section 1) give a discussion of these three approaches].

6.2.3 Optimal Linear Prediction (Kriging) for Dynamical Models

From the kriging equations in this section, it is clear that once the spatio-temporal covariance entries are obtained from the chosen covariance model (see Section 6.1 for examples of such models), kriging does not take notice of the spatio-temporal setting. That is, we might as well be predicting in $\mathbb{R}^{d+1}$, instead of in $\mathbb{R}^d$ (space) $\times \mathbb{R}$ (time). In contrast, spatio-temporal prediction (smoothing, filtering, forecasting) from a dynamical model exploits the sequential nature of the time component. Broadly speaking, a dynamical approach can finesse the need to take the inverse of the $mT \times mT$ covariance matrix Σ_Z. For example, the Kalman filter computes $Y^*(s_0; t_0)$ and $\sigma_{sk}(s_0; t_0)$ from data $Z_1, Z_2, \ldots, Z_{t_0}$, sequentially. At any time step in the sequence, only matrices of order $m \times m$ need to be inverted. This too may be problematic if m is large. Extensive details are given in Section 8.2, and Section 8.4 presents optimal *nonlinear* prediction in the context of dynamical hierarchical statistical models.

6.3 STOCHASTIC DIFFERENTIAL AND DIFFERENCE EQUATIONS

One of the themes of this book is to use scientific, dynamical relationships where possible, when analyzing spatio-temporal data. Incorporating uncertainty into those relationships is another theme, and we saw in the introduction to this chapter how deterministic PDEs can be made stochastic. Processes that solve stochastic PDEs are (by definition) stochastic, and in this section we discuss some of their statistical properties. We also consider difference equations that are discrete-time approximations to the continuous-time PDEs, and we discuss some of their statistical properties. This section is meant to be motivation for a much more complete discussion that can be found in Sections 7.2 and 7.3.

6.3.1 Spatio-Temporal Statistical Properties

A spatio-temporal stochastic process, $\{Y(s; t): s \in D_s, t \in D_t\}$ (continuous time) or $\{Y_t(s): s \in D_s, t = 0, 1, \ldots\}$ (discrete time), is characterized by its finite-dimensional distributions, which are the set of all joint distributions of Y evaluated at any finite subset of $D_s \times D_t$. In practice, it is not easy to derive these joint distributions without further assumptions on the stochastic process. For example, if the process Y is assumed Gaussian, then it is enough to derive just the first two moments of the stochastic process, namely the mean function and the covariance function.

Conversely, if a mean function and a covariance function are specified (Section 6.1), and Y is assumed to be a Gaussian stochastic process with those mean and covariance functions, then obviously any finite-dimensional distribution's mean vector and covariance matrix are fully specified, and that distribution is multivariate Gaussian. This is an example of a valid statistical model that can be used to *describe* spatio-temporal variability.

However, our preference is to *explain* the etiology of the spatio-temporal variability, and we attempt to do this by establishing "physical statistical" relationships. For example, the diffusion-injection model given by (6.1) is a stochastic PDE that could be used to describe the concentration, $Y(s; t)$, of some nutrient in soil at location s and time t. The second derivative with respect to the spatial coordinate represents physical diffusion of the nutrient, which tends to equalize concentration, whereas the term $-\alpha Y(s; t)$ serves to remove nutrient due to oxidation, leaching, or extraction by plants. The "injection" part of the model is given by $\delta(s; t)$, which represents small random additions/removals of the nutrient (Whittle, 1986, p. 431). We shall revisit this model and its statistical properties in Section 6.3.2. Other examples can be found in Ecology, where PDEs are often used; Wikle (2003b) investigates their discrete-time, discrete-space approximations. In this subsection, a more general discussion of the statistical properties of stochastic PDEs and their discrete-time approximations is given.

Here we follow Brown et al. (2000), who give an excellent presentation of how continuous-time models can be limiting cases of discrete-time models. Let $W(\cdot; t)$ denote a continuous-time Brownian motion of spatial processes. That is, W has independent increments in time, and, for any given t, $dW(\cdot; t)$ is a Gaussian spatial process with mean zero and covariance function that we write as $C_\delta(\mathbf{s}, \mathbf{x}) \, dt$; $\mathbf{s}, \mathbf{x} \in D_s \subset \mathbb{R}^d$.

Our intention is to use $W(\cdot; t)$ to describe the noise process in a *stochastic* PDE; formally, we write $dW(\cdot; t) = \delta(\cdot; t) \, dt$. Then $C_\delta(\mathbf{s}, \mathbf{x})$ is the *spatial* covariance function of $\delta(\cdot; \cdot)$. For example, $C_\delta(\mathbf{s}, \mathbf{x}) = \sigma_\delta^2 I(\mathbf{s} = \mathbf{x})$, is a model of spatial white noise that is often used in stochastic PDEs such as (6.1); then δ has the characteristics of white noise in *both* time and space.

Let $\{X(\mathbf{s}): \mathbf{s} \in D_s\}$ denote a spatial process in $D_s \subset \mathbb{R}^d$. Define

$$\frac{\partial X(\mathbf{s})}{\partial \mathbf{s}} \equiv \left(\frac{\partial X(\mathbf{s})}{\partial s_1}, \dots, \frac{\partial X(\mathbf{s})}{\partial s_d} \right)', \quad \text{and}$$

$$\frac{\partial^2 X(\mathbf{s})}{\partial \mathbf{s} \partial \mathbf{s}'} \equiv \left(\frac{\partial X(\mathbf{s})}{\partial s_i \partial s_j} : i = 1, \dots, d; \, j = 1, \dots, d \right),$$

which are, respectively, the d-dimensional vector process of first derivatives and the $d \times d$ matrix process of Hessians. Brown et al. (2000) consider the following stochastic PDE:

$$\frac{\partial Y(\mathbf{s}; t)}{\partial t} = (-1/2)\{A \, Y(\cdot; t)\}(\mathbf{s}) + \delta(\mathbf{s}; t), \quad (6.56)$$

where $\delta(\cdot; \cdot)$ is a Gaussian stochastic process that is temporally "white" (i.e., uncorrelated) and spatially "colored" (i.e., correlated), with covariance function

C_δ; and A is a spatial operator defined as follows:

$$\{A\,X(\cdot)\}(\mathbf{s}) = 2\boldsymbol{\mu}'\frac{\partial X(\mathbf{s})}{\partial \mathbf{s}} - \mathrm{tr}\left\{\frac{\partial^2 X(\mathbf{s})}{\partial \mathbf{s}\partial \mathbf{s}'}\right\}\boldsymbol{\Sigma} + 2\lambda X(\mathbf{s}),$$

depending on parameters $\boldsymbol{\mu}$ (translation rate), $\boldsymbol{\Sigma}$ ("blurring" rate), and λ (decay rate).

The special case of $\boldsymbol{\mu} = \mathbf{0}$, $\boldsymbol{\Sigma} = 2\beta\mathbf{I}$, $\lambda = \alpha$, and $C_\delta(\mathbf{s},\mathbf{x}) = \sigma_\delta^2 I(\mathbf{s}=\mathbf{x})$ gives

$$\frac{\partial Y(\mathbf{s};t)}{\partial t} = \beta\sum_{i=1}^{d}\frac{\partial^2 Y(\mathbf{s})}{\partial s_i^2} - \alpha Y(\mathbf{s};t) + \delta(\mathbf{s};t),$$

which is the d-dimensional version of the diffusion-injection equation (6.1). Other linear stochastic PDEs are given in the introduction to this chapter and in Section 7.2; some nonlinear stochastic PDEs are discussed in Section 7.3.

Brown et al. (2000) show that $Y(\mathbf{s};t)$ given by (6.56) can be written as

$$Y(\mathbf{s};t) = \int_0^\infty \exp(-\lambda v)\phi(\mathbf{s}; v\boldsymbol{\mu}, v\boldsymbol{\Sigma})\circ\delta(\mathbf{s};t-v)\,dv, \tag{6.57}$$

where "$\circ$" denotes the spatial convolution operator,

$$f_1(\mathbf{s})\circ f_2(\mathbf{s}) \equiv \int f_1(\mathbf{x})f_2(\mathbf{s}-\mathbf{x})\,d\mathbf{x};$$

and $\phi(\cdot; v\boldsymbol{\mu}, v\boldsymbol{\Sigma})$ is a d-variate Gaussian density with mean $v\boldsymbol{\mu}$ and covariance matrix $v\boldsymbol{\Sigma}$. They also show that the function

$$G(\mathbf{s};t) \equiv \exp(-\lambda t)\phi(\mathbf{s}; t\boldsymbol{\mu}, t\boldsymbol{\Sigma})I(0\le t<\infty)$$

is the Green's function (or point-spread function) for $Y(\cdot;\cdot)$. Consequently, the covariance function C_Y of Y can be obtained from the covariance function C_δ of the error process δ, as follows.

Suppose that δ is spatially (second-order) stationary (Section 4.1.1), with stationary covariance function $C_\delta(\mathbf{h})$. Then the covariance function of Y is stationary in space and time, and

$$C_Y(\mathbf{h};\tau) = \int_0^\infty \exp\{-\lambda(2v+|\tau|)\}\phi(\mathbf{h}; \tau\boldsymbol{\mu}, (2v+|\tau|)\boldsymbol{\Sigma})\circ C_\delta(\mathbf{h})\,dv. \tag{6.58}$$

In general, $C_Y(\mathbf{h};t) \ne C_Y(\mathbf{h};0)C_Y(\mathbf{0};\tau)/C_Y(\mathbf{0};0)$, reinforcing our earlier statement that separability is not a common occurrence in physically based models. Furthermore, the spectral density of Y is

$$f_Y(\boldsymbol{\omega};\xi) = |f_G(\boldsymbol{\omega};\xi)|^2 f_\delta(\boldsymbol{\omega}), \tag{6.59}$$

where $f_\delta(\omega)$ is the spectral density obtained from $C_\delta(\mathbf{h})$ using Bochner's Theorem (Section 4.1.1), and $f_G(\omega; \xi)$ is the Fourier transform of $G(\mathbf{h}; \tau)$.

In conclusion, Brown et al. (2000) show that if Y satisfies the linear stochastic PDE (6.56), then it can be written as (6.57). Since the error process δ in (6.56) is Gaussian, so too is Y. And if δ is spatially stationary, then Y has covariance function given by (6.58) and spectral density given by (6.59). Brown et al. (2000) derive other expressions for Y and C_Y in terms of the operator A, which we do not present here.

Discrete-time processes can arise from continuous-time processes, due to sampling or aggregation from continuous-time processes, or simply because the process is defined that way (e.g., tree-ring width is a process indexed by a discrete time unit of one year). If, for example, the stochastic PDE (6.56) was discretized in time, then we would obtain the approximation,

$$Y(\mathbf{s}; t) \simeq \{(I - (\Delta_t/2)A_{\Delta_t})Y(\cdot; t - \Delta_t)\}(\mathbf{s}) + \delta(\mathbf{s}; t), \tag{6.60}$$

where here I is the identity operator and A_{Δ_t} is a linear operator defined by

$$\{(I - (\Delta_t/2)A_{\Delta_t})X(\cdot)\}(\mathbf{s}) = \exp(-\lambda\Delta_t) \int \phi(\mathbf{x}; \Delta_t\boldsymbol{\mu}, \Delta_t\boldsymbol{\Sigma})X(\mathbf{s} - \mathbf{x})\,d\mathbf{x}.$$

In the expression above, if the spatial domain is discretized to become $D_s = \{\mathbf{s}_1, \ldots, \mathbf{s}_n\}$, and terms involving boundary effects and discretization error are dropped, then from (6.60) we obtain the multivariate, discrete-time (Markov) process,

$$\mathbf{Y}_t \simeq \mathbf{M}\mathbf{Y}_{t-\Delta_t} + \boldsymbol{\delta}_t, \qquad t = \Delta_t, 2\Delta_t, \ldots, \tag{6.61}$$

where $\mathbf{Y}_t \equiv (Y(\mathbf{s}_1; t), \ldots Y(\mathbf{s}_n; t))'$ is the n-dimensional process vector, $\mathbf{Y}_{t-\Delta_t}$ is independent of $\boldsymbol{\delta}_t$, $\boldsymbol{\delta}_t \sim iid\ Gau(\cdot, \cdot)$, and $\mathbf{M}$ is an $n \times n$ matrix whose entries can be identified from (6.60). In Section 6.3.2 below, we identify $\mathbf{M}$ for the special case of $\boldsymbol{\mu} = \mathbf{0}$, $\boldsymbol{\Sigma} = 2\beta\mathbf{I}$, and $\lambda = \alpha$ in one-dimensional space, and we show that spatio-temporal covariances derived from (6.61) approximate the covariance function (6.58) very well. Other linear and nonlinear stochastic PDEs are discretized in Sections 7.2.4 and 7.3, respectively.

Consider a discrete-time process $\{Y_t(\mathbf{s}): \mathbf{s} \in D_s, t = 0, 1, \ldots\}$. During the time interval from $t - 1$ to t, $Y_{t-1}(\mathbf{x})$ can influence the behavior of $Y_t(\mathbf{s})$, where $\mathbf{x}$ could come from near (local weather) or far (teleconnection). The integration of all these influences over $\mathbf{x}$ leads to an integro-difference equation (IDE):

$$Y_t(\mathbf{s}) = \int_{D_s} m(\mathbf{s}, \mathbf{x}; \boldsymbol{\theta})Y_{t-1}(\mathbf{x})\,d\mathbf{x},$$

where $m(\mathbf{s}, \mathbf{x}; \boldsymbol{\theta})$ represents the "influence" of $Y_{t-1}(\mathbf{x})$ on $Y_t(\mathbf{s})$; see Section 7.2.5, where m is called a redistribution kernel that depends on parameters $\boldsymbol{\theta}$. To make the IDE stochastic, we write

$$Y_t(\mathbf{s}) = \int_{D_s} m(\mathbf{s}, \mathbf{x}; \boldsymbol{\theta}) Y_{t-1}(\mathbf{x}) \, d\mathbf{x} + \eta_t(\mathbf{s}), \qquad \mathbf{s} \in D_s, \qquad (6.62)$$

where, like δ in (6.56), $\{\eta_t(\mathbf{s}): \mathbf{s} \in D_s, t = 1, 2, \ldots\}$ is uncorrelated in time but correlated in space, and it is often assumed to be a stationary Gaussian process.

Here we follow Storvik, Frigessi, and Hirst (2002), who give results that determine when classes of second-order spatio-temporal covariance functions can be represented according to (6.62) with $D_s = \mathbb{R}^d$ and stationary redistribution kernel, $m(\mathbf{x} - \mathbf{s})$, where for convenience dependence on $\boldsymbol{\theta}$ is suppressed. Then (6.62) can be written as

$$Y_t(\mathbf{s}) = \int m(\mathbf{v}) Y_{t-1}(\mathbf{s} + \mathbf{v}) \, d\mathbf{v} + \eta_t(\mathbf{s}), \qquad \mathbf{s} \in D_s. \qquad (6.63)$$

Let $C_\eta(\mathbf{h})$ denote the second-order stationary spatial covariance function of $\eta_t(\cdot)$, and denote its spectral density as $f_\eta(\boldsymbol{\omega})$. Then from (6.63), Y is second-order stationary, and we denote its covariance function as $C_Y(\mathbf{h}; \tau)$. Hold τ fixed and let $f_{Y,\tau}(\boldsymbol{\omega})$ denote the Fourier transform of $C_Y(\mathbf{h}; \tau)$; $\tau = 0, \pm 1, \pm 2, \ldots$. Finally, let $f_m(\boldsymbol{\omega})$ be the Fourier transform of the kernel $m(\mathbf{h})$. Then Storvik, Frigessi, and Hirst (2002) show that, for $\boldsymbol{\omega} \in \mathbb{R}^d$,

$$f_{Y,0}(\boldsymbol{\omega}) = \frac{f_\eta(\boldsymbol{\omega})}{1 - f_m(\boldsymbol{\omega}) f_m(-\boldsymbol{\omega})}$$

and

$$f_{Y,\tau}(\boldsymbol{\omega}) = f_{Y,0}(\boldsymbol{\omega}) \{ f_m(-\boldsymbol{\omega}) \}^{|\tau|}, \qquad \tau = 0, +1, \pm 2, \ldots. \qquad (6.64)$$

Consequently, $C_Y(\mathbf{h}; \tau)$ can be obtained by computing (numerically or analytically) the inverse Fourier transform of the right-hand side of (6.64). In some cases, an analytical result is possible; Storvik, Frigessi, and Hirst (2002) give an example of a spatio-temporal, nonseparable, Matérn-like covariance function for $C_Y(\mathbf{h}; \tau)$, $\mathbf{h} \in \mathbb{R}^d$, $\tau = 0, \pm 1, \pm 2, \ldots$, which they note is also valid when $-\infty < \tau < \infty$.

Perhaps surprisingly, it is possible to start with a valid spatio-temporal covariance function, $\{C_Y(\mathbf{h}; \tau): \mathbf{h} \in \mathbb{R}^d, \tau \in \mathbb{R}\}$ and, under regularity conditions, obtain a spatio-temporal process Y that satisfies the stochastic IDE (6.63). Storvik, Frigessi, and Hirst (2002) show that (i) *if* $f_{Y,\tau}(\boldsymbol{\omega})$ exists for any $\tau \in \mathbb{R}$; (ii) *if* we can write

$$f_{Y,\tau}(\boldsymbol{\omega}) = f_{Y,0}(\boldsymbol{\omega}) \{ f(-\boldsymbol{\omega}) \}^{|\tau|}, \qquad \tau \in \mathbb{R}, \qquad (6.65)$$

where the function $\{f(\boldsymbol{\omega}): \boldsymbol{\omega} \in \mathbb{R}^d\}$ has an inverse Fourier transform $m(\mathbf{h})$, $|f(\cdot)| < 1$, $f_{Y,0}(\cdot) > 0$, and $\int f_{Y,0}(\boldsymbol{\omega})d\boldsymbol{\omega} < \infty$; and (iii) *if* we define

$$f_{\eta}(\boldsymbol{\omega}) \equiv f_{Y,0}(\boldsymbol{\omega})\{(1 - f(\boldsymbol{\omega})f(-\boldsymbol{\omega}))\} \qquad (6.66)$$

and let $\eta_t(\cdot)$ be a temporally white and spatially colored stochastic process with spectral density $f_{\eta}(\cdot)$; *then* there exists a stochastic process $Y(\mathbf{s}; t)$ that satisfies (6.63). They then use this result to give a stochastic IDE representation for a process that has covariance function given by one of the nonseparable examples due to Cressie and Huang (1999).

In conclusion, it is possible to investigate which spatio-temporal covariance functions have a natural, physical interpretation as a stochastic IDE. Essentially, there has to be a "well behaved" function $f(\cdot)$ in (6.65), and the error process $\eta_t(\cdot)$ has to be chosen to satisfy (6.66); in this case, a stochastic IDE can be recovered.

6.3.2 The Diffusion-Injection Equation, Revisited

In this book, we encourage spatio-temporal statistical modelers to build their models from physical/chemical/biological/economic/etc. relationships and to use them to *motivate* various levels of the HM. Here, we choose a homogeneous reaction-diffusion PDE given by (6.2); we give further examples in Sections 6.3.1 and 7.2.4. In what is to follow, the PDE (6.2) is discretized, both temporally and spatially, resulting in the equation, $\mathbf{Y}_{t+\Delta_t} \simeq \mathbf{M}\mathbf{Y}_t$, where the propagator matrix $\mathbf{M}$ is structured (tridiagonal and very sparse). Then the resulting *stochastic* difference equation will be of the VAR(1) type given by (3.98); see also (7.46) and Wikle (2003b).

The PDE (6.2) has a first-order partial derivative in time and a second-order partial derivative in (one-dimensional) space. There is some choice involved in replacing the first-order derivative with a forward or a backward difference and replacing the second-order derivative with a forward, centered, or backward difference; which of these one chooses will make a (hopefully small) difference to the solution meant to approximate the PDE.

Replacing the first-order derivative with a forward difference and the second-order derivative with a centered difference, (6.2), is approximated as

$$\frac{Y(s; t + \Delta_t) - Y(s; t)}{\Delta_t} = \beta \left\{ \frac{Y(s + \Delta_s; t) - 2Y(s; t) + Y(s - \Delta_s; t)}{\Delta_s^2} \right\}$$
$$- \alpha Y(s; t),$$

which reduces to

$$Y(s; t + \Delta_t) = \theta_1 Y(s; t) + \theta_2 Y(s + \Delta_s; t) + \theta_2 Y(s - \Delta_s; t), \qquad (6.67)$$

where $\theta_1 \equiv (1 - \alpha\Delta_t - 2\beta\Delta_t/\Delta_s^2)$, $\theta_2 \equiv \beta\Delta_t/\Delta_s^2$, and recall that $\alpha > 0$ and $\beta > 0$. We shall see below that (6.67) approximates the PDE (6.2) well, provided that $\alpha\Delta_t < 1$ and $2\beta\Delta_t/\Delta_s^2 < 1$.

From (6.67), the next (future) value of Y at s is related to current values at s *and* neighboring spatial locations. Now let $D_s \equiv \{s_0, \ldots, s_{n+1}\}$, where $s_j = s_0 + j \cdot \Delta_s$; $j = 0, 1, \ldots, n+1$. The locations s_0 and s_{n+1} are spatial boundary locations. Then,

$$
\begin{aligned}
Y(s_1; t + \Delta_t) &= \theta_1 Y(s_1; t) &+& \theta_2 Y(s_2; t) &+& \theta_2 Y(s_0; t) \\
Y(s_2; t + \Delta_t) &= \theta_1 Y(s_2; t) &+& \theta_2 Y(s_3; t) &+& \theta_2 Y(s_1; t) \\
&\ \ \vdots & & \ \ \vdots & & \ \ \vdots \\
Y(s_n; t + \Delta_t) &= \theta_1 Y(s_n; t) &+& \theta_2 Y(s_{n+1}; t) &+& \theta_2 Y(s_{n-1}; t).
\end{aligned}
$$

Define $\mathbf{Y}_t \equiv (Y(s_1; t), \ldots, Y(s_n; t))'$ and $\mathbf{Y}_t^{(b)} \equiv (Y(s_0; t), Y(s_{n+1}; t))'$, and so the equations given just above can be written as the (nonstochastic) vector difference equation,

$$ \mathbf{Y}_{t+\Delta_t} = \mathbf{M}\mathbf{Y}_t + \mathbf{M}^{(b)}\mathbf{Y}_t^{(b)}, \tag{6.68} $$

where $\mathbf{M}$ is an $n \times n$ tridiagonal propagator matrix, and $\mathbf{M}^{(b)}$ is an $n \times 2$ boundary propagator matrix:

$$
\mathbf{M} \equiv \begin{bmatrix}
\theta_1 & \theta_2 & 0 & \cdots & \cdots & 0 \\
\theta_2 & \theta_1 & \theta_2 & \cdots & \cdots & 0 \\
0 & \theta_2 & \theta_1 & \ddots & & \vdots \\
\vdots & \vdots & \ddots & \ddots & \ddots & \vdots \\
\vdots & \vdots & & \ddots & \theta_1 & \theta_2 \\
0 & 0 & 0 & \cdots & \theta_2 & \theta_1
\end{bmatrix}, \quad
\mathbf{M}^{(b)} \equiv \begin{bmatrix}
\theta_2 & 0 \\
0 & 0 \\
\vdots & \vdots \\
0 & \theta_2
\end{bmatrix}. \tag{6.69}
$$

Henceforth, let $D_t = \{0, 1, 2, \ldots\}$, in units of Δ_t. Then, from a given initial condition $\mathbf{Y}_0$ and boundary conditions $\{\mathbf{Y}_t^{(b)} : t = 0, 1, \ldots\}$, we can obtain a numerical solution to the difference equation (6.67), which is an approximation to the PDE (6.2). The sparseness of $\mathbf{M}$ helps with computation, but restrictions on Δ_t, Δ_s, α, and β are still needed to avoid unstable solutions of the difference equation. These restrictions ensure that the maximum absolute eigenvalue of $\mathbf{M}$ is less than 1, and they are

$$ \alpha\Delta_t < 1 \quad \text{and} \quad 2\beta\Delta_t/\Delta_s^2 < 1. $$

For example, $\alpha = 1$, $\beta = 20$, $\Delta_t = .01$, and $\Delta_s = 1$ satisfy these inequalities (see Figure 6.1a).

Now add a mean-zero, random error component, $\boldsymbol{\delta}_{t+1}$, to the right-hand side of (6.68):

$$\mathbf{Y}_{t+1} = \mathbf{M}\mathbf{Y}_t + \mathbf{M}^{(b)}\mathbf{Y}_t^{(b)} + \boldsymbol{\delta}_{t+1}, \qquad t = 0, 1, \ldots, \tag{6.70}$$

where $\{\boldsymbol{\delta}_t\}$ are *iid*. This is a *stochastic* spatio-temporal difference equation [which, following Whittle (1986), might be called a *diffusion-injection difference equation*] corresponding to the stochastic PDE (6.1). Since the boundary term, $\mathbf{M}^{(b)}\mathbf{Y}_t^{(b)}$, is given, this stochastic difference equation can be recognized as a multivariate first-order autoregressive model, or VAR(1) model, already considered in Section 3.4.7. Assuming temporal stationarity of the covariance function, we see from a generalization of equation (3.101) that for any nonnegative integer k the $n \times n$ covariance matrix, $\boldsymbol{\Sigma}_Y^{(k)} \equiv \text{cov}(\mathbf{Y}_{t+k}, \mathbf{Y}_t)$, satisfies

$$\boldsymbol{\Sigma}_Y^{(k)} = \mathbf{M}^k \boldsymbol{\Sigma}_Y, \qquad k = 0, 1, 2, \ldots, \tag{6.71}$$

where $\boldsymbol{\Sigma}_Y \equiv \boldsymbol{\Sigma}_Y^{(0)} = \text{var}(\mathbf{Y}_t)$. Consider the spatio-temporal stationary covariance function $C(h; \tau)$ in (6.3), obtained from the stochastic PDE (6.1), where $h > 0$, $\tau > 0$. For a given temporal lag τ, choose k_τ to be the integer part of τ/Δ_t. Furthermore, for a given spatial lag h, choose ℓ_h to be the integer part of h/Δ_s, and since D_s is fixed, n is $O(1/\Delta_s)$. Then the $(i, i + \ell_h)$th element of $\boldsymbol{\Sigma}_Y^{(k_\tau)}$ should approximate $C(h, \tau)$, as we now discuss.

Define $\boldsymbol{\Sigma}_\delta \equiv \text{var}(\boldsymbol{\delta}_t)$, which is the $n \times n$ covariance matrix of the random errors, and evaluate $\text{var}(\mathbf{Y}_{t+1})$ in (6.70):

$$\boldsymbol{\Sigma}_Y = \mathbf{M}\boldsymbol{\Sigma}_Y\mathbf{M}' + \boldsymbol{\Sigma}_\delta. \tag{6.72}$$

For $\mathbf{M}$ and $\boldsymbol{\Sigma}_\delta$ known, we are able to solve for $\boldsymbol{\Sigma}_Y$ using (6.72); hence, from (6.71), we obtain $\{\boldsymbol{\Sigma}_Y^{(k)} : k = 0, 1, \ldots\}$, which fully specifies the discrete-time, discrete-space spatio-temporal covariance function. The solution for $\boldsymbol{\Sigma}_Y$ is given by

$$\text{vec}(\boldsymbol{\Sigma}_Y) = \{\mathbf{I} - \mathbf{M} \otimes \mathbf{M}\}^{-1}\text{vec}(\boldsymbol{\Sigma}_\delta), \tag{6.73}$$

where recall that $\text{vec}(\cdot)$ is the operator on a matrix that strings its columns one underneath the other, and $\otimes$ denotes the Kronecker product such that $\mathbf{A} \otimes \mathbf{B}$ is a matrix whose (i, j)th block is $a_{ij}\mathbf{B}$. Consequently, $\text{vec}(\boldsymbol{\Sigma}_Y)$ and $\text{vec}(\boldsymbol{\Sigma}_\delta)$ are $n^2 \times 1$ vectors, and $\mathbf{I}$ and $\mathbf{M} \otimes \mathbf{M}$ above are $n^2 \times n^2$ matrices. Thus, the spatio-temporal covariance of the stochastic difference equation (that approximates the stochastic PDE) is completely determined by θ_1, θ_2, and $\boldsymbol{\Sigma}_\delta$ (more precisely, by Δ_t, Δ_s, α, β, and $\text{cov}(\boldsymbol{\delta}_t)$).

Recall that $D_s = \{s_0, s_1, \ldots, s_n, s_{n+1}\}$, where $s_j = s_0 + j \cdot \Delta_s$; $j = 0, 1, \ldots, n + 1$. Let $\{Y_t(\mathbf{s}_j) : j = 0, 1, \ldots, n+1, t = 0, 1, \ldots\}$ be the

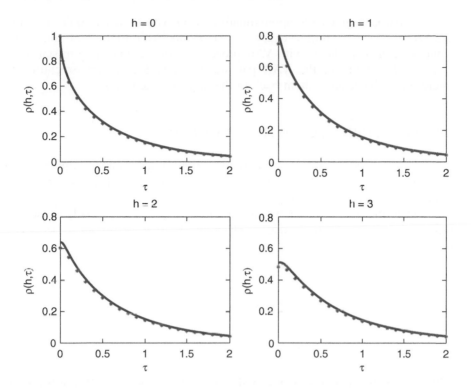

Figure 6.16 Comparison of the discretized correlation function given in (6.75) with the continuous correlation function given in (6.3), as a function of temporal lag τ for several choices of spatial lag h. Here $\alpha = 1$, $\beta = 20$, $\Delta_s = 1$, and $\Delta_t = 0.01$. The red dots display discretized correlation values obtained from (6.75) at time intervals of $10\Delta_t = 0.1$, and the blue line displays the continuous correlation function obtained from (6.3).

spatio-temporal process that solves the discrete-time, discrete-space stochastic difference equation (6.70). Then,

$$\text{cov}(Y_t(s_j), Y_{t+k}(s_{j+\ell})) = (\Sigma_Y^{(k)})_{j,j+\ell}, \tag{6.74}$$

where $\Sigma_Y^{(k)}$ is evaluated from (6.71) and (6.73). Now let $j = [n/2]$, and recall that $\ell_h = [h/\Delta_s]$ and $k_\tau = [\tau/\Delta_t]$ ([x] denotes the integer part of x), where $\Delta_t = .01$ and $\Delta_s = 1$. Figure 6.16 shows plots of

$$\tilde{\rho}(h; \tau) \equiv (\Sigma_Y^{(k_\tau)})_{j,j+\ell_h} / \{(\Sigma_Y)_{jj} \cdot (\Sigma_Y)_{j+\ell_h, j+\ell_h}\}^{1/2}, \tag{6.75}$$

as functions of τ for several choices of h. On those plots is superimposed the continuous spatio-temporal correlation function (6.3) shown in Figure 6.3. The agreement between (6.74) and (6.3) is very good and will get better for smaller Δ_t and Δ_t/Δ_s^2.

The approach given for approximating (6.1) with (6.70) is quite general; see Section 7.2.4 for further examples. Thus, stochastic PDEs with intractible solutions can be replaced with VAR processes that are amenable to statistical analysis. Furthermore, the VAR parameters (here θ_1, θ_2) are scientifically interpretable by relating them back to the approximated PDE.

6.4   TIME SERIES OF SPATIAL PROCESSES

In Section 6.3, we saw how a continuous-time model can be approximated upon introducing a small time-increment, Δ_t. There, $D_t = [0, \infty)$ is replaced with $D_t = \{0, 1, 2, \ldots\}$, in units of Δ_t.

Henceforth, in this section, we choose $D_t = \{0, 1, 2, \ldots\}$, namely a discrete-time model. Since the time index is discrete, the spatio-temporal process can be written as

$$Y_0(\cdot) \equiv \{Y(\mathbf{s}; 0): \mathbf{s} \in D_s\},$$

$$Y_1(\cdot) \equiv \{Y(\mathbf{s}; 1): \mathbf{s} \in D_s\},$$

$$\ldots$$

$$Y_t(\cdot) \equiv \{Y(\mathbf{s}; t): \mathbf{s} \in D_s\}, \tag{6.76}$$

which could be generalized (but will not be in this section) by allowing the spatial index set D_s in (6.76) to depend on the time point t. That is, in (6.76), we have approximated the spatio-temporal process, $Y(\cdot; \cdot)$, as a *time series of spatial processes*:

$$\{Y_t(\cdot): t = 0, 1, \ldots\}. \tag{6.77}$$

We note here and below that one could take the conjugate point of view, namely that the spatio-temporal process could be thought of as a spatial process of time series. That is, think of the spatio-temporal process as a multivariate spatial process, where the multivariate dependencies are in fact inherited from temporal dependencies that may vary with spatial location (e.g., Bennett, 1979; Sansó, Schmidt, and Nobre, 2008).

In the subsections that follow, we consider both continuous-space and discrete-space models for (6.77).

6.4.1   Continuous Spatial Index (Geostatistical Processes)

Formally speaking, the continuous-spatial-index case is defined by $|D_s| > 0$, where recall that for $A \subset \mathbb{R}^d$, $|A| \equiv \int_A d\mathbf{s}$ is the volume (or Lebesgue measure) of A. In the purely spatial context, models for $\{Y(\mathbf{s}): \mathbf{s} \in D_s\}$ have been called *geostatistical processes* (Cressie, 1993, Chapter 2). Thus, our interest here is in time series of geostatistical processes given by (6.77).

In Chapter 3, an example of a dynamical model for a time series of random variables $\{Y_t : t = 0, 1, \dots \}$ was given as

$$Y_t = \mathcal{M}_t(Y_{t-1}) + \delta_t, \qquad t = 0, 1, \dots, \tag{6.78}$$

where $\mathcal{M}_t(\cdot)$ is a possibly nonlinear function that may depend on t, δ_t is an additive error term independent of Y_{t-1}, and $\{\delta_t : t = 0, 1, \dots \}$ are mutually independent. Using (6.78) as motivation, we could define a time series of geostatistical processes through

$$Y_t(\mathbf{s}) = \mathcal{M}_t(\mathbf{s}, Y_{t-1}(\cdot)) + \delta_t(\mathbf{s}), \qquad \mathbf{s} \in D_s, \qquad t = 0, 1, \dots, \tag{6.79}$$

where the spatial process $\delta_t(\cdot)$ is independent of the spatial process $Y_{t-1}(\cdot)$, and $\{\delta_t(\cdot) : t = 0, 1, \dots \}$ are mutually independent processes. For example, Wikle and Cressie (1999) considered models of the form of (6.79), where $\delta_t(\cdot)$ was a spatially colored error process with mean zero, and $\mathcal{M}_t$ did not depend on t. That is, they considered

$$Y_t(\mathbf{s}) = \mathcal{M}(\mathbf{s}, Y_{t-1}(\cdot)) + \delta_t(\mathbf{s}),$$

where

$$\mathcal{M}(\mathbf{s}, f(\cdot)) \equiv \int_{\mathbb{R}^d} m(\mathbf{s}, \mathbf{x}) f(\mathbf{x}) \, d\mathbf{x}, \qquad \mathbf{s} \in D_s, \tag{6.80}$$

for $f(\cdot)$ any function in $\mathbb{R}^d$ such that the integral on the right-hand side of (6.80) exists. The weight function $m(\mathbf{s}, \mathbf{x})$ in (6.80) controls which parts of, and by how much, the process $Y_{t-1}(\cdot)$ influences the current value $Y_t(\mathbf{s})$. Notice that $\{\delta_t(\cdot) : t = 0, 1, \dots \}$ is a time series of error processes that are independent in time; however, each error process can exhibit spatial dependence. Figure 6.17 shows a schematic diagram of the dynamical structure found in (6.79) and (6.80). The diagram is meant to show intuitively how dependencies are transmitted through time and space; in fact, it could be formally interpreted as an acyclic-directed graph (Section 2.4). Further discussion of dynamical models like (6.80) can be found in Section 7.2.5.

There is a lot of flexibility in (6.79), to generate nonstationary spatio-temporal processes; that is, the action of the function $\mathcal{M}_t(\mathbf{s}, \cdot)$ may vary with $\mathbf{s}$ and t. In order to visualize some possibilities, we consider the same spatio-temporal domain as in Figure 6.8, and we divide $D_s = [0, 40]$ and $D_t = [0, 0.8]$ into 40 (i.e., $\Delta_s = 1$) and 80 (i.e., $\Delta_t = .01$) intervals, respectively. That is, we are considering a fine grid on (continuous one-dimensional space) $\times$ (time) that has $40 \times 80 = 3200$ pixels. Then the continuous function $\mathcal{M}_t(s, \cdot)$; $s \in D_s$, $t \in D_t$, can be discretized onto the fine grid by a sequence of 40×40 matrices, $\{\mathbf{M}_t : t = \Delta_t, 2\Delta_t, \dots, 80\Delta_t\}$.

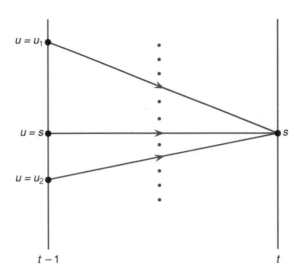

Figure 6.17 Schematic diagram (directed graph) of the dynamic structure found in (6.79) and (6.80); $D_s \subset \mathbb{R}^1$.

For example, consider,

$$\mathbf{M}_t \equiv h_t \cdot \mathbf{M} \equiv h_t \cdot \begin{bmatrix} \mathbf{M}_1 & \mathbf{0} \\ \mathbf{0} & \mathbf{M}_2 \end{bmatrix}, \tag{6.81}$$

where the 20×20 matrices $\mathbf{M}_1$ and $\mathbf{M}_2$ are given by

$$\mathbf{M}_1 \equiv \begin{bmatrix} .90 & .01 & 0 & \cdots & 0 \\ .01 & .90 & 0 & \cdots & 0 \\ 0 & 0 & \ddots & & \vdots \\ \vdots & \vdots & & .90 & .01 \\ 0 & 0 & \cdots & .01 & .90 \end{bmatrix}, \qquad \mathbf{M}_2 \equiv \begin{bmatrix} .20 & .01 & 0 & \cdots & 0 \\ .01 & .20 & 0 & \cdots & 0 \\ 0 & 0 & \ddots & & \vdots \\ \vdots & \vdots & & .02 & .01 \\ 0 & 0 & \cdots & .01 & .20 \end{bmatrix}$$

and

$$h_t \equiv \begin{cases} 1, & \text{if } 1 \leq t \leq 30\Delta_t, \\ -1, & \text{if } 31\Delta_t \leq t \leq 60\Delta_t, \\ 1, & \text{if } 61\Delta_t \leq t \leq 80\Delta_t. \end{cases}$$

Clearly, in $D_s \times D_t$, there are six distinct regions, corresponding to weak/strong spatial dependence $\times$ positive/negative/positive temporal dependence. In spite of these heterogeneities, it is possible to define a $Y_t(\cdot)$ so that it has the same spatial covariance structure for each t, as we shall now demonstrate.

In terms of the grid of 3200 pixels, the geostatistical process $Y_t(\cdot)$ at any given t becomes $\mathbf{Y}_t \equiv (Y_t(1), \ldots, Y_t(40))'$, and the error process $\delta_t(\cdot)$ becomes $\delta_t \equiv (\delta_t(1), \ldots, \delta_t(40))'$; $t = .01, .02, \ldots, .8$. Then, in terms of vectors and matrices, the time series of geostatistical processes can be written in its discretized form as

$$\mathbf{Y}_t = \mathbf{M}_t \mathbf{Y}_{t-1} + \delta_t, \qquad (6.82)$$

where we define

$$\text{var}(\mathbf{Y}_t) \equiv \mathbf{\Sigma}_{Y,t} \quad \text{and} \quad \text{var}(\delta_t) \equiv \mathbf{\Sigma}_{\delta,t}.$$

Clearly, (6.82) could also be used to define a time series of lattice processes, but in this example we have in mind a geostatistical process for which Δ_t and Δ_t/Δ_s^2 are small, such as for the diffusion-injection model considered in Section 6.3.2.

From (6.82), we have a generalization of (6.71) and (6.72):

$$\mathbf{\Sigma}_{Y,t} = \mathbf{M}_t \mathbf{\Sigma}_{Y,t-1} \mathbf{M}_t' + \mathbf{\Sigma}_{\delta,t},$$

and

$$\text{cov}(\mathbf{Y}_{t+\tau}, \mathbf{Y}_t) = \mathbf{M}_{t+\tau} \mathbf{M}_{t+\tau-1} \cdots \mathbf{M}_{t+1} \mathbf{\Sigma}_{Y,t}.$$

In the example, we choose

$$\mathbf{\Sigma}_{Y,t} \equiv \mathbf{\Sigma} \equiv (\exp(-|i - j|/10)) + 4 \cdot \mathbf{I}_{40}, \qquad (6.83)$$

where the expression in parentheses on the right-hand side of (6.83) gives the (i, j)th entry of the 40×40 matrix. Notice that (6.83) does not depend on t. Consequently, if the error process is generated according to $\delta_t \sim Gau(\mathbf{0}, \mathbf{\Sigma}_{\delta,t})$, where

$$\mathbf{\Sigma}_{\delta,t} \equiv \mathbf{\Sigma} - \mathbf{M}_t \mathbf{\Sigma} \mathbf{M}_t', \qquad t = \Delta_t, 2\Delta_t, \ldots,$$

and the initial value in the time series of the geostatistical processes is generated according to $\mathbf{Y}_0 \sim Gau(\mathbf{0}, \mathbf{\Sigma})$, then the recursion given by (6.82) results in a spatio-temporal process, $\mathbf{Y}_{\Delta_t}, \mathbf{Y}_{2\Delta_t}, \ldots$, with homogeneous $\text{var}(\mathbf{Y}_{\Delta_t}) = \text{var}(\mathbf{Y}_{2\Delta_t}) = \cdots = \mathbf{\Sigma}$. This gives a valid spatio-temporal process because $\mathbf{\Sigma} - \mathbf{M}_t \mathbf{\Sigma} \mathbf{M}_t'$ is positive-definite, and this occurs if the eigenvalues of $\mathbf{M}_t \mathbf{M}_t'$ are all strictly less than 1. The model (6.81) satisfies this condition. Figure 6.18 shows three realizations of the spatio-temporal process, where the six regions we referred to earlier are clearly visible.

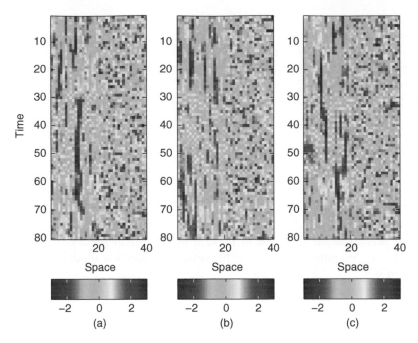

Figure 6.18 Three independent realizations of a non-stationary spatio-temporal process, constructed from (6.81) and (6.82). In the figure, there are six spatio-temporal domains that exhibit different behavior: $\{1, \ldots, 20\} \times \{1, \ldots, 30\}$; $\{1, \ldots, 20\} \times \{31, \ldots, 60\}$; $\{1, \ldots, 20\} \times \{61, \ldots, 80\}$; $\{21, \ldots, 40\} \times \{1, \ldots, 30\}$; $\{21, \ldots, 40\} \times \{31, \ldots, 60\}$; $\{21, \ldots, 40\} \times \{61, \ldots, 80\}$.

The cross-covariances are generally nonstationary. In Figure 6.19, we show various $\text{corr}(Y(s; t), Y(x; r))$, obtained from its covariance-matrix form:

$$\text{cov}(\mathbf{Y}_{t+\tau}, \mathbf{Y}_t) = \mathbf{M}_{t+\tau} \mathbf{M}_{t+\tau-1} \cdots \mathbf{M}_{t+1} \mathbf{\Sigma}, \qquad (6.84)$$

where $\mathbf{M}_t$ is given by (6.81) and $\mathbf{\Sigma}$ is given by (6.83).

From an alternative perspective, a spatial process of time series might be modeled through a temporally stationary covariance function $C_s(\tau)$, $\tau = 0, \pm 1, \pm 2, \ldots$, where here the subscript indexes the *location* of the time series. Then the theorem of Cressie and Huang (1999) that was stated in Section 6.1.6 could be used to construct a coherent spatio-temporal covariance for $s \in D_s$ and $t = 0, 1, 2, \ldots$.

Our focus in this subsection has been on dynamical models of geostatistical processes, even if practical considerations force a discretization of D_s into a collection of small finite elements. Philosophically, the spatial index is continuous, reflected by the possibility that the finite elements might be made larger or smaller, *and* that the geostatistical process $Y_t(\cdot)$ will not be observed at every spatial location $s \in D_s$. One of the opening examples of this chapter was a spatio-temporal process of air pressure anywhere in the earth's atmosphere and at any time. Then, for this example, the spatial index set D_s is clearly

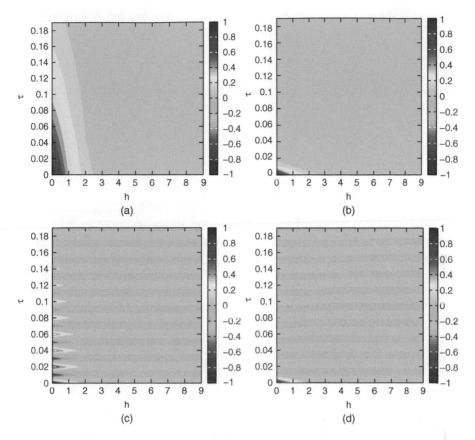

Figure 6.19 (a) Contour plot of corr($Y(1; 1), Y(1 + h; 1 + \tau)$), exhibiting strong positive correlation. (b) Contour plot of corr($Y(21; 1), Y(21 + h; 1 + \tau)$), exhibiting weak positive correlation. (c) Contour plot of corr($Y(1; 31), Y(1 + h; 31 + \tau)$), exhibiting strong oscillatory correlation. (d) Contour plot of corr($Y(21; 31), Y(21 + h; 31 + \tau)$), exhibiting weak oscillatory correlation.

continuous. Another opening example was based on yearly breast-cancer incidence in the 88 counties of Ohio, for which D_s is clearly discrete and is an instance of a time series of *lattice* processes.

6.4.2 Discrete Spatial Index (Lattice Processes)

When D_s is finite or countable, its Lebesgue measure is zero; that is, $|D_s| = 0$. An example of a countable $D_s \subset \mathbb{R}^d$ is the d-dimensional grid of integers, $\{0, 1, \dots\}^d$. In practice, such grids are usually truncated and made finite. For the rest of this subsection, we assume

$$D_s = \{s_1, s_2, \dots, s_n\}, \tag{6.85}$$

a *finite* collection of locations in space. Notice that we are not interested in any other locations in $\mathbb{R}^d$; the spatio-temporal process Y is

$$\{Y_t(\mathbf{s}_i): i = 1, \ldots, n \,;\, t = 0, 1, \ldots\}, \tag{6.86}$$

and we expect that $Y_t(\cdot)$ could be observed at every one of the n locations in D_s. Since D_s is finite, $Y_t(\cdot)$ in (6.77) can be written as

$$\mathbf{Y}_t \equiv (Y_t(\mathbf{s}_1), \ldots, Y_t(\mathbf{s}_n))', \qquad t = 0, 1, \ldots. \tag{6.87}$$

That is, for $t = 1, \ldots, T$, (6.87) can be written as the *n-variate time series*,

$$\mathbf{Y}_0, \mathbf{Y}_1, \ldots, \mathbf{Y}_T. \tag{6.88}$$

Additional discussion of multivariate time series models can be found in Sections 3.4.7 and 7.4. Underlying the approach of using (6.88) for spatio-temporal modeling is the notion that the temporal dependence is more natural to model than the spatial dependence. For example, the Markov model for (6.88),

$$[\mathbf{Y}_t|\mathbf{Y}_0, \ldots, \mathbf{Y}_{t-1}] = [\mathbf{Y}_t|\mathbf{Y}_{t-1}], \qquad t = 1, 2, \ldots, \tag{6.89}$$

does not overtly recognize the spatial context. Much of the spatial modeling of $\mathbf{Y}_t$ has used SAR models (see below), although CAR models are equally appropriate (e.g., Allcroft and Glasbey, 2003).

Modeling through (6.88) is in contrast to modeling $\{Y_t(\mathbf{s}_i)\}$ as a spatial process of time series, namely $\{\mathbf{Y}(\mathbf{s}_i): i = 1, \ldots, n\}$, where $\mathbf{Y}(\mathbf{s}_i) \equiv (Y_0(\mathbf{s}_i), \ldots, Y_T(\mathbf{s}_i))'$; see Sansó, Schmidt, and Nobre (2008). One could also think of the spatio-temporal dependence in terms of a $(T + 1)$-variate spatial lattice process [using, for example, models such as those presented by Sain and Cressie (2007)].

Vector Autoregressive Models

Without simplifying assumptions, the number of parameters specifying the distribution of (6.88) can be enormous. The model (6.89), say, uses the temporal dimension to achieve a more parsimonious model. By recognizing spatial "neighborhood" relationships, we can use the spatial dimension to achieve further parsimony. These ideas are all discussed in Chapter 7, and we give a simple example in the next paragraph.

A special case of (6.89) is the VAR(1) model of dimension n (Section 3.4.7):

$$\mathbf{Y}_t = \mathbf{M}\mathbf{Y}_{t-1} + \boldsymbol{\eta}_t, \tag{6.90}$$

where, in its full generality, $\mathbf{M}$ has n^2 parameters and $\boldsymbol{\Sigma}_\eta = \mathrm{var}(\boldsymbol{\eta}_t)$ has $O(n^2)$ parameters. The spatial context can be used to reduce the number of parameters drastically. For example, suppose that we assume the (i, j)th entry of $\mathbf{M}$, $(\mathbf{M})_{ij} = 0$, unless $\|\mathbf{s}_i - \mathbf{s}_j\| \leq h$. Then the current value at $\mathbf{s}_i$ is related

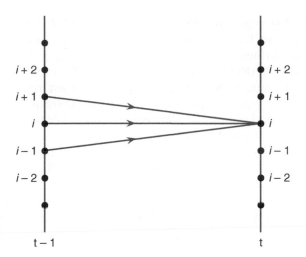

Figure 6.20 Schematic diagram (directed graph) of the dynamic structure found in (6.90) when **M** is defined spatially.

to those immediate-past values at s_i and nearby s_j (within a radius of h). Figure 6.20 shows a schematic diagram (i.e., a directed graph) of the dynamic structure in (6.90) when **M** is defined spatially, here in $\mathbb{R}^1$ with D_s a subset of the integers and $h = 1$. Thus, rather than **M** being made up of n^2 parameters, the parameter space has been reduced by making **M** sparse through spatial proximities of locations in D_s; in Figure 6.20, $(\mathbf{M})_{ij} = 0$, unless $|i - j| \leq 1$. A similar modeling strategy that allows further reduction in the size of the parameter space would choose $\boldsymbol{\Sigma}_\eta$ to be sparse (a geostatistical-type model; see Section 4.1) or $\boldsymbol{\Sigma}_\eta^{-1}$ to be sparse (a lattice-type model; see Section 4.2). A complete discussion of parsimonious parameterization of models like (6.90) is given in Sections 7.2 and 7.3.

We remark that the model (6.90) refers to the entirety of locations; however, the model does not allow inference on an $(n+1)$th location **s**. Consequently, a spatio-temporal statistical model that is defined by an n-dimensional multivariate time series, such as (6.90), cannot handle the problem of off-site predictions.

The VAR(1) model given by (6.90) is a special case of the spatio-temporal autoregressive moving-average (STARMA) model. It is generally true that for these and other multivariate time series, the number of parameters can be potentially enormous, and an important skill of the modeler is to reduce drastically the size of the parameter space. We believe that this is best achieved through recognizing and preserving any known spatio-temporal interactions (e.g., from a PDE) for the underlying process $Y(\cdot; \cdot)$; see Sections 6.3 and 7.2.4. In the absence of such knowledge, other approaches, such as those described throughout Chapter 7, can be taken.

Space–Time Autoregressive Moving-Average (STARMA) Models

In Section 6.3, we have seen how a spatio-temporal stochastic PDE can be discretized and written as a multivariate time series, $\{\mathbf{Y}_t\}$, that can be modeled dynamically as a VAR(1) process. One could look for even more generality in the temporal domain, by assuming higher orders of autoregression as well as a moving-average type of dependence. This would correspond to higher-order temporal partial derivatives and nonspecific temporal dependence in the noise term $\delta(\cdot; \cdot)$ of the stochastic PDE.

Define the *spatio-temporal autoregressive moving-average (STARMA)* model (Ali, 1979; Pfeifer and Deutsch, 1980; and Cressie, 1993, p. 450) as

$$\mathbf{Y}_t = \sum_{k=0}^{p} \left(\sum_{j=1}^{\lambda_k} f_{kj} \mathbf{U}_{kj} \right) \mathbf{Y}_{t-k} + \sum_{\ell=0}^{q} \left(\sum_{j=1}^{\mu_\ell} g_{\ell j} \mathbf{V}_{\ell j} \right) \mathbf{W}_{t-\ell}, \qquad t = 0, 1, \ldots,$$
$$(6.91)$$

where $\{\mathbf{U}_{kj}\}$ and $\{\mathbf{V}_{\ell j}\}$ are known weight matrices; p and q are the orders of the autoregressive part and moving-average part, respectively; $\{f_{kj}\}$ and $\{g_{\ell j}\}$ are parameters of the model; and $\{\mathbf{W}_t\}$ are *iid* random vectors with mean $\mathbf{0}$ and covariance matrix $\mathbf{\Sigma}_w$. In (6.91), the index j is used to denote substructures, although including them makes the number of parameters potentially enormous. Upon reparameterizing, we obtain

$$\mathbf{Y}_t = \sum_{k=0}^{p} \mathbf{B}_k \mathbf{Y}_{t-k} + \sum_{\ell=0}^{q} \mathbf{E}_\ell \mathbf{W}_{t-\ell}, \qquad (6.92)$$

where, without loss of generality, $\mathbf{\Sigma}_w = \sigma_w^2 \mathbf{I}$, and, for identifiability reasons, $\mathbf{B}_0$ has zero entries down the diagonal. We assume henceforth that $(\mathbf{I} - \mathbf{B}_0)$ is invertible.

The number of parameters in (6.92) is still very large. Consider several simple cases. First, $p = 0$ and $q = 0$ reduces (6.92) to a sequence of purely spatial processes without any temporal dependence linking them:

$$\mathbf{Y}_t = \mathbf{B}_0 \mathbf{Y}_t + \mathbf{E}_0 \mathbf{W}_t, \qquad t = 0, 1, \ldots.$$

Upon rewriting this expression, we obtain,

$$\mathbf{Y}_t = (\mathbf{I} - \mathbf{B}_0)^{-1} \mathbf{E}_0 \mathbf{W}_t, \qquad t = 0, 1, 2, \ldots, \qquad (6.93)$$

and since $\{\mathbf{W}_0, \mathbf{W}_1, \ldots\}$ are mutually independent, we see that the time series $\{\mathbf{Y}_t\}$ given by (6.93) has no temporal dependence. When $\mathbf{E}_0 = \mathbf{I}$, these random vectors are *iid* mean-zero simultaneous autoregressions (SARs); see Section 4.2.5.

The second case is $p = 1$ and $q = 0$, and recall that $\mathbf{B}_0$ has all-zero diagonal entries. Then,

$$\mathbf{Y}_t = \mathbf{B}_0 \mathbf{Y}_t + \mathbf{B}_1 \mathbf{Y}_{t-1} + \mathbf{E}_0 \mathbf{W_t}, \qquad t = 0, 1, \dots .$$

Given $\mathbf{Y}_{t-1}$, $\mathbf{Y}_t$ has spatial statistical dependence that is of the SAR form. From Cressie (1993, p. 409), a SAR can be written as a CAR, which is a Markov random field with simple *conditional* probability dependencies (Section 4.2.5). These dependencies are captured by an undirected graph (see Section 4.2.2). The equation just above can be written equivalently as,

$$\mathbf{Y}_t = (\mathbf{I} - \mathbf{B}_0)^{-1}\mathbf{B}_1 \mathbf{Y}_{t-1} + (\mathbf{I} - \mathbf{B}_0)^{-1}\mathbf{E}_0 \mathbf{W}_t$$
$$\equiv \mathbf{M}\mathbf{Y}_{t-1} + \boldsymbol{\eta}_t , \qquad (6.94)$$

where $\mathbf{M} \equiv (\mathbf{I} - \mathbf{B}_0)^{-1}\mathbf{B}_1$ and $\{\boldsymbol{\eta}_t\}$ are *iid* with mean zero and $\mathrm{var}(\boldsymbol{\eta}_t) = \sigma_w^2 \boldsymbol{\Sigma}_\eta (\mathbf{I} - \mathbf{B}_0)^{-1}\mathbf{E}_0\mathbf{E}_0'(\mathbf{I} - \mathbf{B}_0')^{-1}$. The matrix $\mathbf{B}_0$ represents "instantaneous" spatial dependence (see below).

Another way to achieve the model in the same form, is the case $p = 1$, $q = 0$, *and* $\mathbf{B}_0 \equiv \mathbf{0}$. Then,

$$\mathbf{Y}_t = \mathbf{B}_1 \mathbf{Y}_{t-1} + \mathbf{E}_0 \mathbf{W}_t , \qquad t = 0, 1, \dots ,$$

which is equivalent to

$$\mathbf{Y}_t = \mathbf{M}\mathbf{Y}_{t-1} + \boldsymbol{\eta}_t , \qquad (6.95)$$

where now $\mathbf{M} \equiv \mathbf{B}_1$, and $\{\boldsymbol{\eta}_t\}$ are *iid* with mean zero and $\mathrm{var}(\boldsymbol{\eta}_t) = \sigma_w^2 \mathbf{E}_0 \mathbf{E}_0'$. This is also a VAR(1) model.

One might then ask, "What is the purpose of $\mathbf{B}_0$?" Figure 6.21 gives a schematic diagram of the type of spatio-temporal dependence in (6.94), for which D_s is a subset of the integers in $\mathbb{R}^1$ and $\mathbf{B}_0$ is tridiagonal. In Figure 6.21a, notice the three directed edges from sites $i + 1, i, i - 1$ at time $t - 1$ to site i at time t. Notice also the four undirected edges at time t between site i and its neighbors at sites $i + 2$, $i + 1$, $i - 1$, and $i - 2$ (corresponding to instantaneous spatial dependence); this could be considered to define a chain graph, with a combination of directed and undirected edges (e.g., Lauritzen, 1996). Compare this to Figure 6.20, which in fact gives a schematic diagram of the spatio-temporal dependence in (6.95), for which $\mathbf{B}_0 = \mathbf{0}$ (no instantaneous spatial dependence). If we multiply out $(\mathbf{I} - \mathbf{B}_0)^{-1}\mathbf{B}_1$, where recall that $\mathbf{B}_0$ is tridiagonal, we obtain $\mathbf{M}$ in (6.94) that is generally *not* sparse. The graphical structure of (6.94) where $\mathbf{M}$ is not sparse, is shown in Figure 6.21b; notice that there are directed edges from *all* sites at time $t - 1$ to site i at time t. Even though Figures 6.21a and 6.21b represent the same type of model, the parameterization required for Figure 6.21a is much simpler.

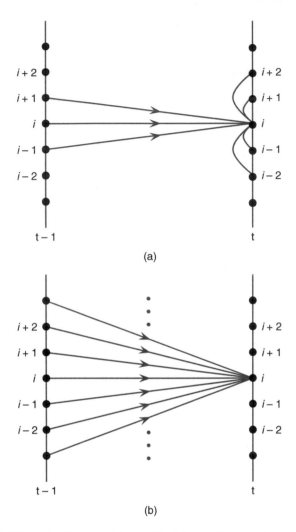

Figure 6.21 (a) Schematic diagram (chain graph) of the spatio-temporal dependence in (6.94), which includes instantaneous spatial dependence. (b) Schematic diagram (directed graph) of the spatio-temporal dependence structure with edges from all sites, which is equivalent to the spatio-temporal dependence exhibited in (a).

There are clearly a number of different ways to arrive at the same type of model. The difference between them lies in their parameterizations. When possible, we should look for a sparse but appropriate parameterization by considering the role each parameter plays in the physical model. One way to think of $\mathbf{B}_0$ is that it captures the variability at time steps much smaller than the unit of time specified for the autoregression. Small-temporal-scale dynamics, which may be important and unwise to ignore, are collected together into the matrix $\mathbf{B}_0$ that models *instantaneous spatial dependence* (Cressie, 1993,

p. 450). Thus, it is an approximation of dynamical structure running at time scales much smaller than the unit of time in the autoregression. Other interpretations are possible. Therefore, although the case of nonzero $\mathbf{B}_0$ in (6.94) and the case of $\mathbf{B}_0 = \mathbf{0}$ in (6.95) both lead to VAR(1) models, their interpretation is very different.

Now, consider the case $p = 1$, $q = 0$, $\mathbf{B}_0 = \mathbf{0}$, $\mathbf{E}_0 = \mathbf{I}$, and $\mathbf{B}_1 = \text{diag}\{b_1, \ldots, b_n\}$. Then, the STARMA model reduces to

$$Y_t(\mathbf{s}_i) = b_i Y_{t-1}(\mathbf{s}_i) + W_t(\mathbf{s}_i), \qquad i = 1, \ldots, n, \, t = 0, 1, \ldots, \qquad (6.96)$$

which is a collection of uncorrelated (in space) first-order autoregressive time series at each location $\{\mathbf{s}_i : i = 1, \ldots, n\}$. In this case, prediction of values of the process at pixels where there are no data cannot "borrow strength" from observations at (nearby) pixels. Fortunately, the spatial context usually means that $\mathbf{B}_1$ is *not* a diagonal matrix, which makes this last case an unlikely one. Notice that if the "forcing matrix," $\mathbf{E}_0$, is *not* the identity in the case discussed just above, $\mathbf{Y}_t$ *is* spatially dependent.

In the simple model (6.96), there is an opportunity to show the flexibility of conditional-probability modeling. Think of $\mathbf{b} \equiv (b_1, \ldots, b_n)'$ in (6.96) as given; that is, the model (6.96) is

$$[\mathbf{Y}_t | \mathbf{Y}_{t-1}, \mathbf{b}] = \prod_{i=1}^{n} [Y_t(\mathbf{s}_i) | Y_{t-1}(\mathbf{s}_i), b_i], \qquad t = 0, 1, \ldots, \qquad (6.97)$$

where the right-hand side specifies *spatial* (conditional) independence. Now think of the autoregressive coefficients $\mathbf{b}$ as a spatial process with distribution $[\mathbf{b}]$. Then, marginally,

$$[\mathbf{Y}_t | \mathbf{Y}_{t-1}] = \int \left\{ \prod_{i=1}^{n} [Y_t(\mathbf{s}_i) | Y_{t-1}(\mathbf{s}_i), b_i] \right\} [\mathbf{b}] \, d\mathbf{b}. \qquad (6.98)$$

From the conditional model (6.98), $Y_t(\mathbf{s}_i)$ generally depends on all entries of $\mathbf{Y}_{t-1}$, which was not the case for the conditional model (6.96). Thus, through simple (conditional) models at successive levels of a hierarchy, complex (unconditional) structure can be captured. Wikle, Berliner, and Cressie (1998) used four levels of a hierarchical statistical model to model complex spatio-temporal dependence in meteorological data (Section 6.6). This hierarchical statistical approach to modeling spatio-temporal processes can be found in Chapter 7 and is applied to substantive problems in Chapter 9.

6.5   SPATIO-TEMPORAL POINT PROCESSES

Recall from Section 4.3 the definition of a spatial point process in a bounded subset D_s of $\mathbb{R}^d$ as a stochastic counting process defined on all Lebesgue measurable subsets of D_s. It is a simple matter to extend the definition to a bounded subset, $D_{s,t}$, of $\mathbb{R}^d \times \mathbb{R}$. Let T denote the largest time in that subset; then there exists a bounded subset D_s of $\mathbb{R}^d$ such that $D_{s,t} \subset D_s \times [0, T]$. Hereafter, we write $D_{s,t} = D_s \times [0, T]$, and hence we can think about a spatio-temporal point process either as a point process in $\mathbb{R}^{d+1}$ (descriptive) or as a temporal process of spatial point processes (dynamical). Note that in some circumstances, a spatial point process of temporal processes might be a sensible model, but it is less likely and we do not pursue it here.

In this section, we consider only simple point processes (i.e., almost surely, either no event or a single event occurs at any point in space×time). Let $Z(A)$ denote the number of events in $A \subset D_s \times [0, T]$; if $Z(A)$ is (almost surely) finite for all such A, then $\{Z(A) : A \subset D_s \times [0, T]\}$ characterizes the point process. To emphasize the presence of spatial and temporal components, we sometimes refer to the point process as $Z(\cdot\,; \cdot)$. Indeed, from a dynamical perspective, $\{Z(\cdot\,; t) : t \in [0, T]\}$ and $\{Z_t(\cdot) : t = 0, 1, \dots\}$ represent, respectively, a continuously evolving and a discretely evolving class of spatial point processes.

Definitions for the (first-order) intensity, $\{\lambda(\mathbf{s}; t) : \mathbf{s} \in D_s, t \in [0, T]\}$, and higher-order moment measures follow in the same manner as in Section 4.3. In this brief presentation of spatio-temporal point processes, we go from the specific to the general. First, the *spatio-temporal (homogeneous) Poisson point process* Z has constant intensity λ^o, $Z(A) \sim Poi(\lambda^o|A|)$, where $|A|$ is the $(d + 1)$-dimensional volume of A, and for $A_1 \cap A_2 = \emptyset$, $Z(A_1)$ and $Z(A_2)$ are independent. The *inhomogeneous Poisson point process* is obtained by replacing λ^o with $\lambda(\cdot\,; \cdot)$, so that $Z(A) \sim Poi(\int_A \lambda(\mathbf{x}; r)d\mathbf{x}dr)$. For example, suppose

$$\lambda(\mathbf{s}; t) = \lambda^o(t), \qquad \mathbf{s} \in D_s, \ t \in [0, T].$$

Then for fixed $t \in [0, T]$, $Z(\cdot\,; t)$ is a homogeneous Poisson process with constant (over space) intensity $\lambda^o(t)$.

It is straightforward to extend the definitions in Section 4.3 to define spatio-temporal versions of the *pair-correlation function*, the *K function*, and the *L function* (e.g., Gabriel and Diggle, 2009). It is also possible to extend the models in Section 4.3 to the spatio-temporal equivalent of *dependent (spatial Markov) point processes* and *marked point processes*. However, it is important to remember here that the time dimension is ordered and, where possible, point processes should respect the evolutionary nature of the phenomena they are modeling.

Spatial point processes generally do not have directionality associated with them (for an exception to this, see Section 4.3.5 where Directed Markov Point Processes are discussed). Hence, in the spatial setting, the notion of *conditional intensity*, conditional on "the past," is not natural. Conditional intensities are attractive, because, as will be seen below, the point process' likelihood function is straightforward to write down.

A simple point process can be characterized uniquely by its conditional intensity (Fishman and Snyder, 1976). The formal definition requires the notions of σ-algebras, a filtration, and a martingale (e.g., Daley and Vere-Jones, 2003); in what follows, we give an intuitive presentation of the conditional intensity function in the spatio-temporal setting. Think about the entire "history," $\mathcal{H}_t$, of a spatio-temporal point process up to time t. Then the conditional intensity, $\psi(\mathbf{s}; t)$, is the frequency with which events are expected to occur at $(\mathbf{s}; t)$, *given* $\mathcal{H}_t$. Formally,

$$\psi(\mathbf{s}; t) \equiv \lim_{\substack{|ds| \to 0 \\ dt \to 0}} \frac{E(Z(ds; dt)|\mathcal{H}_t)}{|ds|\,|dt|}, \tag{6.99}$$

where recall that ds is a small region located at $\mathbf{s}$, and likewise dt is a small time interval at t. We write the parameterized conditional intensity as $\psi(\mathbf{s}; t; \boldsymbol{\theta})$.

Let the events of Z be written as $\{(\mathbf{s}_i; t_i): i = 1, \ldots, N\}$, where $N = Z(D_s \times [0, T])$. Then the loglikelihood function (up to an additive constant) is (e.g., Daley and Vere-Jones, 2003),

$$\sum_{i=1}^{n} \log \psi(\mathbf{s}_i; t_i \boldsymbol{\theta}) - \int_0^T \int_{D_s} \psi(\mathbf{x}; r; \boldsymbol{\theta})\,d\mathbf{x}dr. \tag{6.100}$$

This attractive expression belies the difficulty sometimes encountered in evaluating the integral in (6.100), as well as in interpreting the conditional intensity back in terms of the physical/chemical/biological/economic/etc. phenomenon originally being modeled. In its full generality, a spatio-temporal point process has a likelihood analogous to the rather complicated expression (4.186) in the spatial case; see the discussion surrounding this expression in Section 4.3.3. Yet, (6.100) is equally the (log)likelihood and appears to be in a much simpler form. Thus, the evolutionary aspect of the temporal component allows conceptual simplification. Of course, once a conditional intensity is fitted to the available data, it then needs to be interpreted properly, as a quantification of the *conditional* properties of the process.

A simple example of a joint specification of a spatio-temporal point process can be given through the inhomogeneous Poisson point process, which was defined at the beginning of this section. This process *is* characterized by the first-order intensity function, $\lambda(\mathbf{s}; t)$, but recall that it has a rather strong independence property for counts in nonintersecting sets A_1 and A_2. However, some flexibility is achieved by making the first-order intensity random; that is, $\{\lambda(\mathbf{s}; t): \mathbf{s} \in D_s, t \in [0, T]\}$ is assumed to be a spatio-temporal *stochastic* process. This results in a spatio-temporal *Cox process* (Section 4.3.1), an example of which is the *log-Gaussian Cox process* (Møller, Syversveen, and Waagepetersen, 1998). Here, $\lambda(\mathbf{s}; t) = \exp\{Y(\mathbf{s}; t)\}$, where $\{Y(\mathbf{s}; t): \mathbf{s} \in \mathbb{R}^d, t \in [0, T]\}$ is a Gaussian process whose behavior could be captured by any of the models discussed in Sections 6.1, 6.3, and 6.4.1 and in Chapter 7.

As an HM, the log Gaussian Cox process has a data model and process model given by:

Data model: $[Z(\cdot; \cdot)|Y(\cdot; \cdot)]$ is an inhomogeneous Poisson process with
                   intensity function, $\exp\{Y(\cdot; \cdot)\}$.

Process model: $[Y(\cdot; \cdot)|\mu_Y, C_Y]$ is a (possibly nonstationary) Gaussian pro-
                   cess with mean function μ_Y and covariance function C_Y.

At the third level of the hierarchy, a parameter model would put a prior distribution on (the parameters of) μ_Y and C_Y. Clearly, once the randomness of
the event locations/times is handled by the data model, the next levels of the
HM can exploit the power of the DSTMs given in Chapter 7 (i.e., the process
models presented in Sections 7.2, 7.3, and 7.4, and the parameter models presented in Section 7.5). Of course, because the data model for point processes
is fundamentally different from those presented in Section 7.1, the posterior
distributions will be too.

The goal of an HM approach is to obtain the posterior distribution
of all unknowns, given the spatio-temporal event locations $\{(s_i; t_i): i =
1, \ldots, N\}$ and the number of such events, $N = Z(D_s \times [0, T])$. Møller
and Waagepetersen (2004, Sec. 9.3) discuss Bayesian inference briefly, in
the spatial context, Diggle, Rowlingson, and Su (2005) use spatio-temporal
Bayesian inference to identify clusters, and Frcalová, Beneš, and Klement
(2010) present Bayesian nonlinear filtering of evolving spatial point patterns.
It is clear that modeling, implementation, and inference for HMs for
spatio-temporal point patterns, particularly dynamical ones, is an area that is
just beginning to develop.

There is a growing literature on spatio-temporal point processes; Diggle
(2007) gives an informative review, and Illian et al. (2008, Section 6.10) has
a section discussing different ways the temporal component could be used to
augment spatial-point-process modeling. Most of the models in the literature
are based on a "marginal probability" approach; that is, a point process model,
$[Z|\boldsymbol{\theta}]$, is fitted to data, $\{(s_i; t_i): i = 1, \ldots, N\}$ and $N = Z(D_s \times [0, T])$,
where Z might be defined dynamically or nondynamically through either the
intensity function or the conditional intensity function (e.g., Rodrigues and
Diggle, 2010).

An example of a nondynamical point process model is given in the paper
by Møller and Díaz-Avalos (2010), where the log-intensity function of a
log-Gaussian Cox process has a spatio-temporal shot-noise component that
depends spatially on nearby events and temporally on both past and future
events. A dynamical model may be as simple as a (log) regression of an
intensity function on a covariate that itself is varying with time (and possibly space); for example, see Peng, Schoenberg, and Woods (2005). Or, it may
involve an intensity function that is "self-exciting," such as for modeling epicenters of earthquakes and their aftershocks; for example, see Ogata (1998)
and Schoenberg (2003). Or, it may be a log-Gaussian Cox process that has a
dynamical intensity function; for example, see Brix and Diggle (2001).

Finally, spatio-temporal *marked* point processes have an analogous definition to that given in the purely spatial case (Section 4.3.3). Here, a point process

is combined with a geostatistical process to model such things as location *and* size of trees in a natural forest; in the spatio-temporal context, an important application is to the locations/times/magnitudes of earthquakes in $D_s \times [0, T]$ (e.g., Ogata, 1998; Schoenberg, 2003; Ogata, 2004). Särkkä and Renshaw (2006) can be consulted for discussion of the general area and an application to a pine-forest dataset; an updated discussion with emphasis on physical-statistical modeling of the mark process can be found in Renshaw (2010).

6.6 SPATIO-TEMPORAL COMPONENTS-OF-VARIATION MODELS

We saw in Section 6.1 how components-of-variation models can be used to motivate different spatio-temporal covariance functions. A very general components-of-variation model for the spatio-temporal process, $\{Y(\mathbf{s}; t): \mathbf{s} \in D_s, t \in D_t\}$, takes the form (Wikle, 2003a),

$$Y(\mathbf{s}; t) \equiv \mu(\mathbf{s}; \boldsymbol{\theta}_t) + \gamma(t; \boldsymbol{\theta}_\mathbf{s}) + \kappa(\mathbf{s}; t; \boldsymbol{\theta}_{\mathbf{s};t}) + \delta(\mathbf{s}; t), \qquad (6.101)$$

where space and time could be continuous or discrete. A slightly more general formulation posits the same additive components of variation for a *transformed* process, $g(Y(\mathbf{s}; t))$. This is a straightforward approach to spatio-temporal modeling, where the spatial, temporal, and spatio-temporal variabilities are separated into additive components, and where a great deal of generality is achieved by allowing parameters to vary also.

The first term on the right-hand side of (6.101), $\mu(\mathbf{s}; \boldsymbol{\theta}_t)$, represents a *spatial* trend surface with parameters that may vary with time. Similarly, the second term on the right-hand side, $\gamma(t; \boldsymbol{\theta}_\mathbf{s})$, represents a temporal trend that may have spatially varying parameters. The third term, $\kappa(\mathbf{s}; t; \boldsymbol{\theta}_{\mathbf{s},t})$, typically represents a complicated (usually nonseparable) spatio-temporal random process that could be a dynamical process (e.g., a process defined by the diffusion-injection equation discussed in the introduction to this chapter and in Section 6.3.1). The last term, $\delta(\mathbf{s}; t)$, represents micro-scale spatio-temporal variation that we model as a mean-zero uncorrelated process in $D_s \times D_t$. We are thinking of at least the components κ and δ as being random and, depending on circumstances, μ and γ could be too; all random effects are assumed independent of each other. The result is a spatio-temporal mixed-effects model.

Obviously, (6.101) may not be identifiable unless substantial prior knowledge is used in determining the form of, and the distributions for μ, γ, κ, and δ. For example, is it better to represent $Y(\mathbf{s}; t)$ as a spatial process with temporally varying parameters, or as a temporal process with spatially varying parameters? Our position throughout this book is that the question is very difficult to answer without a physical/chemical/biological/economic/etc. process to guide the choice.

There are two ways to consider the components-of-variation model (6.101). One is based on marginal probabilities, where probabilities associated with the left-hand side of (6.101) are obtained by convolution calculations of components' probability distributions. The other, which we prefer, is based on a sequence of conditional probabilities, as each random quantity is successively put into the conditioning set of random components. Moreover, the conditional approach allows (6.101) to be generalized to nonadditive (and non-Gaussian) decompositions of spatial, temporal, and spatio-temporal variability.

Example: Spatio-temporal Modeling of Temperatures in the Midwest

An example of the type of modeling motivated by (6.101) was given by Wikle, Berliner, and Cressie (1998), where the spatio-temporal process under study was the monthly average of maximum temperatures in a portion of the U.S. Midwest "corn belt" (centered around Iowa) for 240 months (i.e., 20 years from 1974 through 1993). Thus, space is continuous (over the corn belt) and time is discrete (monthly). From climatological knowledge, they specified the component μ to depend on space only (a Gaussian Markov random field with mean depending linearly on latitude and longitude; see Section 4.2.2 for more details on Markov random fields). The temporal trend γ was used to model an obvious seasonal cycle of temperatures (a linear combination of sine and cosine, each with period 12 months, where the two regression coefficients are themselves linear functions of latitude and longitude). The stochastic spatio-temporal term κ was modeled as being dynamical in time and descriptive in space, where the dynamics captured the month-to-month circulation changes in the atmosphere. This is clearly where a stochastic PDE or a stochastic difference equation, like those presented in Sections 6.3 and 7.2, could be used to model the smaller-scale (in both space and time) variability. Since large-scale weather patterns often exhibit fairly stationary longitudinal wavelike patterns in the mid-latitudes, and such patterns are fairly persistent in time with general west-to-east movement, it is possible that air temperatures at a given location in a given month could be related to air temperatures in regions to the west in the previous month. This suggested that a "lagged nearest neighbor" (Section 7.2.3) parameterization of the propagator matrix was reasonable. Specifically, the parameters corresponding to the neighbors to the east, west, north, and south were distinct, and the parameters corresponding to the same site at the previous time were allowed to vary with space.

Through (6.101), the spatio-temporal variability of temperature in and around Iowa was decomposed into a climatological component, a seasonal component, and a shorter-term dynamical component. An alternative, less satisfying decomposition would be to write the first part of (6.101), $\mu(\mathbf{s}; \boldsymbol{\theta}_t) + \gamma(t; \boldsymbol{\theta}_\mathbf{s})$, as a deterministic trend made up of a linear combination of (mixed) polynomials in space and time. Then, $\kappa(\mathbf{s}; t; \boldsymbol{\theta}_{\mathbf{s};t})$ would be a purely stochastic component with mean zero and covariance function given by, for example, one of the descriptive models presented in Section 6.1. As we mentioned above, there is clearly nonidentifiability associated with the spatio-temporal model (6.101); the extra dimension, time, does not allow one to avoid the difficulty discussed by Cressie (1993, p. 25): "What is one person's ... covariance structure may be another person's mean structure." Which decomposition to use should depend as much as possible on the underlying scientific problem being studied. For example, the model of temperature in the Midwest given earlier, which incorporates climatology, seasonality, and changes in dynamical circulation, has far more explanatory power than a model with deterministic trend plus stationary stochastic error. Both may *describe* the particular spatio-temporal dataset well, but the latter model will generally do much worse in forecasting future temperatures in a spatial domain *similar* to (but different from) Iowa and surroundings. In conclusion, to the extent possible, we advocate choosing scientifically interpretable components of variation, including dynamical terms behaving (approximately) according to accepted physical relationships.

6.6.1 Dimension Reduction in a Dynamical Model

Recall the stochastic difference equation (6.70), which is a dynamical spatio-temporal statistical model. Wikle, Berliner, and Cressie (1998) use a model like this to capture the variability in temperature due to month-to-month circulation changes in the atmosphere. When space is discretized into pixels, $\{\kappa(\mathbf{s}; t; \boldsymbol{\theta}_{\mathbf{s};t}) : \mathbf{s} \in D_s\}$ in (6.101) can be written as the vector $\boldsymbol{\kappa}_t$, where the dimension of the vector is the number of pixels. The parameters $\{\boldsymbol{\theta}_{\mathbf{s};t}\}$ are the elements of propagator matrices, $\{\mathbf{M}_t\}$, and the variance and covariance parameters in the error covariance $\boldsymbol{\Sigma}_\eta$, as we now illustrate.

Let $D_t = \{0, 1, 2, \dots\}$, and assume that the spatio-temporal variability in (6.101) is given by the first-order linear dynamical process,

$$\boldsymbol{\kappa}_t = \mathbf{M}_t \boldsymbol{\kappa}_{t-1} + \boldsymbol{\eta}_t, \qquad t = 1, 2, \dots, \tag{6.102}$$

where $\{\mathbf{M}_t\}$ is a sequence of propagator matrices, $\{\boldsymbol{\eta}_t\}$ is an *iid* sequence of error vectors each with mean $\mathbf{0}$ and covariance matrix $\boldsymbol{\Sigma}_\eta$, and $\boldsymbol{\eta}_t$ is independent of $\boldsymbol{\kappa}_{t-1}$.

When the number of pixels is very large, fitting the model (6.102) may not be possible without some form of *dimension reduction*. Dimension reduction can be achieved relative to the parameter space by using parameterizations suggested by "nearest neighbor," PDE, or IDE models. Alternatively, dimension reduction can be relative to the process itself, for example, through a *spectral representation* (i.e., basis-function expansion),

$$\boldsymbol{\kappa}_t = \boldsymbol{\Phi} \boldsymbol{\alpha}_t, \tag{6.103}$$

where $\boldsymbol{\Phi}$ is a matrix of basis functions, and $\boldsymbol{\alpha}_t$ is a vector of the associated spectral coefficients with *much* lower dimension (p_α, say) than that of $\boldsymbol{\kappa}_t$. As described in Sections 4.1.4 and 7.1.3, we use the word "spectral" rather broadly to refer to general basis-function expansions, and thus there are many different choices available for these basis functions. For example, one might consider these to be orthogonal functions (e.g., Fourier, orthogonal polynomials such as Hermite polynomials, eigenvectors from a specified or estimated covariance function), wavelets, splines, bisquares, discrete kernel convolutions, and so on, depending on the specific application. As an example, the spectral representation (6.103) could be based on truncating an infinite linear combination of a complete class of orthogonal basis functions. The truncation in such an expansion is a source of error that is often ignored; Wikle and Cressie (1999) handle it by assuming instead,

$$\kappa_t = \Phi\alpha_t + \xi_t,\qquad\qquad\qquad (6.104)$$

where ξ_t is independent of α_t, and $\{\xi_t\}$ models all the hitherto-discarded, high-frequency terms through a relatively simple dependence structure, like $\xi_t \sim iid\,Gau(0, \Sigma_\xi)$. In some cases, one might further decompose ξ_t into components associated with "small-scale" spatio-temporal processes and, perhaps, a white-noise process in space and time. In any case, a dynamical model can be fitted to $\{\alpha_t\}$, namely

$$\alpha_t = M_{\alpha,t}\alpha_{t-1} + \gamma_t,$$

in a p_α-dimensional space (e.g., Wikle and Cressie, 1999).

If sufficient information is available, one can allow the basis functions to vary with time, perhaps on a different time-scale than the process of interest. That is, (6.103) could be generalized to

$$\kappa_t = \Phi_t\alpha_t,\qquad\qquad\qquad (6.105)$$

where the columns of Φ_t are given basis functions that depend on t. Then define $var(\alpha_t) \equiv \Sigma_{\alpha,t}$, whose entries are considered to be a subset of the parameters $\{\theta_{s;t}\}$. In the case where these basis functions are estimated, there are potential identifiability concerns with modeling the dynamics of α_t, and hence simple dynamical structures (e.g., random walks) for α_t need to be specified.

If possible, one should account for the truncation associated with the expansion (6.105), analogously to the model given in (6.104):

$$\kappa_t = \Phi_t\alpha_t + \xi_t,\qquad t = 0, 1, \ldots,\qquad\qquad (6.106)$$

where ξ_t is independent of α_t, and assume $\xi_t \sim iid\,Gau(0, \Sigma_\xi)$. Once again, $\{\xi_t\}$ plays the role of modeling residual spatio-temporal or spatial dependence (Section 6.4.2). In some cases, this residual term may just account for variation, but without spatial or temporal dependence; for example, Cressie, Shi, and Kang (2010) use (6.106) with $\Sigma_\xi = \sigma_\xi^2 I$, to capture pixel-scale variability in a model applied to a remote-sensing problem, or Σ_ξ could be diagonal.

If one has sufficient knowledge to specify the time-varying basis functions, then it is possible to consider more complicated dependence in the process α_t. That is, one could consider a first-order dynamical process such as

$$\kappa_t = \Phi_t\alpha_t + \xi_t,$$
$$\alpha_t = M_{\alpha,t}\alpha_{t-1} + \gamma_t,\qquad\qquad\qquad (6.107)$$

where $\mathbf{M}_{\alpha,t}$ is a $p_\alpha \times p_\alpha$ propagator matrix, and $\boldsymbol{\gamma}_t$ is a p_α-dimensional vector independent of $\boldsymbol{\alpha}_{t-1}$ [e.g., see Cressie, Shi, and Kang (2010)]. Such a model implies marginal covariances for $\boldsymbol{\kappa}_t$ that are nonstationary and nonseparable (Sections 6.1.2 and 6.1.3). An example using (6.107) in an EHM is given in Section 9.2.

6.6.2 Hierarchical Spatio-Temporal Statistical Modeling

We close this section with an indication of what is to come in Chapter 7. In Chapter 6, we have made the case for preferring dynamical (conditional-probability-based) spatio-temporal models over descriptive (marginal-probability-based) spatio-temporal models. However, we have not yet shown how the dynamical models fit into a hierarchical statistical structure. Consider observations and potential observations described by $\{Z(\mathbf{s}; t): \mathbf{s} \in D_s, t \in D_t\}$, or $Z(\cdot; \cdot)$. We are careful to distinguish $Z(\cdot; \cdot)$ from $\{Y(\mathbf{s}; t): \mathbf{s} \in D_s, t \in D_t\}$, or $Y(\cdot; \cdot)$, which is the physical/chemical/biological/economic/etc. process of interest.

We observe $Y(\cdot; \cdot)$ imperfectly because the observations are incomplete and noisy. We write the data $\mathbf{Z}$ in a way that emphasizes their spatio-temporal coordinates:

$$\mathbf{Z} \equiv (Z(\mathbf{s}_i; t_i): i = 1, \ldots, m)', \tag{6.108}$$

and we often assume that the error due to measurement is additive, namely

$$Z(\mathbf{s}_i; t_i) = Y(\mathbf{s}_i; t_i) + \varepsilon(\mathbf{s}_i; t_i), \qquad i = 1, \ldots, m, \tag{6.109}$$

where $\varepsilon(\mathbf{s}_i; t_i)$ represents a random measurement-error component, whose probability distribution is specified. For example, if $\boldsymbol{\varepsilon} \equiv (\varepsilon(\mathbf{s}_1; t_1), \ldots, \varepsilon(\mathbf{s}_m; t_m))'$, then suppose that $\boldsymbol{\varepsilon} \sim Gau(\boldsymbol{\mu}_\varepsilon, \boldsymbol{\Sigma}_\varepsilon)$; often, $\boldsymbol{\mu}_\varepsilon = \mathbf{0}$ and $\boldsymbol{\Sigma}_\varepsilon = \sigma_\varepsilon^2 \mathbf{I}$, because the measuring instrument performs unbiasedly, consistently, and independently at each place and time a measurement is taken. The best instruments are built so that $\boldsymbol{\mu}_\varepsilon = \mathbf{0}$ and σ_ε^2 is as small as possible. The assumption (6.109), of additive Gaussian measurement error, is an example of a *data model*. We can generalize the data model by expressing it in terms of conditional probabilities:

$$[\mathbf{Z}|Y(\cdot; \cdot), \boldsymbol{\theta}_D], \tag{6.110}$$

where $\boldsymbol{\theta}_D$ are *parameters* in the data model. This is the *first* level of the HM.

The *second* level of the HM is the *process model*:

$$[Y(\cdot; \cdot)|\boldsymbol{\theta}_P], \tag{6.111}$$

where $\boldsymbol{\theta}_P$ are *parameters* of the process model. In most of the sections of this chapter, we have concentrated on the distribution of the hidden process,

(6.111) and various ways were given to (partially) specify it, either dynamically or descriptively.

Bayes' Theorem tells us that the posterior distribution of $Y(\cdot; \cdot)$ given the data (and the parameters), is

$$[Y(\cdot; \cdot)|\mathbf{Z}, \boldsymbol{\theta}] \propto [\mathbf{Z}|Y(\cdot; \cdot), \boldsymbol{\theta}_D][Y(\cdot; \cdot)|\boldsymbol{\theta}_P], \qquad (6.112)$$

where $\boldsymbol{\theta} \equiv \{\boldsymbol{\theta}_D, \boldsymbol{\theta}_P\}$. From (6.112), we can predict (parts of, or functionals of) the "hidden" process $Y(\cdot; \cdot)$. Notice that the right-hand side of (6.112) is simply the product of the data model (6.110) and the process model (6.111). What should be done about the unknown parameters $\boldsymbol{\theta}$?

The *empirical hierarchical model* (EHM) performs separate estimation of $\boldsymbol{\theta}$, based on the data $\mathbf{Z}$ or other data; the resulting $\widehat{\boldsymbol{\theta}}$ is "plugged into" the posterior distribution given by (6.112); see Section 9.2 for an example. The *Bayesian hierarchical model* (BHM) posits a *third* level of the hierarchy, namely the *parameter model* (or prior),

$$[\boldsymbol{\theta}] = [\boldsymbol{\theta}_D, \boldsymbol{\theta}_P]. \qquad (6.113)$$

Then, Bayes' Theorem allows inference on *all* unknowns, $Y(\cdot; \cdot)$ *and* $\boldsymbol{\theta}$, in the same manner through the posterior distribution:

$$[Y(\cdot; \cdot), \boldsymbol{\theta}|\mathbf{Z}] \propto [\mathbf{Z}|Y(\cdot; \cdot), \boldsymbol{\theta}_D][Y(\cdot; \cdot)|\boldsymbol{\theta}_P][\boldsymbol{\theta}], \qquad (6.114)$$

where now the right-hand side of (6.114) is simply the product of the distributions specified at the first level (data model (6.110)), the second level (process model (6.111)), and the third level (parameter model (6.113)) of the hierarchy. See Sections 9.1, 9.3, and 9.4 for examples. A spatio-temporal HM and the inferences associated with it might seem like a way to do *data assimilation*. In fact, it is (Wikle and Berliner, 2007).

Now, when we think of spatio-temporal statistical models as time series of spatial processes, we can think of optimal smoothing, filtering, and forecasting of the processes. By allowing the (discretized) spatial dimension to define a vector of attributes, $\mathbf{Y}_t$, we see that spatio-temporal prediction (smoothing, filtering, forecasting) can be obtained from a multivariate version of optimal prediction (e.g., Shumway and Stoffer, 2006). As has already been noted, Chapter 9 considers both the EHM and the BHM approaches to spatio-temporal statistical analysis of various real-world phenomena, where dynamical spatio-temporal models are featured.

6.7 BIBLIOGRAPHIC NOTES

General References to Spatio-Temporal Statistics

Books and edited volumes that have contributed to the subject's recent evolution are Le and Zidek (2006), Finkenstädt, Held, and Isham (2007), and Gelfand et al. (2010, Part V). That literature has developed largely from spatial statistics, although Bennett (1979) develops models from time series. Banerjee, Carlin, and Gelfand (2004) and Schabenberger and Gotway (2005) each have a chapter devoted to spatio-temporal modeling, and Cressie (1991, 1993) has a small discussion of spatio-temporal statistics in each of the three parts of his book. Higdon (2007) gives a primer on space-time modeling from a Bayesian perspective; Chen, Fuentes, and Davis (2006) review the literature relevant to the study of environmental processes; Christakos (2000) presents a rather specialized approach from a geostatistical viewpoint; and Renshaw (1991) gives a stochastic processes approach to modeling biological populations in space and time.

Models for Spatio-Temporal Covariance Functions

There has been a little work done on models for spatio-temporal variograms (Fernandez-Casal, González-Manteiga, and Febrero-Bande, 2003). Generally the literature has concentrated on spatio-temporal covariance functions; Sherman (2011) reviews models for spatio-temporal covariance functions. Spectral representations of stationary spatio-temporal covariance functions are another way to describe the spatio-temporal dependence; see the review by Fuentes, Guttorp, and Sampson (2007).

Separable spatio-temporal models were used in early studies of spatio-temporal statistics; their convenience (positive-definiteness and efficient computations) outweighed their obvious lack of flexibility. Since 1999, there has been substantial work done to understand separability, to understand full symmetry, and to construct quite general classes of nonseparable spatio-temporal covariance functions (Cressie and Huang, 1999; Kyriakidis and Journel, 1999; De Iaco, Myers, and Posa, 2002; Gneiting, 2002; Stein, 2005; Genton, 2007; Gneiting, Genton, and Guttorp, 2007; and Jun and Stein, 2007). Mathematically speaking, one seeks functions of spatial lag **h** and temporal lag τ that are non-negative definite and *not* of product form. There have been some ingenious constructions, although only a few of them have been fitted to spatio-temporal data (De Cesare, Myers, and Posa, 2001; Ma, 2003, 2005; Stein, 2005; Porcu, Gregori, and Mateu, 2006; Porcu, Mateu, and Saura, 2008). Nonseparable, nonstationary, spatio-temporal covariance functions have been considered by Fuentes, Chen and Davis (2008) and Cressie, Shi, and Kang (2010).

Spatio-Temporal Kriging

Kriging typically involves the inverse of the data covariance matrix. A general difficulty with inversion of this matrix has led to simplifying assumptions about spatio-temporal covariance functions, such as separability and additivity. Separability is discussed in the previous paragraph. A model that adds a purely spatial covariance to a purely temporal covariance was considered by Bilonick (1985) and Rouhani and Hall (1989), although for certain data configurations the covariance matrix can be singular. One could use spatio-temporal neighborhoods to reduce the order of the kriging equations (Haas, 1995, 2002). Models for spatio-temporal kriging do not have to be dynamical (e.g., Cressie and Majure, 1997; Hartfield and Gunst, 2003; Huang and Hsu, 2004; Lophaven, Carstensen, and Rootzen, 2004; Augustin et al., 2009; Bodnar and Schmid, 2010).

Stochastic Partial Differential Equations

A physical system defined by a stochastic PDE in space and time implies a spatio-temporal covariance function. Whittle (1963, 1986) has been a major contributor to this area; he is also acknowledged by Heine as having suggested the problem solved in the seminal paper of Heine (1955).

Spatio-Temporal Models Based on Conditional Probabilities

Decomposition of complex spatio-temporal processes can often be decomposed into relatively simple conditional-probability-based models. Early examples of this include the articles by Handcock and Wallis (1994), Brown, Le, and Zidek (1994), Waller et al. (1997), Knorr-Held and Besag (1998), and Wikle, Berliner, and Cressie (1998). It is natural to assume that the immediate-past state of the process affects the current state (e.g., Guttorp, Meiring, and Sampson, 1994; Huang and Cressie, 1996; Mardia et al., 1998; Wikle and Cressie, 1999; Wikle et al., 2001; Stroud, Müller, and Sansó, 2001). Brown et al. (2000) discuss stochastic PDEs and their discretization, as do Wikle (2003b), Xu and Wikle (2007), Wikle and Hooten (2006), and Hooten and Wikle (2008). Stochastic IDEs were proposed by Wikle and Cressie (1999), Storvik, Frigessi, and Hirst (2002), Wikle (2002a), and Xu, Wikle, and Fox (2005).

Times Series of Spatial Processes

Before we review this area, we would like to point to an alternative approach to modeling spatio-temporal data, namely as a spatial process of time series (Bennett, 1979; Rouhani and Wackernagel, 1990; Sansó, Schmidt, and Nobre, 2008).

When considering time series of spatial processes, the choice is generally between time series of geostatistical processes or time series of lattice processes. Many spatio-temporal studies address problems in the environmental sciences, for which geostatistical processes evolving in time are usually chosen (e.g., Haslett et al., 2006; Lemos and Sansó, 2009; and Hering and Genton, 2010). These are the predominant class of models studied in Chapter 7, and hence for these we refer the reader to the Bibliographic Notes in Section 7.8. Nevertheless, there are two reviews of the field that should be mentioned here, namely Kyriakidis and Journel (1999) and Chen, Fuentes, and Davis (2006).

For studies in the social sciences in general, and for Public Health studies in particular, spatio-temporal data are usually aggregated spatially to small areas (often for confidentiality reasons). Hence, lattice processes evolving in time are usually chosen [Pavía, Larraz, and Montero (2008), is an exception to this]. Examples include Waller et al. (1997), Knorr-Held and Besag (1998), Knorr-Held (2000), Lagazio, Dreassi, and Biggeri (2001), Assunção, Reis, and Oliveira (2001), Mugglin, Cressie, and Gemmell (2002), Carlin and Banerjee

(2003), and Norton and Niu (2009). However, there are studies in the environmental sciences that have also used lattice processes (particularly Markov random fields) evolving in time to capture dependence on discretized space (e.g., Rathbun and Cressie, 1994; Lavine and Lozier, 1999; Allcroft and Glasbey, 2003; Zhu, Huang, and Wu, 2005; Daniels, Zhou, and Zou, 2006; Zhang and Zhu, 2008; Zhu et al., 2008; Ugarte, Goicoa, and Militino, 2010).

Spatio-Temporal Point Processes

A number of references were already given in Section 6.5. The use of an HM is not all that common in the literature, although obviously a Cox process can be thought of this way. Much of the modeling and inference has been based on a model that we express here generically as $[Z|\theta]$. Even for the Cox process, marginalization has often been carried out through, $[Z|\theta] = \int [Z|Y][Y|\theta] \, dY$, where $\lambda \equiv e^Y$ (for example) is the intensity of the inhomogeneous Poisson process, $Z|Y$. Estimation of θ through maximum likelihood (Veen and Schoenberg, 2008) or "pseudo" likelihood (Schoenberg, 2005; Baddeley and Turner, 2006; Diggle, 2006) are the predominant methods proposed. There has been some Bayesian inference (e.g., Brix and Diggle, 2001; Brix and Møller, 2001; Diggle, Rowlingson, and Su, 2005) in the literature, and it is clear that this will be an area of growth in the future.

Identifying clusters in spatio-temporal point patterns is important for disease surveillance and defending against bio-terrorism. This has attracted considerable interest since 2001; for example, see Clark and Lawson (2002), Diggle, Rowlingson, and Su (2005), Kulldorf et al. (2005), and Assunção and Correa (2009).

In the area of spatio-temporal marked point processes, there have been innovative contributions to modeling atmospheric precipitation through stochastic rainfall models (e.g., see Gupta and Waymire, 1979; Smith and Karr, 1985; Rodriguez-Iturbe and Eagleson, 1987; Velghe et al., 1994). When the mark process is based on random sets, stochastic models of biological growth can be built that are very flexible and interpretable (e.g., Cressie and Hulting, 1992; Chiu and Quine, 2001; Jensen et al., 2007; and the sequence of random-set models presented in Figures 4.19b, 4.20b, and 4.20d).

CHAPTER 7

Hierarchical Dynamical Spatio-Temporal Models

As described in Chapter 6, it is often natural to model spatio-temporal processes dynamically. In this chapter, we consider statistical models for such processes and refer to these models as *dynamical spatio-temporal models* (DSTMs). We shall consider both linear and nonlinear DSTMs, as well as data, process, and parameter models that could be Gaussian or non-Gaussian.

The essence of a DSTM is the hierarchical state-space framework described in Section 3.6. Specifically, we recognize that it is impossible to observe any process perfectly, and thus we require a mapping that relates a set of observations to the true process of interest. As mentioned previously, this is just the data-model level in a hierarchical framework. At the next level, we specify a model for this true (hidden/latent/state) process. In the context of DSTMs, this model typically assumes some sort of Markovian-dependence structure in time. As in the case of purely spatial (Chapter 4) or purely temporal (Chapter 3) processes, a prior distribution might be put on the collection of parameters used in the model specification at these two levels, to create a third level (BHM), or it may be decided to estimate them (EHM).

We can write the general DSTM schematically in terms of a data model, process model, and possibly parameter (prior) model as follows.

Data Models
The distribution of data can be generally written as

$$[\{Z(\mathbf{x}; r): \mathbf{x} \in D_s, r \in D_t\} | \{Y(\mathbf{s}; t): \mathbf{s} \in \mathcal{N}_x, t \in \mathcal{N}_r\}, \boldsymbol{\theta}_D], \qquad (7.1)$$

where $Z(\mathbf{x}; r)$ is an (actual or potential) observation at spatial location $\mathbf{x}$ and time r, $Y(\mathbf{s}; t)$ represents the (hidden or latent) process of interest at spatial location $\mathbf{s}$ and time t, and $\boldsymbol{\theta}_D$ refers to data-model parameters that may also vary in space and/or time. Note that the observation locations (in space and time) and their relative supports and/or alignments may be different than those for the process. In addition, we represent the "spatial neighborhood" of $\mathbf{x}$ as $\mathcal{N}_x$ and, similarly, the "past neighborhood" of r as $\mathcal{N}_r$. Thus, equation (7.1) simply gives the distribution of observations at possibly different supports, conditional on values of the true process of interest at some other locations/levels of support and some parameters. Usually, the data are conditionally independent, yielding a data model that is a product of univariate conditional distributions. In the absence of conditional independence, the data model involves the joint (conditional) distribution of all observations given by (7.1).

The form of the DSTM data model given in (7.1) is really too general to be of much use. One can imagine an infinite number of formulations for data models that could be used in various spatio-temporal applications. Rather than continue to generalize, we find it more useful to discuss specific types of models that have proven useful for spatio-temporal models and that illustrate the power of the conditional framework. Thus, in Section 7.1, we present a discussion of the data model for a number of specific cases. Critical in the formulation of such models in practice is the parameterization of change of support, as well as dimension reduction. In the case of the latter, this corresponds to the notion that the true underlying (hidden) dynamical process is operating on a lower-dimensional manifold than physical space. Other issues of importance have to do with the distributional nature of the observations—for example, deciding whether the data, conditional on the process, are Gaussian or non-Gaussian, and deciding whether the observations are not conditionally independent (given the hidden process).

Process Model

The DSTM process distribution (i.e., process model) that we shall use can generally be written as

$$[Y(\mathbf{s}; t)|\{Y(\mathbf{w}; t - \tau_1): \mathbf{w} \in \mathcal{N}_s^{(1)}\}, \ldots, \{Y(\mathbf{w}; t - \tau_p): \mathbf{w} \in \mathcal{N}_s^{(p)}\}, \boldsymbol{\theta}_P],$$
$$(7.2)$$

where $\mathcal{N}_s^{(1)}, \ldots, \mathcal{N}_s^{(p)}$ are neighborhoods of the spatial location $\mathbf{s}$, corresponding to the time lags $0 < \tau_1 < \ldots < \tau_p$, and $\boldsymbol{\theta}_P$ refers to the process-model parameters that may vary with space and/or time. Going from conditional distributions (7.2) to a joint distribution for the whole process $Y(\cdot; \cdot)$ requires the same type of theory developed in the spatial-only case in Section 4.2.3. This form of the DSTM process model is too general to be of much use. In Sections 7.2 and 7.3, we shall discuss specific formulations of linear and non-linear dynamical-process specifications, respectively. Then, in Section 7.4, we discuss multivariate processes in the context of the DSTM framework.

One of the critical aspects of using DSTMs is the curse of dimensionality. Specifically, we recognize that in many disciplines where spatio-temporal data are available, the number of time points at which there are data can be relatively few. In such situations, specifying interactions of the process across space and time is problematic, unless one can efficiently reduce dimensionality of either the process or the parameters. These issues are even more pronounced in the case of nonlinear-evolution operators.

Parameter Models

In general, the parameter-model distribution is represented as

$$[\theta_D, \theta_P | \theta_h], \tag{7.3}$$

where θ_h refers to "hyperparameters." Again, this framework is quite general, and ultimately it is more useful to consider specific examples; these will obviously depend on choices made at higher levels of the hierarchy. In many cases, one assumes (conditional) independence in the parameter distributions; for example, $[\theta_D, \theta_P | \theta_h] = [\theta_D | \theta_h][\theta_P | \theta_h]$. It is important to reiterate that in certain instances, it may be sufficient to estimate or specify either the data parameters or the process parameters (or hyperparameters), rather than model them at this third level of the hierarchy. Furthermore, we recognize that we might need even lower levels in complicated modeling scenarios. It is often the case that the choice of these prior distributions is driven by the underlying scientific problem.

It is important to note that it is not always possible to distinguish clearly between process and parameters. Indeed, just as one person's mean structure is another's correlation structure, so it is with processes and parameters. In many cases, the underlying Science makes the distinction clear. However, it really doesn't matter, as long as one has plausible conditional probability structures. The general hierarchical model is not intended to be a rigid structure, but rather a framework for developing conditional-probability models to model complex problems.

7.1   DATA MODELS FOR THE DSTM

As with all hierarchical formulations, the power of the data model for DSTMs comes from conditioning. That is, the specification of the spatio-temporal data distribution given the true process of interest is typically much simpler than the unconditional distribution of the data. Specifically, if the data are $\mathbf{Z}_1, \ldots, \mathbf{Z}_T$, it is exceedingly difficult to specify the joint distribution $[\mathbf{Z}_1, \ldots, \mathbf{Z}_T]$. However, in most cases, the dependence in the data comes from the hidden process $\{\mathbf{Y}_t\}$, and not typically the measurement process. Thus, the conditional distribution of data given the process is often simplified greatly. For example, the data model might be

$$[\mathbf{Z}_1, \ldots, \mathbf{Z}_T | \mathbf{Y}_1, \ldots, \mathbf{Y}_T, \theta_D] = \prod_{t=1}^{T} [\mathbf{Z}_t | \mathbf{Y}_t, \theta_D], \tag{7.4}$$

where we have included dependence on parameters θ_D. The main point here is the assumption that the data are conditionally independent in time, given the hidden process.

Conditioning also plays a very important role in how multiple sources of information are handled. Indeed, one of the most powerful features of hierarchical models is their ability to accommodate multiple datasets (e.g., Section 2.1.5). For example, say we have observations $\mathbf{Z}_t^{(1)}$ and $\mathbf{Z}_t^{(2)}$ (perhaps at different supports or from different instruments) of some process $\mathbf{Y}_t$. In this case, we seek a model for the joint distribution of both data vectors, conditional upon the process $\mathbf{Y}_t$. It is often the case that, conditional on the hidden process, the two datasets are independent. That is, the errors in measurement (or aggregation, etc.) in the two datasets are not related, given one knows the true process. This implies the following simplifying assumption in the data model:

$$[\mathbf{Z}_t^{(1)}, \mathbf{Z}_t^{(2)}|\mathbf{Y}_t, \theta_D] = [\mathbf{Z}_t^{(1)}|\mathbf{Y}_t, \theta_D^{(1)}][\mathbf{Z}_t^{(2)}|\mathbf{Y}_t, \theta_D^{(2)}], \qquad (7.5)$$

where $\theta_D \equiv \{\theta_D^{(1)}, \theta_D^{(2)}\}$ are parameters associated with the two data models. Clearly, the benefit of such an assumption is that for each dataset we can use one of the data models presented below, and we do not have to specify the joint dependencies in the datasets directly. Of course, the common dependence of $\mathbf{Z}_t^{(1)}$ and $\mathbf{Z}_t^{(2)}$ on $\mathbf{Y}_t$ would induce marginal dependence between $\mathbf{Z}_t^{(1)}$ and $\mathbf{Z}_t^{(2)}$.

Data models of this sort arise when one has multiple observation sources for a given process, including remotely sensed observations (e.g., from satellites or radars), deterministic model output (such as from numerical weather/climate models), and *in situ* observations. For example, Wikle et al. (2001) consider observations for tropical winds, as given by satellite-based scatterometers, as well as "observations" from numerical-weather-forecast models. This latter source may seem somewhat unusual since the "observations" from such models are not direct observations. However, such models assimilate observations from other sources and produce output that can be thought of as interpolated or smoothed observations of the hidden process. As such, it is information regarding the true state and can certainly be included as "data" in a hierarchical framework.

The hierarchical framework can be used with multiple datasets and multiple processes as well (e.g., Section 2.1.5). That is, assume that associated with each dataset $\mathbf{Z}_t^{(1)}$ and $\mathbf{Z}_t^{(2)}$ are (hidden) processes $\mathbf{Y}_t^{(1)}$ and $\mathbf{Y}_t^{(2)}$, respectively. Again, it is often reasonable to assume that the two datasets are conditionally independent, conditional on knowing the true states of the processes:

$$[\mathbf{Z}_t^{(1)}, \mathbf{Z}_t^{(2)}|\mathbf{Y}_t^{(1)}, \mathbf{Y}_t^{(2)}, \theta_D] = [\mathbf{Z}_t^{(1)}|\mathbf{Y}_t^{(1)}, \theta_D][\mathbf{Z}_t^{(2)}|\mathbf{Y}_t^{(2)}, \theta_D]. \qquad (7.6)$$

In addition to characterizing the distributional nature of measurement error in such data models, differences in support/alignment and other transformations between the observations and the hidden process can also be accounted for. In the remainder of this section, we describe a variety of different parameterizations of the data model that account for such transformations.

7.1.1 Linear Mappings with Equal Dimensions

The simplest data model occurs when observation locations and process locations coincide (i.e., there are no missing data), and measurement errors are additive and conditionally independent in space and time. That is,

$$Z(\mathbf{s}; t) = Y(\mathbf{s}; t) + \epsilon(\mathbf{s}; t), \tag{7.7}$$

where the measurement errors $\epsilon(\mathbf{s}; t)$ have zero mean, common variance σ_ϵ^2, are independent of $Y(\cdot; \cdot)$, and are independent across time and space. Although not necessary, it is often the case that a reasonable distributional assumption on the measurement errors is that they are Gaussian. Thus, for spatial locations $\mathbf{s}_1, \ldots, \mathbf{s}_n$, the data model implies that

$$\mathbf{Z}_t = \mathbf{Y}_t + \boldsymbol{\varepsilon}_t, \qquad \boldsymbol{\varepsilon}_t \sim iid\ Gau(\mathbf{0}, \sigma_\epsilon^2 \mathbf{I}), \tag{7.8}$$

where $\mathbf{Z}_t \equiv (Z(\mathbf{s}_1; t), \ldots, Z(\mathbf{s}_n; t))'$, $\mathbf{Y}_t \equiv (Y(\mathbf{s}_1; t), \ldots, Y(\mathbf{s}_n; t))'$, and $\boldsymbol{\varepsilon}_t \equiv (\epsilon(\mathbf{s}_1; t), \ldots, \epsilon(\mathbf{s}_n; t))'$ is independent of $\mathbf{Y}_t$. The obvious advantage of this model is that it only contains one parameter, σ_ϵ^2. Despite its simplicity, such a model can be quite useful, since there is often interest in modeling at the same locations/resolutions as the observations, and the conditionally independent error structure is reasonable in many real-world applications. If the measuring instruments are properly calibrated and the calibration results are available, measurement-error variances might be assumed known.

Perhaps the next level of sophistication is to make the same assumptions as above, with the further possibility of additive and multiplicative bias in the observations. For example, consider

$$Z(\mathbf{s}; t) = a + hY(\mathbf{s}; t) + \epsilon(\mathbf{s}; t), \tag{7.9}$$

where a and h represent the additive and multiplicative bias terms, respectively. Notice that in this formulation, any bias has been taken out of the error term $\varepsilon(\mathbf{s}; t)$, leaving it with zero mean. In principle, it might be the case that the biases in (7.9) could vary with space and time; for spatial locations $\mathbf{s}_1, \ldots, \mathbf{s}_n$, this would imply that

$$\mathbf{Z}_t = \mathbf{a}_t + \text{diag}(\mathbf{h}_t)\mathbf{Y}_t + \boldsymbol{\varepsilon}_t, \qquad \boldsymbol{\varepsilon}_t \sim iid\ Gau(\mathbf{0}, \sigma_\epsilon^2 \mathbf{I}), \tag{7.10}$$

where $\mathbf{a}_t \equiv (a(\mathbf{s}_1; t), \ldots, a(\mathbf{s}_n; t))'$, $\mathbf{h}_t \equiv (h(\mathbf{s}_1; t), \ldots, h(\mathbf{s}_n; t))'$, and recall that diag($\mathbf{h}$) is a matrix with the elements of $\mathbf{h}$ down the diagonal and zeros elsewhere. One can see that in this scenario it could be very difficult to estimate these spatially (and potentially temporally) varying parameters. In cases where there is prior knowledge about this bias structure, $\{\mathbf{a}_t\}$ and $\{\mathbf{h}_t\}$ could be further modeled (e.g., parameterized in terms of covariates or modeled in terms of some correlated random process). This could be captured through a parameter model for $\{\mathbf{a}_t\}$ and $\{\mathbf{h}_t\}$ (see Section 7.5).

A logical extension to (7.10) is to consider mappings that relate the observations to linear combinations of the complete process:

$$\mathbf{Z}_t = \mathbf{a}_t + \mathbf{H}_t \mathbf{Y}_t + \boldsymbol{\varepsilon}_t, \qquad \boldsymbol{\varepsilon}_t \sim iid \ Gau(\mathbf{0}, \sigma_\epsilon^2 \mathbf{I}), \qquad (7.11)$$

where $\mathbf{H}_t$ is an $n \times n$ matrix. Obviously, it would be very difficult to estimate these time-varying coefficients without further assumptions. In fact, such a general framework is most often considered in the case where the dimension of the data and process vectors are not equal, as discussed in Section 7.1.2.

Perhaps more important is the case where the observations, after conditioning on the process (and bias/transformation corrections), have heterogeneous measurement errors in time and/or space. For example, satellite observations of an atmospheric quantity might be affected by the presence of clouds, so that measurements in cloudy regions have a different measurement-error variance than those in clear regions. In this case, the model is written as in (7.10) or (7.11), except we assume that $\boldsymbol{\varepsilon}_t \sim ind. \ Gau(\mathbf{0}, \mathrm{diag}(\mathbf{v}_t))$, where $\mathbf{v}_t \equiv (v(\mathbf{s}_1; t), \ldots, v(\mathbf{s}_n; t))'$ and $v(\mathbf{s}_i; t)$ corresponds to the variance associated with the i-th location at time t. Again, these spatially and temporally explicit variances could be difficult to estimate without further assumptions (that could be captured through a parameter model). For example, these might be modeled as spatially varying GARCH or stochastic volatility processes (e.g., Section 3.4.8).

The final extension to the basic scenario, with observations at the same locations as the process, is to relax the assumption of (conditional) spatial independence for the observations. In this case, the model is again as written in (7.10) or (7.11), except that now, $\boldsymbol{\varepsilon}_t \sim ind. \ Gau(\mathbf{0}, \mathbf{R}_t)$, again with the possibility that the covariance matrix is changing in time. Even in the case where $\mathbf{R}_t$ does not vary with time, estimation is typically problematic without further assumptions on the structure of the covariance matrix. In fact, for fixed t, $\mathbf{R}_t$ can be determined from a typical spatial model of dependence as discussed in Chapter 4. Clearly, the assumption of temporal independence may be relaxed, and all manner of time series models (see Chapter 3) could "in principle" be applied. Or, if one has both spatially and temporally correlated measurement errors, one might use a spatio-temporal covariance model such as discussed in Chapter 6.

7.1.2 Linear Mappings with Unequal Dimensions

Assume now a data model for DSTMs, where the observation dimension is different from the state-process dimension, n. For example, assume

$$\mathbf{Z}_t = \mathbf{H}_t \mathbf{Y}_t + \boldsymbol{\varepsilon}_t, \qquad (7.12)$$

where $\mathbf{Z}_t$ is m_t-dimensional, indicating that there are observations at m_t spatial locations; $\mathbf{Y}_t$ is n-dimensional, representing the n-dimensional state process of interest; $\boldsymbol{\varepsilon}_t$ is m_t-dimensional with zero mean and covariance matrix $\mathbf{R}_t$; $\boldsymbol{\varepsilon}_t$ and $\mathbf{Y}_t$ are independent; and $\mathbf{H}_t$ is of dimension $m_t \times n$. It is usual to assume that $\boldsymbol{\varepsilon}_1, \boldsymbol{\varepsilon}_2, \ldots$ are mutually independent. This form is quite general and encompasses many different scenarios in spatio-temporal modeling, as described below. Of course, we could also include bias corrections as discussed in Section 7.1.1, but to keep the presentation simple, we leave it as an exercise for the reader.

In many cases we "know" the form of $\mathbf{H}_t$. Often this is because we have a good scientific sense of the measurement process. For example, in the case of satellite retrievals, it is often the case that this observation matrix corresponds to some representation of radiative transfer that maps the radiance measurements to the process. We consider below some special cases where the form of $\mathbf{H}_t$ is assumed known (in the sense that it is a deterministic function of where and when we have observations).

Incidence Matrix

Often, the observations at certain locations are associated with the process at a different set of locations. In Section 7.1.1, each observation is associated with one state-process element; then $\mathbf{H}_t$ is simply an *incidence matrix*, which is a matrix of zeros with the exception of a single one in each row (corresponding to the element that matches the observation with the process location).

The same 0–1 structure holds when $m_t > n$ or $m_t < n$, and it is certainly reasonable to allow an incidence matrix to vary temporally to account for different observation locations through time. As an example of how an incidence matrix works in this context, consider the case where we have three observation locations $\{\mathbf{x}_i : i = 1, 2, 3\}$ and two process locations $\{\mathbf{s}_1, \mathbf{s}_2\}$, such that observations at $\mathbf{x}_1$ and $\mathbf{x}_2$ are associated with the process at location $\mathbf{s}_1$ and the observation at $\mathbf{x}_3$ is associated with the process at location $\mathbf{s}_2$. That is, $m_t > n$.

In this case, the incidence matrix is given by

$$\mathbf{H}_t \equiv \begin{pmatrix} 1 & 0 \\ 1 & 0 \\ 0 & 1 \end{pmatrix}. \tag{7.13}$$

The implication of using (7.13) for $\mathbf{H}_t$ in (7.12) is that $Z(\mathbf{x}_1; t)$ and $Z(\mathbf{x}_2; t)$ are replicate observations with mean $Y(\mathbf{s}_1; t)$ and variance σ_ϵ^2. An example of when we might consider such a data model is if we are predicting $Y(\cdot; t)$ at spatial locations on a grid or lattice, and we have (possibly) multiple observations at smaller spatial resolution than the process of interest. For example, there might be two point-support observations associated with a process' gridbox value (e.g., Wikle, Berliner, and Cressie, 1998).

The case where m_t is less than n occurs when there are missing data. For example, say we have observations $\mathbf{Z}_t = (Z(\mathbf{s}_1; t), Z(\mathbf{s}_3; t))'$ and the process $\mathbf{Y}_t = (Y(\mathbf{s}_1; t), Y(\mathbf{s}_2; t), Y(\mathbf{s}_3; t))'$. Then the incidence matrix is given by

$$\mathbf{H}_t \equiv \begin{pmatrix} 1 & 0 & 0 \\ 0 & 0 & 1 \end{pmatrix}, \tag{7.14}$$

which accommodates the missing observation for $Y(\mathbf{s}_2; t)$.

Change-of-Support

The incidence-matrix form for $\mathbf{H}_t$ suggests more general possibilities by which one might assign observations to process locations. For example, if $\mathbf{Z}_t = (Z(\mathbf{x}_1; t), Z(\mathbf{x}_2; t), Z(\mathbf{x}_3; t))'$ and $\mathbf{Y}_t = (Y(\mathbf{s}_1; t), Y(\mathbf{s}_2; t))'$, then consider

$$\mathbf{H}_t = \begin{pmatrix} h_{11} & h_{12} \\ h_{21} & h_{22} \\ h_{31} & h_{32} \end{pmatrix}, \tag{7.15}$$

where $h_{ij} > 0$ $(i = 1, \ldots, m_t; \; j = 1, \ldots, n)$ is the weight associated with the observation at location $\mathbf{x}_i$ and the process at location $\mathbf{s}_j$, and $\sum_j h_{ij} = 1$. The obvious question is how should these weights be selected.

A situation where one might know $\{h_{ij}\}$ is with the change-of-support problem. With a slight abuse of notation, assume that locations $\mathbf{x}_i$ and $\mathbf{s}_j$ correspond to areal support, where the areas are given by $|\mathbf{x}_i|$ and $|\mathbf{s}_j|$, respectively. Furthermore, consider the possibility that $|\mathbf{x}_i| \neq |\mathbf{s}_j|$. That is, perhaps the observations are at larger or smaller levels of spatial support than the process of interest (e.g., if observations are from satellites with a resolution smaller than the prediction grid, then $|\mathbf{x}_i| < |\mathbf{s}_j|$). As described briefly in Section 4.1.3, Wikle and Berliner (2005) show that, with minor assumptions, the weights in this case are

$$h_{ij} = |\mathbf{x}_i \cap \mathbf{s}_j| / |\mathbf{x}_i|, \tag{7.16}$$

for $i = 1, \ldots, m_t; \; j = 1, \ldots, n$. These weights simply reflect the intersection (area of overlap) between the observation and process support locations. In particular, they account directly for change-of-support, as well as change in alignment between observation and process locations. Note that many of the weights will be zero, since the intersection of most data-support and process-support locations is null.

In addition, change-of-support has implications for the measurement covariance matrix ($\mathbf{R}_t$, defined above) as well. Again, this is described briefly in Section 4.1.3. Suppressing the temporal index t, assume

$$Y(\mathbf{r}) = Y(\mathbf{s}_j) + \gamma(\mathbf{r}), \tag{7.17}$$

for any (point-support) location $\mathbf{r} \in \mathbf{s}_j$ in the spatial domain of interest, where $\{\gamma(\mathbf{r})\}$ is a correlated process with spatial covariance function $C_\gamma(\mathbf{r}, \mathbf{r}')$, independent of $\{Y(\mathbf{s}_j): j = 1, \ldots, n\}$.

In this illustration, assume that the data supports, $\{|\mathbf{x}_i|: i = 1, \ldots, m\}$, involve smaller areas than the desired prediction supports, $\{|\mathbf{s}_j|: j = 1, \ldots, n\}$, and recall that block support for some arbitrary block R is defined as

$$Y(R) = \frac{1}{|R|} \int_R Y(\mathbf{r}) d\mathbf{r}, \qquad |R| > 0, \tag{7.18}$$

where $|R| \equiv \int_R d\mathbf{r}$. Then, using (7.17) and (7.18), we obtain

$$Y(\mathbf{x}_i) = \frac{1}{|\mathbf{x}_i|} \sum_{j=1}^{n} \left(\int_{\mathbf{x}_i} Y(\mathbf{s}_j) d\mathbf{r} \right) + \frac{1}{|\mathbf{x}_i|} \int_{\mathbf{x}_i} \gamma(\mathbf{r}) d\mathbf{r}$$

$$= \mathbf{h}_i' \mathbf{Y} + \frac{1}{|\mathbf{x}_i|} \int_{\mathbf{x}_i} \gamma(\mathbf{r}) d\mathbf{r}, \tag{7.19}$$

where $\mathbf{Y} \equiv (Y(\mathbf{s}_1), \ldots, Y(\mathbf{s}_n))'$, $\mathbf{h}_i \equiv (h_{i1}, \ldots, h_{in})'$, and h_{ij} is defined by (7.16). Now, for $\mathbf{Y}^{(x)} \equiv (Y(\mathbf{x}_1), \ldots, Y(\mathbf{x}_m))'$, which is the process corresponding to the data supports, we have

$$\mathbf{Y}^{(x)} | \mathbf{Y}, \boldsymbol{\Sigma}_\gamma \quad \sim \quad Gau(\mathbf{HY}, \boldsymbol{\Sigma}_\gamma), \tag{7.20}$$

where the matrix $\mathbf{H}$ has (i, j)th element h_{ij}, and the (p, q)th element of $\boldsymbol{\Sigma}_\gamma$ is given by

$$\frac{1}{|\mathbf{x}_q||\mathbf{x}_p|} \int_{\mathbf{x}_p} \int_{\mathbf{x}_q} C_\gamma(\mathbf{r}, \mathbf{r}') d\mathbf{r} d\mathbf{r}'. \tag{7.21}$$

Given the measurement-error model,

$$\mathbf{Z} | \mathbf{Y}^{(x)}, \boldsymbol{\Sigma}_Z \quad \sim \quad Gau(\mathbf{Y}^{(x)}, \boldsymbol{\Sigma}_Z), \tag{7.22}$$

one can use (7.20) and (7.22) to show that

$$\mathbf{Z} | \mathbf{Y}, \boldsymbol{\Sigma}_\gamma, \boldsymbol{\Sigma}_Z \quad \sim \quad Gau(\mathbf{HY}, \boldsymbol{\Sigma}_\gamma + \boldsymbol{\Sigma}_Z). \tag{7.23}$$

Thus, as noted in Section 4.1.3, change-of-support has induced a correlated structure, $\boldsymbol{\Sigma}_\gamma + \boldsymbol{\Sigma}_Z$, in the data model. Note that similar structures for this covariance matrix and $\mathbf{H}$ arise if the support of the data is larger than the desired prediction support. For a more complete discussion, see Wikle and Berliner (2005).

Finally, we mention that in many problems where this approach to change of spatial support is used in a spatio-temporal framework, it is possible that the weights $\mathbf{H}_t$ will change with time, due to differing observation locations or missing observations. Furthermore, the change-of-support can be given in terms of temporal aggregation as well.

7.1.3 Dimension Reduction

Characterizing the dependence structures in the hidden (state) process can be problematic, due to the curse of dimensionality. It is often necessary in such cases to reduce the effective dimensionality of the (spatial) state vector. In many cases, this is reasonable, since the true dynamical process exists on a lower-dimensional manifold, or at least it is reasonably approximated by the assumption that it does (e.g., see the discussion of dynamical systems in Section 3.2).

Recall, in the linear, additive-error data model (with no additive bias or transformation), we might assume, $Z_t = H_t Y_t + \varepsilon_t$, where Z_t and ε_t are both m_t-dimensional vectors, Y_t is n-dimensional, and ε_t is independent of Y_t. Now, let us assume that the process Y_t can be decomposed as

$$Y_t = \Phi \alpha_t + v_t, \qquad (7.24)$$

where the lower-dimensional process is p_α-dimensional, $\alpha_t \equiv (\alpha_t(1), \ldots, \alpha_t(p_\alpha))'$, Φ is an $n \times p_\alpha$ matrix with $p_\alpha << n$, and v_t is an n-dimensional vector accounting for the residual process not included in $\Phi \alpha_t$. Note that α_t may not be "spatially referenced" but $\Phi \alpha_t$ is. The model (7.24) is a "process model" in the usual HM nomenclature (see Sections 7.2 and 7.3). However, if the modeling focus is on α_t rather than Y_t, it can be convenient to rewrite the data model in terms of α_t. In this case,

$$Z_t = H_t \Phi \alpha_t + H_t v_t + \varepsilon_t, \qquad (7.25)$$

where H_t can take any of the forms described previously, and one may find it useful to combine the error processes into a single (more complicated) process; for example, write $\gamma_t = H_t v_t + \varepsilon_t$. If one does this combining, one loses the ease of predicting Y_t in order to concentrate on predicting α_t or, equivalently, $\Phi \alpha_t$.

The key here is the dimension-reduction matrix Φ. We often refer to this as a matrix of basis functions (e.g., see Section 4.1.4) or the "spectral transformation matrix" (e.g., see Section 3.5). Now Φ is (often) assumed known, does not have to have orthogonal columns, and serves to relate the process vector Y_t to the reduced-dimensional vector α_t. As was seen in Section 6.6, we refer to the decomposition (7.24) as a *spectral representation*, where we use the word "spectral" rather broadly to refer to general basis function expansions. In that sense, α_t can be called a vector of spectral coefficients.

There are many possible choices for the spectral transformation matrix Φ, and "novel" formulations of spatio-temporal dynamical models have often (and continue to be) proposed by suggesting a different choice for Φ. Such novelty is perhaps overstated, but the concept is powerful. Some specific choices for Φ are described in the following subsections.

Finally, it is certainly the case that v_t could be further decomposed in an additional expansion; for example, write

$$v_t = \Psi \xi_t + \omega_t,$$

where ω_t is an error process, ξ_t is a p_ξ-dimensional coefficient vector associated with the $n \times p_\xi$ matrix of basis functions Ψ, which typically are not of the same form as $\boldsymbol{\Phi}$. The vector $\boldsymbol{\xi}_t$ may be allowed to vary dynamically in the process model, similarly to $\boldsymbol{\alpha}_t$. Why would we need to have two different spectral components for the $\{\mathbf{Y}_t\}$ process? One reason would be if we were attempting to capture the variability associated with spatio-temporal processes on different spatial scales (and with different dynamical properties). For example, Wikle et al. (2001) consider such a case, where $\boldsymbol{\Phi}$ corresponds to normal modes of a deterministic dynamical system for atmospheric winds, and $\boldsymbol{\Psi}$ are wavelet basis functions that accommodate the multiresolutional nature of turbulent scaling relationships in atmospheric winds. In this case, the associated spectral coefficients, $\boldsymbol{\alpha}_t$ and $\boldsymbol{\xi}_t$, follow first-order dynamical process models (although, with substantially different parameterizations). Overall, the model, $\mathbf{Y}_t = \boldsymbol{\Phi}\boldsymbol{\alpha}_t + \boldsymbol{\Psi}\boldsymbol{\xi}_t + \boldsymbol{\omega}_t$, provides a flexible and powerful decomposition of a spatio-temporal process. Of course, additional decompositions (e.g., of $\boldsymbol{\omega}_t$) can be specified if there is sufficient scientific justification.

Pure Spectral Decomposition

For motivation, we discuss first the case where we have spectral operators for $\boldsymbol{\Phi}$, and $p_\alpha = n$. In this case, $\mathbf{Y}_t \equiv \boldsymbol{\Phi}\boldsymbol{\alpha}_t$, and $\boldsymbol{\alpha}_t$ is n-dimensional. That is, there is a simple linear transformation of $\boldsymbol{\alpha}_t$ that gives $\mathbf{Y}_t$, with no explicit dimension reduction of the process (i.e., $\boldsymbol{\Phi}$ is an $n \times n$ matrix and $\boldsymbol{v}_t = \mathbf{0}$ for all t). One may ask why this is considered "dimension reduction," and what the advantage is of such an assumption. One advantage is that the parameterization of the process at the next level of the HM is often simpler. That is, for certain basis functions such as the Fourier, wavelet, and EOF bases, the implied process $\boldsymbol{\alpha}_t$ is simpler, since the spectral transformation acts as a *decorrelator* (see Section 3.5). Thus, in this case, "dimension reduction" refers to the implied reduction in the number of process-model *parameters*, even if the dimension of the process itself has not been reduced.

As an example, consider the simple case where $\mathbf{Y}_t \sim Gau(\mathbf{0}, \mathbf{R})$. Then, it follows that $\boldsymbol{\alpha}_t \sim Gau(\mathbf{0}, \mathbf{R}_\alpha)$, where $\mathbf{R}_\alpha \equiv (\boldsymbol{\Phi}'\boldsymbol{\Phi})^{-1}\boldsymbol{\Phi}'\mathbf{R}\boldsymbol{\Phi}(\boldsymbol{\Phi}'\boldsymbol{\Phi})^{-1}$, for $\boldsymbol{\Phi}'\boldsymbol{\Phi}$ nonsingular. Notice that if $\boldsymbol{\Phi}$ is orthogonal such that $\boldsymbol{\Phi}'\boldsymbol{\Phi} = \mathbf{I}$, then $\mathbf{R}_\alpha = \boldsymbol{\Phi}'\mathbf{R}\boldsymbol{\Phi}$. Recall that, for second-order stationary processes, it is often the case that $\mathbf{R}_\alpha$ is reasonably well approximated by a diagonal matrix, $\mathbf{R}_\alpha = \text{diag}(\mathbf{d})$, where $\mathbf{d}$ is a p_α-dimensional vector of variances (see Section 3.5). Furthermore, for known classes of valid spatial covariance functions, $\mathbf{R}(\boldsymbol{\theta})$ depends on parameters $\boldsymbol{\theta}$ (e.g., the Matérn class considered in Section 4.1.1). If there is an analytical form for the spectral transform (e.g., Fourier), one can parameterize the elements of $\mathbf{d}$; we write it here as $\mathbf{d}(\boldsymbol{\theta})$. In addition to the likely simplification in the dynamics at the process level, this suggests powerful computational advantages for spatial prediction over large domains with large numbers of spatial grid points, even in the hierarchical-Bayesian-model case where $\boldsymbol{\theta}$ is given a prior distribution (see Wikle, 2002b; Royle and Wikle, 2005; Paciorek, 2007). Similar computational savings can be shown when multiresolution wavelet basis functions are used (e.g., Nychka, Wikle, and Royle, 2002).

These have the additional advantage of easily accounting for nonstationarity, but they are limited in that, typically, analytical forms for $\mathbf{R}_\alpha$ are not available.

A criticism of these spectral-transformation approaches is that the process has to be modeled on some regular grid in order to take advantage of the computational efficiencies of the spectral operator. However, in all but the rarest cases, we can deal with this by specifying a very-high-resolution grid such that each observation location corresponds to a unique process location. Alternatively, we can use one of the formulations of $\mathbf{H}_t$ given above to account for a regular process-model grid.

It should also be mentioned that many processes, especially those in the atmospheric sciences, are studied theoretically and via data analysis, in the spectral domain. In such cases, process modeling in the spectral domain is not only simpler in terms of model structures and computation, but conceptually as well.

Empirical Orthogonal Functions

Empirical orthogonal functions (EOFs; see Sections 4.1.4 and 5.3) have often been used as the spectral basis functions in $\mathbf{\Phi}$ for dimension reduction. That is, if we had access to the first p_α eigenvectors of a stationary covariance matrix for the process $\{\mathbf{Y}_t\}$ (typically an estimated or "empirical" covariance matrix calculated from $\{\mathbf{Z}_t\}$, or from some other source of information such as a deterministic numerical model), then the process model, $\mathbf{Y}_t = \mathbf{\Phi}\boldsymbol{\alpha}_t + \boldsymbol{\nu}_t$ [see (7.24)], is somewhat simplified, in that $\boldsymbol{\alpha}_t$ has a diagonal covariance matrix with diagonal elements given by the eigenvalues of the original covariance matrix used to generate the EOFs. However, the dynamics of $\boldsymbol{\alpha}_t$ may suggest more complicated structures than implied by the EOF decomposition.

Typically, one only considers the first p_α EOFs that account for some significant portion of $\text{var}(\mathbf{Y}_t)$. Since EOFs typically decrease in spatial scale with decreasing variance explained, it is often reasonable in such cases to assume that $\boldsymbol{\nu}_t \sim Gau(\mathbf{0}, \sigma_\nu^2 \mathbf{I})$. Consequently, σ_ν^2 and σ_ϵ^2 (the measurement-error variance) are not identifiable without additional (prior) information.

In cases where p_α is selected such that a reasonable amount of spatial structure is left in $\boldsymbol{\nu}_t$, one can model it by either choosing a valid spatial covariance function (see Chapter 4) or using a portion of the remaining EOFs to characterize the covariance matrix of $\boldsymbol{\nu}_t$, say $\boldsymbol{\Sigma}_\nu$. That is, one could simply assume

$$\boldsymbol{\Sigma}_\nu = c\mathbf{I} + \sum_{k=p_\alpha+1}^{p_\alpha+p_\nu} \lambda_k \mathbf{\Phi}_k \mathbf{\Phi}_k', \qquad (7.26)$$

where c is an unknown constant, and λ_k and $\mathbf{\Phi}_k$, for $k = p_\alpha + 1, \ldots, p_\alpha + p_\nu$, are the next p_ν (after p_α) eigenvalues and eigenvectors, respectively, of the EOF decomposition. The constant c must be estimated (EHM) or given a prior distribution (BHM) to account for the extra variability lost in the EOF truncation and to ensure that Σ_ν is positive-definite. It may be the case that $\{\lambda_k\}$ in (7.26) are estimated or given prior distributions as well.

Despite their prevalence (especially in atmospheric/ocean science applications) and their success as a means of dimension reduction, there are several issues that can make the EOF basis function less appealing in some situations. First, if we have no missing data and many more time replicates (T) than spatial locations (n), then from the empirical covariance matrix based on $\mathbf{Z}_t$, EOF basis functions can be used to approximate var($\mathbf{Y}_t$). However, when $T < n$, as is often the case in practice, we can only get T EOFs, and they are sometimes of dubious quality due to the sampling variability caused by small T. Furthermore, when data are missing, or interest is in predicting at locations where there are no observations, we cannot get EOFs directly without some sort of data smoothing (e.g., Wikle and Cressie, 1999). This pre-smoothing is less than appealing, given that smoothing is often the goal of the spatio-temporal analysis in the first place, and it is not always clear how much the final predictions are influenced by the pre-smoothing operation. A more rigorous framework for building EOFs in this case makes use of localized basis functions (e.g., Obled and Creutin, 1986; Wikle, 1996), but this can be a computational and practical burden. Alternatively, one can shrink the empirical covariance estimates to some parametric-based covariance matrix (Nott and Dunsmuir, 2002).

Other issues that influence the EOF basis functions concern the sensitivity of EOFs to the geometry of the spatial domain upon which the data are defined. For example, as discussed in Sections 4.1.4 and 5.3, it can be shown that EOFs can be thought of as a discretization of the Karhunen–Loève integral equation. Such a discretization must account for the area of influence of each observation (around its spatial location) if the locations of observations are not on a regular grid (Cohen and Jones, 1969; Buell, 1972; Karl, Koscielny, and Diaz, 1982). In addition, Buell (1975) showed that the EOF basis functions (patterns) are heavily influenced by the shape of the spatial domain where the observations were taken (see Jolliffe, 2002, p. 297, for an in-depth discussion of this issue).

Perhaps a more critical concern is that, although it is the case that the truncated set of EOF basis functions are optimal in the sense of describing the most variance among any orthogonal set of p_α basis functions, they are not necessarily optimal in terms of representing the spatio-temporal dynamics of the process. This was clearly demonstrated in Aubry, Lian, and Titi (1993), who gave an example of an EOF decomposition that accounted for 99.9995% of the variation in the process, but it could not adequately model the dynamics of a particular process. In that case, the process was nonlinear; from a "chaos" perspective (Section 3.2.4), it is perhaps not surprising that a component that represents such a small part of the overall variation can play an important role in the dynamics. This is particularly problematic when the process includes abrupt transitions between different regimes. A statistical approach that can help with this problem is to select the reduced set of EOF basis functions stochastically, rather than by the amount of variation explained. For example, Wikle and Holan (2011) used the stochastic search variable selection methodology of George and McCulloch (1993) to choose the appropriate basis functions for a hierarchical DSTM. However, it is also the case that, in general, the EOF basis may not provide the best low-order reduction for *representing the dynamics* of even linear systems.

Despite these concerns, our experience is that EOFs are one of the better sets of basis functions to use, when the degree of dimension reduction and the computational simplicity are factored in. If nothing else, the EOF set of basis functions should be the standard by which other sets of basis functions are judged.

Alternative System-Reduction Approaches

There is a substantial literature in Control Theory and Fluid Dynamics that addresses alternative sets of basis functions for dimension reduction in dynamical systems [e.g., see Antoulas (2005) for an overview]. As discussed in Sections 7.2 and 7.3, the spatio-temporal behavior of a process is governed by its dynamical operator and its noise-forcing covariance matrix. Thus, it is not surprising that optimal reduction strategies for spatio-temporal systems typically consider one or both of these components. This is one of the motivations for principle oscillation patterns (POPs) as discussed in Section 5.5.

As an example of a different approach to POPs, consider the notion of stochastic optimal analysis (SOA) as described, for example, in Farrell and Ioannou (2001). In order to perform SOA, one must know the form of the governing dynamics. For example, as discussed in Sections 3.4.7 and 6.4.2, consider the vector autoregressive (VAR) process of order one:

$$\mathbf{Y}_t = \mathbf{M}\mathbf{Y}_{t-1} + \boldsymbol{\eta}_t \,;\, t = 1, 2, \ldots,$$

where $E(\boldsymbol{\eta}_t) = \mathbf{0}$, $\mathrm{var}(\boldsymbol{\eta}_t) \equiv \mathbf{Q}_\eta$, and $\boldsymbol{\eta}_t$ is independent of $\mathbf{Y}_{t-1}$, for $t = 1, 2, \ldots$. Furthermore, assume that $E(\mathbf{Y}_t) = \mathbf{0}$ and $\mathrm{var}(\mathbf{Y}_t) \equiv \boldsymbol{\Sigma}_Y$, for all t. Recall from Section 3.4.7 that we can write this VAR(1) process as an infinite-order MA process:

$$\mathbf{Y}_t = \sum_{i \geq 0} \mathbf{M}^i \boldsymbol{\eta}_{t-i},$$

which implies that

$$\boldsymbol{\Sigma}_Y = \sum_{i \geq 0} \mathbf{M}^i \mathbf{Q}_\eta (\mathbf{M}')^i .$$

These series converge if all eigenvalues of $\mathbf{M}$ are less than 1 in absolute value. Now, consider the expected total variation in $\mathbf{Y}_t$:

$$E(\mathbf{Y}_t'\mathbf{Y}_t) = E(tr(\mathbf{Y}_t\mathbf{Y}_t'))$$
$$= tr(\boldsymbol{\Sigma}_Y)$$
$$= tr\left(\sum_{i \geq 0} \mathbf{M}^i \mathbf{Q}_\eta (\mathbf{M}')^i\right).$$

Let $\mathbf{Q}_\eta = \mathbf{FF}'$, so that

$$
\begin{aligned}
E(\mathbf{Y}'_t\mathbf{Y}_t) &= tr\left(\sum_{i\geq0}\mathbf{M}^i\mathbf{FF}'(\mathbf{M}')^i\right)\\
&= \sum_{i\geq0}tr(\mathbf{F}'(\mathbf{M}')^i\mathbf{M}^i\mathbf{F})\\
&= tr\left(\mathbf{F}'\left\{\sum_{i\geq0}(\mathbf{M}')^i\mathbf{M}^i\right\}\mathbf{F}\right).
\end{aligned}
$$

Now, SOA is concerned with the eigenvectors and eigenvalues in the diagonalization of

$$
\mathbf{B} \equiv \sum_{i\geq0}(\mathbf{M}')^i\mathbf{M}^i.
$$

The resulting eigenvectors are (spatial) basis functions that correspond to the dominant patterns of *forcing* that maximize the total variation of the system *response*. Compare this to EOFs, which are the basis functions that diagonalize $\boldsymbol{\Sigma}_Y = \sum_{i\geq0}\mathbf{M}^i\mathbf{Q}(\mathbf{M}')^i$ and correspond to the spatial structures that exhibit the most variation (over time). Obviously, when the noise forcing is "unitary" (i.e., $\mathbf{Q}_\eta = \mathbf{I}$) and the transition matrix is "normal" (i.e., $\mathbf{MM}' = \mathbf{M}'\mathbf{M}$), then the EOFs and *stochastic optimals* (SOs) are identical. However, these assumptions would rarely hold in practice.

Analogous to the solution for the *observability Gramian* in discrete-time linear systems theory (e.g., Kailath, 1980), $\mathbf{B}$ can be found by solving the Lyapunov equation:

$$
\mathbf{M}'\mathbf{BM} - \mathbf{B} + \mathbf{I} = 0, \tag{7.27}
$$

which can be obtained numerically, for example, by the Schur decomposition method of Kitagawa (1977). As an example, say we have

$$
\mathbf{M} = \begin{pmatrix} 0.4 & 0.01 \\ 4.0 & 0.1 \end{pmatrix}. \tag{7.28}
$$

In this case, the Schur decomposition method gives

$$
\mathbf{B} = \begin{pmatrix} 22.5467 & 0.5387 \\ 0.5387 & 1.0135 \end{pmatrix}, \tag{7.29}
$$

and the eigenvectors (SOs) and eigenvalues of the decomposition of $\mathbf{B}$ are, respectively,

$$
\mathbf{E}_B = \begin{pmatrix} 0.9997 & -0.0250 \\ -0.0250 & 0.9997 \end{pmatrix} \quad \text{and} \quad \boldsymbol{\lambda}_B = \begin{pmatrix} 22.56 \\ 1.00 \end{pmatrix}. \tag{7.30}
$$

Thus, the first SO is the eigenvector associated with the largest eigenvalue, 22.56, and is given by $(0.9997, -0.0250)'$. This SO is responsible for *producing* most (its eigenvalue is 95.8% of the sum of eigenvalues) of the variation in the dynamical system. The second SO, which is given by $(-0.0250, 0.9997)'$, is orthogonal to the first and is only responsible for *producing* about 4.2% of the dynamical system's variability. In the context of dimension reduction, it seems reasonable to keep only the first SO and to project the full-dimensional process onto this basis function.

Now, consider the EOFs associated with the dynamical system defined by **M** as in (7.28) above, and let $\mathbf{Q}_\eta = \mathbf{I}$. Note that we can obtain the marginal covariance matrix $\mathbf{\Sigma}_Y$ from (6.73), or by recognizing that this can be obtained by solving the discrete Lyapunov equation:

$$\mathbf{M\Sigma}_Y\mathbf{M}' - \mathbf{\Sigma}_Y + \mathbf{Q}_\eta = \mathbf{0}. \tag{7.31}$$

In this case,

$$\mathbf{\Sigma}_Y = \begin{pmatrix} 1.2135 & 2.1347 \\ 2.1347 & 22.3467 \end{pmatrix}, \tag{7.32}$$

and the associated eigenvectors (EOFs) and eigenvalues are, respectively:

$$\mathbf{E}_Y = \begin{pmatrix} -0.9950 & 0.0995 \\ 0.0995 & 0.9950 \end{pmatrix} \quad \text{and} \quad \mathbf{\lambda}_Y = \begin{pmatrix} 1.00 \\ 22.56 \end{pmatrix}. \tag{7.33}$$

Here, the EOF, $(0.0995, 0.9950)'$, corresponding to the largest eigenvalue, 22.56, *accounts for* most (its eigenvalue is 95.8% of the sum of eigenvalues) of the variance in the dynamical system. If we truncated the expansion at this first EOF, we might expect that it would represent the dynamics reasonably well. However, this EOF is quite similar in structure (first element near zero, second element near one) to the second SO in (7.30), and recall that the second SO is responsible for *producing* only a small portion (4.2%) of the variation in the system response. Correspondingly, the first SO is responsible for *producing* most of the variation in the system response, and it is very similar in structure to the second EOF, which only *accounts for* a relatively small amount of the variance of $\mathbf{Y}_t$. This suggests that the system would not be well approximated by projecting on *either* the first EOF *or* the first SO. Note the seemingly subtle distinction between "accounting for" variation and "producing" variation; from a dynamical-systems perspective, they can be quite different. Recall from the discussion just above about how the SO provides structures that, when forced, lead to the system response. Thus, they are much more related to the mechanism of dynamical evolution. On the other hand, EOFs simply correspond to the spatial (not dynamical) structures that exhibit variation in the system.

A natural development is to find basis functions that simultaneously diagonalize $\mathbf{\Sigma}_Y$ and **B**. In the control literature, this is related to the notion of finding a *balanced truncation* (e.g., Moore, 1981; Farrell and Ioannou, 2001). We note that there are many additional approaches to model reduction, and this is an active area of research [e.g., see the introduction to Crommelin and Majda (2004); also see Antoulas (2005)]. Most of these approaches have not made their way into the Statistics literature. The most likely impediment to this lack of technology transfer is the "jargon differential" between researchers in Control Theory and Fluid Dynamics and researchers in Statistics.

We note that these dimension-reduction approaches do assume specific dynamical models. This may be unappealing to some practitioners, and it partially explains why (dynamically) nonoptimal basis functions such as EOFs and smoothing kernels (see just below) are so popular. In addition, dynamically based optimal dimension-reduction procedures can be much more difficult to compute.

Smoothing-Kernel Parameterizations

Although more difficult to justify from a dynamical perspective, a useful, statistically motivated choice for Φ is based on smoothing kernels. That is, the process $\{Y_t\}$ (or often, the observations $\{Z_t\}$) is approximated by some hidden low-dimensional dynamical process $\{\alpha_t\}$, such that Y_t is just a smoothed version of the individual elements of α_t. For example, consider the process model,

$$Y_t(s_i) = \int_{D_s} \phi(s_i, x; \theta)\alpha_t(x)\,dx + \nu_t(s_i), \tag{7.34}$$

where $\phi(s_i, x; \theta)$ is a smoothing kernel for location s_i, $i = 1, \ldots, n$, applied to locations x in spatial domain D_s and depends on kernel parameters θ (that could also depend on spatial location s_i). Note that we have included an error term $\nu_t(s_i)$ in (7.34) to account for model error associated with the smoothing assumption. This error might exhibit spatial dependence, but typically we assume that it is independent across time.

Practically, it is more common to select some reference locations $\{x_j : j = 1, \ldots, p_\alpha\}$, and thus we discretize (7.34) to obtain

$$Y_t(s_i) = \sum_{j=1}^{p_\alpha} \phi_{ij}(\theta)\alpha_t(x_j) + \nu_t(s_i), \tag{7.35}$$

for $i = 1, \ldots, n$ and $j = 1, \ldots, p_\alpha$ (where θ may depend on i or j as well). Note, as suggested in Section 7.2.6, one can also effectively perform a discretization of (7.34) by expanding the kernel and process in terms of some basis functions. In vector notation, we can write (7.35) as

$$Y_t = \Phi(\theta)\alpha_t + \nu_t, \tag{7.36}$$

where $\Phi(\theta)$ is an $n \times p_\alpha$ matrix depending on kernel parameters θ. Often, θ is assumed fixed and known. However, depending on the assumed structure of the process $\{\alpha_t\}$, these parameters might be estimated (EHM) or given prior distributions (BHM). As discussed below, in general one has to be careful about identifiability related to inference on $\boldsymbol{\theta}$.

One can imagine complicated modeling situations, where $\boldsymbol{\theta}$ is allowed to vary in space (e.g., Higdon, 1998) and/or time. However, we have to be careful in characterizing just where the dynamics are to be modeled in this case. For example, say that the smoothing kernels are spatially varying and represented by relatively high-dimensional vectors $\{\boldsymbol{\theta}_t\}$. Even in the case where the kernels are described by only one (spatially varying) parameter, $\boldsymbol{\theta}_t$ is n-dimensional. If we allowed this to vary with time, for example, in a Markovian fashion, then we would have to model the conditional distributions $\{[\boldsymbol{\theta}_t|\boldsymbol{\theta}_{t-1}]: t = 1, 2, \ldots\}$, which depend on their own set of parameters. This might be a viable model if $\{\boldsymbol{\alpha}_t\}$ were assumed to be white noise. However, we would effectively be replacing a relatively low-dimensional spatio-temporal process $\{\boldsymbol{\alpha}_t\}$ with a high-dimensional one, $\{\boldsymbol{\theta}_t\}$, of (most likely) equal or greater complexity.

General Parameterization of Dimension Reduction

It is intuitively appealing simply to estimate $\boldsymbol{\Phi}$ in (7.24) (or the product $\boldsymbol{\Phi}_H \equiv \mathbf{H}\boldsymbol{\Phi}$) without the basis function or kernel assumptions described in previous sections. However, in the high-dimensional spatio-temporal context, it is difficult to imagine enough data to adequately estimate $\boldsymbol{\Phi}$ (or $\boldsymbol{\Phi}_H$). In addition, there are well known identifiability issues with trying to estimate these matrices in the presence of an unknown dynamical model propagator and covariance matrix. These are, in many respects, just the typical identifiability concerns that one experiences with traditional factor analysis (e.g., Johnson and Wichern, 2007). Without strong assumptions on the structure of $\boldsymbol{\Phi}$ (or $\boldsymbol{\Phi}_H$) or the parameters associated with the process $\{\boldsymbol{\alpha}_t\}$, it is not possible to identify both the data-model parameters and the process-model parameters.

A property of the Bayesian paradigm is that strong prior information mitigates this lack of identifiability. Thus, one can imagine putting an informative prior on the matrix $\boldsymbol{\Phi}$ (or $\boldsymbol{\Phi}_H$), say $[\boldsymbol{\Phi}]$. In fact, this issue has received substantial attention in recent years. In the problem of "blind source separation" found in the engineering literature, one has several different source signals, but the observations of the system are typically unknown mixtures of these sources. In the linear case, understanding these mixtures is just the problem of doing inference on $\boldsymbol{\Phi}$. Specific algorithms have been developed, based on process assumptions [e.g., Independent Component Analysis (Hyvärinen, Karhunen, and Oja, 2001)], and it is known that some of these algorithms can be derived from the Bayesian perspective by the appropriate choice of a matrix prior, $[\boldsymbol{\Phi}]$. For example, Knuth (1999) discusses the prior,

$$[\boldsymbol{\Phi}|\sigma] = \frac{1}{\sqrt{2\pi\sigma^2}} \exp\left\{ -\frac{\|\mathbf{I} - \boldsymbol{\Phi}'\boldsymbol{\Phi}\|_F^2}{2\sigma^2} \right\}, \tag{7.37}$$

where $\mathbf{I}$ is the identity matrix, $\|\cdot\|_F$ represents the Frobenius norm, and σ accounts for uncertainty regarding the orthogonality of $\boldsymbol{\Phi}$. Alternative prior formulations for the "mixing matrix" $\boldsymbol{\Phi}$ are formulated by Knuth (2005).

As an example of prior structure in the DSTM data model, Lopes, Salazar, and Gamerman (2008) put a Gaussian (spatial) random field prior on each column of $\boldsymbol{\Phi}$ (or $\boldsymbol{\Phi}_H$). This is motivated by the dynamical factor models for multiple time series discussed by Aguilar and West (2000). In this case, vague priors for these fields require strong priors for the hidden dynamical process $\{\boldsymbol{\alpha}_t\}$, to ensure identifiability [see also Calder (2007) for a similar implementation in the context of multivariate DSTMs; and see Section 7.4.2]. Similarly, Sansó, Schmidt, and Nobre (2008) consider a dynamic specification of the linear model of coregionalization (see Section 4.1.5 for a discussion in the context of spatial processes), which models $\boldsymbol{\Phi}$ as the lower-triangular matrix decomposition of a covariance matrix. The parameters of this matrix can then be inferred, with appropriate limitations on the process dynamics.

7.1.4 Nonlinear Mappings

In many problems, it may be more appropriate for observations to be thought of as

$$Z(\mathbf{s}_i; t) = h_{i,t}(\mathbf{Y}_t) + \varepsilon(\mathbf{s}_i; t) \,, \tag{7.38}$$

where $h_{i,t}(\cdot)$ is a *nonlinear* mapping of the process $\{\mathbf{Y}_t\}$ and $\varepsilon(\mathbf{s}_i; t)$ is an additive error process (typically, assumed to be Gaussian), for $i = 1, \ldots, m_t$. In most cases, the functional form for $h_{i,t}(\cdot)$ is known, at least up to some parameters. When the parameters are not known, the nonlinearity complicates process prediction in both the EHM (e.g., Kalman filter) and BHM (e.g., particle filter or MCMC) settings (see Chapter 8).

If the functional form of $h_{i,t}(\cdot)$ is known, it is sometimes the case that a Taylor-series-based linearization of the measurement function is considered. In this approach, a first-order expansion about some estimate of the process, $\widehat{\mathbf{Y}}_t$, gives

$$h_{i,t}(\mathbf{Y}_t) = h_{i,t}(\widehat{\mathbf{Y}}_t) + (\mathbf{h}'_{i,t}) \cdot (\mathbf{Y}_t - \widehat{\mathbf{Y}}_t) + \text{higher-order terms},$$

where

$$\mathbf{h}_{i,t} \equiv \left(\frac{\partial h_{i,t}(\mathbf{Y}_t)}{\partial \mathbf{Y}_t} \right) \Bigg|_{\mathbf{Y}_t = \widehat{\mathbf{Y}}_t}$$

is an n-dimensional vector. Then, assuming the first-order truncation is reasonable, the data model is given by

$$\mathbf{Z}_t = \boldsymbol{\mu}_t(\widehat{\mathbf{Y}}_t) + \mathbf{H}_t \mathbf{Y}_t + \boldsymbol{\varepsilon}_t \,,$$

where

$$\mathbf{H}_t \equiv \begin{pmatrix} \mathbf{h}'_{1,t} \\ \vdots \\ \mathbf{h}'_{m_t,t} \end{pmatrix}$$

is an $m_t \times n$ matrix, and

$$\mu_t(\widehat{\mathbf{Y}}_t) \equiv \begin{pmatrix} h_{1,t}(\widehat{\mathbf{Y}}_t) \\ \vdots \\ h_{m_t,t}(\widehat{\mathbf{Y}}_t) \end{pmatrix} - \mathbf{H}_t \widehat{\mathbf{Y}}_t .$$

In this case, the error process, $\{\boldsymbol{\varepsilon}_t\}$, is assumed to account for effects due to measurement error, as well as Taylor-series truncation error. Clearly, higher-order approximations could be considered if necessary.

There are numerous choices for $\widehat{\mathbf{Y}}_t$ in such a parameterization. For example, these might include forecasts (e.g., the mean of $[\mathbf{Y}_t | \mathbf{Z}_{t-1}, \mathbf{Z}_{t-2}, \ldots]$), the prior mean $E(\mathbf{Y}_t)$, estimates from some other model (e.g., a deterministic model of the process), or some average based on an extended dataset (e.g., climatology in the case of a meteorological process).

Perhaps the simplest form of a nonlinear data model extends (7.9) to include a power transformation. For instance, if $\{\mathbf{Y}_t\}$ were positive and transformed in the sense of a Box–Cox transformation (Box and Cox, 1964), the general data model could be written as:

$$Z(\mathbf{s}; t) = a(\mathbf{s}; t) + h(\mathbf{s}; t)Y(\mathbf{s}; t)^{b(\mathbf{s};t)} + \epsilon(\mathbf{s}; t), \qquad (7.39)$$

where $-\infty < b(\mathbf{s}; t) < \infty$, and $\epsilon(\cdot; \cdot)$ is measurement error independent of the process $Y(\cdot; \cdot)$. For example, Sansó and Guenni (1999) used such a data model in the context of modeling a precipitation process. As is the case for a and h, if one allows b to vary with space and/or time, then inference on $Y(\cdot; \cdot)$ might be problematic without strong prior information on b in the parameter-model level of the hierarchical model.

Clearly, the discussion above focuses on the case where at least the functional form of the nonlinear measurement function is known. Alternatively, one might consider semiparametric or nonparametric functions in this context, as is often done in the time-series literature (e.g., Fan and Yao, 2005).

7.1.5 Non-Gaussian Data Models

One of the advantages of the increase in computational power over the last several decades, and the associated development of efficient numerical estimation procedures, is that non-Gaussian data models can now be accounted for readily in most problems encountered in practice. As mentioned previously, the key benefit from the hierarchical formulation of the data model comes if we can justify the *conditional-independence* assumption. Such a formulation is not surprising in data models, particularly in the linear, Gaussian setting where we simply have additive errors. In non-Gaussian settings, this assumption is absolutely critical. It is exceedingly difficult to work with multivariate non-Gaussian distributions, but it is not so difficult to work with a product of a large number of univariate non-Gaussian (conditional) distributions.

In general, we consider the exponential class of data models, conditional on the true process. Specifically, let $\mathbf{Z}_t$ denote the m_t-dimensional vector of data at time t and assume

$$[\mathbf{Z}_t|\boldsymbol{\gamma}_t] \propto \exp\{\boldsymbol{\gamma}_t'\mathbf{Z}_t - b_t(\boldsymbol{\gamma}_t) - c_t(\mathbf{Z}_t)\}, \tag{7.40}$$

where $E(\mathbf{Z}_t|\boldsymbol{\gamma}_t) \equiv \boldsymbol{\mu}_t$ and $\boldsymbol{\gamma}_t$ are m_t-dimensional natural parameters that will depend on the process $\{\mathbf{Y}_t\}$ and the parameters $\boldsymbol{\theta}_D$.

Given the usual regularity conditions for exponential families (e.g., McCulloch and Searle, 2001), the link function $g(\cdot)$ is given in its general form by

$$g(\boldsymbol{\mu}_t) = \mathbf{X}_t\boldsymbol{\beta} + \mathbf{H}_t(\boldsymbol{\theta}_h)\mathbf{Y}_t + \boldsymbol{\nu}_t, \tag{7.41}$$

where $\mathbf{H}_t(\boldsymbol{\theta}_h)$ is the $m_t \times n$ observation matrix, which is often assumed known but may be parameterized in terms of hyperparameters $\boldsymbol{\theta}_h$; $\mathbf{X}_t$ is a matrix of potential covariates (assumed known), with associated (unknown) parameters $\boldsymbol{\beta}$; and $\mathbf{Y}_t$ and $\boldsymbol{\nu}_t$ are independent for all t. As before, there are many options regarding assumptions on the components of variation in (7.41). For example, we may neither need, nor be able to justify, the additive error term $\boldsymbol{\nu}_t$, nor will we always have covariates $\mathbf{X}_t$. Similarly, $\boldsymbol{\beta}$ and/or $\boldsymbol{\theta}_h$ may be time-varying, and we may relate the process $\{\mathbf{Y}_t\}$ to a lower-dimensional dynamical process, as described in (7.24). As an example, a typical model for spatio-temporal counts might assume

$$\mathbf{Z}_t|\boldsymbol{\gamma}_t \sim ind. \; Poi(\boldsymbol{\gamma}_t), \tag{7.42}$$

$$\log(\boldsymbol{\gamma}_t) = \mathbf{X}_t\boldsymbol{\beta} + \boldsymbol{\Phi}\boldsymbol{\alpha}_t + \boldsymbol{\nu}_t, \tag{7.43}$$

where $\boldsymbol{\Phi}$ could represent one of the types of dimension-reduction basis functions described above, $\{\boldsymbol{\nu}_t\}$ are independent Gaussian with mean zero, and $\boldsymbol{\nu}_t$ is independent of $\boldsymbol{\alpha}_t$, for all t. In this case, note that $\boldsymbol{\gamma}_t$ has a non-Gaussian distribution. Typically, in this setting the random components would be assigned distributions at the next level of the hierarchical model; for example, $\{\boldsymbol{\alpha}_t\}$ would be a DSTM. The general framework in (7.41) could be referred to as a generalized linear dynamical mixed model (GLDMM). However, we prefer to indicate specifically that the process is *spatio-temporal* and refer to this model as a generalized linear dynamical spatio-temporal model (GLDSTM). In this case, the process $\{\boldsymbol{\nu}_t\}$ is assumed to have no temporal structure, but it could be modeled as having (independent across time) spatial structure.

In problems with missing data, or different supports, (7.42) can be modified to explicitly account for it, as follows:

$$\mathbf{Z}_t|\boldsymbol{\gamma}_t \sim ind. \; Poi(\mathbf{H}_t\boldsymbol{\gamma}_t), \tag{7.44}$$

where $\mathbf{H}_t$ is an $m_t \times n$ measurement matrix, and $\boldsymbol{\gamma}_t$ is now n-dimensional. In this case, the matrix $\mathbf{H}_t$ accounts for the mapping of the mean process to observation locations as described in (7.11) for Gaussian models. Here, a Gaussian assumption for $\{\boldsymbol{\gamma}_t\}$ would be inappropriate, since they are non-negative intensities, although a log Gaussian assumption like (7.43) would be appropriate.

Another common choice within this class of models is the binomial sampling distribution. Now,

$$\mathbf{Z}_t | \boldsymbol{\gamma}_t, \mathbf{p}_t \sim \textit{ind. Bin}(\boldsymbol{\gamma}_t, \mathbf{p}_t), \tag{7.45}$$

where the observations (e.g., counts) are distributed independently as binomial distributions conditioned on the true counts, $\{\boldsymbol{\gamma}_t\}$, and probabilities, $\{\mathbf{p}_t\}$. In the case where neither $\boldsymbol{\gamma}_t$ nor $\mathbf{p}_t$ are known, we cannot identify both components without additional information (e.g., replicate observations or strong priors). This is common in the ecological sciences, where one has observations $\{\mathbf{Z}_t\}$ of some ecological process (e.g., birds) conditional upon the true abundance $\{\boldsymbol{\gamma}_t\}$ and the probability of detection $\{\mathbf{p}_t\}$ at the spatial locations (and times) at which observations were taken (e.g., see Royle and Dorazio, 2008).

7.2 PROCESS MODELS FOR THE DSTM: LINEAR MODELS

As discussed in Section 3.2, a key issue with dynamical processes is specifying how the process transitions from one time to the next. In the spatio-temporal statistical setting, this is relatively complicated due to the curse of dimensionality. As a simple example, assume we have just three spatial locations of interest for the process, $Y(\mathbf{s}_1; t)$, $Y(\mathbf{s}_2; t)$, and $Y(\mathbf{s}_3; t)$. An ideal spatio-temporal model would completely characterize the joint distribution of these process locations for all times, namely $[Y(\mathbf{s}_1; t), Y(\mathbf{s}_2; t), Y(\mathbf{s}_3; t): t \in D_t]$. That is, we would need to characterize the distributional aspects of all possible interactions of $Y(\mathbf{s}_i; t)$ and $Y(\mathbf{s}_j; r)$ for any and all times t and r and spatial locations $i = 1, 2, 3$ and $j = 1, 2, 3$.

The joint specification of such spatio-temporal distributions is difficult, as described in Chapter 6, although there has been much recent work done regarding the development of valid joint spatio-temporal covariance functions (Section 6.1). However, these formulations are often unrealistic for real-world processes, and inference is still burdened by the curse of dimensionality. Recall that many processes in the environmental sciences exhibit high dimensionality (either in prediction locations or data locations), nonstationarity (typically in space), nonseparability, and complicated dynamics with features such as advection, diffusion, repulsion, growth, and so on. In addition, the process may evolve nonlinearly. It can be very difficult to incorporate what is known about such processes into the joint-dependence structure.

As has been suggested throughout this book, most models of real-world spatio-temporal processes are dynamical, in that the state of the process at the current time can be characterized, conditional on the process in the recent past. Incorporating this recognition into the modeling framework leads to dramatic simplifications through conditional-probability specifications about the process. Consider n finite spatial locations $\{s_1, \ldots, s_n\}$ and discrete times $t \in \{0, 1, 2, \ldots, T\}$. Let $\mathbf{Y}_t \equiv (Y_t(s_1), \ldots, Y_t(s_n))'$ be an arbitrary vector representation of the process at the n spatial locations at time t. The joint distribution of the spatio-temporal process can be factored as follows:

$$[\mathbf{Y}_0, \ldots, \mathbf{Y}_T] = [\mathbf{Y}_T | \mathbf{Y}_{T-1}, \ldots, \mathbf{Y}_0][\mathbf{Y}_{T-1} | \mathbf{Y}_{T-2}, \ldots, \mathbf{Y}_0]$$
$$\ldots [\mathbf{Y}_2 | \mathbf{Y}_1, \mathbf{Y}_0][\mathbf{Y}_1 | \mathbf{Y}_0][\mathbf{Y}_0].$$

We can simplify this greatly with Markov-type assumptions. For example, the first-order Markov assumption for $\{\mathbf{Y}_t\}$ is

$$[\mathbf{Y}_t | \mathbf{Y}_{t-1}, \mathbf{Y}_{t-2}, \ldots] = [\mathbf{Y}_t | \mathbf{Y}_{t-1}].$$

Thus, under this assumption, the joint distribution can be written as

$$[\mathbf{Y}_0, \ldots, \mathbf{Y}_T] = [\mathbf{Y}_0] \prod_{t=1}^{T} [\mathbf{Y}_t | \mathbf{Y}_{t-1}].$$

Critical to the specification of this distribution is a model for $[\mathbf{Y}_t | \mathbf{Y}_{t-1}]$. That is, we need some stochastic model that describes the evolution of the process from time $t - 1$ to time t. In general, we can write such a model as

$$\mathbf{Y}_t = \mathcal{M}(\mathbf{Y}_{t-1}, \boldsymbol{\eta}_t; \boldsymbol{\theta}_P),$$

where $\mathcal{M}(\cdot, \cdot; \cdot)$ is some function of the process at the previous time, an error term, and process parameters $\boldsymbol{\theta}_P$ that describe the dynamical transition. This function can be linear or nonlinear, and the associated distribution can be Gaussian or non-Gaussian, with additive or multiplicative errors. More generally, higher-order Markov assumptions could be considered as well, but many of the issues regarding parameterization of dynamical processes can be illustrated with the first-order model; hence, that will be our focus here.

Consider the simple example above, where we were interested in the process at just three locations $\{s_1, s_2, s_3\}$, so $n = 3$. In this case, we need to specify the relationship between $Y_t(s_i)$ and $Y_{t-1}(s_1), Y_{t-1}(s_2), Y_{t-1}(s_3)$, for $i = 1, 2, 3$. For now, just consider the linear relationship

$$\begin{bmatrix} Y_t(s_1) \\ Y_t(s_2) \\ Y_t(s_3) \end{bmatrix} = \begin{bmatrix} m_{11}Y_{t-1}(s_1) + m_{12}Y_{t-1}(s_2) + m_{13}Y_{t-1}(s_3) \\ m_{21}Y_{t-1}(s_1) + m_{22}Y_{t-1}(s_2) + m_{23}Y_{t-1}(s_3) \\ m_{31}Y_{t-1}(s_1) + m_{32}Y_{t-1}(s_2) + m_{33}Y_{t-1}(s_3) \end{bmatrix} + \begin{bmatrix} \eta_t(s_1) \\ \eta_t(s_2) \\ \eta_t(s_3) \end{bmatrix},$$

or

$$\begin{bmatrix} Y_t(s_1) \\ Y_t(s_2) \\ Y_t(s_3) \end{bmatrix} = \begin{bmatrix} m_{11} & m_{12} & m_{13} \\ m_{21} & m_{22} & m_{23} \\ m_{31} & m_{32} & m_{33} \end{bmatrix} \begin{bmatrix} Y_{t-1}(s_1) \\ Y_{t-1}(s_2) \\ Y_{t-1}(s_3) \end{bmatrix} + \begin{bmatrix} \eta_t(s_1) \\ \eta_t(s_2) \\ \eta_t(s_3) \end{bmatrix},$$

where the *redistribution weights* $\{m_{ij}\}$ describe how the process at location j at the previous time influences the process at location i at the current time (i.e., how the process *propagates* or *transitions* from one time to the next). We have also added a contemporaneous noise process $\{\eta_t(\mathbf{s}_i)\}$ to "force" the system, or to account for model uncertainty. In general, the linear-evolution equation with Gaussian errors can be written in matrix form,

$$\mathbf{Y}_t = \mathbf{M}\mathbf{Y}_{t-1} + \boldsymbol{\eta}_t, \qquad \boldsymbol{\eta}_t \sim iid \ Gau(\mathbf{0}, \mathbf{Q}_\eta), \tag{7.46}$$

where the propagator matrix (or transition matrix, or redistribution matrix) $\mathbf{M}$ is an $n \times n$ matrix of typically unknown parameters $\{m_{ij}\}$; $\{\boldsymbol{\eta}_t\}$ is independent over time and Gaussian with mean zero and covariance matrix $\mathbf{Q}_n$ (although other error processes could be considered); and $\boldsymbol{\eta}_t$ is independent of $\mathbf{Y}_{t-1}$. Note, we have assumed that $\{\mathbf{Y}_t\}$ has mean zero in this example. If this is not the case, we can simply rewrite the evolution equation accounting for the mean vector, $\boldsymbol{\mu}_t$:

$$\mathbf{Y}_t - \boldsymbol{\mu}_t = \mathbf{M}(\mathbf{Y}_{t-1} - \boldsymbol{\mu}_{t-1}) + \boldsymbol{\eta}_t, \qquad \boldsymbol{\eta}_t \sim iid \ Gau(\mathbf{0}, \mathbf{Q}_\eta). \tag{7.47}$$

Unless specified otherwise, we shall assume $\{\mathbf{Y}_t\}$ has mean zero throughout this discussion.

Consider the ith element of $\mathbf{Y}_t$ and the associated evolution equation implied by the model (7.46),

$$Y_t(\mathbf{s}_i) = \sum_{j=1}^{n} m_{ij} Y_{t-1}(\mathbf{s}_j) + \eta_t(\mathbf{s}_i),$$

where the redistribution weight m_{ij} corresponds to the ith row and jth column of $\mathbf{M}$. It is seldom the case in real-world problems that one knows the elements of $\mathbf{M}$ with certainty. When n is relatively small, we can estimate $\mathbf{M}$ outright (e.g., see the discussion of DSTM estimation in Section 8.3). But, in realistic spatio-temporal problems with high-dimensional state spaces, this is not possible. Generally speaking, obtaining reliable estimates of the $n \times n$ propagator matrix $\mathbf{M}$ is a challenge, unless $T >> n$, which is seldom the case. Thus, the key issue becomes how $\mathbf{M}$ can be parameterized to capture adequately the dynamics using relatively few parameters. This is the fundamental problem in spatio-temporal dynamical modeling! Furthermore, as difficult as this is in the linear case, it is much more complicated in the nonlinear case, where one must have a strong sense of the underlying dynamics to make efficient and useful parameterizations of the transition operator (see Section 7.3, below).

In the remainder of this section, we consider various approaches to parameterizing the propagator matrix for first-order, linear DSTMs. Similar approaches will apply to higher-order models (i.e., models with higher lags). Note that higher-order VAR models can always be reparameterized and written as first-order models [e.g., see equations (3.38) and (3.39) in Section 3.1.1; and see

Lütkepohl (2005, p. 15)]. However, this does not reduce dimensionality of the parameter space.

Ultimately, we must parameterize the propagator (or transition) matrix $\mathbf{M}$ in terms of some parameters $\boldsymbol{\theta}_P$ that have dimensionality significantly less than the n^2 required to estimate $\mathbf{M}$ directly. There are several strategies that one can use, many of which are motivated by the underlying dynamical process. The following subsections describe various types of model specifications for first-order linear models, starting from the very simple and increasing in complexity.

7.2.1 Spatio-Temporal Random Walk

Perhaps the simplest parameterization of the DSTM process model is the multivariate extension of the random walk (see Section 3.4.2). That is,

$$\mathbf{Y}_t = \mathbf{Y}_{t-1} + \boldsymbol{\eta}_t, \qquad \boldsymbol{\eta}_t \sim iid\, Gau(\mathbf{0}, \mathbf{Q}_\eta).$$

In this case, the process value at location $\mathbf{s}_i$ and time t is just the value of the process at the same location $\mathbf{s}_i$ at the previous time $(t-1)$, plus some noise. Clearly, in this case, $\mathbf{M} = \mathbf{I}$. However, there is the possibility that the forcing term $\boldsymbol{\eta}_t$ is spatially dependent. The obvious advantage of this parameterization is that there are very few parameters (there are none in the transition matrix, since it is just the identity matrix). The disadvantage is that it is nonstationary in time (leading to increasing variance with time) and cannot directly accommodate dynamical interactions across space and time. In this sense, the parameterization is not very realistic for most spatio-temporal processes (at least those on relatively large spatial and temporal scales).

An obvious way to introduce stationarity in this model is to allow a single autoregressive parameter in the transition operator:

$$\mathbf{Y}_t = m\mathbf{Y}_{t-1} + \boldsymbol{\eta}_t, \qquad \boldsymbol{\eta}_t \sim iid\, Gau(\mathbf{0}, \mathbf{Q}_\eta),$$

where $|m| < 1$. That is, for each spatial location, the transition between the past state and the current state is determined by a parameter m, which is homogeneous across space. Of course, this is still a very-low-dimensional parameterization, but it is probably not all that realistic for most spatio-temporal processes. In both of these models, spatial dependence in $\mathbf{Q}_\eta$ does imply quite interesting marginal spatio-temporal covariance structure for the process $\{\mathbf{Y}_t\}$, but it does not allow dynamical interaction, which is needed for, say, forecasting.

7.2.2 Spatial Autoregressive Model

An obvious extension of the simple autoregressive model given above, is to allow the AR parameters to vary heterogeneously across space. For example, in the three-location example,

$$
\begin{bmatrix} Y_t(\mathbf{s}_1) \\ Y_t(\mathbf{s}_2) \\ Y_t(\mathbf{s}_3) \end{bmatrix} = \begin{bmatrix} m_{11}Y_{t-1}(\mathbf{s}_1) \\ m_{22}Y_{t-1}(\mathbf{s}_2) \\ m_{33}Y_{t-1}(\mathbf{s}_3) \end{bmatrix} + \begin{bmatrix} \eta_t(\mathbf{s}_1) \\ \eta_t(\mathbf{s}_2) \\ \eta_t(\mathbf{s}_3) \end{bmatrix},
$$

or, for general n,

$$
\mathbf{Y}_t = \text{diag}(\mathbf{m})\mathbf{Y}_{t-1} + \boldsymbol{\eta}_t, \qquad \boldsymbol{\eta}_t \sim iid\, Gau(\mathbf{0}, \mathbf{Q}_\eta), \qquad (7.48)
$$

where $\mathbf{m} \equiv (m(\mathbf{s}_1), \dots, m(\mathbf{s}_n))'$. Again, the advantages of this model are that there are relatively few parameters, that it is nonseparable (provided $\mathbf{Q}_\eta$ is not diagonal), and that it is fairly easy to estimate (or model) the parameters. That is, one might have strong prior assumptions for $\mathbf{m}$, and their distribution could be specified at the parameter-model level of the hierarchy (e.g., $\mathbf{m}$ could be represented as a spatial random field). The complicated spatial dependencies in $\mathbf{m}$ will be reflected in the marginal distribution of $\{\mathbf{Y}_t\}$, and hence the spatio-temporal dependencies can be quite rich in this setting. However, this model obviously cannot handle direct interaction between space and time for multiple spatial locations. As such, many processes that are of interest to physical and biological scientists, such as advection and diffusion, cannot be accommodated directly in (7.48).

7.2.3 "Lagged Nearest-Neighbor" Model

Now consider the case where we let $\mathbf{M}$ be parameterized such that only the m_{ij} corresponding to the location $\mathbf{s}_i$ and its nearest neighbors $\{\mathbf{s}_j; j \in \mathcal{N}_i\}$ at the previous time are important (e.g., Wikle, Berliner, and Cressie, 1998). This model assumes that we have a reasonable way to characterize the nearest neighbors. This might be in the context of a process with areal support (say county-level data), or it might be for processes on a regular grid, with point or areal support. This model is written as

$$
Y_t(\mathbf{s}_i) = \sum_{j \in \mathcal{N}_i} m_{ij}Y_{t-1}(\mathbf{s}_j) + \eta_t(\mathbf{s}_i), \qquad (7.49)
$$

where $\mathcal{N}_i$ refers to a prespecified "neighborhood" of $\mathbf{s}_i$, $i = 1, \dots, n$. We typically assume that the errors are Gaussian: $\boldsymbol{\eta}_t \sim iid\, Gau(\mathbf{0}, \mathbf{Q}_\eta)$. These models are relatively sparse, in the sense that many of the elements of $\mathbf{M}$ are zero, yet lagged-neighbor interaction can accommodate a very large class of dynamical processes (as will be shown below). However, even in this case, with relatively large numbers of process locations, the estimation of the nonzero m_{ij} can be difficult, if not impossible, given typical datasets. This suggests that further parameterization is needed. The specification for parameterized neighbor interactions is not necessarily simple, but it can often be facilitated by using scientific theory related to the process of interest. An example of this, based on partial-differential-equation dynamics, is given in the next subsection.

We note that one is tempted to consider this model a special case of the space–time autoregressive (STAR) models outlined in Section 6.4.2. Recall that, as shown in (6.94), $\mathbf{M} \equiv (\mathbf{I} - \mathbf{B}_0)^{-1}\mathbf{B}_1$ for STAR models, where the matrix $\mathbf{B}_0$ has zeros down the main diagonal (representing "instantaneous" spatial dependence). Thus, even if $\mathbf{B}_0$ and $\mathbf{B}_1$ are formulated in terms of the first-order (nearest) neighbors, $\mathbf{M}$ does not have such a diagonal structure due to the typically unbanded nature of $(\mathbf{I} - \mathbf{B}_0)^{-1}$. However, this is an interesting approach for *parameterizing* $\mathbf{M}$ in terms of $\mathbf{B}_0$ and $\mathbf{B}_1$, since each is parameterized in terms of only a few parameters. Obviously, if $\mathbf{B}_0 = \mathbf{0}$, then $\mathbf{M}$ and $\mathbf{B}_1$ are equivalent.

Of course, as in all of the dynamical models presented in this section, higher-order lags in time can be considered if desired.

7.2.4 PDE-Based Parameterizations

For many environmental processes, the underlying spatio-temporal process may follow partial differential equations (PDEs) or ordinary differential equations (ODEs). In the case of linear PDEs, standard finite differencing implies linear Markov spatio-temporal models and suggests parameterizations of the propagator matrix $\mathbf{M}$ as described above (e.g., Section 6.3; Wikle, 2003b; Wikle and Hooten, 2010). For example, consider the general PDE,

$$\frac{\partial Y}{\partial t} = \mathcal{M}(Y, w, \boldsymbol{\theta}),$$

where $\mathcal{M}$ is some function of the variable of interest, Y, other potential variables, w, and process-model parameters, $\boldsymbol{\theta}$. As a process model, it is deterministic.

Simple finite-difference representations (e.g., see Haberman, 1987) suggest an approximate difference-equation model,

$$\mathbf{Y}_t - m(\mathbf{Y}_{t\ \Delta_t}, \mathbf{w}_t, \boldsymbol{\theta}) + \boldsymbol{\eta}_t,$$

where an independent noise term, $\boldsymbol{\eta}_t$, has been added to account for the error of discretization and/or stochastic forcing. Note that it is also reasonable (and probably more appropriate) to consider this error term to include model errors, in the sense that the original PDE should be made stochastic to reflect that it is only an approximation of the real process of interest.

As an example, consider a simple spatio-temporal process $Y(x; t)$ in one-dimensional space, $0 \le x \le L$ (i.e., $D_s = [0, L]$), and time t. We assume a *diffusion equation* to be an approximate representation of the true process:

$$\frac{\partial Y}{\partial t} = \frac{\partial}{\partial x}\left(b(x)\frac{\partial Y}{\partial x}\right),$$

where (for now) the diffusion coefficients, $b(x)$, the boundary conditions, $Y(0; t) = Y_0$ and $Y(L; t) = Y_L$, and the initial condition, $\{Y(x; 0) : 0 \leq x \leq L\}$, are known. This PDE is different from the diffusion-injection equation considered in the introduction to Chapter 6.

Now, as in traditional numerical analysis, we approximate the partial derivatives by finite differences. For example, we might use a centered difference,

$$\frac{\partial Y}{\partial x} \simeq \frac{Y(x + \Delta_x; t) - Y(x - \Delta_x; t)}{2\Delta_x},$$

along with a second-order difference given by

$$\frac{\partial^2 Y}{\partial x^2} \simeq \frac{Y(x + \Delta_x; t) - 2Y(x; t) + Y(x - \Delta_x; t)}{\Delta_x^2}.$$

For an approximation of the time derivative, we could use a forward difference:

$$\frac{\partial Y}{\partial t} \simeq \frac{Y(x; t + \Delta_t) - Y(x; t)}{\Delta_t}.$$

Thus, using a forward difference in time and centered differences in space, we obtain the finite-difference approximation of the one-dimensional diffusion equation:

$$\frac{Y(x; t + \Delta_t) - Y(x; t)}{\Delta_t} \simeq b(x) \left(\frac{Y(x + \Delta_x; t) - 2Y(x; t) + Y(x - \Delta_x; t)}{\Delta_x^2} \right)$$

$$+ \left(\frac{Y(x + \Delta_x; t) - Y(x - \Delta_x; t)}{2\Delta_x} \right)$$

$$\left(\frac{b(x + \Delta_x) - b(x - \Delta_x)}{2\Delta_x} \right),$$

which can be rewritten as

$$Y(x; t + \Delta_t) \simeq \left(1 - \frac{2b(x)\Delta_t}{\Delta_x^2} \right) Y(x; t) + Y(x + \Delta_x; t)$$

$$\left(\frac{\Delta_t}{\Delta_x^2} [b(x) + \{b(x + \Delta_x) - b(x - \Delta_x)\}/4] \right)$$

$$+ Y(x - \Delta_x; t) \left(\frac{\Delta_t}{\Delta_x^2} [b(x) - \{b(x + \Delta_x) - b(x - \Delta_x)\}/4] \right).$$

Collecting terms in the finite-difference representation, we obtain

$$Y(x; t + \Delta_t) \simeq \theta_1(x)Y(x; t) + \theta_2(x)Y(x + \Delta_x; t) + \theta_3(x)Y(x - \Delta_x; t),$$

where $\{\theta_i(x) : i = 1, 2, 3\}$ are functions of Δ_x, Δ_t, $b(x)$, $b(x - \Delta_x)$, and $b(x + \Delta_x)$. It is critical to note that $\theta_1(\cdot)$, $\theta_2(\cdot)$, and $\theta_3(\cdot)$ play the role of the m_{ij} from before. Thus, this is analogous to the "lagged-nearest-neighbor" structure mentioned in Section 7.2.3. However, now the diffusion PDE suggests the parameterization. In particular, we see that if we know the spatially varying $b(x)$ and the discretization parameters, then we know the structure of the nearest-neighbor interactions. Then, just as in Section 6.3 for the diffusion-injection equation, we can write this in matrix form.

As a simple example, consider $n = 3$ equally spaced locations $s_1 = x_1$, $s_2 = x_2$, $s_3 = x_3$, and boundary points $s_0 = x_0 = 0$ and $s_4 = x_4 = L$. We can then write

$$
\begin{bmatrix} Y(x_1; t + \Delta_t) \\ Y(x_2; t + \Delta_t) \\ Y(x_3; t + \Delta_t) \end{bmatrix} \simeq \begin{bmatrix} \theta_1(x_1)Y(x_1; t) + \theta_2(x_1)Y(x_2; t) + \theta_3(x_1)Y(x_0; t) \\ \theta_1(x_2)Y(x_2; t) + \theta_2(x_2)Y(x_3; t) + \theta_3(x_2)Y(x_1; t) \\ \theta_1(x_3)Y(x_3; t) + \theta_2(x_3)Y(x_4; t) + \theta_3(x_3)Y(x_2; t) \end{bmatrix} ,
$$

which can be written as

$$
\begin{bmatrix} Y(x_1; t + \Delta_t) \\ Y(x_2; t + \Delta_t) \\ Y(x_3; t + \Delta_t) \end{bmatrix} \simeq \begin{bmatrix} \theta_1(x_1) & \theta_2(x_2) & 0 \\ \theta_3(x_2) & \theta_1(x_2) & \theta_2(x_2) \\ 0 & \theta_3(x_3) & \theta_1(x_3) \end{bmatrix} \begin{bmatrix} Y(x_1; t) \\ Y(x_2; t) \\ Y(x_3; t) \end{bmatrix}
$$

$$
+ \begin{bmatrix} \theta_3(x_1) & 0 \\ 0 & 0 \\ 0 & \theta_2(x_3) \end{bmatrix} \begin{bmatrix} Y_0 \\ Y_L \end{bmatrix} .
$$

In general matrix form, this is

$$
\mathbf{Y}_{t+\Delta_t} \simeq \mathbf{M}(\boldsymbol{\theta})\mathbf{Y}_t + \mathbf{M}^{(b)}(\boldsymbol{\theta})\mathbf{Y}_t^{(b)},
$$

where $\mathbf{M}^{(b)}(\boldsymbol{\theta})$ is the boundary propagator matrix, and $\mathbf{Y}_t^{(b)} \equiv (Y_0, Y_L)'$ is the boundary condition. In the HM framework, a prior distribution can be placed on the boundary process, which can simplify computation tremendously (see Wikle, Berliner, and Milliff, 2003).

In the one-dimensional case with general n, $\mathbf{M}(\boldsymbol{\theta})$ is tridiagonal with elements on the three main diagonals, and zeros elsewhere. This sparseness is of great benefit, both computationally and with regard to parameter estimation, due to the reduction in dimensionality of the parameter space. In higher spatial dimensions, the matrix is still relatively sparse, with just a few nonzero diagonals [e.g., for two-dimensional space, the diffusion equation has five diagonals corresponding to the five nearest neighbors; see Wikle (2003b)].

Given an initial condition, the discretized PDE can then be "integrated" forward by iteration from 0 to Δ_t, from Δ_t to $2\Delta_t$, and so on. The initial condition, $\{Y(x; 0) : x \in D_s\}$, is assumed to be known, but again we could put a prior distribution on it.

The model above is now made stochastic to account for discretization error and uncertainty concerning model misspecification. This is most easily done by adding an error term:

$$
\mathbf{Y}_{t+\Delta_t} = \mathbf{M}(\boldsymbol{\theta})\mathbf{Y}_t + \mathbf{M}^{(b)}(\boldsymbol{\theta})\mathbf{Y}_t^{(b)} + \boldsymbol{\eta}_{t+\Delta_t},
$$

where typically, $\boldsymbol{\eta}_t \sim iid\, Gau(\mathbf{0}, \mathbf{Q}_\eta)$.

In most problems, we know neither the diffusion coefficients, $\mathbf{b} \equiv (b(x_1), \ldots, b(x_n))'$, nor the covariance parameters, $\mathbf{Q}_\eta$, that control the noise. These must be estimated or modeled. This is not easy in general, but it is simplified greatly by a hierarchical representation where these parameters are given distributions at the next level of the hierarchy. For pure numerical integration, various conditions on the parameters guarantee the stability of the integration; see also Section 6.3. For example, in the simple diffusion equation above with $b(x) \equiv b$, the condition

$$\left| \frac{2\Delta_t b}{\Delta_x^2} \right| < 1$$

must be satisfied or the solution will be unstable [grow without bound; e.g., see Haberman (1987)]. Now, such stability issues are less critical in the presence of random effects and data, as the data act to stabilize the integration for the posterior distribution. However, in that case, the diffusion coefficients adjust to fit the data, and they may lose their interpretability.

Of course, the simple diffusion equation presented above is just one of a very large number of linear PDEs that could be used to motivate a dynamical spatio-temporal process. For example, if we were interested in a process in which the quantity of concern (e.g., a pollutant) is propagating due to the influence of some velocity field (e.g., wind), then a linear advection-diffusion equation would be an appropriate PDE to motivate the process model. For example, in two spatial dimensions (say, $\mathbf{s} = (x, y) \in D_s \subset \mathbb{R}^2$), this would be

$$\frac{\partial Y}{\partial t} = c_1(x, y) \frac{\partial Y}{\partial x} + c_2(x, y) \frac{\partial Y}{\partial y} + \frac{\partial}{\partial x} \left(b(x, y) \frac{\partial Y}{\partial x} \right) + \frac{\partial}{\partial y} \left(b(x, y) \frac{\partial Y}{\partial y} \right),$$
(7.50)

where the first two and last two terms on the right-hand side correspond to the advection and diffusion portions of the process, respectively, and it is understood that Y is a function of (x, y) and t. As an illustration, consider the numerical simulations of the advection-diffusion process shown in Figure 7.1. The left panels in this plot show a simulation of the process with advection coefficients that are zero (i.e., $c_i(x, y) \equiv 0$, for $i = 1, 2$). One can see that, from an initial state in the center, the process spreads ("diffuses") with time, consequently lowering its magnitude. The center panels of this figure show the advection-diffusion simulation with an advection term that is a (nonzero) constant, such that the process is advected to the lower right corner of the image through time. Observe that, in addition to obvious movement with time, there is a spread with time as well. Finally, the right panels in this figure show the simulated advection-diffusion process with advection parameters that are varying with space as shown in Figure 7.2. In this case, as the object propagates, it is affected by the spatially varying advection in a way that makes it propagate at different velocities, thereby changing over time the propagation direction, shape, and orientation of the object.

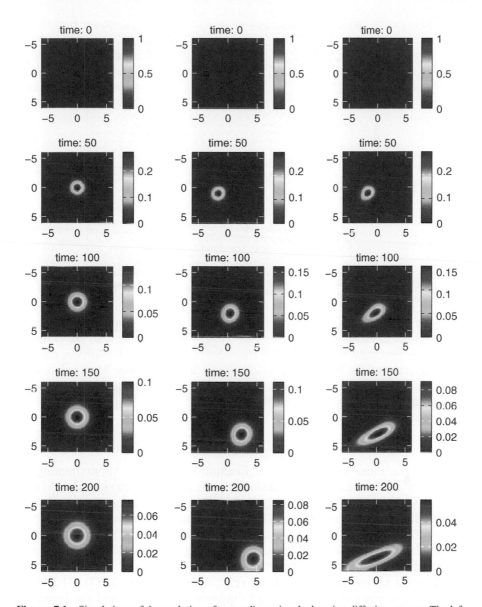

Figure 7.1 Simulations of the evolution of a two-dimensional advection-diffusion process. The left column shows the evolving process with the advection parameter set to zero across the spatial domain (i.e., a pure diffusion process). The center column shows the evolving process with a constant (in space) advection parameter that advects the process toward the lower-right corner. The right column shows an evolving process with spatially varying advection coefficients as given in Figure 7.2.

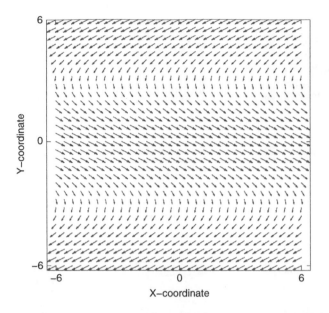

Figure 7.2 Graphical representation of spatially varying advection coefficients associated with the simulation of the two-dimensional advection-diffusion equation shown in the right column of Figure 7.1. The process is advected in the direction shown by the arrows in this plot.

The form of the PDE might also suggest a higher-order Markovian structure in the discretized dynamics. For example, consider the hyperbolic wave equation,

$$\frac{\partial^2 Y}{\partial t^2} = \frac{\partial}{\partial x}\left(d(x)\frac{\partial Y}{\partial x}\right),$$

where it is understood that Y is a function of x and t. Approximating this equation with centered finite differences suggests a second-order Markov (e.g., VAR(2)) statistical model due to the second-order time derivative. Note also that higher-order differencing schemes can imply higher-order discretized model forms as well. Indeed, it is certainly the case that other discretization schemes can be used, including higher-order finite-difference methods, finite-element methods, and Runge–Kutta methods. These might be explicit or implicit formulations (e.g., see Haberman, 1987). The choice is largely dependent on the type of equations considered and the inferential goals at hand. It is important to note that each of these discretization schemes implies a different statistical-model parameterization.

7.2.5 IDE-Based Dynamics

To capture dynamical interactions in space–time that are realistic for many processes (especially those in ecology), the propagator matrix **M** must contain nonzero off-diagonal elements beyond just the nearest neighbors. That is, long-range dependence can sometimes be important in the dynamics. This might suggest using a general form of $\mathbf{M}$, which we have already discounted as impractical when the number of process locations n is large. However, a general non-sparse $\mathbf{M}$ can be parameterized so that the true number of parameters necessary to describe $\mathbf{M}$ is much smaller than n^2. One way to consider such a parameterization again comes from a theoretical deterministic framework, in particular integro-difference equations (IDEs).

Consider the deterministic IDE model, used in population ecology (e.g., Kot, Lewis, and van den Driessche, 1996) when time is discrete and space is continuous. In the case of linear dynamics, the IDE model is simply

$$Y_t(\mathbf{s}) = \int_{D_s} m(\mathbf{s}, \mathbf{x}; \boldsymbol{\theta}) Y_{t-1}(\mathbf{x}) \, d\mathbf{x}, \qquad \mathbf{s} \in D_s, \tag{7.51}$$

where $m(\mathbf{s}, \mathbf{x}; \boldsymbol{\theta})$ is the redistribution kernel, which depends on parameters $\boldsymbol{\theta}$. One could think of this process as simply redistributing in space the process from the previous time, where the redistribution is controlled by the kernel m. In particular, $m(\mathbf{s}, \mathbf{x}; \boldsymbol{\theta})$ gives the redistribution weight for the process at location $\mathbf{x}$ at the previous time, relative to the location $\mathbf{s}$ at the current time. The simple addition of a random noise term, independent of $Y_{t-1}(\cdot)$, then gives a stochastic IDE model:

$$Y_t(\mathbf{s}) = \int_{D_s} m(\mathbf{s}, \mathbf{x}; \boldsymbol{\theta}) Y_{t-1}(\mathbf{x}) \, d\mathbf{x} + \eta_t(\mathbf{s}), \qquad \mathbf{s} \in D_s, \tag{7.52}$$

where the error process $\{\eta_t(\cdot)\}$ is independent in time but may be correlated in space.

It has been shown that this redistribution kernel can model diffusive wave fronts (e.g., Kot, Lewis, and van den Driessche, 1996), where the shape and speed of diffusion depends on kernel width and tail behavior (i.e., kernel dilation). For example, Figure 7.3a and Figure 7.4a show simulations of one-dimensional spatial deterministic IDE processes based on Gaussian kernels $m(||\mathbf{s} - \mathbf{x}||; \sigma^2)$ with standard deviations $\sigma = 1$ and $\sigma = 3$, respectively. Note how much more quickly the initial disturbance disperses when the variance (width) of the kernel is larger. Figures 7.3b and 7.4b shows simulations from the respective stochastic IDE processes with an additive Gaussian white-noise error process $\eta_t(\cdot)$, in which $\text{var}(\eta_t(\mathbf{s})) = 1$.

In addition, so-called nondiffusive propagation (e.g., advection) can be modeled via the relative displacement of the kernel (i.e., translation from its initial location $\mathbf{s}$), which is manifested as skewness; see Wikle (2002a). Figure 7.5a and Figure 7.6a show simulated one-dimensional spatial, deterministic IDE processes with a "skewed-Gaussian" kernel with skewness (i.e., displacement) parameter equal to 0.2 and -0.5, respectively. Note that, in the case of a positively skewed kernel (Figure 7.5), the propagation through time is to the right; when the kernel is negatively skewed (Figure 7.6), the propagation is to the left. Figure 7.5b and Figure 7.6b show the simulations from the respective stochastic IDE with an additive Gaussian white-noise (in space and time) error

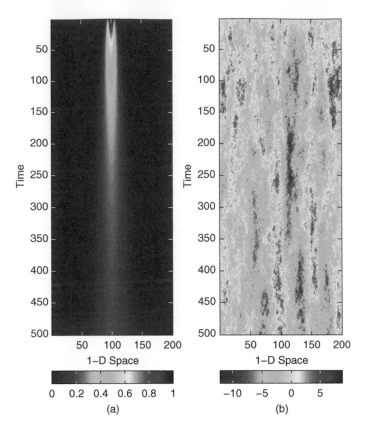

Figure 7.3 Simulation of a one-dimensional IDE process with a symmetric Gaussian transition kernel that has standard deviation, 1. **(a)** The deterministic IDE given in equation (7.51). **(b)** The stochastic IDE given in equation (7.52), with white noise (in space and time) variance, 1.

process $\eta_t(\cdot)$, in which $var(\eta_t(\mathbf{s})) = 1$. This methodology is even more powerful when the kernel translation and dilation parameters are allowed to vary with spatial location (e.g., Wikle, 2002a; Xu, Wikle, and Fox, 2005). Also, nonlinear forms of IDE models are important for spatio-temporal growth processes (e.g., Lewis, 2000; Wikle and Holan, 2011).

The advantage of an IDE dynamical model is that it can accommodate complicated spatio-temporal dynamics with relatively few parameters. For example, discretizing the integral in (7.52) gives

$$Y_t(\mathbf{s}_i) = \sum_{j=1}^{n} m_{ij}(\boldsymbol{\theta})Y_{t-1}(\mathbf{s}_j) + \eta_t(\mathbf{s}_i). \tag{7.53}$$

Thus, this discretized version suggests potential parameterizations of $\mathbf{M}$ in terms of relatively few kernel parameters $\boldsymbol{\theta}$. Such parameterizations include nonzero off-diagonal elements, and typically the propagator matrix is not symmetric (i.e., $m_{ij}(\boldsymbol{\theta}) \neq m_{ji}(\boldsymbol{\theta})$). This is most useful when knowledge of

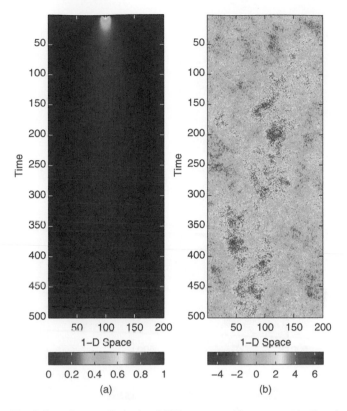

Figure 7.4 Simulation of a one-dimensional IDE process with a symmetric Gaussian transition kernel that has standard deviation, 3. **(a)** The deterministic IDE given in equation (7.51). **(b)** The stochastic IDE given in equation (7.52), with white noise (in space and time) variance, 1.

qualitative features in the dynamics (e.g., diffusion, advection) is presumed, rather than explicit forms.

Disadvantages of this approach have to do with implementation. For example, even if θ is known, the dimensionality of $\mathbf{M}$ can still be problematic from a computational perspective, if n is large. This is compounded by the non-sparse structure of $\mathbf{M}$. Furthermore, estimation of θ can be difficult in general, although the hierarchical Bayesian paradigm simplifies this greatly. That is, one can put a prior on θ at the next stage of the hierarchy. In addition, the choice of the appropriate kernel is not always clear. Hopefully, some *a priori* information regarding the qualitative aspects of the dynamics are available to help with this. Alternatively, mixtures of kernels can allow more complicated long-range dependencies. In addition, it is certainly possible to let the kernel parameters vary with space and time, as suggested above. This can accommodate complicated dynamics but, again, care must be taken not to replace one complicated spatio-temporal model by several complicated spatio-temporal models elsewhere in the hierarchy!

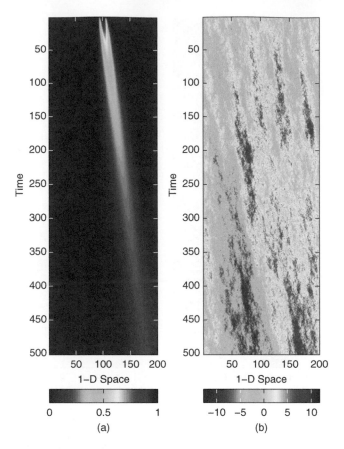

Figure 7.5 Simulation of a one-dimensional IDE process with a skewed-Gaussian transition kernel with standard deviation, 1, and skewness parameter, 0.2, implying propagation to the right. **(a)** The deterministic IDE given in equation (7.51). **(b)** The stochastic IDE given in equation (7.52) with white noise variance (in space and time), 1.

We note that an alternative implementation, which can be more efficient, consists of writing the IDE model in its spectral form. This will be illustrated in Section 7.2.6.

7.2.6   Spectral Parameterizations

As mentioned above, it is often convenient to consider spectral representations for dimension reduction and/or to facilitate scientific interpretation. Such transformations can simplify the parameterization of high-dimensional spatio-temporal processes in different ways. Several of these approaches are discussed here.

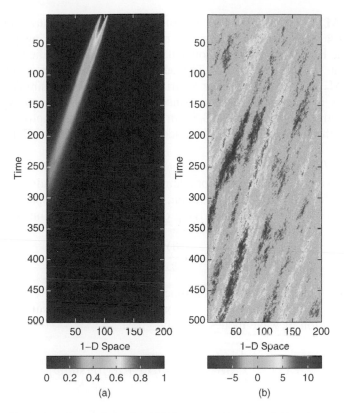

Figure 7.6 Simulation of a one-dimensional IDE process with a skewed-Gaussian transition kernel with standard deviation, 1, and skewness parameter, -0.5, implying propagation to the left. **(a)** The deterministic IDE given in equation (7.51). **(b)** The stochastic IDE given in equation (7.52) with white noise (in space and time) variance, 1.

Consider the general linear DSTM:

$$\mathbf{Y}_t = \mathbf{M}\mathbf{Y}_{t-1} + \boldsymbol{\eta}_t.$$

Now, expanding $\mathbf{Y}_t$ in terms of some complete class of spatial spectral basis vectors, given by the columns of $\boldsymbol{\Phi}$, we obtain

$$\mathbf{Y}_t = \boldsymbol{\Phi}\boldsymbol{\alpha}_t,$$

where $\boldsymbol{\alpha}_t$ are the associated spectral coefficients (Section 7.1.3). Note that at this point we are not assuming any truncation, but rather a simple linear transformation of the spatial process at time t into the spectral domain. One can show (e.g., Wikle and Cressie, 1999) that this suggests the equivalent dynamical relationship:

$$\boldsymbol{\alpha}_t = \mathbf{M}_\alpha \boldsymbol{\alpha}_{t-1} + \boldsymbol{\gamma}_t, \tag{7.54}$$

where $\mathbf{M}_\alpha \equiv (\mathbf{\Phi}'\mathbf{\Phi})^{-1}\mathbf{\Phi}'\mathbf{M}\mathbf{\Phi}$ is the spectral propagator matrix, and $\boldsymbol{\gamma}_t = (\mathbf{\Phi}'\mathbf{\Phi})^{-1}\mathbf{\Phi}'\boldsymbol{\eta}_t$ is the spectrally transformed noise-forcing process. Note that if the basis vectors are orthogonal, then (7.54) is simplified, since we can choose $\mathbf{\Phi}$ such that $\mathbf{\Phi}'\mathbf{\Phi} = \mathbf{I}$. The advantage of the spectral representation is that $\mathbf{M}_\alpha$ and the covariance matrix for $\boldsymbol{\gamma}_t$ are often simpler than their analogues in the spatial domain, since the spectral transform typically acts as a decorrelator (see Section 3.5). In addition, spectral approaches can also facilitate the implementation of science-based (e.g., PDE and IDE) models.

A Simple PDE

Suppose we are interested in a problem in which a simple advection-diffusion equation (for simplicity of illustration, in one-dimensional space) is a reasonable approximation of the underlying dynamics. This equation is given by

$$\frac{\partial Y}{\partial t} = c\frac{\partial Y}{\partial x} + b\frac{\partial^2 Y}{\partial x^2},$$

where it is understood that Y is a function of $x \in D_s$ and $t \in D_t$. Notice that this is just the one-dimensional version of (7.50). Now, assume solutions are a superposition of wave modes, namely,

$$Y_t(x) = \sum_{j=1}^{J}[\alpha_{1j}(t)\cos(\omega_j x) + \alpha_{2j}(t)\sin(\omega_j x)],$$

where $\omega_j = 2\pi j/|D_s|$ is the spatial frequency of a sinusoid over spatial domain D_s with spatial wave number $j = 1, \ldots, J$ (e.g., see Pedlosky, 1987 for similar derivations). Thus, for all spatial locations of interest, we have $\mathbf{Y}_t = \mathbf{\Phi}\boldsymbol{\alpha}_t$, where $\mathbf{\Phi}$ is made up of the Fourier basis functions, and $\{\boldsymbol{\alpha}_t\}$ is the collection of all spectral coefficients.

The deterministic solution gives formulas for $\alpha_{1j}(t)$ and $\alpha_{2j}(t)$, which are exponentially decaying sinusoids in time. For $j = 1, \ldots, J$, we have

$$\alpha_{1j}(t) = \exp(-b\omega_j^2 t)\sin(c\omega_j t),$$

$$\alpha_{2j}(t) = \exp(-b\omega_j^2 t)\cos(c\omega_j t).$$

Deterministic linear wave theory suggests

$$\boldsymbol{\alpha}_j(t + \Delta_t) = \mathbf{G}_j\boldsymbol{\alpha}_j(t), \qquad j = 1, \ldots, J,$$

where $\boldsymbol{\alpha}_j(t) \equiv (\alpha_{1j}(t)\ \alpha_{2j}(t))'$. For this example, we have

$$\begin{bmatrix} e^{-b\omega_j^2(t+\Delta_t)}\sin\{\omega_j(t+\Delta_t)\} \\ e^{-b\omega_j^2(t+\Delta_t)}\cos\{\omega_j(t+\Delta_t)\} \end{bmatrix} = \mathbf{G}_j \begin{bmatrix} e^{-b\omega_j^2 t}\sin\{\omega_j t\} \\ e^{-b\omega_j^2 t}\cos\{\omega_j t\} \end{bmatrix},$$

where

$$\mathbf{G}_j = \begin{bmatrix} e^{-b\omega_j^2 \Delta_t} \cos\{\omega_j \Delta_t\} & e^{-b\omega_j^2 \Delta_t} \sin\{\omega_j \Delta_t\} \\ -e^{-b\omega_j^2 \Delta_t} \sin\{\omega_j \Delta_t\} & e^{-b\omega_j^2 \Delta_t} \cos\{\omega_j \Delta_t\} \end{bmatrix}.$$

Now, we do not expect the true process to behave *exactly* as the linear wave theory suggests. Rather, we let this be the motivation for the DSTM. In particular, we let $\alpha_{1j}(t)$ and $\alpha_{2j}(t)$ be *stochastic* and add the noise term $\boldsymbol{\gamma}_j(t)$ to account for uncertainty. Finally, we let the propagator matrix be $\mathbf{M}_j$ with *prior mean* $\mathbf{G}_j$. That is, conditional on $\mathbf{M}_j$, we obtain

$$\boldsymbol{\alpha}_j(t + \Delta_t) = \mathbf{M}_j \boldsymbol{\alpha}_j(t) + \boldsymbol{\gamma}_j(t + \Delta_t), \qquad j = 1, \ldots, J.$$

Collecting these equations together, we obtain

$$\boldsymbol{\alpha}_{t+1} = \mathbf{M}\boldsymbol{\alpha}_t + \boldsymbol{\gamma}_{t+1},$$

where $\boldsymbol{\alpha}_t \equiv (\boldsymbol{\alpha}_1'(t) \ \ldots \ \boldsymbol{\alpha}_J'(t))'$; $\boldsymbol{\gamma}_t \equiv (\boldsymbol{\gamma}_1'(t), \ldots, \boldsymbol{\gamma}_J'(t))'$; $\mathbf{M}$ is block diagonal with blocks $\{\mathbf{M}_j : j = 1, \ldots, J\}$, and we have assumed that $\Delta_t = 1$. This idea of using spectral basis functions motivated by the deterministic PDE is a powerful modeling framework, and it can be applied to much more complicated PDE dynamical systems (Wikle et al., 2001).

Reduced Dimensionality in the Spectral Domain

The effective dimensionality of $\boldsymbol{\alpha}_t$ is often much less than that of $\mathbf{Y}_t$, since much of the variability of $\mathbf{Y}_t$ can be captured by relatively few spectral modes (see Chapter 3). This is often critical for estimation and implementation. In the simplest cases, the dimensionality of $\boldsymbol{\alpha}_t$ is so reduced ($p_\alpha << n$) that it is possible to estimate the propagator (in linear systems) directly if $p_\alpha << n < T$. This proceeds as with traditional state-space models (see Section 8.3).

There are also cases where dimension reduction is helpful in the spectral domain, when motivated by science-based deterministic models. In particular, this has been applied to the PDE and IDE models, as described in Wikle and Cressie (1999), Wikle (2002a), Wikle et al. (2001), and Xu, Wikle, and Fox (2005). This approach is sketched out below.

Assume the process $\{Y_t(\mathbf{s}) : \mathbf{s} \in D_s, t \in D_t\}$ can be decomposed as

$$Y_t(\mathbf{s}) = Y_t^P(\mathbf{s}) + v_t(\mathbf{s}),$$

where $\{Y_t^P(\mathbf{s})\}$ is assumed to be dynamical, and $v_t(\mathbf{s})$ is a nondynamical process (i.e., it does not exhibit Markovian dependence). Furthermore, assume that $\{Y_t^P(\mathbf{s})\}$ follows a stochastic IDE model, such as (7.52):

$$Y_t^P(\mathbf{s}) = \int_{D_s} m(\mathbf{s}, \mathbf{x}) Y_{t-1}^P(\mathbf{x}) \, dx + \xi_t(\mathbf{s}), \tag{7.55}$$

where $m(\mathbf{s}, \mathbf{x})$ is a transition kernel that maps the process $Y_{t-1}^P(\cdot)$ at the previous time, over the domain D_s, to the process at the current time at location $\mathbf{s}$. For notational simplicity, we do not show the parameters used to specify $m(\cdot, \cdot)$.

Now, assume that the dynamical process can be expanded in terms of p_α basis functions $\{\phi_i(\mathbf{s}): i = 1, \ldots, p_\alpha\}$:

$$Y_t^P(\mathbf{s}) = \sum_{i=1}^{p_\alpha} \alpha_t(i)\phi_i(\mathbf{s}). \tag{7.56}$$

In addition, expand the transition kernel in terms of the basis set $\{\psi_j(\mathbf{x}): j = 1, \ldots, n_J\}$:

$$m(\mathbf{s}, \mathbf{x}) = \sum_{j=1}^{n_J} b_j(\mathbf{s})\psi_j(\mathbf{x}), \tag{7.57}$$

where the basis functions $\phi_i(\cdot)$ and $\psi_i(\cdot)$ are often the same. Substituting (7.56) and (7.57) into (7.55) and assuming that the basis functions are biorthonormal (for simplicity), namely

$$\int_{D_s} \phi_i(\mathbf{x})\psi_j(\mathbf{x})\, dx = \begin{cases} 1, & i = j, \\ 0, & i \neq j, \end{cases} \tag{7.58}$$

we obtain

$$Y_t^P(\mathbf{s}) = \sum_{i=1}^{p_\alpha} b_i(\mathbf{s})\alpha_t(i) + \xi_t(\mathbf{s})$$

$$= \mathbf{b}(\mathbf{s})'\boldsymbol{\alpha}_t + \xi_t(\mathbf{s}), \tag{7.59}$$

where $p_\alpha \leq n_J$, $\mathbf{b}(\mathbf{s}) \equiv (b_1(\mathbf{s}), \ldots, b_{p_\alpha}(\mathbf{s}))'$ and $\boldsymbol{\alpha}_t \equiv (\alpha_t(1), \ldots, \alpha_t(p_\alpha))'$. Note that $\mathbf{Y}_t^P = \boldsymbol{\Phi}\boldsymbol{\alpha}_t$, where the $n \times p_\alpha$ basis function matrix is

$$\boldsymbol{\Phi} \equiv \begin{pmatrix} \phi(\mathbf{s}_1)' \\ \vdots \\ \phi(\mathbf{s}_n)' \end{pmatrix},$$

and $\phi(\mathbf{s}_i) \equiv (\phi_1(\mathbf{s}_i), \ldots, \phi_{p_\alpha}(\mathbf{s}_i))'$; $i = 1, \ldots, n$. In addition, define the $n \times p_\alpha$ matrix

$$\mathbf{B} \equiv \begin{pmatrix} \mathbf{b}(\mathbf{s}_1)' \\ \vdots \\ \mathbf{b}(\mathbf{s}_n)' \end{pmatrix}$$

and the n-dimensional vector, $\boldsymbol{\xi}_t \equiv (\xi_t(\mathbf{s}_1), \ldots, \xi_t(\mathbf{s}_n))'$. Then, after combining all n process locations, we can write

$$\boldsymbol{\alpha}_t = (\boldsymbol{\Phi}'\boldsymbol{\Phi})^{-1}\boldsymbol{\Phi}'\mathbf{B}\boldsymbol{\alpha}_{t-1} + (\boldsymbol{\Phi}'\boldsymbol{\Phi})^{-1}\boldsymbol{\Phi}'\boldsymbol{\xi}_t \tag{7.60}$$

$$\equiv \mathbf{M}_\alpha \boldsymbol{\alpha}_{t-1} + \boldsymbol{\eta}_t, \tag{7.61}$$

where the p_α-dimensional error vector is given by $\boldsymbol{\eta}_t \equiv (\boldsymbol{\Phi}'\boldsymbol{\Phi})^{-1}\boldsymbol{\Phi}'\boldsymbol{\xi}_t$, and the $p_\alpha \times p_\alpha$ propagator matrix is given by $\mathbf{M}_\alpha \equiv (\boldsymbol{\Phi}'\boldsymbol{\Phi})^{-1}\boldsymbol{\Phi}'\mathbf{B}$. Finally, we note the obvious simplification in $\mathbf{M}_\alpha$ and $\boldsymbol{\eta}_t$ if the basis functions $\boldsymbol{\Phi}$ are orthogonal (i.e., $\boldsymbol{\Phi}'\boldsymbol{\Phi} = \mathbf{I}$), in which case $\mathbf{M}_\alpha = \boldsymbol{\Phi}'\mathbf{B}$ and $\boldsymbol{\eta}_t = \boldsymbol{\Phi}'\boldsymbol{\xi}_t$.

Clearly, the spectral truncation (7.56) leads to a reduced-dimension dynamical process (choose $p_\alpha << n$). One would still have to estimate the $n \times p_\alpha$ kernel-transition matrix $\mathbf{B}$ and the $p_\alpha \times p_\alpha$ covariance matrix associated with $\boldsymbol{\eta}_t$, in order to proceed. One distinct advantage of the IDE formulation is that the kernel, $m(\mathbf{s}, \mathbf{x})$, can be parameterized explicitly in terms of just a few critical parameters, namely, $m(\mathbf{s}, \mathbf{x}; \boldsymbol{\theta})$. For example, as discussed in Section 7.2.5, $\boldsymbol{\theta}$ might control the width (diffusion) and skewness (advection) of the kernel. In this case, one might even be able to select appropriate basis functions $\{\psi_j(\mathbf{s}) : j = 1, \ldots, J\}$, so that the expansion coefficients for the kernel are also given (analytically) in terms of the parameters $\boldsymbol{\theta}$. An example is the Fourier basis set, where the Fourier transform of the kernel gives the characteristic function (i.e., Wikle, 2002a; Xu, Wikle, and Fox, 2005). The advantage of this approach is seen when the parameters are allowed to vary with spatial location (i.e., $\boldsymbol{\theta}(\mathbf{s})$ replaces $\boldsymbol{\theta}$), and these spatially varying parameters are then modeled as random fields at the next level of the hierarchy. In this case, the matrix $\mathbf{B}(\boldsymbol{\theta}_s)$ is given in terms of the parameter vector $\boldsymbol{\theta}(\mathbf{s})$, and thus $\mathbf{M}_\alpha$ is completely determined by $\boldsymbol{\theta}(\mathbf{s})$ (since the basis functions $\boldsymbol{\Phi}$ are assumed to be known).

In the PDE and IDE examples presented above, the obvious choices for basis functions were Fourier modes. This is not always the case, as discussed above in Section 7.1. Thus, one has to put considerable care into the choice of basis functions, whether they be Fourier, wavelet, EOF, bisquare, spline, smoothing kernel, and so on. Furthermore, one must decide if the expansion should be truncated (implying dimension reduction of the state process), or whether the parameter space is sufficiently reduced by a complete expansion. One must also be concerned with boundary (edge) effects, as well as implementation on nonregular grids.

At this point, it is instructive to discuss the relationship between the IDE framework and the smoothing-kernel framework presented in Section 7.1.3. The smoothing-kernel formulation given in (7.34) is similar to the IDE formulation given in (7.52), but clearly the main difference is that in (7.34) interest is in smoothing a latent process (i.e., $\{\alpha_t(\cdot)\}$) that is distinct from the process of interest (i.e., $\{Y_t(\cdot)\}$). In contrast, the IDE kernel operates on past values of the Y-process. This distinction is also evident in the discretized version of both formulations given in (7.35) and (7.53). However, the differences blur when we consider the spectral formulation of the IDE model. In this case, the IDE-based HM includes a process model such as given by (7.24), which is similar to the vector form of the kernel smoothing data model given in (7.36). The distinction is then that this spectral matrix $\boldsymbol{\Phi}$ is parameterized in terms of the kernel parameters in (7.36), but in the IDE context this matrix is assumed *known* (e.g., Fourier basis vectors). More critically, the IDE model then allows the kernels to play a role in the dynamical propagator on the process model for $\{\boldsymbol{\alpha}_t\}$, whereas the kernel-smoothing approach typically assumes a simple structure on the dynamics of $\{\boldsymbol{\alpha}_t\}$ (to satisfy identifiability concerns). Thus, the IDE framework is designed to give the modeler much more flexibility in modeling the *dynamics* of the process, while the kernel-smoothing framework places the modeling emphasis on representing the spatial structure of the process at various times, with much less regard for the underlying dynamics. As we have emphasized repeatedly in this book, we believe that, when possible, the modeling emphasis should be placed on the dynamics, since it is closer to the etiology of the real-world spatio-temporal phenomenon being modeled. That being said, there are situations where one simply does not know much about the underlying process dynamics, and it can be useful to take a kernel-smoothing approach.

7.2.7 Multiresolution DSTMs

In many respects, the spectral-basis-function expansion suggested in Section 7.2.6 does, in fact, lead to a multiresolution DSTM. This is because many basis-function expansions (e.g., EOF, Fourier, wavelet, bisquare) are inherently "multiresolutional" in the sense that the basis functions vary by spatial scale. Alternatively, one can consider a tree-structured approach to capture the multiresolution behavior explicitly.

One approach to modeling tree-structured multiresolution DSTMs was given by Johannesson, Cressie, and Huang (2007), in which they extend a multiresolution spatial model (e.g., Chou, Willsky, and Nikoukhah, 1994; Huang and Cressie, 2001; Huang, Cressie, and Gabrosek, 2002) to the dynamic spatio-temporal setting by allowing temporal dynamics on the coarsest scale. Since all scales are linked, the marginal-dependence structure of the process includes dynamics. To illustrate this in more detail, recall from Section 4.1.6 that levels of resolution are defined by partitioning the spatial domain, say D_s, into subdomains at the rth resolution:

$$\{D(i,r): \ i = 1, \ldots, n_r\},$$

where $r = 0, \ldots, R$ are the spatial resolutions of D_s (with $r = 0$ the coarsest resolution), and n_r corresponds to the number of cells at the rth level of resolution. We require $\{D(i,r)\}$ to be disjoint, $D_s = \bigcup_i D(i,r)$, and $D(i,r) = \bigcup_{j=1}^{m_r} D(ch_j(i,r))$, where $ch_j(i,r)$ is the index for the jth child node (cell) of the cell at (i,r); $j = 1, \ldots, m_r$.

Now, consider the spatio-temporal process,

$$\{Y_t(\mathbf{s}): \ \mathbf{s} \in D_s, t = 1, 2, \ldots\},$$

and define the *aggregated* spatio-temporal process as

$$Y_t(i,r) \equiv \frac{1}{|D(i,r)|} \int_{D(i,r)} Y_t(\mathbf{s}) \, d\mathbf{s}.$$

The process model is then defined as follows:

$$\mathbf{Y}_t(ch(i,r)) = \mathbf{1}\, Y_t(i,r) + \boldsymbol{\omega}_t(ch(i,r)),$$

where

$$\mathbf{Y}_t(ch(i,r)) \equiv (Y_t(ch_1(i,r)), \ldots, Y_t(ch_{m_r}(i,r))',$$

$$\boldsymbol{\omega}_t(ch(i,r)) \equiv (\omega_t(ch_1(i,r)), \ldots, \omega_t(ch_{m_r}(i,r)))',$$

and $\boldsymbol{\omega}_t(ch(i,r)) \sim ind.\,Gau(\mathbf{0}, \sigma^2 \mathbf{W}(ch(i,r)))$. Critically, the temporal dynamics are induced through a dynamical linear model on the coarsest scale:

$$\mathbf{Y}_t(0) = \mathbf{M}_t \mathbf{Y}_{t-1}(0) + \boldsymbol{\eta}_t,$$

where $\mathbf{Y}_t(0) \equiv (Y_t(1,0), \ldots, Y_t(n_0, 0))'$, $\{\mathbf{M}_t\}$ are the propagator matrices, and $\boldsymbol{\eta}_t \sim ind.\,Gau(\mathbf{0}, \sigma^2 \mathbf{Q}_t)$.

The implementation of this model (given a suitable data model) makes use of the *change-of-resolution Kalman filter* (see Chou, Willsky, and Nikoukhah, 1994; Fieguth et al., 1995; Huang and Cressie, 2001). An advantage of this approach, beyond computational efficiency, is that one can capture spatial nonstationarity through the covariance matrices, $\{\mathbf{W}(ch(i,r))\}$, although these must be specified, estimated, or given a prior distribution, depending on the implementation at hand. In addition, the propagator and covariance matrices associated with the coarse-resolution dynamics must be specified or estimated. In principle, any of the parameterization approaches for the dynamics described above could be considered here as well. It should be noted that, typically, one wants to constrain the propagator matrices in multiresolution models to satisfy conditions of *nonnegativity*, *mass balance*, and *constant mean* (e.g., Gelpke and Künsch, 2001). Finally, extending the dynamical model to finer scales and interactions between them, results in a breakdown of computational efficiency, although the model may be more appropriate for the phenomenon under study.

7.3 PROCESS MODELS FOR THE DSTM: NONLINEAR MODELS

Linear dynamics, as discussed in Section 7.2, can be quite useful in applications. However, many processes in nature are governed by nonlinear spatio-temporal interactions. For example, in ecological population dynamics, processes are encountered that show state-dependent (i.e., "density-dependent") growth as given, for example, by

$$\frac{\partial Y}{\partial t} = Y g(Y; \boldsymbol{\theta}),$$

for some nonlinear growth function g and where it is understood that Y is a function of $\mathbf{s} \in D_s$ and $t \in D_t$. Similarly, in geophysics one encounters processes that exhibit what is often referred to as *nonlinear advection*. For example, in the one-dimensional spatial setting,

$$\frac{\partial Y}{\partial t} = Y \frac{\partial Y}{\partial x},$$

where again it is understood that Y is a function of $x \in D_s$ and $t \in D_t$. Nonlinear advection comes from fluid dynamics, where Y might be one of the velocity components that make up the flow. Thus, there is a nonlinear interaction between the velocity component and how that component of the flow is advected downstream. In the case of spatio-temporal hierarchical statistical modeling, we must have process models that can accommodate these types of processes, as well as many others. Just like with linear dynamical models, the key is that the nonlinear behavior in spatio-temporal processes generally comes from *interactions* across a variety of spatio-temporal scales of variability and even across multiple processes. Hence, nonlinear DSTMs should reflect this.

As we have noted, the issues of dimensionality and efficient parameterization present the most significant challenges for statistical modeling of linear DSTMs. Perhaps not surprisingly, these issues are even more critical for nonlinearly evolving spatio-temporal dynamical processes. Indeed, we live in a nonlinear world, and sooner or later the nonlinearity has to be modeled in order to capture the essence of the true dynamics. In addition, for forecasting, we know from chaos theory that seemingly insignificant events can make a huge difference in the time evolution of a process (see Section 3.2.4). That is, uncertainties in initial and boundary conditions can affect dramatically our ability to predict such processes. For these reasons, from a parametric perspective, the modeler must have an even stronger sense of the basic nonlinear dynamical form in order to perform scientific inference and/or prediction.

Currently, the Statistics literature that considers nonlinear spatio-temporal processes is somewhat sparse. However, by borrowing information from nonlinear statistical time series analysis and other disciplines (e.g., atmospheric science, ecology, etc.) we can begin to formulate classes of nonlinear DSTMs. We note the distinction between nonlinearity in the state variables and in the parameters. In hierarchical nonlinear DSTMs, both parameter and process nonlinearities are possible. It is often the case in spatio-temporal dynamics that one is interested in predicting (or forecasting) at a finite set of points in space. Thus, we focus our discussion on the vector-valued process, $\{\mathbf{Y}_t : t = 1, 2, \ldots\}$, as defined previously. This discussion follows closely that in Wikle and Hooten (2010).

A general class of nonlinear dynamical models is the *nonlinear autoregressive model*:

$$\mathbf{Y}_t = \mathcal{M}(\mathbf{Y}_{t-1}, \boldsymbol{\eta}_t; \boldsymbol{\theta}_t); \quad t = 1, 2, \ldots, \tag{7.62}$$

where $\mathcal{M}$ is a nonlinear function operating on elements of the processes $\{\mathbf{Y}_t\}$ and $\{\boldsymbol{\eta}_t\}$, and $\{\boldsymbol{\theta}_t\}$ are parameters that control the process' evolution. Although this model is conceptually quite simple, without a specified form for the operator $\mathcal{M}$, (7.62) is not particularly useful for statistical modeling, other than to indicate that there is first-order Markov dependence. We should mention that higher-order temporal lag terms in the process could be considered as well, but for simplicity we focus here on first-order lag dependence. (The curse of dimensionality can make the higher-order case much more difficult to implement in practice.) In the remainder of this section, we consider several specific formulations of (7.62); however, these are not an exhaustive set of possible models that could be considered.

7.3.1 Local Linear Approximations

A long-standing approach for modeling nonlinear systems is simply to linearize the process. That is, the nonlinear evolution operator is approximated by a locally linear function. Specifically, we can expand the process in a Taylor series about some value of the state process. This value is typically an estimate of the current state or its mean. For example, consider the nonlinear first-order AR model:

$$\mathbf{Y}_t = \mathcal{M}(\mathbf{Y}_{t-1}) + \boldsymbol{\eta}_t, \tag{7.63}$$

where $\mathcal{M}(\cdot)$ is some known nonlinear function, $\mathcal{M}(\cdot) \equiv (m_1(\cdot), \ldots, m_n(\cdot))'$, with $m_i(\cdot)$ a scalar-valued nonlinear function. Now, let $\hat{\mathbf{Y}}_{t-1}$ be an estimate of the mean of $\mathbf{Y}_{t-1}$, and consider the Taylor series expansion:

$$\mathcal{M}(\mathbf{Y}_t) = \mathcal{M}(\hat{\mathbf{Y}}_{t-1}) + \mathbf{M}_t \cdot (\mathbf{Y}_{t-1} - \hat{\mathbf{Y}}_{t-1}) + \ldots, \tag{7.64}$$

where we use the $\cdot$ notation in this section to emphasize the product operator and avoid ambiguity with the functional argument. The ellipses in (7.64) refer to higher-order terms in $(\mathbf{Y}_{t-1} - \hat{\mathbf{Y}}_{t-1})$, and $\mathbf{M}_t$ is an $n \times n$ matrix of first partial derivatives of $\mathcal{M}(\cdot)$, evaluated at $\mathbf{Y}_{t-1} = \hat{\mathbf{Y}}_{t-1}$. That is, the (i, j)th element of $\mathbf{M}_t$ is

$$(\mathbf{M}_t)_{i,j} = \left. \frac{\partial m_i(\mathbf{Y}_t)}{\partial Y_t(\mathbf{s}_j)} \right|_{\mathbf{Y}_t = \hat{\mathbf{Y}}_{t-1}}. \tag{7.65}$$

Thus, for $\mathbf{M}_t$ to be defined, we require that $m_i(\cdot)$ be at least once-differentiable with respect to its vector argument, $\mathbf{Y}_{t-1}$, for each $i = 1, \ldots n$. Typically, we assume that the higher-order terms are negligible or can be absorbed into $\boldsymbol{\eta}_t$ (however, see Section 7.3.3 for the quadratic case), and thus

$$\mathbf{Y}_t = \mathbf{c}_t + \mathbf{M}_t \mathbf{Y}_{t-1} + \boldsymbol{\eta}_t, \tag{7.66}$$

where

$$\mathbf{c}_t \equiv \mathcal{M}(\hat{\mathbf{Y}}_{t-1}) - \mathbf{M}_t \hat{\mathbf{Y}}_{t-1}. \tag{7.67}$$

This setting is analogous to the linear DSTM and, thus one can use similar estimation and inference approaches for the process $\{\mathbf{Y}_t\}$. Note also that we might wish to expand the Taylor series around some quantity other than $\hat{\mathbf{Y}}_{t-1}$. For example, we might use a forecasted value (from this model, or from a deterministic model), historical values (e.g., climatology), $E(\mathbf{Y}_{t-1})$, or some other state vector. Such methods have a long history in the Kalman-filtering literature and are known as *extended Kalman filters* (e.g., see Grewal and Andrews, 1993). Note that we have assumed that we know the functional form, $\mathcal{M}(\cdot)$. However, in spatio-temporal statistical problems it is often the case that we do not know the form of this operator, or it would be too complicated to work with directly (e.g., numerical weather-forecasting models). In this case, $\mathbf{c}_t$ and $\mathbf{M}_t$ would have to be estimated, and the same difficulties described for linear DSTMs would apply, with the additional complication of the time-varying, state-dependent nature of these quantities.

7.3.2　State-Dependent Processes

One way to simplify the general nonlinear first-order AR process model (7.62) is by considering the *nonlinear state-dependent model*:

$$\mathbf{Y}_t = \mathbf{M}(\mathbf{Y}_{t-1}; \boldsymbol{\theta}_t^M) \cdot \mathbf{Y}_{t-1} + \boldsymbol{\eta}_t, \tag{7.68}$$

where the propagator matrix $\mathbf{M}(\cdot; \cdot)$ depends on the state process at the previous time, in addition to (possibly) time-varying parameters $\{\boldsymbol{\theta}_t^M\}$. This model is certainly not new in the time-series literature [e.g., see Section 3.4.8 and overviews in Priestley (1988), Tong (1990), and Fan and Yao (2005)], but it is somewhat less common in the spatio-temporal statistics literature.

Such state-dependent models are powerful and include many nonlinear models as special cases. For example, one might consider exponential autoregressive models, bilinear models, and threshold autoregressive models from this perspective (e.g., Tong, 1990). As an example, consider the threshold AR model:

$$\mathbf{Y}_t = \mathbf{M}_t(\mathbf{Y}_{t-1}) \cdot \mathbf{Y}_{t-1} + \boldsymbol{\eta}_t \equiv \begin{cases} \mathbf{M}_1 \mathbf{Y}_{t-1} + \boldsymbol{\eta}_{1,t}, & \text{if } f_1(\gamma_t) \in c_1 \\ \vdots & \vdots \\ \mathbf{M}_K \mathbf{Y}_{t-1} + \boldsymbol{\eta}_{K,t}, & \text{if } f_K(\gamma_t) \in c_K, \end{cases} \tag{7.69}$$

where $f_k(\gamma_t)$ is a function of a time-varying parameter γ_t, and $f_k(\gamma_t) \in c_k$; $k = 1, \ldots K$, is the condition under which the kth equation is to be followed. Although written as a scalar here, this process $\{\gamma_t\}$ could be multivariate, and it might depend on the state process $\mathbf{Y}_{t-1}$ or other processes and parameters. In summary, through dependence on the value of the (typically hidden) process γ_t, the model uses a different linear evolution operator and, potentially, a different error process. This is related to the state-dependent model (7.68) in the situation where γ_t is a function of $\mathbf{Y}_{t-1}$. An example of such a model is given by Berliner, Wikle, and Cressie (2000), with regard to long-lead forecasting of tropical Pacific sea surface temperature; see Chapter 5 and Section 8.1.

As is often the case in spatio-temporal problems, the state dimension n can be quite large, leading to difficulties in parsimonious parameter specifications [e.g., the matrices $\{\mathbf{M}_k\}$ in (7.69)]. Furthermore, there are often specific types of process behavior, known *a priori*, that one wishes to include in the process model (e.g., advection, diffusion, repulsion, density-dependent growth, etc.). In this case, parameterizing the state-dependent transition matrices, so that they are consistent with these processes (as with the PDE and IDE examples shown previously for the linear case), leads to more efficient inferences. As is always the case in the hierarchical context, these parameterizations can often be simplified by modeling complicated dependence at lower levels of the HM hierarchy.

We thus specify the following, rather general, nonlinear DSTM:

$$\mathbf{Y}_t = \mathbf{M}(\mathbf{Y}_{t-1}; \boldsymbol{\theta}_t^M) \cdot \mathbf{Y}_{t-1} + \mathbf{F}(\mathbf{Y}_{t-1}; \boldsymbol{\theta}_t^F) \cdot \boldsymbol{\eta}_t, \tag{7.70}$$

where $\mathbf{M}(\mathbf{Y}_{t-1}; \boldsymbol{\theta}_t^M)$ is an evolution matrix depending on the state $\mathbf{Y}_{t-1}$ and some (possibly time-varying) parameters $\boldsymbol{\theta}_t^M$, and the "noise forcing matrix" $\mathbf{F}(\mathbf{Y}_{t-1}; \boldsymbol{\theta}_t^F)$ likewise may depend on the state process and some forcing parameters $\boldsymbol{\theta}_t^F$. Here, $\{\boldsymbol{\theta}_t^M\}$ and $\{\boldsymbol{\theta}_t^F\}$ are components of the process-model parameters, $\boldsymbol{\theta}_P$. Our focus here is on parameterization of $\mathbf{M}(\cdot; \cdot)$. We write

$$\mathbf{M}(\mathbf{Y}_{t-1}; \boldsymbol{\theta}_t^M) = \mathbf{A}(\boldsymbol{\theta}_t^A) + \mathbf{B}(\boldsymbol{\theta}_t^B) \cdot \mathbf{G}(\mathbf{Y}_{t-1}; \boldsymbol{\theta}_t^G) \cdot \mathbf{C}(\boldsymbol{\theta}_t^C), \tag{7.71}$$

where $\boldsymbol{\theta}_t^M \equiv \{\boldsymbol{\theta}_t^A, \boldsymbol{\theta}_t^B, \boldsymbol{\theta}_t^C, \boldsymbol{\theta}_t^G\}$. The form of this matrix is quite general and can model realistically the behavior of many nonlinear dynamical processes (Wikle and Hooten, 2010). Examples of special cases include:

- $\mathbf{M}(\mathbf{Y}_{t-1}; \boldsymbol{\theta}_t^M) = \mathbf{A}(\boldsymbol{\theta}^A)$: In this case, the model is simply the basic first-order linear DSTM. An example is a system of linear difference equations, or a linear advection-diffusion PDE discretized by finite differences. In the latter case, $\mathbf{A}$ is quite sparse as shown in Section 7.2.4 (with a diagonal band corresponding to the discretization "stencil"; e.g., there are five nonzero diagonals for the typical two-dimensional finite-difference case).

- $\mathbf{M}(\mathbf{Y}_{t-1}; \boldsymbol{\theta}_t^M) = \mathbf{B}(\boldsymbol{\theta}^B) \cdot \mathbf{G}(\mathbf{Y}_{t-1}; \boldsymbol{\theta}^G)$: In this case, the model reduces to the spatio-temporal "matrix model" (Caswell, 2001; Hooten et al., 2007; and Section 9.3) or the discretized nonlinear IDE model. Here, $\mathbf{G}$ accounts for growth, and $\mathbf{B}$ accounts for diffusion or spread. Typically, $\mathbf{B}$ is parameterized in terms of a kernel function (e.g., Hooten et al., 2007), and the functional form of the the growth process that defines $\mathbf{G}$ is known and typically nonlinear.

- $\mathbf{M}(\mathbf{Y}_{t-1}; \boldsymbol{\theta}_t^M) = \mathbf{A}(\boldsymbol{\theta}^A) + \mathbf{G}(\mathbf{Y}_{t-1}; \boldsymbol{\theta}^G)$: In this case, the model accommodates discretized linear PDE dynamics with a nonlinear growth term; typically, $\mathbf{G}(\mathbf{Y}_{t-1}; \boldsymbol{\theta}^G)$ is diagonal.

- $\mathbf{M}(\mathbf{Y}_{t-1}; \boldsymbol{\theta}_t^M) = \mathbf{A}(\boldsymbol{\theta}^A) + \mathbf{G}(\mathbf{Y}_{t-1}; \boldsymbol{\theta}^G) \cdot \mathbf{C}(\boldsymbol{\theta}^C)$: In this case, the model accomodates a discretized PDE with nonlinear advection.

7.3.3 General Quadratic Nonlinearity (GQN)

We focus on a special case of (7.70) and (7.71), characterized by what Wikle and Hooten (2010) refer to as *general quadratic nonlinearity* (GQN):

$$Y_t(\mathbf{s}_i) = \sum_{j=1}^n a_{ij} Y_{t-1}(\mathbf{s}_j) + \sum_{k=1}^n \sum_{l=1}^n b_{i,kl} Y_{t-1}(\mathbf{s}_k) g(Y_{t-1}(\mathbf{s}_l); \boldsymbol{\theta}^G) + \eta_t(\mathbf{s}_i),$$

$$(7.72)$$

for $i = 1, \ldots, n$, where there are linear terms and quadratic interactions. We note that, although (7.72) is not written that way, the coefficients could also depend on t. The first term on the right-hand side of (7.72) contains a linear combination of process values at the previous time, and the second term on the right-hand side includes interactions between different locations of the process at the previous time. The term "general" is due to the function $g(Y_{t-1}(s_l); \boldsymbol{\theta}^G)$, which is included in the quadratic interaction. There are $O(n^3)$ parameters in this model, which could be quite large for the typical number of process locations n that one might see in applications.

There are several different ways this model could be written in matrix notation. We consider two forms that will be useful below. First, define the $n \times n$ matrix,

$$\mathbf{B}_i \equiv (b_{i,kl}), \tag{7.73}$$

where $b_{i,kl}$ is defined in (7.72) and is put in the (k, l)th entry of the matrix, $\mathbf{B}_i$, for $i = 1, \ldots, n$. Then,

$$\mathbf{Y}_t = \mathbf{A}\mathbf{Y}_{t-1} + (\mathbf{I}_n \otimes \mathcal{G}(\mathbf{Y}_{t-1}; \boldsymbol{\theta}^G)')\mathbf{B}\mathbf{Y}_{t-1} + \boldsymbol{\eta}_t, \tag{7.74}$$

where $\otimes$ denotes the Kronecker product, $\mathcal{G}(\mathbf{Y}_{t-1}; \boldsymbol{\theta}^G) \equiv (g(Y_{t-1}(\mathbf{s}_1); \boldsymbol{\theta}^G), \ldots, g(Y_{t-1}(\mathbf{s}_n); \boldsymbol{\theta}^G))'$, and the $n^2 \times n$ matrix $\mathbf{B}$ is given by

$$\mathbf{B} \equiv \begin{pmatrix} \mathbf{B}_1 \\ \mathbf{B}_2 \\ \vdots \\ \mathbf{B}_n \end{pmatrix}. \tag{7.75}$$

In the context of the general state-dependent model presented in (7.68), we have

$$\mathbf{M}(\mathbf{Y}_{t-1}; \boldsymbol{\theta}^M) = \mathbf{A} + (\mathbf{I}_n \otimes \mathcal{G}(\mathbf{Y}_{t-1}; \boldsymbol{\theta}^G)')\mathbf{B}, \tag{7.76}$$

where the parameters are $\boldsymbol{\theta}^M \equiv \{\mathbf{A}, \mathbf{B}, \boldsymbol{\theta}^G\}$. Although it is possible to allow these parameters to vary with time, we suppress that notation here for simplicity.

Alternatively, we can also write the model as

$$\mathbf{Y}_t = \mathbf{A}\mathbf{Y}_{t-1} + \mathbf{B}_v \cdot (\mathbf{Y}_{t-1} \otimes \mathcal{G}(\mathbf{Y}_{t-1}; \boldsymbol{\theta}^G)) + \boldsymbol{\eta}_t, \qquad (7.77)$$

where the $n \times n^2$ matrix $\mathbf{B}_v$ is given by

$$\mathbf{B}_v = \begin{pmatrix} \text{vec}(\mathbf{B}_1)' \\ \text{vec}(\mathbf{B}_2)' \\ \vdots \\ \text{vec}(\mathbf{B}_n)' \end{pmatrix}, \qquad (7.78)$$

and the $n^2 \times 1$ vector $\mathbf{Y}_{t-1} \otimes \mathcal{G}(\mathbf{Y}_{t-1}; \boldsymbol{\theta}^G)$ is given by

$$(\mathbf{Y}_{t-1} \otimes \mathcal{G}(\mathbf{Y}_{t-1}; \boldsymbol{\theta}^G))' = (Y_{t-1}(\mathbf{s}_1)g(Y_{t-1}(\mathbf{s}_1); \boldsymbol{\theta}^G), \dots,$$
$$Y_{t-1}(\mathbf{s}_1)g(Y_{t-1}(\mathbf{s}_n); \boldsymbol{\theta}^G), Y_{t-1}(\mathbf{s}_2)g(Y_{t-1}(\mathbf{s}_1); \boldsymbol{\theta}^G), \dots,$$
$$Y_{t-1}(\mathbf{s}_n)g(Y_{t-1}(\mathbf{s}_n); \boldsymbol{\theta}^G)),$$

which contains all of the pair-wise interaction terms. We refer to these as *dyadic* interactions.

It is not surprising that for many spatio-temporal processes, $\mathbf{A}$ and $\mathbf{B}$ have too many parameters to permit reliable estimation; however, these matrices could be parameterized in terms of $\boldsymbol{\theta}^A$ and $\boldsymbol{\theta}^B$, namely $\mathbf{A}(\boldsymbol{\theta}^A)$ and $\mathbf{B}(\boldsymbol{\theta}^B)$, respectively. In the case of the linear portion of the propagator, $\mathbf{A}(\boldsymbol{\theta}^A)$, the types of parameterizations discussed previously are still relevant. What about $\mathbf{B}(\boldsymbol{\theta}^B)$? First, note that if $\mathcal{G}(\mathbf{Y}_{t-1}; \boldsymbol{\theta}^G) = \mathbf{Y}_{t-1}$, then we have only $n(n+1)/2$ unique dyadic interactions. Although this greatly simplifies the model, it may limit the appropriateness of the parameterization. We consider some special cases and motivating models in the examples below.

Example: Second-Order Taylor Expansion

If the form of the nonlinearity is known (i.e., the propagator is known), then a common approach to approximating the nonlinearity is to construct a local-linear approximation as discussed in Section 7.3.1. To improve accuracy, the associated Taylor expansion can be extended to second-order terms (e.g., Jazwinski, 1970; West and Harrison, 1997). Such an expansion is a special case of the GQN model presented here.

Recall the deterministic vector-valued nonlinear function:

$$\mathbf{Y}_t = \mathcal{M}(\mathbf{Y}_{t-1}), \qquad (7.79)$$

where $\mathcal{M}(\mathbf{Y}_{t-1}) \equiv (m_1(\mathbf{Y}_{t-1}), \ldots, m_n(\mathbf{Y}_{t-1}))'$, with $\{m_i\}$ being scalar-valued (nonlinear) functions. A second-order Taylor expansion about some specified vector $\hat{\mathbf{Y}}_t$ can then be written:

$$\mathcal{M}(\mathbf{Y}_t) = \mathcal{M}(\hat{\mathbf{Y}}_t) + \mathbf{M}_t \cdot (\mathbf{Y}_t - \hat{\mathbf{Y}}_t)$$

$$+ \frac{1}{2}(\mathbf{I}_n \otimes (\mathbf{Y}_t - \hat{\mathbf{Y}}_t)') \cdot \mathbf{H}_t \cdot (\mathbf{Y}_t - \hat{\mathbf{Y}}_t) + \ldots, \qquad (7.80)$$

where recall that we use the $\cdot$ notation to emphasize the product operator; $\mathbf{M}_t$ is the matrix of first partial derivatives of $\mathcal{M}(\mathbf{Y}_t)$ evaluated at a given $\mathbf{Y}_t = \hat{\mathbf{Y}}_t$, as given in equation (7.65) in Section 7.3.1; and

$$\mathbf{H}_t \equiv \mathbf{H}_t(\hat{\mathbf{Y}}_t) = \left.\begin{pmatrix} \mathbf{H}_{1t}(\mathbf{Y}_t) \\ \vdots \\ \mathbf{H}_{nt}(\mathbf{Y}_t) \end{pmatrix}\right|_{\mathbf{Y}_t = \hat{\mathbf{Y}}_t}, \qquad (7.81)$$

where $\{\mathbf{H}_{it}(\mathbf{Y}_t) : i = 1, \ldots, n\}$ are the Hessian matrices (i.e., matrices of second-partial derivatives) of $\mathcal{M}(\cdot)$, evaluated at a given $\mathbf{Y}_t = \hat{\mathbf{Y}}_t$. For $i = 1, \ldots, n$, the (k, l)th element of $\mathbf{H}_{it}(\hat{\mathbf{Y}}_t)$ is

$$(\mathbf{H}_{it}(\hat{\mathbf{Y}}_t))_{kl} = \left.\frac{\partial^2 m_i(\mathbf{Y}_t)}{\partial Y_t(\mathbf{s}_k)\partial Y_t(\mathbf{s}_l)}\right|_{\mathbf{Y}_t = \hat{\mathbf{Y}}_t}, \qquad k, l = 1, \ldots, n. \qquad (7.82)$$

This equation fits into the GQN form (with respect to $\mathbf{Y}_t - \hat{\mathbf{Y}}_t$), where $\mathbf{M}_t$ and $\mathbf{H}_t$ correspond to $\mathbf{A}$ and $\mathbf{B}$, respectively. As mentioned previously, such an implementation requires complete knowledge of the nonlinear functions (i.e., $m_i(\mathbf{Y}_t)$), which is not typically available for most spatio-temporal processes that require statistical modeling.

Example: Reaction-Diffusion (Growth) Models

Many processes in population ecology are motivated by a reaction-diffusion equation. For example, invasive species tend to spread (diffuse) and grow proportional to the current abundance, so long as the environmental carrying capacity has not been obtained. Such processes can be modeled by a variety of approaches, depending on whether time and space are continuous or discrete. In the context of continuous space and continuous time, a reaction-diffusion PDE provides a good description of the potential spread of the invasive species. For example, consider the PDE:

$$\frac{\partial Y}{\partial t} = \frac{\partial}{\partial x}\left(\delta(x, y)\frac{\partial Y}{\partial x}\right) + \frac{\partial}{\partial y}\left(\delta(x, y)\frac{\partial Y}{\partial y}\right)$$

$$+ \gamma_0(x, y)Y \exp\left(1 - \frac{Y}{\gamma_1(x, y)}\right), \qquad (7.83)$$

where $\mathbf{s} \equiv (x, y)'$; and the diffusion coefficient δ, growth parameter γ_0, and carrying capacity γ_1 are, in general, spatially varying. The growth (i.e., reaction) process in (7.83) follows a logistic formulation. A simple finite-difference discretization of this PDE suggests the following multivariate difference equation:

$$\mathbf{Y}_t \simeq \mathbf{A}(\boldsymbol{\delta})\mathbf{Y}_{t-1} + \mathbf{B}_v(\mathbf{Y}_{t-1} \otimes \mathcal{G}(\mathbf{Y}_{t-1}; \boldsymbol{\gamma}_0, \boldsymbol{\gamma}_1)), \qquad (7.84)$$

where $\mathbf{A}(\boldsymbol{\delta})$ is a sparse $n \times n$ matrix containing five non-zero diagonals with elements from $\boldsymbol{\delta}$ (representing the diffusion component of the model, as discussed in Section 7.2.4 for the linear DSTM); $\mathbf{B}_v$ is a very sparse matrix in which the submatrices $\mathbf{B}_i$ each contain zeros except for a 1 in the (i, i)th location; and the ith element of $\mathcal{G}(\cdot)$ is $\gamma_0(\mathbf{s}_i) \exp\{1 - Y_{t-1}(\mathbf{s}_i)/\gamma_1(\mathbf{s}_i)\}$.

As an example, Figure 7.7 shows a simulation of this deterministic two-dimensional reaction-diffusion process with logistic growth; see (7.83). The left panels show five snapshots of the simulation assuming a constant diffusion coefficient ($\delta = 4$) across the domain, as well as a constant growth rate ($\gamma_0 = .55$) and constant carrying capacity ($\gamma_1 = 2$). The right panels show an analogous simulation, but with a nonhomogeneous diffusion rate ($\delta = .1$ on the left half of the domain, and $\delta = 4$ on the right half of the domain), a nonhomogeneous growth rate ($\gamma_0 = .2$ on the lower half of the domain, and $\gamma_0 = .55$ on the upper half of the domain), and constant carrying capacity ($\gamma_1 = 2$). In both simulations, the process initially decays in its intensity, as with a diffusion process (see Figure 7.1), then increases in its intensity, and it is starting to reach its carrying capacity by the last time shown (400 time steps). The nonhomogeneous diffusion rate in the right panels clearly suggests much stronger spread to the right than to the left. Similarly, the upper-lower variation in the growth rate gives much greater intensities in the upper portion of the domain than in the lower portion. One could imagine these parameters varying spatially for a real-world invasive species, perhaps according to habitat preference.

In our context, (7.84) could serve as "motivation" for a *statistical* model that would typically have an additive or multiplicative error process and random parameters $\{\boldsymbol{\delta}, \boldsymbol{\gamma}_0, \boldsymbol{\gamma}_1\}$, whose distributions (e.g., spatial random fields) would be given at the next level of the HM. An example of this hierarchical approach applied to the prediction of the spread of the invasive Eurasian Collared Dove is given in Wikle and Hooten (2006) and Hooten and Wikle (2008). Of course, other growth functions could be used in this context (e.g., see Wikle and Hooten, 2010).

Example: Nonlinear Process in Geophysics

Consider the case of a dynamical process motivated by a one-dimensional nonlinear advection equation:

$$\frac{\partial Y}{\partial t} = Y\frac{\partial Y}{\partial x}, \qquad (7.85)$$

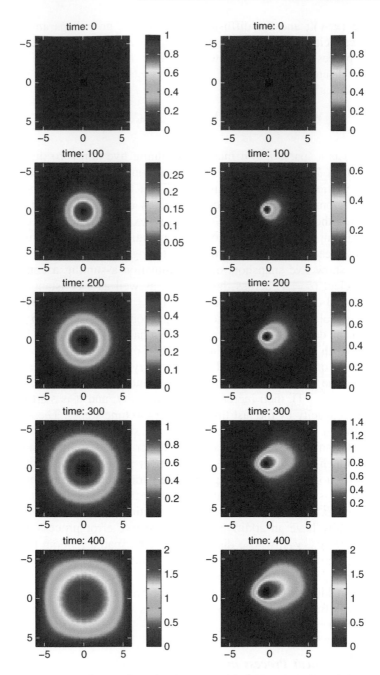

Figure 7.7 Simulation of a two-dimensional reaction-diffusion process with logistic growth as in (7.83). The left panels show the simulated process at five times ($t = 0, 100, 200, 300, 400$) assuming a constant diffusion coefficient ($\delta = 4$) across the domain, as well as a constant growth rate ($\gamma_0 = .55$) and constant carrying capacity ($\gamma_1 = 2$). The right panels show an analogous simulation but with nonhomogeneous diffusion rate ($\delta = .1$ on the left half of the domain, and $\delta = 4$ on the right half of the domain), nonhomogeneous growth rate ($\gamma_0 = .2$ on the lower half of the domain, and $\gamma_0 = .55$ on the upper half of the domain), and constant carrying capacity ($\gamma_1 = 2$).

such as occurs in geophysical fluid dynamics. A basic finite-difference discretization of (7.85) gives

$$Y_t(x) \simeq Y_{t-\Delta_t}(x) + \frac{\Delta_t}{2\Delta_x} Y_{t-\Delta_t}(x) Y_{t-\Delta_t}(x + \Delta_x)$$

$$- \frac{\Delta_t}{2\Delta_x} Y_{t-\Delta_t}(x) Y_{t-\Delta_t}(x - \Delta_x). \tag{7.86}$$

For simplicity of presentation, assume that $\Delta_t = 1$, and also that we have regularly spaced grid points along x given by $x_0, x_1, x_2, \ldots, x_n, x_{n+1}$. Furthermore, let $b \equiv \Delta_t/2\Delta_x$, and assume that boundary values $Y_t(x_0)$ and $Y_t(x_{n+1})$ are zero in this simple example. We can then write (7.86) as the vector equation,

$$\mathbf{Y}_t \simeq \mathbf{A}\mathbf{Y}_{t-1} + (\mathbf{I}_n \otimes \mathbf{Y}'_{t-1})\mathbf{B}\mathbf{Y}_{t-1}, \tag{7.87}$$

where $\mathbf{A} = \mathbf{I}_n$, and $\mathbf{B}$ is given by (7.75). Here, $\mathbf{B}_1$ has b as the (row, column) element $(2, 1)$ and zeros elsewhere; $\{\mathbf{B}_i : i = 2, \ldots, n - 1\}$ are zero matrices with the exception of having b as the element $(i + 1, i)$ and $-b$ as the element $(i - 1, i)$; and $\mathbf{B}_n$ has $-b$ in matrix location $(n, n - 1)$ and zeros elsewhere.

Note that by writing (7.86) as (7.87), we obtain a very sparse matrix $\mathbf{B}$. Thus, the vector form of (7.86) can be written more directly as

$$\mathbf{Y}_t \simeq (\mathbf{I} + \text{diag}(\mathbf{Y}_{t-1})\widetilde{\mathbf{B}})\mathbf{Y}_{t-1}, \tag{7.88}$$

where $\widetilde{\mathbf{B}}$ is a matrix of zeros except for b down the first diagonal above the main diagonal and $-b$ down the first diagonal below the main diagonal.

Of course, using this as motivation for a statistical model, an additive error term in (7.88) would be included, and the parameters would be modeled at a lower level of the HM (BHM) or would be estimated directly (EHM). Obviously, more complicated models for geophysical processes could be considered. For example, a very complex process model for so-called *quasi-geostrophic* flow in the ocean (see Section 7.4) is given in Berliner, Milliff, and Wikle (2003), and this is shown by Wikle and Hooten (2010) to fit into the GQN framework.

Example: Reduced-Dimension State Process
Certainly, there are many situations where the underlying dynamics of a process are not known well enough to motivate it by specific deterministic forms. Or,

it may be that the underlying dynamics are known to some degree, but they are just too complicated to be used as the foundation for a process model in an HM. In addition, it may be the case that in a spectral setting we have no clear prior scientific understanding of how best to truncate the expansion. In such cases, one might consider dimension reduction of the state process itself. Recall the dimension reduced form given in (7.24), where $\boldsymbol{\alpha}_t$ is p_α-dimensional and $p_\alpha << n$. In this case, (7.72) for $\{\boldsymbol{\alpha}_t\}$ yields

$$\alpha_t(i) = \sum_{j=1}^{p_\alpha} a_{ij}\alpha_{t-1}(j) + \sum_{k=1}^{p_\alpha}\sum_{l=1}^{p_\alpha} b_{i,kl}\alpha_{t-1}(k)g(\alpha_{t-1}(l); \boldsymbol{\theta}_g) + \eta_t(i), \quad (7.89)$$

for $i = 1, \ldots, p_\alpha$. Recall that there are $O(p_\alpha^3)$ parameters in this formulation. If p_α is very small, we can proceed by estimating all of the parameters directly. However, in most cases, p_α is not small enough for the amount of data available. Thus, we have to make additional simplifying assumptions and/or perform model selection to choose particular interactions that are important [e.g., see de Luna and Genton (2005) for an example in the linear case and Wikle and Holan (2011) for a GQN example]. Another alternative is to simplify using a dimension-reduction technique called *scale analysis*, where the consequence of recognizing an additional scale is analyzed.

First, assume it is reasonable to decompose the process as

$$\mathbf{Y}_t = \boldsymbol{\Phi}^{(1)}\boldsymbol{\alpha}_t^{(1)} + \boldsymbol{\Phi}^{(2)}\boldsymbol{\alpha}_t^{(2)} + \boldsymbol{\nu}_t, \qquad (7.90)$$

where $\boldsymbol{\alpha}_t^{(i)}$ is $p_{\alpha,i}$-dimensional and where $p_{\alpha,i} << n$; $i = 1, 2$. Typically, the spectral coefficients $\boldsymbol{\alpha}_t^{(1)}$ correspond to "large-scale" basis functions in some sense, and $\boldsymbol{\alpha}_t^{(2)}$ correspond to "small-scale" basis functions. Let $\boldsymbol{\alpha}_t = (\boldsymbol{\alpha}_t^{(1)\prime}, \boldsymbol{\alpha}_t^{(2)\prime})'$ satisfy the GQN model (7.89). Motivated loosely by the concept of "Reynolds averaging" in turbulence theory (e.g., see Holten, 2004, Chapter 5), we want the pairwise interactions between components of $\boldsymbol{\alpha}_t^{(1)}$ to be explicit and described by $\boldsymbol{\alpha}_t^{(1)}$ substituted for $\boldsymbol{\alpha}_t$ in (7.89), but we want those among the "small-scale" components $\boldsymbol{\alpha}_t^{(2)}$ to be in some sense "noise," and the interactions between the components of $\boldsymbol{\alpha}_t^{(1)}$ and $\boldsymbol{\alpha}_t^{(2)}$ to suggest *random* coefficients in a linear combination of the large-scale basis functions (Wikle and Hooten, 2010).

As a simple example, consider a situation where $g(x) = x$ is the *identity function*, $\boldsymbol{\alpha}_t^{(1)} \equiv (\alpha_t^{(1)}(1), \alpha_t^{(1)}(2))'$, and $\boldsymbol{\alpha}_t^{(2)} \equiv (\alpha_t^{(2)}(1), \alpha_t^{(2)}(2), \alpha_t^{(2)}(3))'$. In this case, there are three "resolved" dyadic interactions corresponding to the three quadratic combinations of $\alpha_t^{(1)}(i)$, for $i = 1, 2$. In addition, the six unique pairwise interactions between the large-scale $\alpha_t^{(1)}(i)$ and the small-scale $\alpha_t^{(2)}(j)$; $i = 1, 2$, $j = 1, 2, 3$, coefficients imply linear terms in the large-scale components, with the small-scale components giving rise to unknown but *random* coefficients (i.e., $\{a_{ij}\}$ in (7.89)). Finally, the six dyadic interactions between the small scales $\{\alpha_t^{(2)}(j) : j = 1, 2, 3\}$, are assumed to correspond to the noise process, and because they are quadratic combinations, it suggests that they can be absorbed into the additive error process in the GQN (7.89), resulting in a dependent error process.

More generally (still assuming the function $g(\cdot)$ is the identity function), the GQN model for $\alpha_t^{(1)}$ can be written as

$$\alpha_t^{(1)} = \mathbf{A}\alpha_{t-1}^{(1)} + \left(\mathbf{I}_{p_1} \otimes \alpha_{t-1}^{(1)\prime}\right)\mathbf{B}\alpha_{t-1}^{(1)} + \eta_t ; \quad \eta_t \sim iid\,Gau(\mathbf{0}, \mathbf{Q}). \quad (7.91)$$

These models have not been explored extensively in the spatio-temporal statistics literature, but they have also been considered in other disciplines (see the Bibliographic Notes in Section 7.8). The challenge in this setting is still the choice of meaningful, science-based parameterizations. In addition, we could certainly consider higher-order (e.g., triad) interactions (e.g., Wikle and Holan, 2011), and we could motivate truncations in a similar way to that considered in the turbulence literature (e.g., Lesieur, 2008). However, the curse of dimensionality is so dominant in this case, that the hierarchical statistical modeler must really have a strong science-based approach for parameterization and truncation.

7.3.4 Agent-Based Models

A relatively new approach to statistical modeling of nonlinear and non-Gaussian spatio-temporal dynamical processes comes from *agent-based* models. Such models have been used in a variety of disciplines to mimic the behavior of natural processes. Agent-based procedures model complicated large-scale behavior by focusing on intuitive rules for the process at the smallest scales. In this way, agent-based models can be equated to *cellular automata* (CA) algorithms (e.g., Wolfram, 1984). Basically, an automata can be thought of as a collection of entities or agents whose states are determined by a simple set of rules. Automata are most often defined in a deterministic paradigm, in which the state of the "neighborhood" of an agent determines the future state of the agent. This can be generalized to allow specified probabilities to determine the future state of the agent. Traditionally, such models are used in a simulation context and statistical implementations are less common. However, as shown in Hooten and Wikle (2010), agent-based models can be formulated in a spatio-temporal hierarchical statistical context to characterize processes such as the spread of an epidemic. They show that such a model can be based on an intuitive parameterization of the system dynamics, and it can accommodate features such as long-distance and directionally varying dispersal, as well as spatial heterogeneity.

Consider a deterministic CA that is defined, in general, as

$$\mathbf{Y}_t = \mathcal{M}(\mathbf{Y}_{t-1}, \mathcal{R}, \mathcal{N}), \quad (7.92)$$

where $\mathcal{M}$ is an evolution function that depends on a set of neighborhoods, $\mathcal{N} \equiv \{\mathcal{N}_i : i = 1, \dots, n\}$, and a set of rules $\mathcal{R}$. Specifically, each element $Y_{i,t}$ (the automata) of the state vector $\mathbf{Y}_t \equiv (Y_{1,t}, \dots, Y_{n,t})'$ is a result of the function $\mathcal{M}$ and the previous set of neighboring automata, $\mathbf{Y}_{\mathcal{N}_i,t-1} \equiv (Y_{j,t-1} : j \in \mathcal{N}_i)'$, where it is possible here that $i \in \mathcal{N}_i$ (unlike for Markov random fields, described in Section 4.2.2). At first glance, this does not seem all that different from the neighbor-based vector autoregressive models (linear or nonlinear) described previously. The difference is in how the function $\mathcal{M}$ is defined, which is now made up of a set of rules, defining the map from all possible states of the set $\mathbf{Y}_{\mathcal{N}_i,t-1}$ to the possible states of $Y_{i,t}$. A CA defined in this simple way can exhibit very complex dynamical behavior (e.g., Wolfram, 1984).

The rules that govern the CA system are critical. However, the space of potential rules can be quite large, even for relatively small neighborhoods. For example, in a simple binary-state automaton (i.e., $Y_{i,t} \in \{0, 1\}$), a mapping function $\mathcal{M}$ over a simple first-order neighborhood in one dimension has $2^3 = 8$ possible neighborhood states, which leads to $2^8 = 256$ possible rules for the binary automaton $Y_{i,t}$. In general, for such a binary-state model, with $|\mathcal{N}_i|$ neighbors (including i), there will be $2^{2^{|\mathcal{N}_i|}}$ possible rules; the rules may or may not be automaton-dependent. As an example of how cumbersome this could be, consider a binary CA on a two-dimensional regular grid of cells and a "Queen's neighborhood" (i.e., the eight nearest neighbors in a cell to which the Queen could move one space in a game of chess), for which $|\mathcal{N}_i| \equiv 9$. In this case, the number of possible rules is 1.34×10^{154}. Thus, if the rules are not known *a priori*, it would not be feasible to do an exhaustive search in order to infer which is governing the observed binary data. Instead, we could consider a stochastic or probabilistic CA.

In essence, a stochastic or probabilistic CA consists of random variables for the cells' states that are conditioned on the neighborhood's variables at the previous time. In this context, the usual vector autoregressive models for time series are stochastic CAs. The conditional distribution describing the probabilistic CA can be written as

$$Y_{i,t} | \mathbf{Y}_{\mathcal{N}_i,t-1} \sim [Y_{i,t} \mid \mathcal{M}(\mathbf{Y}_{\mathcal{N}_i,t-1})], \qquad i = 1, \dots, n. \tag{7.93}$$

As an example, for binary automata, the distribution in (7.93) could be a Bernoulli distribution, in which the Bernoulli probabilities are a function of the neighborhood at the previous time, along with some parameters. An obvious advantage of this probabilistic specification over the deterministic one, is that, from a statistical perspective, it is easier to search the space of probability rules. However, it might be viewed that a disadvantage of the probabilistic approach is that the evolution from the previous state to the current state is no longer completely predictable. Note that there is a strong similarity between these models and so-called auto-logistic models (e.g., Zhu, Huang, and Wu, 2005; Royle and Dorazio, 2008).

Example: Modeling a Racoon Rabies Epidemic

As a simple illustration of how one might apply a stochastic CA, consider the model presented in Hooten and Wikle (2010). The authors were interested in modeling the spread of the racoon rabies epidemic on the east coast of the United States during the early 1990s [for more discussion of such epidemics, see, e.g., Nettles et al. (1979) and Smith et al. (2002)]. The process in this case is binary ($Y_{i,t} = 1$, corresponding to the presence of rabies in the ith grid box at a time t, and $Y_{i,t} = 0$, corresponding to no rabies present). It is assumed that data and process here are equivalent, and hence the HM consists of the following process model:

$$Y_{i,t}|\mathbf{Y}_{t-1} \sim Ber(\theta_{i,t}), \tag{7.94}$$

where the Bernoulli probability, $\theta_{i,t}$, that the disease is present in the ith grid cell at time t is modeled as

$$\theta_{i,t} = \phi Y_{i,t-1} + (1 - Y_{i,t-1})(I_{\mathcal{N}_{i,t-1}})\bar{p}_{i,t} + (1 - I_{\mathcal{N}_{i,t-1}})\psi, \tag{7.95}$$

for all i and t in the spatio-temporal support of the data. In (7.95),

$$I_{\mathcal{N}_{i,t-1}} \equiv \begin{cases} 1, & \sum_{j \in \mathcal{N}_i} Y_{j,t-1} > 0, \\ 0, & \sum_{j \in \mathcal{N}_i} Y_{j,t-1} = 0, \end{cases} \tag{7.96}$$

and $\mathcal{N}_i$ is the spatial neighborhood of grid cell i (assumed to be a Queen's neighborhood, made up of the eight neighbors immediately adjacent to cell i, *as well as* cell i).

There are three disjoint situations represented on the right-hand side of (7.95):

- $Y_{i,t-1}$: Cell i has rabies present (i.e., is "occupied" at time $t - 1$),
- $(1 - Y_{i,t-1})(I_{\mathcal{N}_{i,t-1}})$: At least one of the neighbors of the ith cell is occupied at time $t - 1$, but cell i is not occupied; and
- $1 - I_{\mathcal{N}_{i,t-1}}$: No cell in $\mathcal{N}_i$ (including cell i) is occupied at time $t - 1$.

Then the parameter ϕ in (7.95) is the probability that, once the phenomenon is present in cell i, it is present in that cell at the next time. Correspondingly, ψ is the probability of "out-of-neighborhood dispersal," meaning that ψ is the probability that the phenomenon will jump to cell i without occupying any neighborhood cell in $\mathcal{N}_i$. The neighborhood dispersal in this model is handled by the second term on the right-hand side of (7.95), which is controlled by the probability parameter $\bar{p}_{i,t}$. There are many possible specifications for this probability, depending on the spatial domain, level of realistic detail desired, and ease of estimation. Hooten and Wikle (2010) consider

$$\bar{p}_{i,t} = 1 - \exp((\mathbf{Y}_{\mathcal{N}_{i,t-1}})' \log(\mathbf{1} - \mathbf{p})), \tag{7.97}$$

where $\mathbf{Y}_{\mathcal{N}_i, t-1}$ consists of ones and zeros corresponding to the state of the neighborhood of the ith cell, $\mathbf{1}$ is a vector whose entries are all 1s, and $\mathbf{p} \equiv (p_1, p_2, \ldots, p_{|\mathcal{N}_i|})'$ is a vector of transition probabilities to cell i from each of its $|\mathcal{N}_i|$ neighbors, which they assumed did not depend on i. As shown in Hooten and Wikle (2010), this specification considers the probability of presence at time t, for a cell that has been previously unoccupied to be the union of transition probabilities from occupied neighbors. To be clear, the model (7.95)–(7.97) assumes that the neighborhood-based dispersal is dynamically anisotropic (unequal $\{p_i\}$) but homogeneous ($\{p_i\}$ do not depend on t). This model has been extended to the case of heterogeneous transition probabilities, dependent on some environmental conditions, by Hooten and Wikle (2010).

In a BHM, the parameters ϕ, ψ, and $\mathbf{p}$ would be given distributions at the next level of the hierarchy. For example, ϕ and ψ could each be given a beta prior distribution, and $\mathbf{p}$ could be given a Dirichlet prior distribution, possibly dependent on hyperparameters (Hooten and Wikle, 2010).

7.4 PROCESS MODELS FOR THE DSTM: MULTIVARIATE MODELS

Just as most real-world processes are not linear, most processes do not exist in isolation from other processes. For example, although we could consider *surface ozone* as a spatio-temporal process, a model for its behavior would surely be better if its relationship with *ambient air temperature* were included. One might just think of temperature as a covariate in this case, since typically surface ozone responds to temperature, and not so much the other way around (although this is not the case in the upper atmosphere). What about temperature and pressure? These are physically related, and one may think about their (statistical) dependence jointly, or in a conditional-probability setting, depending on the circumstances. Obviously, modeling joint statistical dependence could be extended to more meteorological processes (e.g., wind, pressure, temperature, density, water vapor, etc.). In this section, we consider both joint and conditional formulations for multivariate DSTM process models.

7.4.1 Augmenting the State Process (Multivariate DSTMs)

From a dynamical perspective, all of the approaches for modeling DSTMs are still applicable in the multivariate context. For example, if we were modeling a system of several processes in which first-order linear dynamics were appropriate, we could simply augment the state variable (by concatenating the various state vectors) and use the models described above: Say we have processes $\mathbf{Y}_t^{(k)}$ of dimension n_k; $k = 1, \ldots, K$. The augmented state variable is $\mathbf{Y}_t = (\mathbf{Y}_t^{(1)'} \ \ldots \ \mathbf{Y}_t^{(K)'})'$, and hence we can use a dynamical model to capture its spatio-temporal variability, such as the linear DSTM:

$$\mathbf{Y}_t = \mathbf{M}\mathbf{Y}_{t-1} + \boldsymbol{\eta}_t; \quad \boldsymbol{\eta}_t \sim iid\, Gau(\mathbf{0}, \mathbf{Q}_\eta), \tag{7.98}$$

which is of dimension $n_+ \equiv \sum_k n_k$. Of course, the nonlinear evolution models discussed in Section 7.3 could also be considered from a multivariate perspective, but we focus here on the linear case.

The propagator matrix $\mathbf{M}$ allows each process at the previous time to have an impact on itself and the others at the current time. Similarly, the error covariance matrix $\mathbf{Q}_\eta$ is in block form, corresponding to the covariance matrix of each process (the diagonal blocks) and the cross-covariance matrices (the off-diagonal blocks). Note that higher-order time lags could be used, and the propagator matrices could vary over time. However, the curse of dimensionality would limit such models, except in very highly parameterized settings. In what follows, we shall focus on the linear, first-order lag structure and non-time-varying propagator matrices, since they are sufficient to illustrate general multivariate-modeling issues.

Obviously, the potential difficulty now concerns dimensionality. If there was concern about dimensionality with just one process, the problems will only be compounded by the extra dimensions coming from the augmentation of the state with more vector-valued processes. Any of the strategies to reduce dimensionality considered previously in Section 7.1 (e.g., neighbor-based parameterization, truncation of spectral representations, etc.) could be used here as well. For example, the discretization (e.g., using finite-difference, finite-element, or spectral methods) of a system of PDEs provides a framework to motivate a model such as (7.98) (or the nonlinear equivalents of it, as suggested in Section 7.3.3). That is, the propagator matrix should be relatively sparse, and the associated parameters could either be estimated directly (EHM) or modeled probabilistically (BHM) at a lower level of the HM.

As an example of how (7.98) can be simplified, consider the spectral decomposition of the process vectors: $\mathbf{Y}_t^{(k)} = \mathbf{\Phi}^{(k)} \boldsymbol{\alpha}_t^{(k)}$, where the $\mathbf{\Phi}^{(k)}$ are $n_k \times n_k$ matrices of spatial basis functions. Then, (7.98) can be written as

$$\boldsymbol{\alpha}_t = \mathbf{M}_\alpha \boldsymbol{\alpha}_{t-1} + \boldsymbol{\eta}_{\alpha,t}, \tag{7.99}$$

where $\boldsymbol{\alpha}_t \equiv (\boldsymbol{\alpha}_t^{(1)\prime}, \ldots, \boldsymbol{\alpha}_t^{(K)\prime})\prime$, $\mathbf{M}_\alpha \equiv (\mathbf{W}'\mathbf{W})^{-1}\mathbf{W}'\mathbf{M}\mathbf{W}$, $\boldsymbol{\eta}_{\alpha,t} \equiv (\mathbf{W}'\mathbf{W})^{-1}\mathbf{W}'\boldsymbol{\eta}_t$ (assuming $(\mathbf{W}'\mathbf{W})^{-1}$ exists), and $\mathbf{W} \equiv (\mathbf{\Phi}^{(1)\prime}, \ldots, \mathbf{\Phi}^{(K)\prime})\prime$. As is the case for univariate spectral representations, one would expect that the dependence structure in $\boldsymbol{\eta}_{\alpha,t}$ would be simpler than that of $\boldsymbol{\eta}_t$ in (7.98), given the decorrelating effects of spectral transformations.

More practically, one would most likely perform dimension reduction by writing $\mathbf{Y}_t^{(k)} = \mathbf{\Phi}^{(k)} \boldsymbol{\alpha}_t^{(k)} + \boldsymbol{v}_t^{(k)}$, where $\boldsymbol{\alpha}_t^{(k)}$ is $p_{\alpha,k}$-dimensional ($p_{\alpha,k} << n_k$), and thus $\mathbf{\Phi}^{(k)}$ has dimension $n_k \times p_{\alpha,k}$; $k = 1, \ldots, K$. Additional computational savings are possible if the basis functions are mutually orthogonal (or, at least, orthogonal for each process, k). Furthermore, one might simply choose to estimate the $p_{\alpha,+} \times p_{\alpha,+}$ propagator matrix $\mathbf{M}_\alpha$ directly, if $p_{\alpha,+} \equiv \sum_k p_{\alpha,k}$ is sufficiently small.

The joint-modeling approach can also be considered in the context of an integro-difference equation (IDE). For example, say we have K spatio-temporal processes in continuous space and discrete time, $\{Y_t^{(k)}(\cdot) : k = 1, \ldots, K\}$. The multivariate version of the linear stochastic IDE process model given in Section 7.2.5 can then be written as

$$Y_t^{(k)}(\mathbf{s}) = \int_{D_s} \sum_{j=1}^{K} m^{(kj)}(\mathbf{s}, \mathbf{x}; \boldsymbol{\theta}) \, Y_{t-1}^{(j)}(\mathbf{x}) \, d\mathbf{x} + \eta_t^{(k)}(\mathbf{s}), \qquad (7.100)$$

for $k = 1, \ldots, K$, and where the kernels $m^{(kj)}(\mathbf{s}, \mathbf{x}; \boldsymbol{\theta})$ are assumed to depend on some parameters $\boldsymbol{\theta}$ (that, in principle, could also be spatially and/or temporally varying). We can write (7.100) in matrix notation as

$$\mathbf{Y}_t(\mathbf{s}) = \int_{D_s} \mathbf{M}(\mathbf{s}, \mathbf{x}; \boldsymbol{\theta}) \mathbf{Y}_{t-1}(\mathbf{x}) \, d\mathbf{x} + \boldsymbol{\eta}_t(\mathbf{s}), \qquad (7.101)$$

where $\mathbf{Y}_t(\mathbf{s}) \equiv (Y_t^{(1)}(\mathbf{s}), \ldots, Y_t^{(K)}(\mathbf{s}))'$, $\mathbf{M}(\mathbf{s}, \mathbf{x}; \boldsymbol{\theta})$ is a $K \times K$ matrix with (k, j)th element given by $m^{(kj)}(\mathbf{s}, \mathbf{x}; \boldsymbol{\theta})$, and $\boldsymbol{\eta}_t(\mathbf{s}) \equiv (\eta_t^{(1)}(\mathbf{s}), \ldots, \eta_t^{(K)}(\mathbf{s}))'$. Notice that $\mathbf{M}$ in (7.101) does not depend on t.

Discretization of (7.101) in space would imply a form such as (7.98), and the usual issues related to the curse of dimensionality could play a role. However, as described in Section 7.2.5, an advantage of the IDE formulation defined by kernels in the dynamical process is that the kernels can be parameterized efficiently to capture specific (qualitative) dynamical behavior (e.g., diffusion, advection, interaction, etc.). In addition, as described in Section 7.2.6, one might expand both the process and the kernels in terms of spectral basis functions and then consider the evolution of the reduced-dimensional spectral coefficients in the dynamical model, analogous to the formulation given in (7.99).

7.4.2   Dependence on Common Processes

An obvious way to build spatio-temporal dependence between processes is to represent these processes in terms of a common process. As with the univariate spectral decomposition discussed in Section 7.2.6, this hidden process is dynamical, but may or may not be spatial, depending on the implementation. For example, as with the multivariate IDE model given in (7.101), consider K spatio-temporal processes, $\{Y_t^{(k)}(\mathbf{s}) : k = 1, \ldots, K\}$. In the spirit of Ver Hoef and Barry (1998), consider the construction of a multivariate spatio-temporal process given by

$$Y_t^{(k)}(\mathbf{s}) = \int_{D_s} \sum_{j=1}^{J} h^{(kj)}(\mathbf{s}, \mathbf{x}; \boldsymbol{\theta}) \, \alpha_t^{(j)}(\mathbf{x}) \, d\mathbf{x} + \gamma_t^{(k)}(\mathbf{s}), \qquad \mathbf{s} \in D_s, \qquad (7.102)$$

for $k = 1, \ldots, K$, and where the kernels $h^{(kj)}(\mathbf{s}, \mathbf{x}; \boldsymbol{\theta})$ are assumed to depend on some parameters $\boldsymbol{\theta}$. Notice that these parameters do not (in general) depend on t and hence do not contribute to the dynamics. In matrix notation, we can write (7.102) as

$$\mathbf{Y}_t(\mathbf{s}) = \int_{D_s} \mathbf{H}(\mathbf{s}, \mathbf{x}; \boldsymbol{\theta})\boldsymbol{\alpha}_t(\mathbf{x})\, d\mathbf{x} + \boldsymbol{\gamma}_t(\mathbf{s}), \qquad \mathbf{s} \in D_s, \qquad (7.103)$$

where $\mathbf{Y}_t(\mathbf{s}) \equiv (Y_t^{(1)}(\mathbf{s}), \ldots, Y_t^{(K)}(\mathbf{s}))'$, $\mathbf{H}(\mathbf{s}, \mathbf{x}; \boldsymbol{\theta})$ is a $K \times J$ matrix with (k, j)th element given by $h^{(kj)}(\mathbf{s}, \mathbf{x}; \boldsymbol{\theta})$, $\boldsymbol{\alpha}_t(\mathbf{x}) \equiv (\alpha_t^{(1)}(\mathbf{x}), \ldots, \alpha_t^{(J)}(\mathbf{x}))'$, and $\boldsymbol{\gamma}_t(\mathbf{s}) \equiv (\gamma_t^{(1)}(\mathbf{s}), \ldots, \gamma_t^{(K)}(\mathbf{s}))'$. That is, a K-dimensional process $\mathbf{Y}_t(\cdot)$ is expressed in terms of a J-dimensional process $\boldsymbol{\alpha}_t(\cdot)$. This has benefit if the hidden dynamical process, $\{\alpha_t^{(j)}(\cdot) : j = 1, \ldots, J\}$, has simplifying structure (e.g., they are a set of J independent AR(1) processes with unit variances). The α-processes induce dependence between the various Y-processes, defined by the smoothing induced from the kernels. In order for this framework for building DSTMs to induce realistic dynamics, one would typically need nontrivial parameterizations of some combination of the propagator and error covariance matrices. Indeed, as described in Section 7.1.3 for the univariate DSTM, without strong assumptions about the structure of the kernels and the dynamical parameters associated with the hidden processes, such models are not typically identifiable. Furthermore, this model can suffer from a serious curse of dimensionality. For example, if we approximate the integrals in (7.102) and (7.103) with summations, then for the kth process we have

$$\int_{D_s} \sum_{j=1}^{J} h^{(kj)}(\mathbf{s}, \mathbf{x}; \boldsymbol{\theta})\, \alpha_t^{(j)}(\mathbf{x})\, d\mathbf{x} \simeq \sum_{i=1}^{p_\alpha} \sum_{j=1}^{J} h^{(kj)}(\mathbf{s}, \mathbf{x}_i; \boldsymbol{\theta})\, \alpha_t^{(j)}(\mathbf{x}_i), \qquad (7.104)$$

where $\{\mathbf{x}_i : i = 1, \ldots, p_\alpha\}$ correspond to a discrete set of locations in D_s. Thus, in matrix notation, a discretized model for (7.103) is given by

$$\mathbf{Y}_t(\mathbf{s}) = \mathbf{H}(\mathbf{s})\boldsymbol{\alpha}_t + \boldsymbol{\gamma}_t(\mathbf{s}), \qquad \mathbf{s} \in D_s, \qquad (7.105)$$

where $\mathbf{Y}_t(\mathbf{s})$ and $\boldsymbol{\gamma}_t(\mathbf{s})$ are defined above in (7.103); $\boldsymbol{\alpha}_t \equiv (\boldsymbol{\alpha}_t^{(1)\prime}, \ldots, \boldsymbol{\alpha}_t^{(J)\prime})'$ with $\boldsymbol{\alpha}_t^{(j)} \equiv (\alpha_t^{(j)}(\mathbf{x}_1), \ldots, \alpha_t^{(j)}(\mathbf{x}_{p_\alpha}))'$; and $\mathbf{H}(\mathbf{s})$ is a $K \times J p_\alpha$ matrix whose kth row is made up of $J p_\alpha$-dimensional vectors, $\{(h^{(kj)}(\mathbf{s}, \mathbf{x}_i; \boldsymbol{\theta}) : i = 1, \ldots, p_\alpha)' : j = 1, \ldots, J\}$.

Now, suppose that in (7.105), we assume $p_\alpha = 1$ and let $\mathbf{x}_1 = \mathbf{s}$. Then (7.105) becomes

$$\mathbf{Y}_t(\mathbf{s}) = \mathbf{H}\tilde{\boldsymbol{\alpha}}_t(\mathbf{s}) + \boldsymbol{\gamma}_t(\mathbf{s}); \quad \mathbf{s} \in D_s, \qquad (7.106)$$

where $\tilde{\boldsymbol{\alpha}}_t(\mathbf{s}) \equiv (\alpha_t^{(1)}(\mathbf{s}), \ldots, \alpha_t^{(J)}(\mathbf{s}))'$ is J-dimensional, and the $K \times J$ matrix $\mathbf{H}$ has (k, j)th entry $h_{kj} \equiv h^{(kj)}(\mathbf{s}, \mathbf{s}; \boldsymbol{\theta})$. Fix t, and suppose the spatial processes, $\alpha_t^{(1)}(\cdot), \ldots, \alpha_t^{(J)}(\cdot)$, are independent. Then (7.106) gives the linear model of coregionalization, with an extra, additive noise term $\gamma_t(\cdot)$ (e.g., Gelfand et al., 2004; Gelfand, Banerjee and Gamerman, 2005; Sansó, Schmidt, and Nobre, 2008; see also Section 4.1.5, for discussion of this model in the spatial context).

Now consider the K processes at common multiple locations, $\{\mathbf{s}_1, \mathbf{s}_2, \ldots, \mathbf{s}_n\}$; that is, $n_1 = \ldots = n_K = n$. Then write $\mathbf{Y}_t^{(k)} \equiv (Y_t^{(k)}(\mathbf{s}_1), \ldots, Y_t^{(k)}(\mathbf{s}_n))'$, which is an n-dimensional vector. (Note that this could be generalized to the case where locations for each process are different, but we do not do so for ease of presentation.) Then define the augmented (Kn)-dimensional spatio-temporal processes, $\mathbf{Y}_t \equiv (\mathbf{Y}_t^{(1)\prime}, \ldots, \mathbf{Y}_t^{(K)\prime})'$. Hence, for multiple locations, the process model (7.105) can be rewritten as

$$\mathbf{Y}_t = \tilde{\mathbf{H}}\tilde{\boldsymbol{\alpha}}_t + \boldsymbol{\gamma}_t, \tag{7.107}$$

where $\tilde{\boldsymbol{\alpha}}_t$ is a (Jn)-dimensional vector given by $\tilde{\boldsymbol{\alpha}}_t \equiv (\tilde{\boldsymbol{\alpha}}_t^{(1)\prime}, \ldots, \tilde{\boldsymbol{\alpha}}_t^{(J)\prime})'$, with $\tilde{\boldsymbol{\alpha}}_t^{(j)} \equiv (\alpha_t^{(j)}(\mathbf{s}_1), \ldots, \alpha_t^{(j)}(\mathbf{s}_n))'$; $\tilde{\mathbf{H}}$ is a $(Kn) \times (Jn)$ matrix (which we could allow to be time-varying, in general); and $\boldsymbol{\gamma}_t$ is a (Kn)-dimensional vector of error processes, $\{\boldsymbol{\gamma}_t^{(k)} : k = 1, \ldots, K\}$.

Now, if $\{\tilde{\boldsymbol{\alpha}}_t\}$ has relatively interesting dynamics, then spatio-temporal dependence will be induced in $\{\mathbf{Y}_t^{(k)} : k = 1, \ldots, K\}$ through the temporal and between-component dependence in $\{\tilde{\boldsymbol{\alpha}}_t\}$ and, critically, through the matrix $\tilde{\mathbf{H}}$. As discussed above, even in the case where this matrix is not time-varying, there is an identifiability issue with estimating the parameters of $\tilde{\mathbf{H}}$ along with any proposed non-trivial dynamical propagator for $\{\tilde{\boldsymbol{\alpha}}_t\}$.

Another special case of (7.105) for multiple locations is given by Calder (2007):

$$\mathbf{Y}_t = (\mathbf{K} \otimes \mathbf{F})\boldsymbol{\alpha}_t + \boldsymbol{\gamma}_t, \tag{7.108}$$

where $\mathbf{K}$ is an $n \times p_\alpha$ matrix; $\mathbf{F}$ is a $K \times J$ matrix; and $\boldsymbol{\gamma}_t = (\boldsymbol{\gamma}_t^{(1)\prime}, \ldots, \boldsymbol{\gamma}_t^{(K)\prime})'$, with $\boldsymbol{\gamma}_t^{(k)} \sim ind. Gau(\mathbf{0}, \lambda_\gamma^{(k)}\mathbf{I}); k = 1, \ldots, K$. This can be rewritten as

$$\mathcal{Y}_t = \mathbf{K}\mathbf{A}_t\mathbf{F}' + \mathbf{G}_t, \tag{7.109}$$

where $\mathcal{Y}_t \equiv (\mathbf{Y}_t^{(1)}, \ldots, \mathbf{Y}_t^{(K)})$ is an $n \times K$ matrix of process vectors, $\mathbf{A}_t \equiv (\boldsymbol{\alpha}_t^{(1)}, \ldots, \boldsymbol{\alpha}_t^{(J)})$ is a $p_\alpha \times J$ matrix of hidden processes, $\mathbf{G}_t \equiv (\boldsymbol{\gamma}_t^{(1)}, \ldots, \boldsymbol{\gamma}_t^{(K)})$ is an $n \times K$ matrix of error processes, and $\mathbf{K}$ and $\mathbf{F}$ are as defined above. In this form, the model is related to dynamical factor models for multiple time series (e.g., Aguilar and West, 2000). Here there are non-trivial dynamics on the hidden processes that make up $\mathbf{A}_t$, and there are identifiability issues to be taken into account. Calder (2007) uses a discrete-kernel convolution matrix for $\mathbf{K}$ and proposes identifiability restrictions on $\mathbf{F}$ based on those given in Aguilar and West (2000). However, the introduction of parameters in the evolution processes $\{\boldsymbol{\alpha}_t^{(j)} : j = 1, \ldots, J\}$ may require further identifiability restrictions.

In certain scientific applications, the hidden process $\{\tilde{\boldsymbol{\alpha}}_t\}$ in (7.107) might correspond to a real-world process, and there might be known relationships between $\tilde{\boldsymbol{\alpha}}_t$ and $\mathbf{Y}_t$ that suggest efficient parameterizations of $\tilde{\mathbf{H}}$. For example, Royle et al. (1999) considered spatial processes given by the east–west and north–south wind components and conditioned them on a hidden spatial process given by atmospheric pressure. Theoretical relationships (e.g., *geostrophy*) suggest that the wind components are proportional to the gradient of pressure, to a first-order approximation, in the mid-latitudes. This, in turn, suggests a low-dimensional parameterization for the matrix $\tilde{\mathbf{H}}$. For more details of such an example in the spatio-temporal context, see Berliner, Milliff, and Wikle (2003) and Milliff et al. (2010). We expand on this notion of scientific-process conditioning in the next section.

7.4.3 Conditional Formulation

Once again, conditioning can be used to help with the reduction of dimensionality, to ensure that valid models are being fitted, and (in many cases) to facilitate the incorporation of scientific information. For example, consider the case where we have two spatio-temporal processes $\{\mathbf{Y}_t^{(1)}\}$ and $\{\mathbf{Y}_t^{(2)}\}$. From the first-order dynamical perspective, we have $[\mathbf{Y}_t^{(1)}, \mathbf{Y}_t^{(2)}|\mathbf{Y}_{t-1}^{(1)}, \mathbf{Y}_{t-1}^{(2)}]$ (where dependence on parameters in the conditional distribution is supressed for notational clarity). Now, we could make use of conditional probabilities and write

$$[\mathbf{Y}_t^{(1)}, \mathbf{Y}_t^{(2)}|\mathbf{Y}_{t-1}^{(1)}, \mathbf{Y}_{t-1}^{(2)}] = [\mathbf{Y}_t^{(2)}|\mathbf{Y}_t^{(1)}, \mathbf{Y}_{t-1}^{(1)}, \mathbf{Y}_{t-1}^{(2)}][\mathbf{Y}_t^{(1)}|\mathbf{Y}_{t-1}^{(1)}, \mathbf{Y}_{t-1}^{(2)}]. \quad (7.110)$$

Hopefully, there would be a good scientific reason for conditioning $\mathbf{Y}_t^{(2)}$ on $\mathbf{Y}_t^{(1)}$; in the example of near-surface ozone and temperature mentioned at the beginning of this section, it would make sense to consider ozone ($\mathbf{Y}_t^{(2)}$, say) conditioned on temperature ($\mathbf{Y}_t^{(1)}$, say), since the production of surface ozone is partially driven by ambient air temperature. Now, it might be the case that there is further scientific insight that allows sensible assumptions to be made about the conditional models on the right-hand side of (7.110). For example, say we believe that (on the given temporal scale) it is reasonable to allow $\mathbf{Y}_t^{(2)}$ to be independent of $\mathbf{Y}_{t-1}^{(1)}$ given $\mathbf{Y}_t^{(1)}$ (often a reasonable assumption), and perhaps we believe that $\mathbf{Y}_t^{(1)}$ is independent of $\mathbf{Y}_{t-1}^{(2)}$ given $\mathbf{Y}_{t-1}^{(1)}$. Then, (7.110) becomes

$$[\mathbf{Y}_t^{(1)}, \mathbf{Y}_t^{(2)}|\mathbf{Y}_{t-1}^{(1)}, \mathbf{Y}_{t-1}^{(2)}] = [\mathbf{Y}_t^{(2)}|\mathbf{Y}_t^{(1)}, \mathbf{Y}_{t-1}^{(2)}][\mathbf{Y}_t^{(1)}|\mathbf{Y}_{t-1}^{(1)}]. \quad (7.111)$$

Of course, this is just one example, and the type of assumptions that would be valid for a given system are certainly problem-dependent and should be justified. The point is that (7.111), which was derived from (7.110), has simplified the model through a conditional-probability specification, for which more scientifically meaningful propagator and covariate parameterizations might be suggested. While this will reduce the number of parameters that need to be estimated/modeled, the curse of dimensionality still needs to be dealt with.

Example: Bayesian Hierarchical Modeling of Air–Sea Interaction

Berliner, Milliff, and Wikle (2003) consider a model for air–sea interaction that is multivariate and includes process models motivated by relatively complex PDE dynamics. The scientific problem considered in this study was to understand the interaction between atmospheric wind forcing and the associated ocean response in the Labrador Sea. The Labrador Sea is a locus of deep convection in the ocean, with processes occurring on relatively short time scales with small spatial footprints. It is an important region, since the deep convection provides a source of deep-water formation and transport, a driving factor in climate-scale ocean circulation. The primary interest in Berliner, Milliff, and Wikle (2003) was in the so-called *preconditioning* phase of the deep convection, in which the coincidence of momentum concentration from the atmosphere and weakened upper-ocean stratification leads to regional surface-buoyancy-forcing events. The study was focused on determining whether a hierarchical model of coupled ocean and atmospheric processes, with relatively sparsely sampled winds and sea-surface heights from satellite-based scatterometry and altimetry, could capture this preconditioning. Our focus here is on the coupled air-sea portion of the process model, although we present some aspects of the full HM to facilitate the motivation.

First, it is helpful to consider the full hierarchical model from a schematic perspective. Let D_a and D_o denote the atmosphere (scatterometer) and ocean (altimeter) data, respectively. Then, the hierarchical model can be written as

Data model: $[D_a, D_o | \text{Atm}, \text{Ocean}, \theta_a, \theta_o]$

Process model: $[\text{Atm}, \text{Ocean} | \eta_a, \eta_{o|a}]$

Parameter model: $[\theta_a, \theta_o, \eta_a, \eta_{o|a}]$

where "Atm" and "Ocean" represent the atmosphere and ocean processes, respectively, and the associated data and process parameters are θ_a, θ_o, η_a, and $\eta_{o|a}$. Efficient modeling in this case is achieved by assuming conditional independence of the atmosphere and ocean observations, as well as a conditional-probability specification of the process model. Thus, the data and process models become

Data model: $[D_a, D_o | \text{Atm}, \text{Ocean}, \theta_a, \theta_o] = [D_a | \text{Atm}, \theta_a][D_o | \text{Ocean}, \theta_o]$

Process model: $[\text{Atm}, \text{Ocean} | \eta_a, \eta_{o|a}] = [\text{Ocean} | \text{Atm}, \eta_{o|a}][\text{Atm} | \eta_a]$

Hence, the air–sea model is a stochastic atmosphere model coupled to a stochastic ocean-conditional-on-atmosphere model. The posterior distribution is then

$$[\text{Atm}, \text{Ocean}, \theta_a, \theta_0, \eta_a, \eta_{o|a} | D_a, D_o],$$

which represents a complete coupling between the atmosphere and ocean processes.

Specifically, the ocean-process model was motivated by *quasigeostrophy* (e.g., see Pedlosky, 1987). That is, if ψ is the ocean streamfunction (a scalar function of two-dimensional fluid motion such that lines of constant streamfunction are everywhere tangent to the local flow), then the quasigeostrophic equation is given by

$$\left(\nabla^2 - \frac{1}{r^2}\right)\frac{\partial \psi}{\partial t} = -J(\psi, \nabla^2\psi) - \beta\frac{\partial \psi}{\partial x} + \frac{1}{\rho H}\,\mathrm{curl}_z\tau - \gamma\nabla^2\psi - a_H\nabla^4\psi,$$

$$(7.112)$$

where $J(a, b) \equiv \partial a/\partial x \cdot \partial b/\partial y - \partial b/\partial x \cdot \partial a/\partial y$ is the Jacobian (nonlinear in ψ); $\mathrm{curl}_z\tau$ is the "wind stress curl" given by $\partial\tau_y/\partial x - \partial\tau_x/\partial y$ (where the wind-stress components τ_y and τ_x are related, respectively, to the integral of the u- and v-wind components through a portion of the atmosphere boundary layer); and $r, \beta, \rho, H, \gamma, a_H$ are parameters related to the flow. Using standard finite-difference approximations to temporal derivatives and spatial derivatives in (7.112), Berliner, Milliff, and Wikle (2003) obtain a *vector* representation of this ocean-conditional-on-atmosphere process model with additive errors. Wikle and Hooten (2010) show that this model, discretized, is a special case of the GQN models discussed in Section 7.3.3.

The atmosphere process model in this HM was similar in spirit to the so-called "stochastic geostrophy" model first outlined in Royle et al. (1999). In that case, the spatio-temporal component-wind processes were conditioned on the spatio-temporal pressure field, and fairly simple data models for the scatterometer and altimeter were considered.

Obviously, the posterior distribution is analytically intractable and must be approximated numerically (e.g., by Monte Carlo methods). Berliner, Milliff, and Wikle (2003) exploit the special conditional nature of this posterior form, and they show that a hybrid-sampling approach using an importance sampler and a Gibbs sampler leads to efficient sampling.

7.5 DSTM PARAMETER MODELS

We begin by reiterating that the distinction between "process" and "parameters" is often quite arbitrary. Indeed, one person's process may be another person's parameters. However, at least in science-based, spatio-temporal hierarchical statistical modeling, at a given level of the hierarchy it is usually possible to distinguish between parameters and processes. A strength of the hierarchical approach is that it allows parameters from one level to be modeled as a stochastic process at the next level. This ability to construct models by exploiting conditional dependence can lead to very flexible joint probability distributions. The spatial, temporal, and spatio-temporal models used to build these conditional distributions have been discussed in Chapters 3, 4, and 6 and this chapter, respectively. This being said, there are usually components of models (e.g., variance–covariance parameters and parameters that control propagation) that most would agree are parameters. We focus on those in this section.

As we have seen, a key consideration when constructing hierarchical spatio-temporal models is efficient parameterization at both the data-model and the process-model levels. In some cases, these levels are sufficiently simple or low-dimensional, so that it is reasonable to estimate the parameters directly (EHM), or to assign them relatively noninformative prior distributions (BHM). We shall explore this in more detail in Chapter 8, and we give examples in Chapter 9.

The more typical case, at least for complex data models and process models, is to model the parameters explicitly in the parameter stage of the hierarchical model. There are myriad choices for such models, with specific choices depending on the data model and the process model employed. Nevertheless, there are some general issues and approaches that are often of importance. We discuss some of these below.

7.5.1   Data-Model Parameters

It is often the case that some prior information is available regarding the measurement-error variance, allowing a fairly informative parameter model to be specified. For example, if we are assuming conditionally independent measurement errors that are $iid\, Gau(0, \sigma_\varepsilon^2)$, then we should specify an informative prior for σ_ε^2. Say we were interested in ambient air temperature, and we saw that the instrument manufacturer's specifications indicated an "error" of $\pm 0.1°C$. Assuming that this "error" corresponds to 2 standard deviations (an assumption that should be checked!), we might then specify σ_ε^2 to have a prior mean of $(0.1/2)^2 = 0.0025$. Because of the instrument manufacturer's specification, we would assume a distribution that had a clearly defined and fairly narrow peak at 0.0025 (e.g., inverse gamma). In fact, we could just fix σ_ε^2 at 0.0025; however, the data-model error may have other components of uncertainty too (Section 7.1). To avoid possible identifiability problems with process-model error, it is *very* important that modelers reduce the uncertainty in σ_ε^2 as much as the Science allows, including doing side studies designed to have replicated data.

Note that the iid error assumption in the data model is not always realistic. For example, when measuring ambient air temperature, it is certainly possible that the instrument error could be greater depending on the true ambient temperature (e.g., very cold or very warm temperatures). Because the data-model variances might change with state, with time, or in space, the data-model error might be modeled as a threshold process, a time series (stationary or nonstationary), or a spatial process. The most common form of dependence considered in DSTM models is spatial. Any of the spatial models discussed in Chapter 4 could be used in this case. Also, as discussed in Sections 7.2.6 and 7.1.3, in the context of EOF expansions, we might be able to parameterize the (spatially dependent) data-model covariance in terms of a noncomplete set of orthogonal basis vectors:

$$\boldsymbol{\Sigma}_\varepsilon = c\mathbf{I} + \sum_{k=1}^{n_\varepsilon} \lambda_k \boldsymbol{\phi}_k \boldsymbol{\phi}_k', \tag{7.113}$$

where c is an unknown constant, $\{\boldsymbol{\phi}_k\}$ are selected orthogonal basis functions, and $\{\lambda_k\}$ are their associated coefficients; these are selected to model small-scale to microscale spatial variations. Clearly, this suggests all manner of covariance-model parameterizations, depending on how c, n_ε, $\{\lambda_k\}$, and $\{\boldsymbol{\phi}_k\}$ are chosen (e.g., see Berliner, Wikle, and Cressie, 2000).

Although the discussion of data-model parameters has focused on variance (and covariance) parameters, the additive and multiplicative bias parameters discussed in Section 7.1 could also be modeled explicitly. One may have some *a priori* knowledge about these parameters or, if not, they may be given vague priors according to the specifics of the application. For example, say we expect the additive bias terms given in (7.10), $\{\mathbf{a}_t\}$, to be dependent on known covariates, $\mathbf{X}_t$. Then, we might assume $\mathbf{a}_t = \mathbf{X}_t \boldsymbol{\beta}$, where we assign a prior distribution to $\boldsymbol{\beta}$ (e.g., a multivariate Gaussian distribution) at this parameter stage. Alternatively, it might make more sense in some applications to let $\mathbf{a}_t$ follow a Gaussian random spatial process; for example, $\mathbf{a}_t \sim iid\, Gau(\boldsymbol{\mu}_a, \boldsymbol{\Sigma}_a)$, as in Chapter 4, or a random spatio-temporal process as in Chapter 6. Similar choices could used for the multiplicative bias terms $\{\mathbf{h}_t\}$ in (7.10). In general, multiple levels of hierarchical specification could be applied, assuming there is relevant data and/or scientific information to inform such specifications. As shown in Wikle, Berliner, and Cressie (1998), considerable flexibility in a DSTM can be obtained by allowing the higher-level model parameters to vary spatially.

7.5.2 Process-Model Parameters

In this subsection, we consider some standard approaches to putting (prior) distributions on the process-model parameters.

Parameters of Process-Model Error
Recall that the covariance matrix of the process error $\{\boldsymbol{\eta}_t\}$ is written as $\mathbf{Q}_\eta$. It is often the case that we assume homogeneous variance, σ_η^2, in which case $\mathbf{Q}_\eta = \sigma_\eta^2 \mathbf{R}_\eta$, where $\mathbf{R}_\eta$ is a correlation matrix. Note that various prior distributions for the process variance σ_η^2 could be specified, although one typically does not have a great deal of *a priori* understanding about this variance. We also note that there is often some knowledge about how σ_η^2 and the data-model variance, σ_ε^2, are related. Thus, in practice, the signal-to-noise ratio, $\xi = \sigma_\eta^2/\sigma_\varepsilon^2$, and σ_ε^2 are often modeled, rather than the individual variances. In addition to a natural interpretation, the signal-to-noise ratio has the advantage of being scale-free.

As will be discussed in Section 8.3, an inverse-Wishart prior distribution is often applied to covariance matrices when implementing dynamical models in a Bayesian framework. Alternatively, in cases where $\mathbf{Q}_\eta$ represents a spatial covariance matrix, one could specify a relevent geostatistical or lattice covariance model (see Chapter 4) as the prior structure. The parameters that characterize those spatial models might also be allowed to vary with time, if there is sufficient justification. Yet another alternative is a covariance model based on a matrix decomposition. We saw a simple example of this in Section 7.5.1. One can also use a Cholesky decomposition,

$$\mathbf{T}\mathbf{Q}_\eta\mathbf{T}' = \mathbf{D},\qquad(7.114)$$

where $\mathbf{T}$ is a lower-triangular matrix, and $\mathbf{D}$ is a diagonal matrix with positive entries, facilitating interpretation and (MCMC) computation (e.g., Pourahmadi, 1999; Chen and Dunson, 2003).

There are also many cases where one might have scientific information about the prior covariance structure. For example, in Wikle et al. (2001), scientific considerations suggested that the tropical ocean winds should follow a turbulent power-law spectrum. This was incorporated by specifying a relationship between spectral scales in $\mathbf{Q}_\eta$.

Parameters of the Propagator Matrix

The parameter model should accommodate scientific understanding of the dynamical process. In the case of low-dimensional processes, the entire propagator matrix $\mathbf{M}$ in the DSTM might be modeled, as will be shown in Section 8.3. This could be done using a matrix prior (e.g., a matrix normal) or, equivalently, by modeling the vectorized form, vec($\mathbf{M}$).

It is more common that the curse of dimensionality has led the modeler to parameterize $\mathbf{M}$ as $\mathbf{M}(\boldsymbol{\theta})$. Prior distributions for $\boldsymbol{\theta}$ would then depend on the particular type of parameterization. Some parameterizations assume that there is spatial dependence in at least some of the $\boldsymbol{\theta}$. For example, the basic spatial univariate AR model given in Section 7.2.2 assumes that $\mathbf{M} = \text{diag}(\mathbf{m})$. In this case, $\mathbf{m}$ might be assumed to follow a Gaussian spatial process, such as discussed in Chapter 4. This is quite powerful, in that the elements of $\mathbf{Y}_t$ might be assumed to be (conditionally) independent (i.e., $\mathbf{Q}_\eta = \sigma_\eta^2\mathbf{I}$) but, if $\mathbf{M}$ exhibits spatial dependence, then the marginal distribution of $\mathbf{Y}_t$ would still show spatial dependence. Of course, these parameters could be allowed to vary with time as well, possibly being dependenton other covariates.

There might also be scientific information to help model $\mathbf{M}(\boldsymbol{\theta})$. For example, if we were modeling an ecological process that exhibited non-isotropic diffusion over time, it might be useful to model the process based on a discretized diffusion PDE, in which the diffusion parameters vary with space. As shown in Section 7.2.4, these diffusion coefficients are included in the off-diagonal entries of $\mathbf{M}(\boldsymbol{\theta})$. It would then be reasonable to model these coefficients as a spatial process, possibly related to habitat covariates (see Wikle, 2003b). In another example, one might have knowledge of advection dynamics, where the relevant parameters $\boldsymbol{\theta}$ could be related to wind fields (e.g., Xu, Wikle, and Fox, 2005), suggesting once again that the parameter model might involve spatial dependence.

Recall from our discussion of vector autoregression models in Section 3.4.7 that the propagator matrix **M** in a linear DSTM must have all of its eigenvalues less than one in modulus to ensure that the process is not explosive. In principle, it is not difficult to enforce such constraints in the implementation of a DSTM. However, depending on the parameterization of **M**, this may or may not be easy to constrain in practice within a hierarchical context. In simple parameterizations it can be done efficiently (e.g., see Sansó, Schmidt, and Nobre, 2008). However, it is not always clear that such constraints should be enforced. For example, if one were using such a linear DSTM to characterize an environmental process, unconstrained estimation that suggested explosive behavior would probably indicate that the linear model is inappropriate and that the process is exhibiting some sort of nonlinear growth, which is reflected in the data driving the parameters into the explosive regime. In this case, one should probably be using a nonlinear process model. Alternatively, in a relatively-short-period forecasting situation (i.e., a *nowcast*), an explosive linear model that is suggested by the recent past might produce a realistic forecast of a process exhibiting growth (e.g., a thunderstorm growing in intensity). Thus, we should be careful employing restrictions on the parameter space, unless we are fairly certain that our statistical model is the "correct" model for the dynamics of the underlying spatio-temporal process.

7.5.3 Deterministic Process Models with Random Parameters

Recall from our discussion in Sections 7.2.4 and 7.3, that we can often motivate dynamical models with deterministic (e.g., PDE and IDE) models. For example, recall (7.62):

$$\mathbf{Y}_t = \mathcal{M}(\mathbf{Y}_{t-1}, \boldsymbol{\eta}_t; \boldsymbol{\theta}_t), \qquad (7.115)$$

where $\mathcal{M}$ is some nonlinear dynamical operator depending on parameters $\boldsymbol{\theta}_t$, that may vary with t. If $\mathcal{M}$ is known and the parameters are allowed to be random, the behavior of the system may be unrealistic if it is not in some way constrained. In relatively simple systems, there may be enough understanding of the process parameters $\{\boldsymbol{\theta}_t\}$ to be able to specify reasonable constraints. Perhaps more importantly, the HM approach allows the data to help *control* the process' behavior.

On the one hand, random parameters allow the process to have much more flexibility (even in the constrained case), but on the other hand these random parameters may not be interpretable in the context of the original process. This interpretability is further complicated when there is model error $\{\boldsymbol{\eta}_t\}$. It is often the case that one simply needs the error process because the deterministic model, even with random parameters, cannot accommodate real-world data. Clearly, there are now two sources trying to account for the unrepresentativeness of the underlying deterministic model, namely the random parameters $\{\boldsymbol{\theta}_t\}$

and the (additive) error process $\{\boldsymbol{\eta}_t\}$. Although the trade-offs between data and process uncertainty, as they relate to system behavior, have long been considered in Control Theory (e.g., Aström, 1970), the interplay between these uncertainties *and* random parameters (in the context of hierarchical spatio-temporal statistical models) is presently under-developed and an active area of research.

7.6 DYNAMICAL DESIGN OF MONITORING NETWORKS

It is not usually possible to sample a spatio-temporal process completely. This section is concerned with choosing where (and when) to sample, through the design of a monitoring network. Typically, political, geographic, or economic factors govern the design, but choosing sampling locations without also taking into account statistical factors will lead to a sub-optimal design. There has been a great deal of work in the Statistics literature related to obtaining optimal designs for spatial processes [e.g., see the overviews in Müller (2000) and Le and Zidek (2006, Chapter 11)]. Indeed, many of these same methodologies are applicable to spatio-temporal processes as well. Most of the work done in this context has been related to finding a fixed design (over time) that considers the joint spatio-temporal dependence when determining the optimal design. However, as demonstrated in Wikle and Royle (1999), substantial efficiencies can be gained in the spatio-temporal context if the design is allowed to change with time (provided such a change is allowed by the monitoring protocol). This is sometimes referred to as targeted design or adaptive design. We prefer the term dynamical design, since it emphasizes the dynamical nature of the design changing with time and the fact that the underlying process is also evolving dynamically.

Wikle and Royle (1999) show that when considering Gaussian data and Gaussian dynamical processes, dynamical designs show greater efficiencies relative to static designs as the temporal correlation increases (their measure of efficiency is based on the average prediction variance across the spatial domain). Such an improvement is no surprise, in that if observations were made at location **s** at time t, then it might be redundant to take observations at this same location at time $t + 1$ when there is strong temporal dependence at location **s**. In addition, there will generally be large improvements in design efficiency if the spatial dependence is strong. Again, this is intuitive, since if there is strong dependence in space between two nearby locations at time t, then at $t + 1$, the monitor could be moved far away from both of these locations.

To illustrate a simple procedure for dynamic spatio-temporal design, consider Gaussian data and Gaussian process models:

$$\mathbf{Z}_t = \mathbf{H}_t \mathbf{Y}_t + \boldsymbol{\varepsilon}_t, \qquad \boldsymbol{\varepsilon}_t \sim ind.\ Gau(\mathbf{0}, \mathbf{R}_t), \tag{7.116}$$

$$\mathbf{Y}_t = \mathbf{M}_t \mathbf{Y}_{t-1} + \boldsymbol{\eta}_t, \qquad \boldsymbol{\eta}_t \sim ind.\ Gau(\mathbf{0}, \mathbf{Q}_t), \tag{7.117}$$

where, as before, $\mathbf{Z}_t$ is an m_t-dimensional data vector, $\mathbf{Y}_t$ is an n-dimensional process vector, $\mathbf{H}_t$ is the $m_t \times n$ data-mapping matrix, $\mathbf{M}_t$ is the $n \times n$

propagator matrix, and $\mathbf{R}_t$ and $\mathbf{Q}_t$ are the data-error and process-error covariance matrices, respectively. Thus, the "design" at a given time is what relates the observations $\mathbf{Z}_t$ to the process $\mathbf{Y}_t$; this is precisely the data-mapping matrix $\mathbf{H}_t$. As discussed in Section 7.1, the form of this matrix can be quite general, so long as it is varying in time and can accommodate different potential observation networks (designs) at each time. For illustration, it is perhaps simplest to think of this as simply the incidence matrix of zeros and ones described in Section 7.1.2. In this case, the process is gridded and the observation locations correspond to a specific grid point. Thus, if a sampling design were proposed, we could easily specify the form of $\mathbf{H}_t$.

Given the measurement equation (7.116) (i.e., the data model) and state equation (7.117) (i.e., the process model), we can obtain the sequential designs quite simply. For now, assume we know (or have estimated) the parameter matrices $\mathbf{M}_t$, $\mathbf{Q}_t$, and $\mathbf{R}_t$. From the discussion of the Kalman filter recursions given in Section 8.2.1, we can obtain the following recursive equations for the prediction-error covariances:

$$\mathbf{P}_{t|t} \equiv \text{var}(\mathbf{Y}_t | \mathbf{Z}_1, \ldots, \mathbf{Z}_t)$$
$$= (\mathbf{H}_t' \mathbf{R}_t^{-1} \mathbf{H}_t + \mathbf{P}_{t|t-1})^{-1}$$
$$- \mathbf{P}_{t|t-1} - \mathbf{P}_{t|t-1} \mathbf{H}_t' (\mathbf{H}_t \mathbf{P}_{t|t-1} \mathbf{H}_t' + \mathbf{R}_t)^{-1} \mathbf{H}_t \mathbf{P}_{t|t-1}, \qquad (7.118)$$

where

$$\mathbf{P}_{t|t-1} \equiv \text{var}(\mathbf{Y}_t | \mathbf{Z}_1, \ldots, \mathbf{Z}_{t-1})$$
$$= \mathbf{M}_t \mathbf{P}_{t-1|t-1} \mathbf{M}_t' + \mathbf{Q}_t. \qquad (7.119)$$

Now, given that $\mathbf{P}_{0|0}$ is specified, we could proceed with the recursion for $t = 1, 2, \ldots$, by first obtaining $\mathbf{P}_{t|t-1}$ from (7.119) and then using it to obtain $\mathbf{P}_{t|t}$ in (7.118). In practice, we need to specify $\mathbf{P}_{0|0}$, $\mathbf{M}_t$, $\mathbf{R}_t$, and $\mathbf{Q}_t$ to implement these recursions. Data may have been collected in a pilot study, from which estimates could be obtained (see Section 8.3 for the case where the matrices are not varying in time).

The recursion in (7.118) and (7.119) provides the mechanism for the dynamic design of spatio-temporal monitoring networks. If, as is typically the case, the parameter matrices are not time-varying, then the only temporal dependence in $\mathbf{P}_{t|t}$ comes from the design matrix $\mathbf{H}_t$. That is, it changes through time only as a function of the observation locations at each time. Thus, by allowing the monitoring locations to change with t, we should be able to find more efficient designs by optimizing some function of $\mathbf{P}_{t|t}$ (the *design criterion*). That is, we can search the space of potential designs to find the "optimal" design. For example, a common design criterion is the spatial average of the prediction error variance, which one would minimize with respect to $\mathbf{H}_t$, for $t = 1, 2, \ldots$.

Typically, it is not possible to search exhaustively the complete design space, but we can make use of algorithms that can find a "nearly optimal" or, at least, a "good" design. For example, one can use an exchange algorithm that evaluates the design criterion successively for different designs, and the design is updated by exchanging "bad" locations for "better" locations. Such algorithms are common in practice, and there are many different variants (e.g., see Cook and Nachtsheim, 1980; Nychka, Yang, and Royle, 1997).

Notice that the procedure described above does not take into account the uncertainty associated with the estimation of the model parameters; in that sense, it is EHM-based. In addition, this approach is greatly simplified by the Gaussian assumptions, since the prediction covariances do not depend on the data, only on the data locations and parameters. If one wants to take into account the parameter estimation and/or account for non-Gaussian or nonlinear structures, then one might consider a Bayesian approach to design [e.g., see Chaloner and Verdinelli (1995) for an overview; also see Diggle and Lophaven (2006)]. For example, the approach suggested by Müller (1999) relies on simulation and is useful for such problems. In essence, a Bayesian-based design seeks to maximize the expected value of some utility function of interest. Finding the design that maximizes this expected utility is typically intractable analytically, and one is forced either to simplify the utility greatly or to approximate the expected-utility maximization by simulation. Such approaches still require very computationally efficient optimization algorithms. Müller (1999) shows that this can be facilitated when augmenting the model by including the design as a random quantity. As in any relatively high-dimensional optimization problem, there is no guarantee to obtain *the* optimal design with this procedure, but it does give "good" designs (which is a huge help in complicated design problems). Royle and Wikle (2005) demonstrate this in the context of dynamical spatio-temporal design with a non-Gaussian data model and a DSTM, where good designs were chosen for the sampling locations associated with annual July brood-count surveys of North American waterfowl.

7.7   SWITCHING THE EMPHASIS OF TIME AND SPACE

This chapter has focused on an HM where a data model relates a vector of spatial observations at a given time either to a true spatial process evolving over time, or to a spectral representation of such a spatial process evolving over time. This perspective is motivated at least in part by our preference that the more natural (i.e., physical, biological, etc.) way to present a spatio-temporal process is for a spatial field to evolve over time. However, from a modeling perspective, it may be more efficient to consider the alternative perspective of a time series varying in space, though this is done at the expense of a "dynamical" interpretation.

Consider a situation in which we have many more time observations than spatial observations (i.e., $m \ll T$). We can define $\mathbf{Z}_i \equiv (Z(\mathbf{s}_i; 1), \ldots, Z(\mathbf{s}_i; T))'$ to be the T-dimensional vector of observations at location $\mathbf{s}_i$, for times $t = 1, \ldots, T$ and $i = 1, \ldots, m$. We could then characterize the temporal behavior functionally in terms of a dimension-reduced (say,

$q < m << T$) set of basis functions:

$$\mathbf{Z}_i = \mathbf{\Psi}\boldsymbol{\beta}_i + \boldsymbol{\varepsilon}_i, \qquad i = 1, \ldots, m,$$

where $\mathbf{\Psi}$ is a $T \times q$ matrix of basis-function coefficients, $\boldsymbol{\beta}_i \equiv (\beta_i(1), \ldots, \beta_i(q))'$ is a q-dimensional vector of coefficients for the ith spatial location, and $\{\boldsymbol{\varepsilon}_i\}$ is a T-dimensional error process. In this case, each basis function (column of $\mathbf{\Psi}$) is a function of time (i.e., a time series). These might be chosen deterministically (e.g, Fourier, wavelets, bisquares) or from the data (e.g., EOFs, splines), just as with the spatially referenced basis functions discussed in Section 7.1.3. Now, it is natural to re-orient the coefficients $\{\boldsymbol{\beta}_i : i = 1, \ldots, m\}$ into spatial processes. For example, fix the jth coefficient and let i vary over $\{1, 2, \ldots, m\}$. Define

$$\boldsymbol{\beta}(j) = (\beta_1(j), \ldots, \beta_m(j))', \qquad j = 1, \ldots, q,$$

which corresponds to an m-dimensional spatial field for the jth basis-function coefficients. In an HM context, we could then specify a spatial process model for each of $\boldsymbol{\beta}(j); j = 1, \ldots, q$ (see Chapter 4). It may even be the case that an additional spectral expansion/dimension reduction could be considered on these spatial fields. For example, write

$$\boldsymbol{\beta}(j) - \mathbf{\Phi}\boldsymbol{\alpha}(j) + \boldsymbol{\nu}(j),$$

where $\mathbf{\Phi}$ is an $m \times p_\alpha$ matrix of spatial-basis-function coefficients, $\boldsymbol{\alpha}(j)$ is the associated p_α-dimensional vector of spectral coefficients, and $\boldsymbol{\nu}(j)$ is an error process that accounts for the variation remaining after the dimension reduction. See Wikle and Anderson (2003) for an implementation of such an approach applied to modeling spatio-temporal distributions of tornado counts given climatological time series. In addition, Sansó, Schmidt, and Nobre (2008) give a discussion of such models from the perspective of the linear model of coregionalization.

To sum up, although switching the modeling emphasis of a spatio-temporal process from time to space can be a very useful modeling strategy, it is not dynamical in the sense of the earlier sections of this chapter. Consequently, it may be difficult to imagine real-world processes whose etiologies are consistent with such a formulation.

7.8 BIBLIOGRAPHIC NOTES

General Hierarchical Formulation

As discussed in the Bibilographic Notes of Chapter 3 (Section 3.7), the motivation for hierarchical modeling has been around in Statistics for quite some time. Almost any modern book on Bayesian Statistics (e.g., Carlin and Louis, 2000; Gelman et al., 2003) cover this topic in detail. Furthermore, modern approaches to time series analysis (e.g., West and Harrison, 1997; Shumway and Stoffer, 2006; Prado and West, 2010) give significant coverage to hierarchical representations. This is also the case with modern treatments of spatial statistics (e.g., Banerjee, Carlin, and Gelfand 2004; Diggle and Ribeiro, 2007). Specific discussion of dynamical linear models in the spatial context can be found in Gamerman and Lopes (2006). Our view of hierarchical modeling is based on the important paper of Berliner (1996), which discusses hierarchical modeling of environmental time series from the perspective of a series of conditional models for "data given process and parameters," "process given parameters," and "parameters." This approach is further developed by Wikle, Berliner, and Cressie (1998), Berliner, Wikle, and Cressie (2000), Wikle et al. (2001), Berliner, Milliff, and Wikle (2003), Wikle (2003a,b), and Wikle and Hooten (2010), among many others discussed here and in other chapters.

Data Models—Incidence Matrices and Change-of-Support

Incidence matrices are essentially design matrices for mapping a spatial process vector to a spatial data vector by using ones and zeros. This perspective is illustrated in Wikle, Berliner, and Cressie (1998), Royle et al. (1999), Wikle and Royle (1999), and Wikle et al. (2001).

Spatial change of support is outlined in Section 4.1.3. An excellent review of this problem and traditional modeling approaches addressing it is given in Gotway and Young (2002). The hierarchical perspective is given in Mugglin, Carlin, and Gelfand (2000) and Gelfand, Zhu, and Carlin (2001). Our perspective, which implies a specific form of the data-mapping matrix in the hierarchical DSTM context, is motivated by Wikle and Berliner (2005). Recent examples of hierarchical change-of-support for spatio-temporal data are given in Berrocal, Gelfand, and Holland (2010) and Sahu, Gelfand, and Holland (2009).

Data Models—Spectral Decomposition

We use the term "spectral decomposition" quite broadly in this book. That is, representation of the spatial process vector for a given time, as the product of a basis function matrix and a random vector (which need not be spatially referenced), is a "spectral" expansion. In this respect, there is a very large literature in which such decompositions are used in DSTMs, with the primary difference being which basis set is being used, and, to a lesser extent, the type of estimation being employed. Examples include empirical orthogonal functions, Fourier series, bisquares, polynomials, splines, and multiresolution wavelets (e.g., Wikle, 1996; Mardia et al., 1998; Wikle and Cressie, 1999; Berliner, Wikle, and Cressie, 2000; Stroud, Müller, and Sansó, 2001; Wikle et al., 2001; Cressie and Wikle, 2002; Xu, Wikle, and Fox, 2005; Johannesson, Cressie, and Huang, 2007; Malmberg et al., 2008; Kang and Cressie, 2011; Cressie, Shi, and Kang, 2010; Kang, Cressie, and Shi, 2010). In these formulations, the spectral coefficients are not typically spatially referenced, but correspond to some hidden process that is transformed into physical space by multiplying by the basis functions. In addition, the basis functions in these settings are typically assumed known. For an overview of these methods, see Wikle (2010b).

Data Models—Parameterized Low-Rank Expansions
An alternative perspective is to allow the random process to correspond to a finite number of "reference" spatial locations and then to build dependence by smoothing these. Indeed, this is the primary motivation behind so-called "process convolution" methods in spatial statistics (e.g., Barry and Ver Hoef, 1996; Ver Hoef and Barry, 1998; Higdon, 1998). In the discrete-convolution setting and the linear model of coregionalization, one can then apply a dynamical linear spatio-temporal process model on the process at the reference locations (e.g., Calder, Holloman, and Higdon, 2002; Sansó, Schmidt, and Nobre, 2008; Lemos and Sansó, 2009). Alternatively, one can consider kernels derived from kriging-based support points, as done for so-called "predictive processes" (Banerjee et al., 2008; Finley et al., 2009). The kernels depend on parameters, which limits the size of datasets that the predictive-process approach can handle.

Rather than fix the basis functions or parameterize the kernels, one could seek to estimate the transformation matrix directly, as with factor analysis in multivariate statistics (e.g., Wang and Wall, 2003; Forni et al., 2005). An example of this in the DSTM setting is given in Calder (2007), Lopes, Salazar, and Gamerman (2008), and Sáfadi and Peña (2008). In this case, as with factor analysis, there are fundamental identifiability issues associated with estimating both the data-mapping matrix and the transition matrix in the dynamical process model; see also Strickland et al. (2011). More generally, this is just the "blind source separation" problem in Engineering (e.g., Jutten, Herault, and Guerin, 1988), and there are many algorithmic approaches to dealing with the problem [e.g., independent component analysis; see Hyvärinen, Karhunen, and Oja (2001)]. Knuth (1999, 2005) considers Bayesian approaches for source separation. For an overview of blind source separation and independent component analysis, see Choi et al. (2005).

Data Models—Alternative System Reduction Approaches
There is a long history in the Control Engineering literature of seeking optimal dimension reduction for dynamical systems (e.g., Kailath, 1980; Moore, 1981). Although not specific to spatio-temporal systems, *per se*, these methods are applicable to the kinds of spatio-temporal processes one encounters in the environmental sciences. For example, Farrell and Ioannou (2001) discuss stochastic optimals, EOFs, and balanced truncation in the context of continuous-time spatio-temporal processes in Atmospheric Science. Crommelin and Majda (2004) compare various optimal basis methodologies for geophysical processes, including principal interaction patterns (PIPs) and optimal persistence patterns (OPPs). More generally, Antoulas (2005) provides an overview of methods that have been used to approximate large-scale dynamical systems.

Data Models—Nonlinear and Non-Gaussian Models
Nonlinear data models are typically specified by the scientific problem at hand. Alternatively, one might include a transformation of the process at this level of the hierarchy (e.g., Sansó and Guenni, 1999). More common is the case of non-Gaussian data. Such models were specified in the spatial statistics literature by Diggle, Tawn, and Moyeed (1998) and have been considered by

numerous authors in the context of state-space models (e.g., Kitagawa, 1987; Fahrmeir and Kaufmann, 1991; Carlin, Polson, and Stoffer, 1992; Fahrmeir, 1992; Gamerman, 1998). The use of such data models in spatio-temporal processes is also common (e.g., Brix and Diggle, 2001; Wikle, 2003b; Wikle and Hooten, 2006; Hooten et al., 2007; Hooten and Wikle, 2008). In each of these contexts, one assumes that the data are from an exponential family and some transformation of the true spatio-temporal dynamical process is Gaussian. There are situations with non-Gaussian data where the usual exponential-family/canonical-link formulations may not be the most realistic, and one has to consider data models that are more appropriate for the process (e.g., Cangelosi and Hooten, 2009).

Basic Linear Process Model Specifications

Linear dynamical process evolution is certainly well characterized in the multivariate time series literature (see Chapter 3 for references). Bennett (1979) and Rouhani and Wackernagel (1990) considered time series at each spatial location and developed models accordingly. In general, these approaches can be included in the DSTM framework as in traditional state-space modeling. The challenges come as one must reduce the dimensionality of the parameter space or the process itself to avoid the curse of dimensionality. Huang and Cressie (1996) considered a simple dynamical parameterization in the DSTM, where the propagator was just a scalar multiplied by the identity matrix. Wikle, Berliner, and Cressie (1998) considered a more complicated hierarchical spatio-temporal model, which included seasonality, trends, and a dynamical process that was parameterized by a lagged-nearest-neighbor propagator. An original feature of this model was the use of spatial processes for parameters, which fits nicely into the hierarchical modeling framework.

PDE-Based Process Parameterizations

The use of PDEs to motivate statistical models is not new (e.g., see Hotelling, 1927). In fact, as outlined in Section 6.3, the connection between stochastic PDEs and spatial and spatio-temporal covariances is fundamental in spatial statistics (e.g., Heine, 1955; Whittle, 1954, 1962; Jones and Zhang, 1997). Mollison discusses diffusion and growth processes to motivate "spatial contact" models. More recently, the use of PDEs to motivate spatial and spatio-temporal statistical models was facilitated by the development of hierarchical Bayesian methods (e.g., Royle et al., 1999; Wikle et al., 2001; Berliner, Milliff, and Wikle, 2003; Wikle, 2003b; Wikle, Berliner, and Milliff, 2003; Hooten and Wikle, 2008; Malmberg et al., 2008; Cangelosi and Hooten, 2009; Stroud et al., 2010; Zheng and Aukema, 2011; Lindgren et al., 2011). Note that statistical fitting (e.g., parameter estimation), as distinct from model motivation, of PDE models in a scientific context is prevalent in several disciplines, including pharmacokinetics (e.g., Gelman, Bois, and Jiang, 1996), virology (e.g., Huang, Liu, and Wu, 2006), and ecology (Haario et al., 2006). A general approach in the context of functional data analysis is presented by Ramsay et al. (2007).

IDE-Based Process Parameterizations

Integro-difference equations (IDEs) have also proven to be a useful framework to motivate dynamical process models. Deterministic forms of IDE models have been useful in population ecology (e.g., Kot, 1992; Kot, Lewis, and van den Driessche, 1996). Spatio-temporal statistical formulations are presented in Wikle (1996), Wikle and Cressie (1999), Wikle (2002a), Huang and Hsu (2004), Xu, Wikle, and Fox (2005), Dewar, Scerri, and Kadirkamanathan (2009), and Scerri, Dewar, and Kadirkamanathan (2009). The implied covariance structure of these models is discussed in Brown et al. (2000) and Storvik, Frigessi, and Hirst (2002).

Reduced-Dimension Process Models

The spectral-representation, low-rank-parameterization, and IDE references listed above generally involve reduced dimensions. Most of them contain fairly simple multivariate-time-series process models, where dimension reduction follows from parameterizations of the process' propagator and covariance matrices. As discussed in Wikle and Cressie (1999), Xu and Wikle (2007), and Chapter 8, it is straightforward to perform estimation and prediction for such processes using Kalman filtering/smoothing, method-of-moments, EM algorithm, or fully Bayesian methodologies.

Multiresolution Process Models

The essence of the change-of-resolution multiresolution models presented here can be found in Chou, Willsky, and Nikoukhah (1994) and Fieguth et al. (1995). The models migrated into the Statistics literature through papers by Gelpke and Künsch (2001), Huang, Cressie, and Gabrosek (2002), Johannesson and Cressie (2004), and Johannesson, Cressie, and Huang (2007). Clearly, many of the spectral approaches described previously are also multiresolution in that the basis functions correspond to different spatial scales. For example, Nychka, Wikle, and Royle (2002) consider multiresolution wavelet basis functions to model spatially nonstationary processes. Such processes can be allowed to vary dynamically as well (Berliner, Wikle, and Milliff, 1999; Wikle et al., 2001). For a more general discussion of Bayesian multiscale modeling, see Ferreira and Lee (2007).

Nonlinear Process Models

Nonlinear statistical process models are most often considered in the time series literature (e.g., Priestley, 1988; Tong, 1990; Young, 2000; Chatfield, 2004; Fan and Yao, 2005). Historically, the papers by Jones (1965, 1978) were very insightful with regard to nonlinear prediction and nonlinear autoregressive processes. State-dependent models are common in spatio-temporal applications (e.g., Hughes and Guttorp, 1994; Berliner, Wikle, and Cressie, 2000). Relatively few examples exist for more general nonlinear spatio-temporal dynamical process models. Wendt, Irwin, and Cressie (2004) give a Bayesian waypoint analysis, where the state is the trajectory of an object moving according to nonlinear equations of motion. Lu et al. (2009) describe a flexible, adaptively varying coefficient model that can accommodate nonlinear spatio-temporal interactions, as well as spatial nonstationarity and non-Gaussian data models. Wikle and Hooten (2010) show that general quadratic nonlinearity (GQN) is present in many real-world processes (e.g., Kondrashov et al., 2005), and this can be used to motivate statistical models (e.g., Wikle, Berliner, and Milliff, 2003; Wikle and Hooten, 2006; Hooten et al., 2007; Hooten and Wikle, 2008). This structure is also present in the multivariate functional coefficient autoregressive formulation for multivariate time series described in Harvill and Ray (2006). Functional polynomial regression models for time series are discussed in Yan and Müller (2010). Wikle and Holan (2011) consider a hierarchical formulation of spatio-temporal polynomial models in an IDE framework with stochastic search variable selection.

There are many fine discussions of nonlinear stochastic models in the geophysics literature, (e.g., Majda and Wang, 2006). For example, Majda, Abramov, and Grote (2005) consider such processes from an information theory perspective, and Majda and Franzke (2009) consider reduced dimensional EOF formulations of stochastic climate models.

Individual- or agent-based models (e.g., Lee et al., 1990; Grimm and Railsback, 2005) for spatio-temporal processes (e.g., Smith et al., 2002) are just now finding their way into the Statistics literature (e.g., Hooten and Wikle, 2010). There are strong connections between these models and models for non-Gaussian spatio-temporal processes (e.g., Zhu, Huang, and Wu, 2005; Royle and Kery, 2007). In a similar spirit, Fewster (2003) builds a spatio-temporal model for species spread, focusing on movement between individual sites.

Nonlinear effects of continuous covariates and temporal trends in spatio-temporal processes can be accommodated through nonparametric and semiparametric models. For example, Fahrmeir, Kneib, and Lang (2004) demonstrate such models using penalized structured additive regression in a Bayesian setting. Augustin et al. (2009) illustrate the use of generalized additive mixed models for spatio-temporal forest health data.

Multivariate Process Models

In many respects, statisticians are a bit "behind the curve" when it comes to formulating and implementing multivariate DSTMs. Note that such models are commonly (and operationally) implemented in the geophysical sciences in the context of data assimilation [e.g., see the overviews in Daley (1991), Ghil and Malanotte-Rizzoli (1991), Talagrand (1997), Bennett (2002), and Kalnay (2003)].

In Statistics, science-driven hierarchical multivariate spatial models were proposed by Royle and Berliner (1999). Although related to the geostatistical concepts of "linear models of coregionalization" [e.g., see the review in Wackernagel (2003); also see Schmidt and Gelfand (2003) and Gelfand et al. (2004)], it differs fundamentally in the emphasis on science-based conditional modeling (see Section 4.1.5). This idea was used in a dynamical process model in Berliner, Milliff, and Wikle (2003), where high-dimensional spatio-temporal dynamical processes (atmosphere and ocean) were coupled. Motivated by the spatio-temporal dynamical model of Tonellato (2001), Shaddick and Wakefield (2002) consider a multivariate DSTM for multiple pollutants. The multivariate process-convolution approach, developed by Ver Hoef and Barry (1998), and the linear model of coregionalization can be used in the hierarchical framework to motivate DSTMs for multivariate processes (e.g., Gelfand, Banerjee, and Gamerman, 2005; Calder, 2007; Sahu and Challenor, 2008). Daniels, Zhou, and Zou (2006) consider the conditional specification of spatio-temporal models, more from a Markov-random-field perspective, although their methodology can be used for geostatistical processes of point or areal support.

Parameter Specifications
The essence of hierarchical modeling for spatio-temporal processes is the specification of parameter models at lower levels of the hierarchy. As illustrated in Wikle, Berliner, and Cressie (1998) and Gelfand et al. (2003), one can easily place spatial process priors on lower levels of the hierarchy for parameters of a dynamical spatio-temporal or purely spatial process. This is the obvious construction in hierarchical modeling and is one of the advantages of taking Berliner's (1996) view of hierarchical modeling of environmental processes.

Perhaps more critical are the distributions one might place on parameters at lower levels of the hierarchy, particularly the choice of hyperparameters. Overviews of these issues relative to hierarchical spatial processes are given in Banerjee, Carlin, and Gelfand (2004), Diggle and Ribeiro (2007), and Wikle (2010a).

Dynamical Design
The design of spatial monitoring networks is well covered in the literature [e.g., see reviews in Müller (2000); also see Le and Zidek (2006), Zimmerman (2006) and Diggle and Ribeiro (2007)]. In addition, ideas related to adaptive spatial designs were presented in Chao and Thompson (2001). Designs for dynamical processes were discussed by Titterington (1980). Bueso, Angulo, and Alonso (1998) use a state-space model to obtain an optimal static spatial design. The notion of choosing the design locations as a function of the underlying dynamical process was proposed in an adaptive-weather-observation context by Berliner, Lu, and Snyder (1999). In a series of papers, Wikle and Royle (1999, 2005) and Hooten et al. (2009) illustrate general dynamical design for monitoring networks for Gaussian and non-Gaussian data with underlying Gaussian dynamical processes.

Switching Time and Space
The formal development of semiparametric statistical models with emphasis on spatially varying time series is considered by Delicado et al. (2010) and Giraldo et al. (2010). This is summarized in the discussion of Mateu (2010), who describes how one might formulate an IDE model that is continuous in time yet discrete in space.

CHAPTER 8

Hierarchical DSTMs: Implementation and Inference

In general, implementation and inference for DSTMs in the context of complicated hierarchical models is problem-specific. However, there are some common approaches that are used in both the EHM and BHM frameworks to find the filtering and forecast posterior distributions of the process and to perform inference on the parameters. We note that implementation approaches for DSTMs are rapidly evolving and still very much the subject of intensive research. Furthermore, these methodologies are linked very closely with the state of computing technology. In this chapter we give an overview, and we point to the many books, book chapters, and papers devoted to these implementation issues in the Bibliographic Notes in Section 8.5.

8.1 DSTM PROCESS: GENERAL IMPLEMENTATION AND INFERENCE

In this section, we (temporarily) assume that all parameters are fixed and *known*, and we focus our general discussion of implementation and inference on the state process. Thus, when denoting conditional distributions, we choose not to feature the parameters unless absolutely necessary.

Generally, the data model is

$$[\{\mathbf{Z}_t : t = 1, \ldots, T\} | \{\mathbf{Y}_t : t = 0, \ldots, T\}],$$

where $\mathbf{Z}_t$ is an m_t-dimensional vector of spatial observations at time t, and $\mathbf{Y}_t$ is an n-dimensional vector representation of the state process for n spatial locations at time t. The models discussed in Section 7.1 provide a rich source of examples.

Statistics for Spatio-Temporal Data, by Noel Cressie and Christopher K. Wikle
Copyright © 2011 John Wiley & Sons, Inc.

At the next level, we specify the state-evolution distributions; in the case where the state process has first-order Markovian evolution, we specify

$$[\mathbf{Y}_0] \quad \text{and} \quad [\mathbf{Y}_t|\mathbf{Y}_{t-1}]; \quad t = 1, \ldots, T.$$

Examples of such evolution distributions are given in Section 7.2. Typically, inference on the state process for such models is performed sequentially, and this will also be our focus here.

8.1.1   Sequential Implementation: General

Before discussing sequential approaches for state-process inference, we establish some useful notation. Let $\mathbf{Z}_{1:t} \equiv \{\mathbf{Z}_1, \ldots, \mathbf{Z}_t\}$ and $\mathbf{Y}_{0:t} \equiv \{\mathbf{Y}_0, \ldots, \mathbf{Y}_t\}$, for $t = 0, 1, \ldots T$. In addition, assume we employ a first-order Markov assumption, such that

$$[\mathbf{Y}_{0:T}] = [\mathbf{Y}_0] \prod_{t=1}^{T} [\mathbf{Y}_t|\mathbf{Y}_{t-1}], \tag{8.1}$$

where $[\mathbf{Y}_t|\mathbf{Y}_{t-1}]$ is the *evolution distribution*, and $[\mathbf{Y}_0]$ is an initial distribution that might in fact be based on all data up to and including $t = 0$, the reference starting time.

As discussed in Section 7.1, we assume that the observations in $\mathbf{Z}_{1:t}$ are conditionally independent, given $\mathbf{Y}_{0:t}$, and that for a fixed t the conditional-probability density functions of $\mathbf{Z}_t$, given $\mathbf{Y}_{0:t}$, in fact only depend on $\mathbf{Y}_t$; $t = 1, 2, \ldots T$. That is, the data model is

$$[\mathbf{Z}_{1:T}|\mathbf{Y}_{0:T}] = \prod_{t=1}^{T} [\mathbf{Z}_t|\mathbf{Y}_t], \tag{8.2}$$

where $[\mathbf{Z}_t|\mathbf{Y}_t]$ is sometimes called the measurement distribution.

Under the evolution-distribution assumptions (8.1) and the data-model assumptions (8.2), Bayes' rule can be used to find filtering and forecast distributions. That is, to predict $\mathbf{Y}_{0:T}$ in (8.1), given the observations $\mathbf{Z}_{1:T}$, we can write the posterior distribution of $\mathbf{Y}_{0:T}$ as

$$[\mathbf{Y}_{0:T}|\mathbf{Z}_{1:T}] \propto [\mathbf{Y}_0] \prod_{t=1}^{T} [\mathbf{Z}_t|\mathbf{Y}_t][\mathbf{Y}_t|\mathbf{Y}_{t-1}]. \tag{8.3}$$

The key to the sequential approach is that, as new data become available, one seeks to update the previous filtering distribution. That is, the posterior distribution based on the data up to time $t - 1$ becomes the prior for the distribution for data up to time t. Specifically, we seek the *forecast distribution*,

$$[\mathbf{Y}_t|\mathbf{Z}_{1:t-1}], \tag{8.4}$$

and the *filtering distribution*,

$$[\mathbf{Y}_t|\mathbf{Z}_{1:t}], \tag{8.5}$$

for $t = 1, \ldots, T$.

The *forecast distribution* (8.4) can be obtained by considering it in terms of the filtering distribution at the previous time:

$$[\mathbf{Y}_t|\mathbf{Z}_{1:t-1}] = \int [\mathbf{Y}_t, \mathbf{Y}_{t-1}|\mathbf{Z}_{1:t-1}]d\mathbf{Y}_{t-1}$$

$$= \int [\mathbf{Y}_t|\mathbf{Y}_{t-1}][\mathbf{Y}_{t-1}|\mathbf{Z}_{1:t-1}]d\mathbf{Y}_{t-1}, \tag{8.6}$$

where the second equality follows from the conditional-independence assumption. The first distribution in the integrand of (8.6) is the process-evolution distribution, and the second distribution is the filtering (posterior) distribution for the state at the previous time. Forecast distributions beyond one time step can be obtained similarly.

Now, the *filtering distribution* can be obtained by Bayes' rule:

$$[\mathbf{Y}_t|\mathbf{Z}_{1:t}] = [\mathbf{Y}_t|\mathbf{Z}_t, \mathbf{Z}_{1:t-1}]$$

$$\propto [\mathbf{Z}_t|\mathbf{Y}_t, \mathbf{Z}_{1:t-1}][\mathbf{Y}_t|\mathbf{Z}_{1:t-1}]$$

$$= [\mathbf{Z}_t|\mathbf{Y}_t][\mathbf{Y}_t|\mathbf{Z}_{1:t-1}], \tag{8.7}$$

where the first distribution on the right-hand side of (8.7) is obtained from the data model, and the second distribution is the forecast distribution (8.6). If we iterate between the filtering distribution and the forecast distribution as new data become available, we obtain the following sequences of distributions: $[\mathbf{Y}_1|\mathbf{Z}_1],[\mathbf{Y}_2|\mathbf{Z}_1],[\mathbf{Y}_2|\mathbf{Z}_{1:2}], \ldots, [\mathbf{Y}_T|\mathbf{Z}_{1:T-1}], [\mathbf{Y}_T|\mathbf{Z}_{1:T}]$. This sequential procedure is known as *filtering*.

The term *smoothing* refers to obtaining $[\mathbf{Y}_t|\mathbf{Z}_{1:T}]$, the distribution of the state at any time $t \in \{1, 2, \ldots, T\}$, given all relevant data from time 1 to T, which includes data collected *after* time t up to time T. Obviously, for $t = T$, the smoothing distribution is just the filtering distribution.

We can write the smoothing distribution as

$$[\mathbf{Y}_t|\mathbf{Z}_{1:T}] = \int [\mathbf{Y}_t|\mathbf{Y}_{t+1}, \mathbf{Z}_{1:T}][\mathbf{Y}_{t+1}|\mathbf{Z}_{1:T}]d\mathbf{Y}_{t+1}. \tag{8.8}$$

The first distribution on the right-hand side of (8.8) can be written as

$$[\mathbf{Y}_t|\mathbf{Y}_{t+1}, \mathbf{Z}_{1:T}] = [\mathbf{Y}_t|\mathbf{Y}_{t+1}, \mathbf{Z}_{1:t}], \tag{8.9}$$

since $\{\mathbf{Z}_{t+1}, \ldots, \mathbf{Z}_T\}$ are independent of $\mathbf{Y}_t$ given $\mathbf{Y}_{t+1}$. Now, note that Bayes' rule gives,

$$[\mathbf{Y}_t|\mathbf{Y}_{t+1}, \mathbf{Z}_{1:t}] \propto [\mathbf{Y}_{t+1}|\mathbf{Y}_t, \mathbf{Z}_{1:t}][\mathbf{Y}_t|\mathbf{Z}_{1:t}] = [\mathbf{Y}_{t+1}|\mathbf{Y}_t][\mathbf{Y}_t|\mathbf{Z}_{1:t}], \qquad (8.10)$$

where the first term on the right-hand side of (8.10) is just the evolution distribution, and the second term is the filtering distribution for time t. Thus, given the filtering and evolution distributions, a *sequential smoothing algorithm* written in pseudo code can be constructed as follows:

For $t = T - 1$ to 1

1. Obtain $[\mathbf{Y}_t|\mathbf{Y}_{t+1}, \mathbf{Z}_{1:t}]$ via (8.10), making use of the filtering distribution, $[\mathbf{Y}_t|\mathbf{Z}_{1:t}]$, and the evolution distribution, $[\mathbf{Y}_{t+1}|\mathbf{Y}_t]$.
2. Obtain the smoothing distribution, $[\mathbf{Y}_t|\mathbf{Z}_{1:T}]$, from (8.8), making use of the smoothing distribution from the subsequent time, $[\mathbf{Y}_{t+1}|\mathbf{Z}_{1:T}]$, obtained for the current time, t.

end

8.2 INFERENCE FOR THE DSTM PROCESS: LINEAR/GAUSSIAN MODELS

In general, it may be difficult to get explicit analytical formulations for the forecast, filtering, and smoothing distributions (8.6), (8.7), and (8.8), respectively. However, in the case of an observation operator that is linear, an evolution operator that is linear, and Gaussian error distributions, we can obtain the forecast, filtering, and smoothing distributions explicitly. This results in the well known *Kalman filter* and *Kalman smoother* recursions.

8.2.1 Kalman Filter

The *Kalman filter* is ideal for sequential updating, where the operators are linear and the error distributions are Gaussian (e.g., Kalman, 1960; Jazwinski, 1970; Anderson and Moore, 1979; West and Harrison, 1997; Wikle and Cressie, 1999). It can be derived from many different perspectives. Here, we use the general Bayesian formulas presented, for example, in Jazwinski (1970), Meinhold and Singpurwalla (1983), and West and Harrison (1997).

Define the conditional expectations for the filtering and forecast distributions as $\mathbf{Y}_{t|t} \equiv E[\mathbf{Y}_t|\mathbf{Z}_{1:t}]$ and $\mathbf{Y}_{t|t-1} \equiv E[\mathbf{Y}_t|\mathbf{Z}_{1:t-1}]$, respectively. Define the conditional error covariance matrices for filtering and forecasting, respectively, as

$$\mathbf{P}_{t|t} \equiv E[(\mathbf{Y}_t - \mathbf{Y}_{t|t})(\mathbf{Y}_t - \mathbf{Y}_{t|t})'|\mathbf{Z}_{1:t}]$$

and

$$\mathbf{P}_{t|t-1} \equiv E[(\mathbf{Y}_t - \mathbf{Y}_{t|t-1})(\mathbf{Y}_t - \mathbf{Y}_{t|t-1})'|\mathbf{Z}_{1:t-1}].$$

Consider the measurement distribution, $[\mathbf{Z}_t|\mathbf{Y}_t]$, given by the model,

$$\mathbf{Z}_t = \mathbf{H}_t\mathbf{Y}_t + \boldsymbol{\varepsilon}_t; \quad \boldsymbol{\varepsilon}_t \sim ind.\,Gau(\mathbf{0}, \mathbf{R}_t), \tag{8.11}$$

where $\mathbf{H}_t$ is the observation operator that maps the process to the observations, and $\mathbf{R}_t$ is the potentially time-varying measurement (or data) error covariance matrix, where the measurement errors are assumed to be independent across time.

Also, consider the evolution (or process) distribution, $[\mathbf{Y}_t|\mathbf{Y}_{t-1}]$, given by the VAR(1) model:

$$\mathbf{Y}_t = \mathbf{M}_t\mathbf{Y}_{t-1} + \boldsymbol{\eta}_t; \quad \boldsymbol{\eta}_t \sim ind.\,Gau(\mathbf{0}, \mathbf{Q}_t), \tag{8.12}$$

where $\mathbf{M}_t$ is the (linear) model operator, or propagator matrix, that maps the evolution of the process in time, and $\mathbf{Q}_t$ is a covariance matrix representing temporally independent stochastic forcing, or features not resolved by the model. Typically, it is assumed that the measurement-error process and the evolution-error process are mutually independent for all time. We have also assumed that all error processes have mean zero. These assumptions of independence and zero means can be relaxed (e.g., Anderson and Moore, 1979).

Using standard conditional-expectation and conditional-variance calculations, the *forecast distribution* is found to be

$$\mathbf{Y}_t|\mathbf{Z}_{1:t-1} \sim Gau(\mathbf{Y}_{t|t-1}, \mathbf{P}_{t|t-1}),$$

with mean vector and covariance matrix given, respectively, by

$$\mathbf{Y}_{t|t-1} = E(E(\mathbf{Y}_t|\mathbf{Y}_{t-1})|\mathbf{Z}_{1:t-1}) = E(\mathbf{M}_t\mathbf{Y}_{t-1}|\mathbf{Z}_{1:t-1}) - \mathbf{M}_t\mathbf{Y}_{t-1|t-1}, \tag{8.13}$$

and

$$\begin{aligned}
\mathbf{P}_{t|t-1} &= E(\mathrm{var}(\mathbf{Y}_t|\mathbf{Y}_{t-1})|\mathbf{Z}_{1:t-1}) + \mathrm{var}(E(\mathbf{Y}_t|\mathbf{Y}_{t-1})|\mathbf{Z}_{1:t-1}) \\
&= E(\mathbf{Q}_t|\mathbf{Z}_{1:t-1}) + \mathrm{var}(\mathbf{M}_t\mathbf{Y}_{t-1}|\mathbf{Z}_{1:t-1}) \\
&= \mathbf{Q}_t + \mathbf{M}_t\mathbf{P}_{t-1|t-1}\mathbf{M}_t'. \tag{8.14}
\end{aligned}$$

In addition, the *filtering distribution* is given by

$$\mathbf{Y}_t|\mathbf{Z}_{1:t} \sim Gau(\mathbf{Y}_{t|t}, \mathbf{P}_{t|t}), \tag{8.15}$$

where

$$\mathbf{Y}_{t|t} = \mathbf{P}_{t|t}(\mathbf{H}'_t\mathbf{R}_t^{-1}\mathbf{Z}_t + \mathbf{P}_{t|t-1}^{-1}\mathbf{Y}_{t|t-1}),\tag{8.16}$$

and

$$\mathbf{P}_{t|t} = (\mathbf{H}'_t\mathbf{R}_t^{-1}\mathbf{H}_t + \mathbf{P}_{t|t-1}^{-1})^{-1}.\tag{8.17}$$

Using the Sherman–Morrison–Woodbury matrix identities (e.g., Henderson and Searle, 1981; Shumway and Stoffer, 2000, p. 317),

$$(\mathbf{A}'\mathbf{B}^{-1}\mathbf{A} + \mathbf{D}^{-1})^{-1} = \mathbf{D} - \mathbf{D}\mathbf{A}'(\mathbf{A}\mathbf{D}\mathbf{A}' + \mathbf{B})^{-1}\mathbf{A}\mathbf{D},\tag{8.18}$$

$$(\mathbf{A}'\mathbf{B}^{-1}\mathbf{A} + \mathbf{D}^{-1})^{-1}\mathbf{A}'\mathbf{B}^{-1} = \mathbf{D}\mathbf{A}'(\mathbf{A}\mathbf{D}\mathbf{A}' + \mathbf{B})^{-1},\tag{8.19}$$

we can write the mean and variance of (8.15) equivalently as

$$\mathbf{Y}_{t|t} = \mathbf{Y}_{t|t-1} + \mathbf{K}_t(\mathbf{Z}_t - \mathbf{H}_t\mathbf{Y}_{t|t-1})\tag{8.20}$$

and

$$\mathbf{P}_{t|t} = (\mathbf{I} - \mathbf{K}_t\mathbf{H}_t)\mathbf{P}_{t|t-1},\tag{8.21}$$

respectively, where $\mathbf{K}_t$ is called the *Kalman gain or gain matrix* and is given by

$$\mathbf{K}_t \equiv \mathbf{P}_{t|t-1}\mathbf{H}'_t(\mathbf{H}'_t\mathbf{P}_{t|t-1}\mathbf{H}_t + \mathbf{R}_t)^{-1}.\tag{8.22}$$

Assuming the parameter matrices, $\mathbf{H}_t$, $\mathbf{M}_t$, $\mathbf{Q}_t$, and $\mathbf{R}_t$ are known, for $t = 1, \ldots, T$, and given initial conditions (or background state) $\mathbf{Y}_{0|0} \equiv \boldsymbol{\mu}_0$, $\mathbf{P}_{0|0} \equiv \boldsymbol{\Sigma}_0$, the following *Kalman filter algorithm* (written in pseudo code) can be used to obtain sequential estimates of the state, along with their mean squared prediction error matrices:

For $t = 1$ to T

1. Obtain the forecast-distribution mean, $\mathbf{Y}_{t|t-1}$, and covariance matrix, $\mathbf{P}_{t|t-1}$, from (8.13) and (8.14), respectively.
2. Obtain the gain, $\mathbf{K}_t$, and the filtering-distribution mean, $\mathbf{Y}_{t|t}$, and covariance matrix, $\mathbf{P}_{t|t}$, from (8.22), (8.20), and (8.21), respectively.

end

For time periods in which there are no observations, the filter-update step is simply skipped, and the filtering-distribution means and covariances are $\mathbf{Y}_{t|t} \equiv \mathbf{Y}_{t|t-1}$ and $\mathbf{P}_{t|t} \equiv \mathbf{P}_{t|t-1}$, respectively.

Example: As a simple example, assume that we have the univariate measurement model:

$$Z_t = Y_t + \epsilon_t, \qquad \epsilon_t \sim iid\,Gau(0, 0.1), \qquad (8.23)$$

where, in the notation introduced above, $R_t \equiv 0.1$ and $H_t \equiv 1$. Also assume we have the process model:

$$Y_t = 0.7Y_{t-1} + \eta_t, \qquad \eta_t \sim iid\,Gau(0, 0.5), \qquad (8.24)$$

where here $Q_t \equiv 0.5$ and $M_t \equiv 0.7$.

Given an initial condition, $Y_0 \sim Gau(0, 1)$, we simulated Y_t and Z_t for $t = 1, \ldots, 100$. In addition, we deleted the data at times 40 to 43 and 80 to 83. The simulated process and data are shown in Figure 8.1. Our goal here is to make inference on the process (or "hidden state") Y_t, using the filtering distribution. That is, we seek the distribution of Y_t given the data $\mathbf{Z}_{1:t}$; $t = 1, \ldots, 100$. The Kalman filter is simple to compute for this univariate example. Figure 8.2 shows the estimate of the state process obtained by filtering, and Figure 8.3 shows the associated filtering-distribution variances, which are clearly larger during time periods where there are missing data.

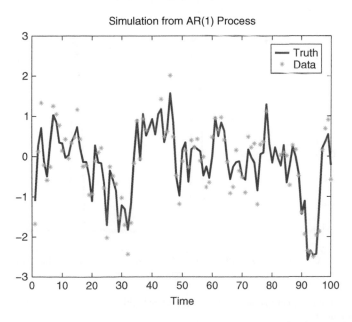

Figure 8.1 Simulated AR(1) process, or "truth" (solid blue line), and "data" (green dots).

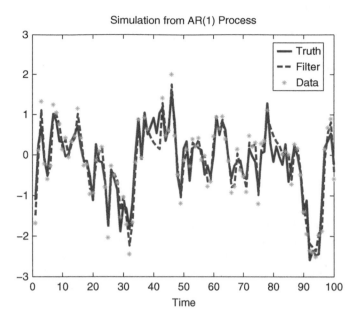

Figure 8.2 Kalman filter estimate of the state process (dashed red line), "truth" (solid blue line), and "data" (green dots).

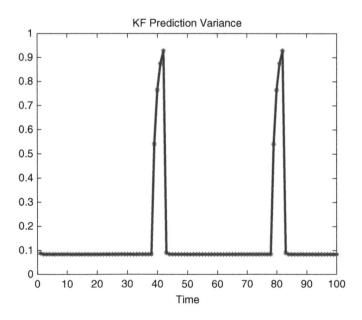

Figure 8.3 Kalman filter variance estimates associated with the simulated AR(1) process and data shown in Figure 8.2.

For more realistic examples featuring spatio-temporal data models and process models, see, for example, Wikle and Cressie (1999) and Kang, Cressie, and Shi (2010).

8.2.2 Kalman Smoother

As mentioned previously, in some situations there is interest in the distribution of $\mathbf{Y}_t$ at time $t \leq T$, given all the data up to T (i.e., both before and after time t), namely $[\mathbf{Y}_t|\mathbf{Z}_{1:T}]$; this is the *smoothing* (posterior) distribution of $\mathbf{Y}_t$. The smoothing distribution is useful for retrospective analyses (i.e., re-analyses) and is not something that one typically does "on-line." As suggested by the general algorithm given in Section 8.1, we can use the Kalman filter and associated backwards-recursion formulas to obtain the smoothing distributions. This procedure, which is sometimes known as the *Kalman smoother*, can be derived from various perspectives. For extensive development, we refer the reader to one of the many excellent texts that discuss filtering and smoothing in detail, listed in the Bibliographic Notes in Section 8.5. We take an EHM approach in this subsection.

As with the Kalman-filter derivation, let $\mathbf{Y}_{t|T} \equiv E(\mathbf{Y}_t|\mathbf{Z}_{1:T})$ and $\mathbf{P}_{t|T} \equiv \mathrm{var}(\mathbf{Y}_t|\mathbf{Z}_{1:T})$. We seek sequential formulas for $[\mathbf{Y}_t|\mathbf{Z}_{1:T}]$ and assume that we have access to the filtering distributions, $\mathbf{Y}_t|\mathbf{Z}_{1:t} \sim Gau(\mathbf{Y}_{t|t}, \mathbf{P}_{t|t})$, and the forecast distributions, $\mathbf{Y}_{t+1}|\mathbf{Z}_{1:t} \sim Gau(\mathbf{Y}_{t+1|t}, \mathbf{P}_{t+1|t})$, for $t = 1, \ldots, T$. These are available from the Kalman-filter algorithm.

First, we can obtain $[\mathbf{Y}_t|\mathbf{Y}_{t+1}, \mathbf{Z}_{1:t}]$ from Bayes' rule, as suggested by (8.10). This density is proportional to the product of two Gaussian densities:

$$[\mathbf{Y}_t|\mathbf{Y}_{t+1}, \mathbf{Z}_{1:t}] \propto Gau(\mathbf{Y}_{t|t}, \mathbf{P}_{t|t}) Gau(\mathbf{M}_{t+1}\mathbf{Y}_t, \mathbf{Q}_{t+1}), \qquad (8.25)$$

where there is a slight abuse of notation by using $Gau(\cdot, \cdot)$ to represent Gaussian densities. By completing the square and using identities (8.18) and (8.19), this distribution is $Gau(\mathbf{u}_t, \mathbf{U}_t)$, where

$$\mathbf{u}_t \equiv \mathbf{Y}_{t|t} + \mathbf{J}_t(\mathbf{Y}_{t+1} - \mathbf{M}_{t+1}\mathbf{Y}_{t|t}), \qquad (8.26)$$

$$\mathbf{U}_t \equiv \mathbf{P}_{t|t} - \mathbf{J}_t\mathbf{M}_{t+1}\mathbf{P}_{t|t}, \qquad (8.27)$$

and

$$\mathbf{J}_t \equiv \mathbf{P}_{t|t}\mathbf{M}'_{t+1}(\mathbf{M}_{t+1}\mathbf{P}_{t|t}\mathbf{M}'_{t+1} + \mathbf{Q}_{t+1}^{-1}) = \mathbf{P}_{t|t}\mathbf{M}'_{t+1}\mathbf{P}_{t+1|t}^{-1}. \qquad (8.28)$$

Next, we obtain the *smoothing distribution* from (8.8). Specifically,

$$\mathbf{Y}_t|\mathbf{Z}_{1:T} \sim Gau(\mathbf{Y}_{t|T}, \mathbf{P}_{t|T}), \qquad (8.29)$$

where

$$\mathbf{Y}_{t|T} = E(E(\mathbf{Y}_t|\mathbf{Y}_{t+1}, \mathbf{Z}_{1:t})|\mathbf{Z}_{1:T})$$
$$= E(\mathbf{u}_t|\mathbf{Z}_{1:T}) = \mathbf{Y}_{t|t} + \mathbf{J}_t(\mathbf{Y}_{t+1|T} - \mathbf{Y}_{t+1|t}) \tag{8.30}$$

and

$$\mathbf{P}_{t|T} = E(\text{var}(\mathbf{Y}_t|\mathbf{Y}_{t+1}, \mathbf{Z}_{1:t})|\mathbf{Z}_{1:T}) + \text{var}(E(\mathbf{Y}_t|\mathbf{Y}_{t+1}, \mathbf{Z}_{1:t})|\mathbf{Z}_{1:T})$$
$$= E(\mathbf{U}_t|\mathbf{Z}_{1:T}) + \text{var}(\mathbf{u}_t|\mathbf{Z}_{1:T})$$
$$= \mathbf{P}_{t|t} - \mathbf{J}_t\mathbf{M}_{t+1}\mathbf{P}_{t|t} + \mathbf{J}_t\text{var}(\mathbf{Y}_{t+1}|\mathbf{Z}_{1:T})\mathbf{J}_t'$$
$$= \mathbf{P}_{t|t} - \mathbf{J}_t\mathbf{P}_{t+1|t}\mathbf{J}_t' + \mathbf{J}_t\mathbf{P}_{t+1|T}\mathbf{J}_t'$$
$$= \mathbf{P}_{t|t} + \mathbf{J}_t(\mathbf{P}_{t+1|T} - \mathbf{P}_{t+1|t})\mathbf{J}_t'. \tag{8.31}$$

Thus, given the forecast and filter estimates (actually, they are "predictions" rather than "estimates," since we are inferring random quantities), $\mathbf{Y}_{t|t}$, $\mathbf{P}_{t|t}$, $\mathbf{Y}_{t+1|t}$, and $\mathbf{P}_{t+1|t}$, for $t = 0, \ldots, T$, the *Kalman smoother algorithm* can be written in pseudo code as follows:

For $t = T - 1$ to 0

　　1. Obtain $\mathbf{J}_t$ from (8.28).
　　2. Obtain $\mathbf{Y}_{t|T}$ from (8.30).
　　3. Obtain $\mathbf{P}_{t|T}$ from (8.31).

end

Note that even when $T = 0$, the algorithm is still well defined because $\mathbf{Y}_{0|0} \equiv \boldsymbol{\mu}_0$ and $\mathbf{P}_{0|0} \equiv \boldsymbol{\Sigma}_0$. This smoothing algorithm is sometimes known as a *fixed-interval smoother*. Other smoothing algorithms (e.g., fixed-lag and fixed-point smoothers) can be implemented "on-line," but they are not considered here (e.g., see Grewal and Andrews, 1993).

8.3   INFERENCE FOR THE DSTM PARAMETERS: LINEAR/GAUSSIAN MODELS

Recall that a critical assumption in the filtering and smoothing algorithms presented in the previous section is that the parameter matrices are known for all time t. Outside of rare engineering applications, this is almost never the case. It is fairly common that the measurement matrix $\mathbf{H}_t$ is known (and possibly the measurement-error covariance matrix, $\mathbf{R}_t$), but it is much less likely that the parameters associated with the evolution distribution are known. In the case where these parameter matrices are not time varying, one can, in principle, *estimate* them. This is the empirical hierarchical modeling (EHM) framework discussed previously. One approach is to use method-of-moments estimates (e.g., Wikle and Cressie, 1999; Kang, Cressie, and Shi, 2010). Another approach is to maximize the likelihood numerically using Newton–Raphson (or similar) methods (e.g, Gupta and Mehra, 1974; Shumway and Stoffer, 2006, Section 6.3). Another likelihood-based approach is to use the Expectation-Maximization (EM) algorithm in this context (e.g., Shumway and Stoffer, 1982, 2006). Alternatively, the Bayesian hierarchical modeling (BHM) framework could be used, in which case the parameters are assumed to be random and are given prior distributions; then, estimation proceeds in a Bayesian fashion via the parameters' posterior distributions. The following subsections consider the EM algorithm for the EHM approach, and a Gibbs sampler for the BHM approach.

8.3.1 EHM Implementation via the EM Algorithm

The basic EM algorithm is used to find maximum likelihood estimates in the presence of missing data (Dempster, Laird, and Rubin, 1977; McLachlan and Krishnan, 1997). In general, let the *complete data*, Z, be the union of the observations, Z_{obs}, and the missing data, Z_{mis}, so that $Z = (Z_{obs}, Z_{mis})$. If θ represents unknown parameters, then the complete data density is $[Z|\theta]$, and we write the complete likelihood as $L(\theta|Z) \equiv [Z|\theta]$; the loglikelihood is $\ln L(\theta|Z)$. Let $\hat{\theta}^{(i-1)}$ be the parameter estimate at the beginning of the ith iteration of the algorithm. Then, the algorithm consists of two steps:

- **E-Step:** Calculate $E(\ln L(\theta|Z)|Z_{obs}, \hat{\theta}^{(i-1)}) \equiv q(\theta|\hat{\theta}^{(i-1)})$.
- **M-Step:** Find θ that maximizes $q(\theta|\hat{\theta}^{(i-1)})$, and call this $\hat{\theta}^{(i)}$.

Thus, given a starting value, $\hat{\theta}^{(0)}$, iterating between the E-step and the M-step yields a sequence of estimates, $\{\hat{\theta}^{(i)} : i = 1, 2, \ldots\}$. The algorithm is stopped when a given convergence criterion is met.

In the state-space setting given by (8.11) and (8.12), assume for illustration that the data-model matrix $\mathbf{H}_t$ is known and that the remainder of the parameters are *not time dependent*. Our exposition follows that of Shumway and Stoffer (2006, Section 6.3), with obvious notational differences. Let $\boldsymbol{\Theta} \equiv \{\boldsymbol{\mu}_0, \boldsymbol{\Sigma}_0, \mathbf{Q}, \mathbf{R}, \mathbf{M}\}$ denote the set of parameters, where recall the initial condition, $\mathbf{Y}_{0|0} \sim Gau(\boldsymbol{\mu}_0, \boldsymbol{\Sigma}_0)$. In this context, the observed data are $\mathbf{Z}_{1:T}$, as before, and the "missing data" refer to the state process, $\mathbf{Y}_{0:T}$, which is, of course, unobservable by definition. The joint density of the complete data is then

$$[\mathbf{Z}_{1:T}, \mathbf{Y}_{0:T}|\boldsymbol{\Theta}] = \left(\prod_{t=1}^{T}[\mathbf{Z}_t|\mathbf{Y}_t]\right)[\mathbf{Y}_0]\prod_{t=1}^{T}[\mathbf{Y}_t|\mathbf{Y}_{t-1}].$$

Thus, the complete-data, negative twice loglikelihood is (up to an additive constant)

$$-2 \ln L(\boldsymbol{\Theta}|\mathbf{Z}_{1:T}, \mathbf{Y}_{0:T}) = \ln|\boldsymbol{\Sigma}_0| + (\mathbf{Y}_0 - \boldsymbol{\mu}_0)'\boldsymbol{\Sigma}_0^{-1}(\mathbf{Y}_0 - \boldsymbol{\mu}_0)$$

$$+ T \ln|\mathbf{Q}| + \sum_{t=1}^{T}(\mathbf{Y}_t - \mathbf{MY}_{t-1})'\mathbf{Q}^{-1}(\mathbf{Y}_t - \mathbf{MY}_{t-1})$$

$$+ T \ln|\mathbf{R}| + \sum_{t=1}^{T}(\mathbf{Z}_t - \mathbf{H}_t\mathbf{Y}_t)'\mathbf{R}^{-1}(\mathbf{Z}_t - \mathbf{H}_t\mathbf{Y}_t).$$

$$(8.32)$$

Now, the E-step of the EM algorithm requires the calculation of the expectation,

$$q(\boldsymbol{\Theta}|\hat{\boldsymbol{\Theta}}^{(i-1)}) \equiv E(-2\ln L(\boldsymbol{\Theta}|\mathbf{Z}_{1:T}, \mathbf{Y}_{1:T})|\mathbf{Z}_{1:T}, \hat{\boldsymbol{\Theta}}^{(i-1)})$$

$$= \ln|\boldsymbol{\Sigma}_0| + \text{tr}\left\{\boldsymbol{\Sigma}_0^{-1}\left[\mathbf{P}_{0|T} + (\mathbf{Y}_{0|T} - \boldsymbol{\mu}_0)(\mathbf{Y}_{0|T} - \boldsymbol{\mu}_0)'\right]\right\} \quad (8.33)$$

$$+ T\ln|\mathbf{Q}| + \text{tr}\{\mathbf{Q}^{-1}[\mathbf{S}_{11} - \mathbf{S}_{10}\mathbf{M}' - \mathbf{MS}_{10}' + \mathbf{MS}_{00}\mathbf{M}']\} + T\ln|\mathbf{R}|$$

$$+ \text{tr}\left\{\mathbf{R}^{-1}\sum_{t=1}^{T}\left[(\mathbf{Z}_t - \mathbf{H}_t\mathbf{Y}_{t|T})(\mathbf{Z}_t - \mathbf{H}_t\mathbf{Y}_{t|T})' + \mathbf{H}_t\mathbf{P}_{t|T}\mathbf{H}_t'\right]\right\},$$

for

$$\mathbf{S}_{11} \equiv \sum_{t=1}^{T}(\mathbf{P}_{t|T} + \mathbf{Y}_{t|T}\mathbf{Y}_{t|T}')$$

$$\mathbf{S}_{00} \equiv \sum_{t=1}^{T}(\mathbf{P}_{t-1|T} + \mathbf{Y}_{t-1|T}\mathbf{Y}_{t-1|T}')$$

$$\mathbf{S}_{10} \equiv \sum_{t=1}^{T}(\mathbf{P}_{t,t-1|T} + \mathbf{Y}_{t|T}\mathbf{Y}_{t-1|T}'),$$

where, in general, $\mathbf{P}_{t_1,t_2|T} \equiv E((\mathbf{Y}_{t_1} - \mathbf{Y}_{t_1|T})(\mathbf{Y}_{t_2} - \mathbf{Y}_{t_2|T})'|\mathbf{Z}_{1:T})$ and $\mathbf{P}_{t|T} \equiv \mathbf{P}_{t,t|T}$. The right-hand side of (8.33) is dependent on $\hat{\boldsymbol{\Theta}}^{(i-1)}$, although for economy of notation this is *not* made explicit. For example, $\mathbf{Y}_{t|T} = E(\mathbf{Y}_t|\mathbf{Z}_{1:T})$ depends on $\boldsymbol{\Theta}$; when it appears on the right-hand side of (8.33), it should be understood that it is evaluated at $\boldsymbol{\Theta} = \hat{\boldsymbol{\Theta}}^{(i-1)}$.

The M-step then proceeds by minimizing $q(\Theta|\hat{\Theta}^{(i-1)})$, as given by (8.33), with respect to the parameters Θ. This gives

$$\hat{\mathbf{M}}^{(i)} = \mathbf{S}_{10}\mathbf{S}_{00}^{-1} \tag{8.34}$$

$$\hat{\mathbf{Q}}^{(i)} = (1/T)(\mathbf{S}_{11} - \mathbf{S}_{10}\mathbf{S}_{00}^{-1}\mathbf{S}_{10}') \tag{8.35}$$

$$\hat{\mathbf{R}}^{(i)} = (1/T)\sum_{t=1}^{T}\left((\mathbf{Z}_t - \mathbf{H}_t\mathbf{Y}_{t|T})(\mathbf{Z}_t - \mathbf{H}_t\mathbf{Y}_{t|T})' + \mathbf{H}_t\mathbf{P}_{t|T}\mathbf{H}_t'\right), \tag{8.36}$$

and

$$\hat{\boldsymbol{\mu}}_0^{(i)} = \mathbf{Y}_{0|T}. \tag{8.37}$$

Although we follow the tradition of estimating $\boldsymbol{\mu}_0$ and fixing $\boldsymbol{\Sigma}_0$ (e.g., Shumway and Stoffer, 2000, p.325), we note that one could update $\boldsymbol{\Sigma}_0$ by setting it equal to $\mathbf{P}_{0|T}$ (e.g., Shumway and Stoffer, 2006, p. 344). Thus, in our case, $\hat{\Theta}^{(i)} \equiv \{\hat{\boldsymbol{\mu}}_0^{(i)}, \hat{\mathbf{Q}}^{(i)}, \hat{\mathbf{R}}^{(i)}, \hat{\mathbf{M}}^{(i)}\}$, and $\boldsymbol{\Sigma}_0$ is fixed. However, before $\hat{\Theta}^{(i)}$ can be calculated, we still have to evaluate $\mathbf{P}_{t,t-1|T}$ in $\mathbf{S}_{10}$, which can be accomplished by the *lag-one covariance smoother* (Shumway and Stoffer, 2006, Property P6.3). Given $\mathbf{K}_t$ defined by (8.22), $\mathbf{J}_t$ defined by (8.28), and $\mathbf{P}_{t|t}$ defined by (8.21) evaluated at $\hat{\Theta}^{(i-1)}$, for $t = 0, \ldots, T$, we first calculate $\mathbf{P}_{T,T-1|T} = (\mathbf{I} - \mathbf{K}_T\mathbf{H}_T)\mathbf{M}\mathbf{P}_{T-1|T-1}$. Then, for $t = T, T-1, \ldots, 2$,

$$\mathbf{P}_{t-1,t-2|T} = \mathbf{P}_{t-1|t-1}\mathbf{J}_{t-2}' + \mathbf{J}_{t-1}(\mathbf{P}_{t,t-1|T} - \mathbf{M}\mathbf{P}_{t-1|t-1})\mathbf{J}_{t-2}'.$$

Then the *EM algorithm* can be written in pseudo code as follows:

Select starting values, $\hat{\Theta}^{(0)} = \{\hat{\boldsymbol{\mu}}_0^{(0)}, \hat{\mathbf{Q}}^{(0)}, \hat{\mathbf{R}}^{(0)}, \hat{\mathbf{M}}^{(0)}\}$, and choose $\boldsymbol{\Sigma}_0$.

For $i = 1, 2, \ldots$ (until convergence)

1. **E-step:** Use $\hat{\Theta}^{(i-1)}$ in the Kalman filter, Kalman smoother, and lag-one covariance smoother to obtain $\mathbf{Y}_{t|T}, \mathbf{P}_{t|T}, \mathbf{P}_{t,t-1|T}$, for $t = 1, \ldots, T$. Use these quantities to calculate $\mathbf{S}_{00}, \mathbf{S}_{11}$, and $\mathbf{S}_{10}$.

2. **M-step:** Update estimates $\hat{\Theta}^{(i)}$, specifically, $\hat{\boldsymbol{\mu}}_0^{(i)}, \hat{\mathbf{Q}}^{(i)}, \hat{\mathbf{R}}^{(i)}$, and $\hat{\mathbf{M}}^{(i)}$, using (8.37), (8.35), (8.36), and (8.34), respectively.

end

We also note that sometimes the M-step update is difficult to obtain; this occurs, for example, in the case of highly parameterized propagator and covariance matrices in state-space models. In this situation, a general EM (GEM) approach can be taken, and the M-step can be replaced with several simple conditional maximization steps (McLachlan and Krishnan, 1997). Alternatively, for scalar parameters, it may be possible to use a Newton–Raphson step within the GEM (McLachlan and Krishnan, 1997). Xu and Wikle (2007) discuss the application of these approaches to structured matrix parameters in DSTMs.

Although we do not explicitly describe algorithms to obtain standard errors for the EHM parameter estimates, they can be computed in various ways. For example, it may be possible to evaluate the Hessian matrix after convergence (Shumway and Stoffer, 2006). Alternatively, it may be possible to obtain the standard errors by perturbing the likelihood function and using numerical differentiation (e.g., Shumway and Stoffer, 2006; Tanner, 1996). However, although the likelihood-based parameter estimates are consistent and asymptotically normal, the asymptotic results may not be applicable in spatio-temporal applications where the sample sizes are relatively small. In that case, a bootstrap procedure may be appropriate, and it is straightforward to implement. For example, Stoffer and Wall (1991) describe a simple bootstrap-sampling algorithm, for parameter estimates in general state-space models, that is appropriate for the spatio-temporal setting discussed here. In addition, Wall and Stoffer (2002) describe how bootstrap resampling in this context can also give appropriate estimates of conditional forecast accuracy.

8.3.2 BHM Implementation via the Gibbs Sampler

Assume the data model:

$$\mathbf{Z}_t = \mathbf{H}_t \mathbf{Y}_t + \boldsymbol{\varepsilon}_t; \quad \boldsymbol{\varepsilon}_t \sim iid\, Gau(\mathbf{0}, \mathbf{R}), \tag{8.38}$$

for $t = 1, \ldots, T$, and the process model:

$$\mathbf{Y}_t = \mathbf{M} \mathbf{Y}_{t-1} + \boldsymbol{\eta}_t; \quad \boldsymbol{\eta}_t \sim iid\, Gau(\mathbf{0}, \mathbf{Q}), \tag{8.39}$$

$$\mathbf{Y}_0 \sim Gau(\boldsymbol{\mu}_0, \boldsymbol{\Sigma}_0). \tag{8.40}$$

Now, since we are considering inference using a BHM, we must specify prior distributions for parameters. For example, assume the parameter model,

$$\mathbf{R}^{-1} \sim W((v_R \mathbf{C}_R)^{-1}, v_R) \tag{8.41}$$

$$\mathbf{Q}^{-1} \sim W((v_Q \mathbf{C}_Q)^{-1}, v_Q) \tag{8.42}$$

$$\mathbf{m} \equiv \text{vec}(\mathbf{M}) \sim Gau(\boldsymbol{\mu}_m, \boldsymbol{\Sigma}_m), \tag{8.43}$$

where $W(\cdot, \cdot)$ denotes a Wishart distribution. For now, we assume that the (hyper)parameters $\boldsymbol{\mu}_0, \boldsymbol{\Sigma}_0, v_R, \mathbf{C}_R, v_Q, \mathbf{C}_Q, \boldsymbol{\mu}_m$, and $\boldsymbol{\Sigma}_m$ are fixed and "known." One advantage of the hierarchical approach is that we could assign prior distributions to these parameters as well. While (8.41), (8.42), and (8.43) are chosen for computational ease, other prior distributions could be chosen (e.g., see West and Harrison, 1997; Section 7.5).

We seek the posterior distribution,

$$[\mathbf{Y}_0, \mathbf{Y}_1, \ldots, \mathbf{Y}_T, \mathbf{M}, \mathbf{Q}, \mathbf{R}|\mathbf{Z}_{1:T}]$$

$$\propto \left(\prod_{t=1}^{T}[\mathbf{Z}_t|\mathbf{Y}_t, \mathbf{R}]\right)[\mathbf{Y}_0]\left(\prod_{t=1}^{T}[\mathbf{Y}_t|\mathbf{Y}_{t-1}, \mathbf{M}, \mathbf{Q}]\right)[\mathbf{R}][\mathbf{Q}][\mathbf{M}], \quad (8.44)$$

where, for convenience, we have assumed that the parameter model is based on independent distributions. Unfortunately, the normalizing constant for (8.44) cannot be found analytically. However, Markov chain Monte Carlo (MCMC) samples from this posterior distribution can be obtained from a Gibbs sampler. This requires the following full conditional distributions:

$$[\mathbf{Y}_0|\cdot] \propto [\mathbf{Y}_1|\mathbf{Y}_0, \mathbf{M}, \mathbf{Q}][\mathbf{Y}_0],$$

$$[\mathbf{Y}_t|\cdot] \propto [\mathbf{Z}_t|\mathbf{Y}_t, \mathbf{R}][\mathbf{Y}_{t+1}|\mathbf{Y}_t, \mathbf{M}, \mathbf{Q}][\mathbf{Y}_t|\mathbf{Y}_{t-1}, \mathbf{M}, \mathbf{Q}], \quad t = 1, \ldots, T - 1,$$

$$[\mathbf{Y}_T|\cdot] \propto [\mathbf{Z}_T|\mathbf{Y}_T, \mathbf{R}][\mathbf{Y}_T|\mathbf{Y}_{T-1}, \mathbf{M}, \mathbf{Q}],$$

$$[\mathbf{R}|\cdot] \propto \prod_{t=1}^{T}[\mathbf{Z}_t|\mathbf{Y}_t, \mathbf{R}][\mathbf{R}],$$

$$[\mathbf{Q}|\cdot] \propto \prod_{t=1}^{T}[\mathbf{Y}_t|\mathbf{Y}_{t-1}, \mathbf{M}, \mathbf{Q}][\mathbf{Q}],$$

$$[\mathbf{M}|\cdot] \propto \prod_{t=1}^{T}[\mathbf{Y}_t|\mathbf{Y}_{t-1}, \mathbf{M}, \mathbf{Q}][\mathbf{M}],$$

where "$\cdot$" in the conditioning set denotes all quantities on the left-hand side of (8.44), except the variable whose conditional distribution we are considering.

All of the full conditional distributions implied by (8.38)–(8.43) are "conjugate," and this greatly simplifies the derivation of these distributions. To illustrate what this means, consider the case where we have an n_w-dimensional Gaussian distribution, $\mathbf{w}|\mathbf{x} \sim Gau(\mathbf{Ax}, \mathbf{\Sigma}_w)$, and an n_x-dimensional Gaussian distribution, $\mathbf{x} \sim Gau(\mathbf{B\mu}, \mathbf{\Sigma}_x)$; we are interested in the conditional distribution, $[\mathbf{x}|\mathbf{w}] \propto [\mathbf{w}|\mathbf{x}][\mathbf{x}]$. First,

$$[\mathbf{x}|\mathbf{w}] \propto \exp\{-(1/2)[(\mathbf{w} - \mathbf{Ax})'\mathbf{\Sigma}_w^{-1}(\mathbf{w} - \mathbf{Ax}) + (\mathbf{x} - \mathbf{B\mu})'\mathbf{\Sigma}_x^{-1}(\mathbf{x} - \mathbf{B\mu})]\}$$

$$\propto \exp\{-(1/2)[\mathbf{x}(\mathbf{A}'\mathbf{\Sigma}_w^{-1}\mathbf{A} + \mathbf{\Sigma}_x^{-1})\mathbf{x}' - 2(\mathbf{w}'\mathbf{\Sigma}_w^{-1}\mathbf{A} + \mathbf{\mu}'\mathbf{B}'\mathbf{\Sigma}_x^{-1})\mathbf{x}]\},$$

where it is understood that here $\mathbf{x} \in \mathbb{R}^{n_x}$ and $\mathbf{w} \in \mathbb{R}^{n_w}$. Now, using the fact that $[\mathbf{v}] \propto \exp\{-1/2(\mathbf{v}'\mathbf{Dv} - 2\mathbf{b}'\mathbf{v})\}$ implies that $\mathbf{v} \sim Gau(\mathbf{D}^{-1}\mathbf{b}, \mathbf{D}^{-1})$, which is obtained by completing the square, the general Gaussian/Gaussian result for the conditional distribution follows:

$$\mathbf{x}|\mathbf{w} \sim Gau\left((\mathbf{A}'\boldsymbol{\Sigma}_w^{-1}\mathbf{A} + \boldsymbol{\Sigma}_x^{-1})^{-1}(\mathbf{w}'\boldsymbol{\Sigma}_w^{-1}\mathbf{A} + \boldsymbol{\mu}'\mathbf{B}'\boldsymbol{\Sigma}_x^{-1})', (\mathbf{A}'\boldsymbol{\Sigma}_w^{-1}\mathbf{A} + \boldsymbol{\Sigma}_x^{-1})^{-1}\right).$$

(8.45)

Similarly, if $\mathbf{x}_i|\boldsymbol{\Sigma}_x \sim Gau(\boldsymbol{\mu}, \boldsymbol{\Sigma}_x)$, for $i = 1, \ldots, T$, and $\boldsymbol{\Sigma}_x^{-1} \sim W((\mathbf{S}v)^{-1}, v)$, then this represents conjugacy, since the following result can be derived:

$$\boldsymbol{\Sigma}_x^{-1}|\mathbf{x}_1, \ldots, \mathbf{x}_T \sim W\left(\left(\sum_{i=1}^{T}(\mathbf{x}_i - \boldsymbol{\mu})(\mathbf{x}_i - \boldsymbol{\mu})' + v\mathbf{S}\right)^{-1}, v + T\right), \quad (8.46)$$

where recall that $W(\cdot, \cdot)$ denotes a Wishart distribution.

Using (8.45), we can obtain the full conditional distributions for the state process as follows:

$$\mathbf{Y}_0|\cdot \sim Gau(\mathbf{V}_0\mathbf{a}_0, \mathbf{V}_0), \qquad (8.47)$$

where

$$\mathbf{V}_0 \equiv (\mathbf{M}'\mathbf{Q}^{-1}\mathbf{M} + \boldsymbol{\Sigma}_0^{-1})^{-1},$$

$$\mathbf{a}_0 \equiv \mathbf{M}'\mathbf{Q}^{-1}\mathbf{Y}_1 + \boldsymbol{\Sigma}_0^{-1}\boldsymbol{\mu}_0;$$

similarly, for $t = 1, \ldots, T - 1$, we have

$$\mathbf{Y}_t|\cdot \sim Gau(\mathbf{V}_t\mathbf{a}_t, \mathbf{V}_t), \qquad (8.48)$$

where

$$\mathbf{V}_t \equiv (\mathbf{H}_t'\mathbf{R}^{-1}\mathbf{H}_t + \mathbf{Q}^{-1} + \mathbf{M}'\mathbf{Q}^{-1}\mathbf{M})^{-1},$$

$$\mathbf{a}_t \equiv \mathbf{H}_t'\mathbf{R}^{-1}\mathbf{Z}_t + \mathbf{Q}^{-1}\mathbf{M}\mathbf{Y}_{t-1} + \mathbf{M}'\mathbf{Q}^{-1}\mathbf{Y}_{t+1};$$

and for $t = T$,

$$\mathbf{Y}_T|\cdot \sim Gau(\mathbf{V}_T\mathbf{a}_T, \mathbf{V}_T), \qquad (8.49)$$

where

$$\mathbf{V}_T \equiv (\mathbf{H}_T'\mathbf{R}^{-1}\mathbf{H}_T + \mathbf{Q}^{-1})^{-1},$$

$$\mathbf{a}_T \equiv \mathbf{H}_T'\mathbf{R}^{-1}\mathbf{Z}_T + \mathbf{Q}^{-1}\mathbf{M}\mathbf{Y}_{T-1}.$$

The full conditional distributions of the covariance matrices can be obtained by using (8.46). Thus,

$$
\mathbf{R}^{-1}|\cdot \sim W\left(\left(\sum_{t=1}^{T}(\mathbf{Z}_t - \mathbf{H}_t\mathbf{Y}_t)(\mathbf{Z}_t - \mathbf{H}_t\mathbf{Y}_t)' + v_R\mathbf{C}_R\right)^{-1}, v_R + T\right), \quad (8.50)
$$

$$
\mathbf{Q}^{-1}|\cdot \sim W\left(\left(\sum_{t=1}^{T}(\mathbf{Y}_t - \mathbf{M}\mathbf{Y}_{t-1})(\mathbf{Y}_t - \mathbf{M}\mathbf{Y}_{t-1})' + v_Q\mathbf{C}_Q\right)^{-1}, v_Q + T\right). \tag{8.51}
$$

The full conditional distribution for $\mathbf{M}$ also makes use of the Gaussian/Gaussian result (8.45), but it is facilitated by rewriting the evolution model (8.39) in a matrix format, as follows. Define $\mathcal{Y}_{1:T} \equiv [\mathbf{Y}_1, \ldots, \mathbf{Y}_T]$, an $n \times T$ matrix. Similarly, define the $n \times T$ matrices, $\mathcal{Y}_{0:T-1} \equiv [\mathbf{Y}_0, \mathbf{Y}_1, \ldots, \mathbf{Y}_{T-1}]$ and $\mathcal{U}_{1:T} \equiv [\boldsymbol{\eta}_1, \ldots, \boldsymbol{\eta}_T]$. Thus, we can rewrite the evolution model (8.39) as $\mathcal{Y}_{1:T} = \mathbf{M}\mathcal{Y}_{0:T-1} + \mathcal{U}_{1:T}$. This, in turn, can be written equivalently as

$$
\text{vec}(\mathcal{Y}_{1:T}) = (\mathcal{Y}'_{0:T-1} \otimes \mathbf{I}_n)\mathbf{m} + \text{vec}(\mathcal{U}_{1:T}), \tag{8.52}
$$

where $\text{var}(\text{vec}(\mathcal{U}_{1:T})) = \mathbf{I}_T \otimes \mathbf{Q} \equiv \tilde{\mathbf{Q}}$, and recall that $\mathbf{m} \equiv \text{vec}(\mathbf{M})$. Now, using (8.43) and (8.52) as well as the Gaussian/Gaussian result (8.45), we obtain the full conditional distribution,

$$
\mathbf{m}|\cdot \sim Gau(\mathbf{V}_m\mathbf{a}_m, \mathbf{V}_m), \tag{8.53}
$$

where

$$
\begin{aligned}
\mathbf{V}_m &\equiv ((\mathcal{Y}'_{0:T-1} \otimes \mathbf{I}_n)'\tilde{\mathbf{Q}}^{-1}(\mathcal{Y}'_{0:T-1} \otimes \mathbf{I}_n) + \boldsymbol{\Sigma}_m^{-1})^{-1}, \\
\mathbf{a}_m &\equiv (\mathcal{Y}'_{0:T-1} \otimes \mathbf{I}_n)'\tilde{\mathbf{Q}}^{-1}\text{vec}(\mathcal{Y}_{1:T}) + \boldsymbol{\Sigma}_m^{-1}\boldsymbol{\mu}_m.
\end{aligned} \tag{8.54}
$$

The *Gibbs sampler algorithm* can be written in pseudo code as follows:

Select hyperparameters: $\boldsymbol{\mu}_0, \boldsymbol{\Sigma}_0, v_R, \mathbf{C}_R, v_Q, \mathbf{C}_Q, \boldsymbol{\mu}_m, \boldsymbol{\Sigma}_m$
Select initial values: $\{\mathbf{Y}_t^{(0)} : t = 0, \ldots, T\}, \mathbf{M}^{(0)}, \mathbf{R}^{(0)}, \mathbf{Q}^{(0)}$
For $i = 1$ to N_{gibbs}

- Sample from $\mathbf{Y}_0^{(i)}|\mathbf{Y}_1^{(i-1)}, \mathbf{M}^{(i-1)}, \mathbf{Q}^{(i-1)}$, using (8.47).
- For $t = 1, \ldots, T - 1$, sample from $\mathbf{Y}_t^{(i)}|\mathbf{Y}_{t-1}^{(i)}, \mathbf{Y}_{t+1}^{(i-1)}, \mathbf{M}^{(i-1)}, \mathbf{Q}^{(i-1)}$, using (8.48).
- Sample from $\mathbf{Y}_T^{(i)}|\mathbf{Y}_{T-1}^{(i)}, \mathbf{M}^{(i-1)}, \mathbf{Q}^{(i-1)}$, using (8.49).
- Sample from $\mathbf{R}^{(i)}|\{\mathbf{Y}_t^{(i)} : t = 0, \ldots, T\}$, using (8.50).
- Sample from $\mathbf{Q}^{(i)}|\{\mathbf{Y}_t^{(i)} : t = 0, \ldots, T\}, \mathbf{M}^{(i-1)}$, using (8.51).
- Sample from $\mathbf{m}^{(i)}|\{\mathbf{Y}_t^{(i)} : t = 0, \ldots, T\}, \mathbf{Q}^{(i)}$, using (8.53)

end

The Gibbs sampler algorithm for the BHM presented in this section can be made more efficient, in the sense of faster convergence, if we sample the state process jointly, rather than individually. We saw in Section 8.2.1 that the basis of the Kalman filter/smoother algorithm gives us the ability to obtain sequentially the joint distribution of the state process at all times, given all observations. Effectively, we can use the Kalman filter algorithms within the Gibbs iterations to obtain the joint distribution of the states as follows (e.g., Shumway and Stoffer, 2006, Section 6.9). First, note that from the Markov assumption, we have

$$[\mathbf{Y}_0, \dots, \mathbf{Y}_T | \mathbf{Z}_{1:T}, \mathbf{\Theta}] = [\mathbf{Y}_0 | \mathbf{Y}_1, \mathbf{\Theta}][\mathbf{Y}_1 | \mathbf{Y}_2, \mathbf{Z}_{1:1}, \mathbf{\Theta}]$$
$$\dots [\mathbf{Y}_{T-1} | \mathbf{Y}_T, \mathbf{Z}_{1:T}, \mathbf{\Theta}][\mathbf{Y}_T | \mathbf{Z}_{1:T}, \mathbf{\Theta}], \quad (8.55)$$

where here $\mathbf{\Theta}$ denotes the parameter matrices $\mathbf{M}$, $\mathbf{R}$, and $\mathbf{Q}$. Thus, starting from the last distribution on the right-hand side of (8.55), we could sample $\mathbf{Y}_T$, and then we could use that to sample $\mathbf{Y}_{T-1}$ from the second-to-last distribution on the right-hand side of (8.55), and so on, until we obtain samples for all $\{\mathbf{Y}_t : t = T, \dots, 0\}$. To do this, we must be able to sample easily from $[\mathbf{Y}_t | \mathbf{Y}_{t+1}, \mathbf{Z}_{1:t}, \mathbf{\Theta}]$, for $t = T - 1, \dots, 0$. Fortunately, this is feasible by making use of results from the Kalman filter/smoother. First, recall from (8.10) that

$$[\mathbf{Y}_t | \mathbf{Y}_{t+1}, \mathbf{Z}_{1:t}, \mathbf{\Theta}] \propto [\mathbf{Y}_{t+1} | \mathbf{Y}_t, \mathbf{Z}_{1:t}, \mathbf{\Theta}][\mathbf{Y}_t | \mathbf{Z}_{1:t}], \quad (8.56)$$

and if the two components are Gaussian distributions, this is precisely (8.25). By completing the square, the distribution is Gaussian with mean and variance given by (8.26) and (8.27), respectively. This can be used in the Gibbs sampler in what is known as the *forward filtering, backward sampling algorithm* (Carter and Kohn, 1994; Frühwirth-Schnatter, 1994). Specifically, rather than sample $\{\mathbf{Y}_t : t = 0, \dots, T\}$ individually in the Gibbs sampler, we would like to sample $[\mathbf{Y}_0, \mathbf{Y}_1, \dots, \mathbf{Y}_T | \cdot]$, which is accomplished by carrying out the following steps:

1. Run the Kalman filter with the current Gibbs samples for $\mathbf{\Theta}$ substituted into $\mathbf{Y}_{t|t}$, $\mathbf{Y}_{t|t-1}$, $\mathbf{P}_{t|t}$, and $\mathbf{P}_{t|t-1}$.

2. Sample $\mathbf{Y}_T^{(i)}$ from $Gau(\mathbf{Y}_{T|T}, \mathbf{P}_{T|T})$.

3. For $t = T - 1, \dots, 0$, sample $\mathbf{Y}_t^{(i)}$ from $Gau(\mathbf{Y}_{t|t} + \mathbf{J}_t(\mathbf{Y}_{t+1}^{(i)} - \mathbf{Y}_{t+1|t})$, $\mathbf{P}_{t|t} - \mathbf{J}_t \mathbf{P}_{t+1|t} \mathbf{J}_t')$, using the most recently sampled $\mathbf{Y}_{t+1}^{(i)}$.

Although using the forward filtering, backward sampling algorithm may seem excessively complicated compared to the basic Gibbs sampler presented previously, typically it produces faster convergence in the sampler if the dependence between $\mathbf{Y}_t$ and $\mathbf{Y}_{t-1}$ is moderate to strong.

Example: As a simple illustration of the Gibbs-sampler algorithm described above, consider the case of simulating noisy data from the AR(1) process given in Section 8.2.1; the data model is given by (8.23) and the process model is given by (8.24). We also specify a prior for the initial condition, namely $Y_0 \sim Gau(0, 1)$. For this illustration, we assume that we "know" the measurement-error variance (i.e., $R = 0.1$), the evolution operator M has prior distribution, $M \sim Unif(-1, 1)$, and the process-model variance has prior distribution, $\sigma_\eta^2 \sim IG(2, 1)$. [The notation, $Unif(u_1, u_2)$, corresponds to a continuous uniform distribution between u_1 and u_2, and $IG(a, b)$ corresponds to an inverse gamma distribution with shape parameter a and scale parameter b.] The MCMC in this case seeks the posterior distributions of M, σ_η^2, and $Y_0, Y_1, \ldots, Y_T$. Then the Gibbs-sampler algorithm is a special case of the more general (matrix/vector) algorithm presented above. Specific formulas for the full-conditional distributions for this example are given in Wikle and Berliner (2007, Section 5.3.1). The algorithm was implemented on the simulated data shown in Figure 8.1, with an MCMC sample of 45,000 after a burn-in period of 5000 iterations. Figure 8.4 shows a histogram of samples from the posterior distributions of M and σ_η^2. Recall that the true values for these parameters used in the simulation were $M = 0.7$ and $\sigma_\eta^2 = 0.5$; clearly, the posterior distributions cover these true values. Figure 8.5 shows the posterior mean of the state process $\{Y_t\}$ as well as the 2.5 percentiles and 97.5 percentiles from the posterior distribution of the state process for each time, which is a way to

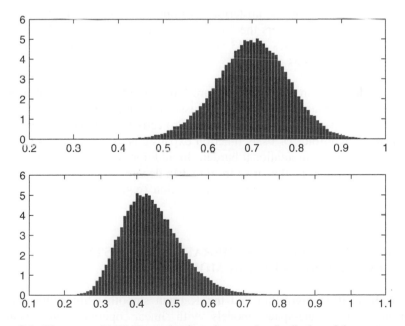

Figure 8.4 Histogram of MCMC samples from the posterior distribution of the parameters. **Top panel:** Evolution operator, M. **Bottom panel:** Process-model variance, σ_η^2.

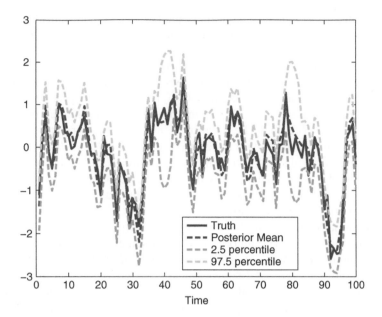

Figure 8.5 Summary of MCMC output for the posterior distribution of the state process, $\{Y_t\}$. Solid blue line: "truth"; dashed red line: posterior mean; dashed green line: lower 2.5 percentiles; dash–dot green line: upper 97.5 percentiles.

measure uncertainty in the posterior distribution. Observe that the posterior distribution generally covers the "truth," and the uncertainty in the time periods with no data (at times 40–43 and 80–83) is much larger than in periods where there are data, as expected.

Although Gaussian linear DSTMs are fairly simple to implement in principle, there can be practical computational issues when the dimension of the state process and/or parameter vectors is high. Projecting these vectors onto lower dimensional manifolds or basis function expansions as described in Chapter 7 can help ease the computational burden. In addition, one can exploit simplifying reparameterizations that arise from matrix decompositions of the parameter matrices, such as the Cholesky decomposition (e.g., Eubank 2006; Lee and Ghosh 2008).

8.4 INFERENCE FOR THE HIERARCHICAL DSTM: NONLINEAR/NON-GAUSSIAN MODELS

The Kalman filter algorithm and the Kalman smoother algorithm are most appropriate for state-space models with linear operators and Gaussian error. Unfortunately, many spatio-temporal statistical models violate these assumptions. In this section, we discuss several options for accommodating more complicated spatio-temporal structures. We refer the reader to the Bibliographic Notes in Section 8.5 for references that give more complete coverage.

8.4.1 Extended Kalman Filter

Consider the general DSTM formulation within an HM: The data model is

$$\mathbf{Z}_t = \mathcal{H}_t(\mathbf{Y}_t; \boldsymbol{\theta}_D) + \boldsymbol{\varepsilon}_t, \tag{8.57}$$

and the process model is

$$\mathbf{Y}_t = \mathcal{M}_t(\mathbf{Y}_{t-1}; \boldsymbol{\theta}_P) + \boldsymbol{\eta}_t, \tag{8.58}$$

where $\mathcal{H}_t(\cdot)$ and $\mathcal{M}_t(\cdot)$ are known, nonlinear functions. While linear and additive combinations of Gaussian random variables have Gaussian distributions, this is not the case for nonlinear transformations. Thus, it is not necessary that the error terms in the data model and the process model be Gaussian—or even additive—although they are additive in (8.57) and (8.58). In general, the errors should be included in the functions $\mathcal{H}_t$ and $\mathcal{M}_t$. However, in the context described here, one assumes that the first two moments are sufficient to describe the state and measurement distributions, and thus additive error terms are often assumed. In this section, we assume that the errors $\boldsymbol{\varepsilon}_t$ and $\boldsymbol{\eta}_t$ in (8.57) and (8.58), respectively, have mean zero and are temporally independent within and between series.

The traditional approach to this problem when equations (8.57) and (8.58) are not far from linear is to employ some sort of linearization (e.g., West and Harrison, 1997, Section 13.2; Grewal and Andrews, 1993, Chapter 5). Primarily, this involves *tangent-linear expansions* of $\mathcal{H}_t$ and $\mathcal{M}_t$. That is, one expands these functions using Taylor series and then truncates, typically considering terms only up to first order (as discussed in Sections 7.1.4 and 7.3.1). Thus, the nonlinear functions are approximated by

$$\mathcal{H}_t \simeq \left[\frac{\partial \mathcal{H}_t(\mathbf{Y}_t)}{\partial \mathbf{Y}_t} \right]_{\mathbf{Y}_t = \hat{\mathbf{Y}}_t} \equiv \tilde{\mathbf{H}}_t, \tag{8.59}$$

$$\mathcal{M}_{t-1} \simeq \left[\frac{\partial \mathcal{M}_t(\mathbf{Y}_{t-1})}{\partial \mathbf{Y}_{t-1}} \right]_{\mathbf{Y}_{t-1} = \hat{\mathbf{Y}}_{t-1}} \equiv \tilde{\mathbf{M}}_{t-1}, \tag{8.60}$$

where $\{\hat{\mathbf{Y}}_t\}$ are suitable state estimates about which to linearize. A common choice is the forecasted trajectory of the state process. These linear approximations are then used in the "update step" to update the filter's state vector and covariance matrices; however, the full nonlinear equations are used in the forecast step. Given the measurement and evolution error covariance matrices, $\mathbf{R}_t$ and $\mathbf{Q}_t$, respectively, and initial values $\mathbf{Y}_{0|0}$ and $\mathbf{P}_{0|0}$, the algorithm, often referred to as the *extended Kalman filter* (EKF), can be written in pseudo code as follows:

For $t = 1$ to T

  1. Obtain the forecast distribution's mean and covariances:

    (a) $\mathbf{Y}_{t|t-1} = \mathcal{M}_t(\mathbf{Y}_{t-1|t-1})$.

    (b) $\mathbf{P}_{t|t-1} = \tilde{\mathbf{M}}_{t-1}\mathbf{P}_{t-1|t-1}\tilde{\mathbf{M}}'_{t-1} + \mathbf{Q}_{t-1}$.

  2. Calculate the gain matrix, $\mathbf{K}_t = \mathbf{P}_{t|t-1}\tilde{\mathbf{H}}'_t(\tilde{\mathbf{H}}'_t\mathbf{P}_{t|t-1}\tilde{\mathbf{H}}_t + \mathbf{R}_t)^{-1}$.

  3. Obtain the filter distribution's mean and covariances:

    (a) $\mathbf{Y}_{t|t} = \mathbf{Y}_{t|t-1} + \mathbf{K}_t(\mathbf{Z}_t - \mathcal{H}_t(\mathbf{Y}_{t|t-1}))$.

    (b) $\mathbf{P}_{t|t} = (\mathbf{I} - \mathbf{K}_t\tilde{\mathbf{H}}_t)\mathbf{P}_{t|t-1}$.

end

Note that one uses the current EKF forecast value for $\hat{\mathbf{Y}}_t$ in this algorithm.

8.4.2 BHM Implementation via MCMC

In principle, the BHM formulation can accommodate nonlinear and non-Gaussian structures. This can be implemented through MCMC or through *importance sampling*. Importance sampling will be discussed in the next subsection. Here, we briefly discuss MCMC-related implementation issues, following Carlin, Polson, and Stoffer (1992) and Shumway and Stoffer (2006, Chapter 6). Note that implementation issues for non-Gaussian data models are typically similar to those found in spatial statistics (e.g., Banerjee, Carlin, and Gelfand, 2004; Diggle and Ribeiro, 2007), since the observations are usually assumed conditionally independent, given the latent spatio-temporal dynamical process.

To illustrate the basic ideas of MCMC for a BHM, we consider several cases. Consider the case where the data model is linear and the evolution model is nonlinear:

$$\mathbf{Z}_t = \mathbf{H}_t\mathbf{Y}_t + \boldsymbol{\varepsilon}_t, \qquad \boldsymbol{\varepsilon}_t \sim iid\,Gau(\mathbf{0}, \mathbf{R}), \qquad (8.61)$$

$$\mathbf{Y}_t = \mathcal{M}(\mathbf{Y}_{t-1}; \boldsymbol{\theta}_P) + \boldsymbol{\eta}_t, \qquad \boldsymbol{\eta}_t \sim iid\,Gau(\mathbf{0}, \mathbf{Q}). \qquad (8.62)$$

Now, assume that the Gibbs sampler is such that we need to sample from the full conditional distribution, $[\mathbf{Y}_t \mid \cdot]$. Thus,

$$[\mathbf{Y}_t \mid \cdot] \propto [\mathbf{Z}_t|\mathbf{Y}_t][\mathbf{Y}_t|\mathbf{Y}_{t-1}][\mathbf{Y}_{t+1}|\mathbf{Y}_t]$$

$$\propto Gau(\mathbf{A}_{1t}\mathbf{a}_{1t}, \mathbf{A}_{1t})[\mathbf{Y}_{t+1}|\mathbf{Y}_t],$$

where once again there is a slight abuse of notation in writing $Gau(\cdot, \cdot)$ instead of its density, and

$$\mathbf{A}_{1t} \equiv (\mathbf{Q}^{-1} + \mathbf{H}'_t\mathbf{R}^{-1}\mathbf{H}_t)^{-1},$$

$$\mathbf{a}_{1t} \equiv \mathbf{Q}^{-1}\mathcal{M}(\mathbf{Y}_{t-1}; \boldsymbol{\theta}_P) + \mathbf{H}'_t\mathbf{R}^{-1}\mathbf{Z}_t.$$

However, note that

$$[\mathbf{Y}_{t+1}|\mathbf{Y}_t] \propto \exp\{-(1/2)[(\mathbf{Y}_{t+1} - \mathcal{M}(\mathbf{Y}_t; \boldsymbol{\theta}_P))'\mathbf{Q}^{-1}(\mathbf{Y}_{t+1} - \mathcal{M}(\mathbf{Y}_t; \boldsymbol{\theta}_P))]\}$$

$$\equiv \gamma_1(\mathbf{Y}_t), \tag{8.63}$$

and since $\mathcal{M}(\mathbf{Y}_t; \boldsymbol{\theta}_P)$ is nonlinear in $\mathbf{Y}_t$ (and $\boldsymbol{\theta}_P$), the full conditional distribution cannot be obtained analytically. One could use a Metropolis–Hastings step to sample this full conditional distribution. The key to using a Metropolis–Hastings step within a Gibbs sampler is to find a good proposal distribution. One such proposal distribution, when the evolution equation is not far from linear, involves using a linearized model distribution in place of $\gamma_1(\mathbf{Y}_t)$, such as suggested by the EKF. By making this Gaussian, the Gaussian/Gaussian result (8.45) can be used to derive an approximate full conditional distribution that is Gaussian. The proposal in the Metropolis–Hastings step is then obtained by sampling from this approximate full conditional distribution. Of course, in high dimensions, the efficiency of this algorithm can be quite low.

Alternatively, as discussed in Shumway and Stoffer (2006, Section 6.9), because $0 \leq \gamma_1(\mathbf{Y}_t) \leq 1$, for all $\mathbf{Y}_t$, the distribution from which we wish to sample is controlled by $Gau(\mathbf{A}_{1t}\mathbf{a}_{1t}, \mathbf{A}_{1t})$, and it is reasonable to use *rejection sampling* (e.g., see Robert and Casella, 2004, Chapter 2) to sample from the desired full conditional distribution. Specifically, we generate $\mathbf{Y}_t^{(i)}$ from $Gau(\mathbf{A}_{1t}\mathbf{a}_{1t}, \mathbf{A}_{1t})$, and we accept it with probability $\gamma_1(\mathbf{Y}_t)$. For $\gamma_1(\mathbf{Y}_t)$ close to zero, rejection sampling will be inefficient, and alternatives, such as adaptive-rejection sampling (e.g., see Robert and Casella, 2004, Chapter 2), should be considered. Often, in the DSTM setting, n is large, and it is thus the case that $\gamma_1(\mathbf{Y}_t)$ is quite small, in which case even adaptive rejection sampling can be very inefficient. Furthermore, in the typical case where the parameters $\boldsymbol{\theta}_P$ are not known *a priori*, they must be sampled as well in the Gibbs sampler. In that case, a Metropolis–Hastings step is typically used.

Now, consider the case where the data model is nonlinear and the evolution model is linear:

$$\mathbf{Z}_t = \mathcal{H}(\mathbf{Y}_t; \boldsymbol{\theta}_D) + \boldsymbol{\varepsilon}_t, \qquad \boldsymbol{\varepsilon}_t \sim iid\, Gau(\mathbf{0}, \mathbf{R}), \tag{8.64}$$

$$\mathbf{Y}_t = \mathbf{M}\mathbf{Y}_{t-1} + \boldsymbol{\eta}_t, \qquad \boldsymbol{\eta}_t \sim iid\, Gau(\mathbf{0}, \mathbf{Q}). \tag{8.65}$$

Analogous to the previous case, the full conditional distribution for $\mathbf{Y}_t$ can be written as

$$[\mathbf{Y}_t \mid \cdot] \propto \gamma_2(\mathbf{Y}_t) Gau(\mathbf{A}_{2t}\mathbf{a}_{2t}, \mathbf{A}_{2t}),$$

where again there is a slight abuse of notation,

$$\mathbf{A}_{2t} \equiv (\mathbf{Q}^{-1} + \mathbf{M}'\mathbf{Q}^{-1}\mathbf{M})^{-1},$$

$$\mathbf{a}_{2t} \equiv \mathbf{Q}^{-1}\mathbf{M}\mathbf{Y}_{t-1} + \mathbf{M}'\mathbf{Q}^{-1}\mathbf{Y}_{t+1},$$

and

$$\gamma_2(\mathbf{Y}_t) \equiv \exp\{-(1/2)(\mathbf{Z}_t - \mathcal{H}(\mathbf{Y}_t; \boldsymbol{\theta}_D))'\mathbf{R}^{-1}(\mathbf{Z}_t - \mathcal{H}(\mathbf{Y}_t; \boldsymbol{\theta}_D))\}.$$

Again, the full conditional distribution cannot be obtained analytically. However, we can use a linearized distribution in place of $\gamma_2(\mathbf{Y}_t)$ in a Metropolis–Hastings step; or we could use a rejection-sampling approach, by sampling from $Gau(\mathbf{A}_{2t}\mathbf{a}_{2t}, \mathbf{A}_{2t})$ and accepting the sample with probability $\gamma_2(\mathbf{Y}_t)$. Again, if $\gamma_2(\mathbf{Y}_t)$ is close to zero (as often happens), this will be inefficient and one must use alternative sampling algorithms (e.g., adaptive-rejection, Metropolis–Hastings, or slice sampling).

Finally, consider the case where both the data model and the evolution model are nonlinear, as given by (8.57) and (8.58), where $\{\boldsymbol{\varepsilon}_t\}$ and $\{\boldsymbol{\eta}_t\}$ are assumed Gaussian. Then the full conditional distribution is

$$[\mathbf{Y}_t| \cdot] \propto \gamma_1(\mathbf{Y}_t)\gamma_2(\mathbf{Y}_t)Gau(\mathcal{M}(\mathbf{Y}_{t-1}; \boldsymbol{\theta}_P), \mathbf{Q}).$$

As before, this suggests that one can use rejection sampling to sample from this distribution; that is, first sample from $Gau(\mathcal{M}(\mathbf{Y}_{t-1}; \boldsymbol{\theta}_P), \mathbf{Q})$, and then accept it with probability $\gamma_1(\mathbf{Y}_t)\gamma_2(\mathbf{Y}_t)$. Such an approach is often inefficient, since $\gamma_1(\mathbf{Y}_t)\gamma_2(\mathbf{Y}_t)$ is typically very small. Then, adaptive-rejection sampling or a Metropolis–Hastings step is often used instead.

8.4.3 Alternative Metropolis–Hastings Algorithms and Approximations

Unfortunately, Metropolis–Hastings updates for high-dimensional nonlinear state-space models with unknown parameters can be difficult to implement and typically require extensive user-informed tuning. Thus, in the spirit of effective model/computation trade-offs (Section 2.5), one might choose to approximate the first-order Markovian dependence using a second-order temporal-dependence model that avoids computational difficulties. For example, the MCMC algorithm employed to fit the GQN ecological reaction-diffusion model described by Hooten and Wikle (2008) contains an approximation to a quadratic evolution equation, where the second-order term, $\theta \cdot \text{diag}(\mathbf{Y}_{t-1})\mathbf{Y}_{t-2}$, is used rather than $\theta \cdot \text{diag}(\mathbf{Y}_{t-1})\mathbf{Y}_{t-1}$ (and θ is a process-model parameter). With Gaussian error assumptions, this slight change in the evolution equation to a second-order equation allows analytical full conditional distributions to be obtained for the state variable $\mathbf{Y}_t$, resulting in more efficient computation via Gibbs sampling. Of course, in many cases, one would not want to change the dependence structure in the process model, but this approach could still be used to generate useful proposals in a block Metropolis-update algorithm. Under the GQN framework discussed in Section 7.3.3, such modifications are only possible when the function $g(\cdot)$ is linear, and thus they are only applicable in specific situations.

Note that many other approximations have been proposed so that the efficiency and robustness of the Gibbs sampler can be assured in the implementation of nonlinear models (e.g., Wakefield et al., 1994), sometimes through additional rejection algorithms (e.g., Carlin, Polson, and Stoffer, 1992; Jungbacker and Koopman, 2007). There has been considerable recent work to develop efficient MCMC algorithms for general, high-dimensional, highly nonlinear models. These include the "differential evolution MCMC" approach of ter Braak (2006), the "delayed rejection adaptive Metropolis" (DRAM) sampling algorithm of Haario et al. (2006), the "multiple very fast simulated annealing" (MVFSA) algorithm of Villagran et al. (2008), the "differential evolution adaptive Metropolis" (DREAM) algorithm of Vrugt et al. (2009), and the "t-walk" general-purpose MCMC sampler of Christen and Fox (2010). All of these methods show promise for increasing efficiency over standard MCMC algorithms for complex model implementations. However, as discussed in the overview of Higdon et al. (2008), although these algorithms (and other similar ones) can be quite effective in improving convergence for nonlinear spatial and spatio-temporal processes, in some cases, relatively simple single-component Metropolis updates can be as efficient as these more complicated sampling algorithms. At this point, our best advice is to evaluate a number of algorithms to see which is best for a specific application.

8.4.4 Importance Sampling Monte Carlo

Importance sampling Monte Carlo is another approach that can be used with a BHM (or an EHM) in the case where models are nonlinear or non-Gaussian (e.g., Robert and Casella, 2004, Section 3.3). We present here a general overview of importance sampling, followed by a special case that is useful for DSTMs, known as sequential importance sampling.

Historically, the primary use of Monte Carlo (MC) has been for the estimation of integrals (i.e., expectations for given probability models). Let g be a possibly multivariate function of the state process, $\mathbf{Y}_0, \dots, \mathbf{Y}_t$; recall that $\mathbf{Z}_{1:t}$ denotes all available data up to and including time t; and suppose we are interested in the conditional expectation,

$$E(g(\mathbf{Y}_{0:t})|\mathbf{Z}_{1:t}) = \int g(\mathbf{Y}_{0:t})[\mathbf{Y}_{0:t}|\mathbf{Z}_{1:t}]d\mathbf{Y}_{0:t}$$

$$= \frac{\int g(\mathbf{Y}_{0:t})[\mathbf{Z}_{1:t}|\mathbf{Y}_{0:t}][\mathbf{Y}_{0:t}]d\mathbf{Y}_{0:t}}{\int [\mathbf{Z}_{1:t}|\mathbf{Y}_{0:t}][\mathbf{Y}_{0:t}]d\mathbf{Y}_{0:t}},$$

assuming the integrals exist. An MC estimate can be obtained through the following *MC integration algorithm* (written in pseudo code):

1. Generate L (pseudo-random) realizations, $\mathbf{Y}_{0:t}^{(l)}$, from $[\mathbf{Y}_{0:t}|\mathbf{Z}_{1:t}]$; $l = 1, \dots, L$.

2. Evaluate g for each realization and compute the arithmetic average of the results, $\hat{E}(g(\mathbf{Y}_{0:t})|\mathbf{Z}_{1:t}) \equiv (1/L) \sum_{l=1}^{L} g(\mathbf{Y}_{0:t}^{(l)})$.

Under independent sampling in 1., this average converges (almost surely) to $E(g(\mathbf{Y}_{0:t})|\mathbf{Z}_{1:t})$ as L tends to infinity, which is a result of the strong law of large numbers. This also holds if realizations are stationary and ergodic, though not necessarily independent (Section 2.3).

We can also approximate the posterior probability density, $p(\cdot|\mathbf{Z}_{1:t}) \equiv [\mathbf{Y}_{0:t}|\mathbf{Z}_{1:t}]$ as follows. Let $\mathbf{y}_{0:t}$ denote a generic argument of $p(\cdot|\mathbf{Z}_{1:t})$. Then define $g(\mathbf{y})$ according to the scaled indicator function,

$$g(\mathbf{y}) \equiv \frac{I(\mathbf{y} \in (\mathbf{y}_{0:t}, \mathbf{y}_{0:t} + \boldsymbol{\Delta}))}{|\Delta_0||\Delta_1| \dots |\Delta_t|},$$

where $\boldsymbol{\Delta} \equiv (\Delta_0, \Delta_1, \dots, \Delta_t)$ is a $(t+1)$-dimensional vector whose components are all nonzero. Define

$$\hat{p}(\mathbf{y}_{0:t}|\mathbf{Z}_{1:t}) \equiv \hat{E}(g(\mathbf{Y}_{0:t})|\mathbf{Z}_{1:t}) = \frac{1}{L} \sum_{l=1}^{L} g(\mathbf{Y}_{0:t}^{(l)}),$$

which is a good approximation to $p(\mathbf{y}_{0:t}|\mathbf{Z}_{1:t})$ as both $\max\{|\Delta_i|\} \to 0$ and $L \to \infty$. In practice, one typically considers kernel-density estimates based on the realizations $\{\mathbf{Y}_{0:t}^{(l)} : l = 1, \dots, L\}$.

Notice that we have introduced the notation, $p(\cdot|\mathbf{Z}_{1:t})$, to emphasize the functional form of the posterior probability density. This notation is also useful when we sample from another density that is not the posterior density. When direct simulation from $p(\mathbf{y}_{0:t}|\mathbf{Z}_{1:t})$ is difficult or impossible, we can use *importance sampling Monte Carlo (ISMC)*. The idea is to consider another density with the same support as $p(\cdot|\mathbf{Z}_{1:t})$, say $q(\cdot|\mathbf{Z}_{1:t})$, that is comparatively easy to sample from. Then, we generate L samples $\{\mathbf{Y}_{0:t}^{(l)} : l = 1, \dots, L\}$ *from the importance density*, $q(\mathbf{y}_{0:t}|\mathbf{Z}_{1:t})$, and evaluate $g(\mathbf{Y}_{0:t}^{(l)})$ for each $l = 1, \dots, L$. However, these samples are not from $p(\cdot|\mathbf{Z}_{1:t})$, so to use these to estimate $E(g(\mathbf{Y}_{0:t})|\mathbf{Z}_{1:t})$, each sample (ensemble) member must be weighted. That is, the estimate is

$$\hat{E}(g(\mathbf{Y}_{0:t})|\mathbf{Z}_{1:t}) \equiv \sum_{l=1}^{L} w_t^{(l)} g(\mathbf{Y}_{0:t}^{(l)}),$$

where the ISMC weights, $\{w_t^{(l)} : l = 1, \dots, L\}$, are given below.

From the ISMC perspective, we have

$$E(g(\mathbf{Y}_{0:t})|\mathbf{Z}_{1:t}) = \int g(\mathbf{y}_{0:t}) \frac{p(\mathbf{y}_{0:t}|\mathbf{Z}_{1:t})}{q(\mathbf{y}_{0:t}|\mathbf{Z}_{1:t})} q(\mathbf{y}_{0:t}|\mathbf{Z}_{1:t}) \, d\mathbf{y}_{0:t}. \tag{8.66}$$

Then $v_t^{(l)}$, the unnormalized weight associated with $\mathbf{Y}_{0:t}^{(l)}$, is given by $p(\mathbf{Y}_{0:t}^{(l)}|\mathbf{Z}_{1:t})/q(\mathbf{Y}_{0:t}^{(l)}|\mathbf{Z}_{1:t})$, $l = 1, \ldots, L$. An intuitive choice for the importance density q in this case is the "prior," or evolution distribution,

$$q(\mathbf{y}_{0:t}|\mathbf{Z}_{1:t}) \equiv p(\mathbf{y}_{0:t}) = p(\mathbf{y}_0) \prod_{k=1}^{t} p(\mathbf{y}_k|\mathbf{y}_{k-1}),$$

which, in fact, does not depend on the data. Thus, given samples from $p(\mathbf{y}_0)$, we could obtain MC samples for all times $k = 1, \ldots, t$, using the evolution model. In this case, the unnormalized weights are just given by the likelihood, since

$$\frac{p(\mathbf{Y}_{0:t}|\mathbf{Z}_{1:t})}{p(\mathbf{Y}_{0:t})} \propto \frac{p(\mathbf{Z}_{1:t}|\mathbf{Y}_{0:t})p(\mathbf{Y}_{0:t})}{p(\mathbf{Y}_{0:t})} = p(\mathbf{Z}_{1:t}|\mathbf{Y}_{0:t}).$$

That is, for a sample, $\mathbf{Y}_{0:t}^{(l)} \equiv \{\mathbf{Y}_0^{(l)}, \mathbf{Y}_1^{(l)}, \ldots, \mathbf{Y}_t^{(l)}\}$, $l = 1, \ldots, L$, generated from the prior, an estimate for $p(\cdot|\mathbf{Z}_{1:T})$ can be obtained by using the *normalized* ISMC weights,

$$w_t^{(l)} = \frac{\prod_{k=1}^{t} p(\mathbf{Z}_k|\mathbf{Y}_k^{(l)})}{\sum_{j=1}^{L} \prod_{k=1}^{t} p(\mathbf{Z}_k|\mathbf{Y}_k^{(j)})}, \qquad l = 1, \ldots, L, \qquad (8.67)$$

where conditional independence, $p(\mathbf{Z}_{1:t}|\mathbf{Y}_{0:t}) = \prod_{k=1}^{t} p(\mathbf{Z}_k|\mathbf{Y}_k)$, is a consequence of (8.2). Specifically, $E(g(\mathbf{Y}_{0:t}|\mathbf{Z}_{1:t}))$ can be approximated by $\sum_{l=1}^{L} w_t^{(l)} g(\mathbf{Y}_{0:t}^{(l)})$, and the posterior density $p(\cdot|\mathbf{Z}_{1:t})$ can be approximated by applying a *weighted* kernel density estimate (with weights $\{w_t^{(l)} : l = 1, \ldots L\}$) to the sample $\{\mathbf{Y}_{0:t}^{(1)}, \ldots, \mathbf{Y}_{0:t}^{(L)}\}$ from the prior.

Now put $t = T$. Then this ensemble-based approach for obtaining samples from the posterior distribution of $\mathbf{Y}_{0:T}$ given $\mathbf{Z}_{1:T}$, is sometimes referred to as an *ensemble smoother*.

Although, in principle, this approach is sound, there are practical issues that limit its use in high dimensions. In particular, as discussed in Berliner and Wikle (2007), consider the case presented here where the importance distribution is the prior and the ISMC weights are proportional to the likelihoods [i.e., equation (8.67)]. Consider a K-variate random vector $\mathbf{d}$ whose distribution is $Gau(\mathbf{a}, \boldsymbol{\Sigma})$, with density written as $p(\mathbf{d}|\mathbf{a}) = c \cdot \exp\{-(1/2)(\mathbf{d} - \mathbf{a})'\boldsymbol{\Sigma}^{-1}(\mathbf{d} - \mathbf{a})\}$, where c is the normalizing constant. From probability theory, we know that the quadratic form, $(\mathbf{d} - \mathbf{a})'\boldsymbol{\Sigma}^{-1}(\mathbf{d} - \mathbf{a})$, has a chi-squared distribution on K degrees of freedom. It can then be shown that $E(\exp\{-(1/2)(\mathbf{d} - \mathbf{a})'\boldsymbol{\Sigma}^{-1}(\mathbf{d} - \mathbf{a})\}) = 2^{-K}$, and the corresponding variance is $3^{-K/2} - 2^{-K}$. A quick calculation of the coefficient of variation shows that it increases exponentially with K. A characteristic of samples from such distributions is that many values are small and one or two are huge. Thus, over the ensemble $\{\mathbf{Y}_{0:t}^{(l)} : l = 1, \ldots, L\}$, where $K = n(t + 1)$, the normalized ISMC weights tend to concentrate on a few (or, just one) ensemble members. This phenomenon is known as *degeneracy*. As will be seen below, degeneracy is also an issue, even in low-dimensional problems where there are multiple time points.

8.4.5   Sequential Monte Carlo

In principle, a general sequential Monte Carlo (MC) algorithm follows from the usual sequential-update distributions, namely the forecast distribution (8.6) and the filtering distribution (8.7). As mentioned in Section 8.4.4, the choice of the prior distribution as the importance distribution gives weights proportional to the likelihood. We note in this case that these weights can be computed iteratively, since from (8.2) we obtain

$$v_t^{(l)} = p(\mathbf{Z}_{1:t}|\mathbf{Y}_{0:t}^{(l)}) = \prod_{k=1}^{t} p(\mathbf{Z}_k|\mathbf{Y}_k^{(l)}) = p(\mathbf{Z}_t|\mathbf{Y}_t^{(l)})v_{t-1}^{(l)} . \tag{8.68}$$

This allows the importance sampler to be implemented sequentially, as we now discuss.

Assume we have L samples (or "particles") from the importance distribution, $q(\cdot|\mathbf{Z}_{1:t})$, which here is the prior $p(\cdot)$, but need not be in general. Associated with each particle, $\mathbf{Y}_{0:t-1}^{(l)}$, is a normalized weight $w_{t-1}^{(l)}$; $l = 1, \ldots, L$. Then from (8.6), the forecast density can be estimated as

$$\hat{p}(\mathbf{y}_t|\mathbf{Z}_{1:t-1}) \equiv \sum_{l=1}^{L} w_{t-1}^{(l)} p(\mathbf{y}_t|\mathbf{Y}_{t-1}^{(l)}) ,$$

where recall that $\mathbf{Y}_{0:t-1}^{(l)} = \{\mathbf{Y}_0^{(l)}, \ldots, \mathbf{Y}_{t-1}^{(l)}\}$, and the conditional density, $p(\mathbf{y}_t|\mathbf{Y}_{t-1}^{(l)})$, on the right-hand side is known from the evolution model. Then, from (8.7) and (8.68), the filtering distribution at time t can be estimated as follows:

$$\hat{p}(\mathbf{y}_t|\mathbf{Z}_{1:t}) \propto p(\mathbf{Z}_t|\mathbf{y}_t) \sum_{l=1}^{L} v_{t-1}^{(l)} p(\mathbf{y}_t|\mathbf{Y}_{t-1}^{(l)}) = \sum_{l=1}^{L} v_t^{(l)} p(\mathbf{y}_t|\mathbf{Y}_{t-1}^{(l)}) ,$$

where, without loss of generality, the unnormalized weights are used.

Unfortunately, the importance weights will eventually degenerate as t increases (i.e., only a few samples, or one sample, will get all of the weight) and the posterior distribution will not be adequately represented by the sample. Various practical solutions to this problem have been considered; the primary one considered here is *particle filtering*.

8.4.6 Particle Filtering

In the presentation given in the previous subsections, the "particles" have been deemphasized, in favor of obtaining kernel estimates of the desired posterior distributions. In this subsection, the L particles, $\{\mathbf{Y}_{0:t}^{(1)}, \ldots, \mathbf{Y}_{0:t}^{(L)}\}$, which are generated from the posterior distribution, $p(\mathbf{y}_{0:t}|\mathbf{Z}_{1:t})$, are featured. It is conventional in the particle-filtering literature to represent the "density" by $\hat{p}(\mathbf{y}_{0:t}|\mathbf{Z}_{1:t}) = (1/L) \sum_{l=1}^{L} \delta_{\mathbf{Y}_{0:t}^{(l)}}$, where $\delta_{\mathbf{y}}$ is the Dirac delta function centered at $\mathbf{y}$. A comprehensive overview of the particle-filtering literature can be found in Doucet, de Freitas, and Gordon (2001). Overcoming the degeneracy-of-weights problem mentioned in Section 8.4.5 is crucial for practical implementation of such approaches.

There are many other approaches to dealing with the particle-filter degeneracy problem, and it remains an active area of research. Perhaps the most basic of these algorithms is the sampling importance resampling (SIR) or *bootstrap filter* (Doucet, de Freitas, and Gordon, 2001; Gordon, Salmond, and Smith, 1993). This algorithm accentuates the importance of particles with large weights and neglects the particles with small weights at each time step. The basic *SIR algorithm* can be written in pseudo code as follows:

1. Initialization at $t = 0$
   - For $l = 1, \ldots L$, sample $\mathbf{Y}_{0|0}^{(l)} \sim p(\mathbf{y}_0)$ and set $t = 1$.
2. Importance-sampling step
   - For $l = 1, \ldots, L$, sample $\tilde{\mathbf{Y}}_t^{(l)} \sim p(\mathbf{y}_t|\mathbf{Y}_{t-1}^{(l)})$, and set $\tilde{\mathbf{Y}}_{0:t}^{(l)} = \{\mathbf{Y}_{1:t-1}^{(l)}, \tilde{\mathbf{Y}}_t^{(l)}\}$.
   - For $l = 1, \ldots, L$, evaluate the importance weights, $\tilde{w}_t^{(l)} = p(\mathbf{Z}_t|\tilde{\mathbf{Y}}_t^{(l)})$. (Note that in this algorithm these weights are *not* proportional to the weights at the previous time, $t - 1$, due to the resampling in step 3 below, which induces equal weights on the resample.)
   - Normalize the IS weights.
3. Resampling step
   - Resample, with replacement, L particles $\{\mathbf{Y}_{0:t}^{(l)} : l = 1, \ldots, L\}$ from the set $\{\tilde{\mathbf{Y}}_{0:t}^{(l)} : l = 1, \ldots, L\}$ using the importance weights for the resampling.
   - Set $t = t + 1$ and go to step 2.

The resampling step in the SIR algorithm reduces the effects of sample degeneracy. However, since particles with large weights are selected many times, there can be a loss of diversity among the particles, leading to "sample impoverishment" (Arulampalam et al., 2002). Pitt and Shepard (1999) considered a variant of the basic bootstrap filter, which they called "auxiliary sampling importance resampling" (ASIR), to address this problem. The basic idea is that one seeks to augment "good" particles such that the associated predictive likelihoods are large for these particles. Thus, the ASIR filter reduces the cost of sampling by resampling less frequently, particles that have small likelihoods. In the actual ASIR implementation, an auxiliary variable is introduced that allows the filter to adapt to the data more efficiently. Such filters, although an improvement, still suffer degeneracy in high-dimensional problems and when the process noise is relatively large. The incorporation of Markov chain moves into the importance sampling algorithm is an alternative approach to improving the degeneracy issues in traditional particle filters. The primary goal is to reduce the variability of the importance weights by attempting more accurate moves at each time step (e.g., Berzuini et al., 1997; MacEachern, Clyde, and Liu, 1999; Godsill and Clapp, 2001; Polson, Stroud, and Müller, 2008).

The extension of the particle filter to parameter estimation is nontrivial. One approach is to model the parameters as a random walk and then augment the state space with the parameters. A limitation with this approach is that it assumes that the state and the parameters have the same conditional-distributional form (e.g., Gaussian), where in reality certain parameters may be constrained in ways to suggest different distributions are more appropriate. Another limitation of this method is that it implies an increase in the variance of the parameters with time, resulting in posteriors that are more diffuse than the actual ones; shrinkage kernels can be used to address this, where the variance of parameters is based on particles from previous time points (Liu and West, 2001). Berliner and Wikle (2007) consider a number of approaches that can help when performing parameter and state process estimation with importance sampling. These include dimension reduction approaches that project processes and parameters into lower dimensional spaces, as well as the use of sufficient statistics and various approximations. Carvalho et al. (2010) describe a promising approach that also exploits the use of sufficient statistics. One can also use Markov chain Monte Carlo moves to facilitate parameter estimation (e.g., Polson, Stroud, and Müller, 2008). In particular, the hybrid sequential Monte Carlo and MCMC approaches of Andrieu, Doucet, and Holenstein (2010) appear to allow construction of efficient proposal distributions for high-dimensional, highly correlated processes using sequential importance sampling within the MCMC algorithm, in a manner that ensures convergence.

8.4.7 Ensemble Kalman Filtering

Although the algorithms and approaches described above help with the degeneracy issue, experience has shown that in high-dimensional situations, like one might encounter in real-world spatio-temporal problems, degeneracy is still problematic for sequential-importance-sampling methodologies. A closely related idea is to use MC in the context of the Kalman filter. Such methods are typically referred to as *ensemble Kalman filters*.

The ensemble Kalman filter (EnKF) was originally developed by Evensen (1994), Evensen and van Leeuven (1996), and Houtekamer and Mitchell

(1998). The basic approach uses Monte Carlo samples from Gaussian distributions to *approximate* the forecast distribution, while, critically, still using the nonlinear process-evolution model. In particular, one estimates the prior (forecast) means and covariance matrices with the Monte Carlo sample (ensemble). This is then used in the linear KF update formulas to obtain the filter distribution. In general, the EnKF algorithm is like the particle filter, with a set of particles being propagated forward with the dynamic model. However, instead of computing weights and resampling, the state-process vectors are updated using the Kalman gain matrix (as in traditional Kalman filtering), but with the forecast sample mean and sample covariance matrix from the ensemble of particles. Importantly, calculation of the sample covariance matrix must be "regularized" (in some way) to accommodate the relatively small number of particles used in its estimation. Although EnKF algorithms are typically stable for high-dimensional state variables, and they do not have the same sample impoverishment problems as the traditional particle filter, they are approximations and still often require parameter-estimation procedures that are disjoint from state estimation. Stroud et al. (2010) provide a discussion of such methods applied to sediment transport modeling in Lake Michigan using an advection-diffusion model (which fits into the nonlinear GQN framework discussed in Section 7.3.3) to motivate the latent dynamical process. In addition, more details can be found in the overview presented in Wikle and Berliner (2007) and Berliner and Wikle (2007), where an example of the EnKF on a simulated AR(1) dataset (similar to that presented in Section 8.2.1) can be found.

Berliner and Wikle (2007) also discuss many other approximate importance sampling algorithms, particularly those focused on exploiting reduced dimensionality.

8.4.8 Integrated Nested Laplace Approximation (INLA)

Finally, a method for implementing latent Gaussian models that has potential in the DSTM context is based on the integrated nested Laplace approximation (i.e., INLA; Rue and Held, 2005; Rue, Martino, and Chopin, 2009; Ruiz-Cárdenas, Krainski, and Rue, 2010). The INLA approach is a numerically implemented analytical solution for approximating posterior marginals in hierarchical models with latent Gaussian processes. The advantages of INLA over Monte Carlo-based solutions (e.g., importance sampling, MCMC) are primarily that INLA algorithms can be orders of magnitude faster and automatic, thus reducing the need for algorithm tuning and making it easier (and quicker) to build and check models. In practice, INLA methods appear to be accurate and, due to the availability of INLA software (e.g., Martino and Rue, 2009), a wide selection of models that meet the INLA criteria can be easily fitted using a suite of previously developed "black box" codings. For models that have a large number of non-Gaussian hyperparameters, process nonlinearities, or spatial structures that cannot be coerced into a GMRF, it is not yet clear if INLA methods will be directly helpful. However, new extensions are being rapidly developed and incorporated into existing INLA software.

We are hopeful that, in the near future, a combination of analytical/computational and Monte Carlo procedures will be available for implementing DSTMs within a hierarchical statistical model, where the models are more and more nonlinear and increasingly non-Gaussian.

8.5　BIBLIOGRAPHIC NOTES

Implementation and inference for DSTMs is rapidly evolving, given its reliance on MCMC and importance sampling algorithms. We fully realize that almost anything said here will be out of date by the time the book is published. However, there are some fundamental implementation details that have stood the test of time, and we have referred to many of them in this chapter. Because of space limitations, not a lot of detail can be given; for that, we refer the reader to many of the excellent books that deal with modern implementations of dynamical models, as well as more general sequential and MCMC implementations. Specifically, we recommend Shumway and Stoffer (2006) for an overview of state-space implementations of various types. We also note that Barndorff-Nielsen, Cox, and Klüppelberg (2001), Robert and Casella (2004) and Robert and Casella (2010) give comprehensive overviews of general Monte Carlo approaches, and Doucet, de Freitas, and Gordon (2001) give an overview of practical sequential Monte Carlo approaches. West and Harrison (1997), Gamerman and Lopes (2006), Marin and Robert (2007), Kitagawa (2010) and Prado and West (2010) give modern perspectives on Bayesian implementation of dynamical models. Banerjee, Carlin, and Gelfand (2004), Clark and Gelfand (2006), Le and Zidek (2006), Diggle and Ribeiro (2007), and Finkenstädt, Held, and Isham (2007) give specific implementational details for various spatial and spatio-temporal models. In addition, we recommend Clark (2007) as an excellent introduction to various inference approaches to modeling complicated data and processes. Finally, we highly recommend the book by Royle and Dorazio (2008), which contains a similar hierarchical modeling approach as that presented in our book, and it gives a variety of detailed examples at various levels, along with specific implementation details.

Sequential Process Estimation
Many of the references for statistical time series analysis given in Chapter 3 discuss sequential estimation to various degrees. Our presentation follows that given in Shumway and Stoffer (2000, 2006). However, the seminal works of Kalman (1960), Jazwinski (1970), Anderson and Moore (1979), West and Harrison (1997), and Doucet, de Freitas, and Gordon (2001) are also excellent references. For the Bayesian perspective, we rely on Jazwinski (1970), Meinhold and Singpurwalla (1983), West and Harrison (1997), and Doucet, de Freitas, and Gordon (2001). We have also found the books by Grewal and

Andrews (1993), Eubank (2006), Kitagawa (2010) and Prado and West (2010) particularly helpful.

Parameter Estimation in Sequential Implementations
Parameter estimation in sequential implementations is covered in many classic texts, but in this chapter we focus on Gupta and Mehra (1974), Carter and Kohn (1994), Frühwirth-Schnatter (1994), West and Harrison (1997), Shumway and Stoffer (1982, 2000, 2006), Doucet, de Freitas, and Gordon (2001), Robert and Casella (2004), Xu and Wikle (2007), and Katzfuss and Cressie (2011).

Particle Filtering
Particle filtering (and its various derivatives) is a rapidly developing area of research. We have presented just the basics in this chapter, motivated by Gordon, Salmond, and Smith (1993), Pitt and Shephard (1999), and Doucet, de Freitas, and Gordon (2001). Irwin, Cressie, and Johannesson (2002) give a comparative review of the Unscented Particle Filter and the Extended Kalman Filter. We also discussed, briefly, the ensemble Kalman filter, which is an approximate sequential importance sampling approach developed in the atmospheric and oceanographic sciences. This is also a rapidly developing area, and we have cited a few of the fundamental references in the area: Evensen (1994), Evensen and van Leeuven (1996), Houtekamer and Mitchell (1998), Evensen (2009), and Stroud et al. (2010). We have also borrowed notation and examples from the tutorial paper by Wikle and Berliner (2007).

Combined MCMC/ISMC
The combined use of MCMC and ISMC may be very useful in nonlinear and non-Gaussian DSTMs, as suggested by the work of Andrieu, Doucet, and Holenstein (2010). Historically, there have been several approaches to combining MCMC and ISMC. Berzuini et al. (1997) consider Markov chain Monte Carlo (MCMC) moves within the particle filter, which they call the Metropolis–Hastings Importance Resampling (MHIR) method. MacEachern, Clyde, and Liu (1999) incorporated Markov chain transitions into a sequential importance sampling algorithm for a nonparametric Bayes model. Berliner, Milliff, and Wikle (2003) proposed a hybrid MCMC/ISMC algorithm for a multivariate spatio-temporal process for the ocean/atmosphere system. In this case, MCMC samples were used from the atmospheric portion of the model within the ISMC ocean model, with a final re-weighting of the atmospheric samples based on the importance weights from the ocean model. Godsill and Clapp (2001) proposed a method to incorporate MCMC resampling ideas into the particle filter by making the MCMC traverse a sequence of "bridging densities" that lie between the forecast density [see (8.4)] and the filtering density [see (8.5)]. Polson, Stroud, and Müller (2008) proposed an approach to Bayesian filtering and sequential parameter learning in general state-space models that relies on a rolling-window MCMC algorithm; the algorithm approximates the target posterior distribution by a mixture of lag-k smoothing distributions.

MCMC Implementations of Nonlinear DSTMs

It is worth noting that one can develop more efficient "block" updates of the state process and the parameters for Metropolis–Hastings implementations of nonlinear (nonconjugate) models. A very useful example is the so-called "differential evolution MCMC" approach of ter Braak (2006), the "delayed rejection adaptive Metropolis" approach of Haario et al. (2006), and the "differential evolution adaptive Metropolis" algorithm of Vrugt et al. (2009). These algorithms and others are evaluated in Higdon et al. (2008).

Alternative Implementations

In terms of other useful methods for fitting nonlinear models, such as the GQN models in Section 7.3.3, when only characteristics of posterior distributions are of interest, specific numerical-optimization procedures have been developed to estimate posterior modes in the nonlinear state-space-modeling framework (So, 2003). Another approach that may prove to be useful is referred to as variational Bayesian learning (e.g., Raiko et al., 2007). These methods, which are largely dependent on additive Gaussian error in both the data model and the process model, can be employed in situations where there exist significant nonlinearities in the mean of the HM components. In essence, these methods work by approximating the intractable posterior distribution of interest with a tractable parametric distribution, and then the estimation is corrected through the use of a cost function that is based on the discrepancy or misfit between the distributions (often Kullback–Leibler divergence). Such methods have proven valuable in applications involving Control Theory (e.g., Raiko and Tornio, 2009) and, as they continue to develop, they may prove to be useful for general DSTMs. In addition, Laplace approximations can provide fast approximate state process estimates in some nonlinear and non-Gaussian settings (Koyama et al. 2010).

CHAPTER 9

Hierarchical DSTMs: Examples

The earlier chapters of this book have focused primarily on (hierarchical statistical) *models* for temporal, spatial, and spatio-temporal processes. In this chapter, we demonstrate, by way of example, the central role these models play in an "inference engine" that allows us to convert observations and information into knowledge. We do this for four examples based on spatio-temporal data and an underlying DSTM. Beyond these examples, the references given throughout this book contain many excellent applications of spatio-temporal statistical modeling. We encourage the reader to look at those sources to appreciate how much has been accomplished in quantifying and exploiting spatio-temporal variability in scientific applications.

Each of the four examples in this chapter was chosen to show different aspects of modeling, implementation, and inference. None of them represents a complete case study, although they are drawn from articles where the full details (from exploratory data analyses, to model building, to computation, to inference) are available. In Section 9.1, the example of long-lead forecasting of tropical Pacific sea surface temperatures is chosen to illustrate how a dimension-reduced BHM that includes a *linear DSTM* contrasts with the same for a particular *nonlinear DSTM*. The latter was built to account for possibly different transitions to and from "warm," "normal," and "cool" sea-surface-temperature regimes. Inferences based on the two BHMs' posterior forecast distributions are used to compare their performances.

Section 9.2 presents a remote-sensing example, where very large datasets of aerosol measurements from the MISR instrument on NASA's Terra satellite are analyzed. In this case, an EHM that includes a *linear DSTM* is fitted to the data, which compares directly to the case in Section 8.1 where a BHM with a linear DSTM is considered. Both use *dimension reduction*, but the computational aspects are quite different. The EHM requires parameters to be *estimated* separately, and in this section we give a method-of-moments estimator. Computing the EHM's posterior means and variances is extremely fast, relative to comparable BHM implementations, but inferences can be too liberal.

In Section 9.3, we consider an example of an invasive species, the Eurasian Collared Dove, that has been invading North America over the last several decades. This example was chosen to illustrate how a *non-Gaussian data model* can be paired with a *nonlinear DSTM* (process model) to obtain a scientifically motivated BHM of the species' invasion. Crucially, the parameter model in the BHM incorporates scientific information to account for uncertain probabilities of detection and landscape-scale variation in the spread and growth of the invasive-species population through time.

Finally, in Section 9.4, an example is considered of predicting and forecasting near-surface winds over the Mediterranean Sea based on remotely sensed scatterometer observations. The purpose of these predictions and forecasts is to provide realistic wind-forcing distributions for an operational ocean forecast model. We chose this example to illustrate how PDE-based scientific knowledge can be used to motivate a *multivariate linear DSTM*. In particular, we demonstrate how such a multivariate model can be built by conditioning on a common process. Another striking feature of this example is that it illustrates how the uncertainty captured in the BHM makes a *scientifically meaningful impact* on ocean forecasts.

This last example is a fitting conclusion to the last chapter, since we believe that the real potential of Statistics for spatio-temporal data can be found in modeling the *interaction of several (or many) variables* in space and time. The future of Statistics, in quantifying uncertainty realistically through multivariate hierarchical models and facilitating the ascent of the knowledge pyramid in Science, is bright!

9.1 LONG-LEAD FORECASTING OF TROPICAL PACIFIC SEA SURFACE TEMPERATURES

The process governing sea surface temperatures (SSTs) in the tropical Pacific Ocean is complex and influenced by interactions between the atmosphere and the ocean on a variety of temporal and spatial scales. In particular, its variability on interannual and interdecadal time scales is related strongly to changes in global-scale atmospheric processes (e.g., see the overview in Philander, 1990). On interannual time scales, the dominant features in this process are the so-called El Niño and La Niña phenomena, which are characterized by quasi-periodic warming and cooling that occurs with periods of approximately 3–5 years. In recent years, as observational networks and data-assimilation approaches have improved, the ability to forecast SSTs with lead times of 6–12 months has improved dramatically. Indeed, due to its complexity and uncertainties related to the fundamental physical mechanisms that drive these phenomena, SST is one of the few processes in oceanography in which "statistical" long-lead forecast models perform as well as or better than deterministic models (e.g., Barnston, Glantz, and He, 1999; van Oldenborgh et al., 2005).

State-space models in a reduced-dimensional space (e.g., based on EOF projections) have proven to be effective long-lead prediction models for quite some time (e.g., Penland and Magorian, 1993). Nevertheless, there is strong evidence that the dynamics of El Niño and La Niña are not linear (e.g., Hoerling, Kumar, and Zhong, 1997; Burgers and Stephenson, 1999; Kondrashov et al., 2005). In this regard, several nonlinear statistical models for SSTs have been developed in recent years, and their forecast performance has generally been comparable to or better than linear models, at least in terms of capturing the magnitude of the El Niño and La Niña events (e.g., Tangang et al., 1998; Berliner, Wikle, and Cressie, 2000; Tang et al., 2000; Timmermann, Voss, and Pasmanter, 2001; Kondrashov et al., 2005).

Given that SST observations have been used to illustrate many of the exploratory methods for spatio-temporal data in Chapter 5, it is appropriate to follow up in this chapter with long-lead forecasting models for SSTs based on hierarchical modeling. In what is to follow, we compare BHM implementations of linear and nonlinear DSTMs. In particular, our goal will be to forecast, six months in advance, tropical Pacific SST anomalies from current and past monthly averages. The data used in these examples are monthly averaged SST anomalies (where the anomalies are with respect to a January 1970–December 1985 climatology) on a $2° \times 2°$ resolution grid over the tropical Pacific Ocean from $29°$ S–$29°$ N latitude and $124°$ E–$70°$ W longitude. In reality, they are the result of combining *in situ* observations (e.g., buoys, ship tracks, etc.) with satellite observations and interpolating them onto the $2° \times 2°$ resolution grid; see (2.11) for a generic way to express this. We consider data for the period January 1970–January 1999 (349 consecutive months). There are 2261 oceanic locations in this dataset giving a total of 789,089 (2261×349) spatio-temporal data—a high-dimensional dataset. Figure 5.4 shows image plots for these data from February 1998 through January 1999. These plots illustrate the latter part of the extreme 1997 El Niño event, followed by the transition into the extreme 1998 La Niña event. For a more complete description of these data, see Chapter 5 and Berliner, Wikle, and Cressie (2000), *hereafter BWC*. In this section, we build a BHM based on a reduced-dimensional linear DSTM, and we compare it to one based on a reduced-dimensional nonlinear DSTM. We note that BWC chose a seven-month-ahead forecast to allow a month for the SST data to become available and for the forecast model to be run; in this section, we use six months lead time, in line with other forecasts.

9.1.1   Reduced-Dimension Linear DSTM

In this subsection, we consider a BHM for a reduced-dimension *linear* DSTM, to perform long-lead (six month) forecasting of monthly SST anomalies. Let the data be represented by $\mathbf{Z}_t \equiv (Z_t(\mathbf{s}_1), \dots, Z_t(\mathbf{s}_m))'$ for $m = 2261$ oceanic grid cells, and $t = 1, \dots, T = 349$ months. We let the underlying latent SST process be represented by $\mathbf{Y}_t \equiv (Y_t(\mathbf{s}_1), \dots, Y_t(\mathbf{s}_n))'$, where in this case $n = m = 2261$. Critically, we assume that the dynamics can be captured exclusively by the reduced-dimensional process $\{\boldsymbol{\alpha}_t\}$, where

$$\mathbf{Y}_t = \boldsymbol{\Phi}\boldsymbol{\alpha}_t + \boldsymbol{\gamma}_t,$$

and $\boldsymbol{\Phi}$ is an $n \times p_\alpha$ matrix of the first p_α EOFs of the empirical spatial covariance matrix of the data. The exploratory spatio-temporal data analysis in Chapter 5 was an important precursor to building this model; see the discussion in Section 5.3 and the associated plots of the first four EOFs in Figures 5.17 and 5.18. For simplicity, in this example we shall assume (somewhat unrealistically) that the error process has white-noise structure; that is, $\boldsymbol{\gamma}_t \sim iid\,Gau(\mathbf{0}, \sigma_\gamma^2 \mathbf{I})$. We seek to forecast the smoothed process, $\mathbf{Y}_{t+\tau}^P \equiv \boldsymbol{\Phi}\boldsymbol{\alpha}_{t+\tau}$, given data through time t (i.e., $\mathbf{Z}_{1:t} \equiv \{\mathbf{Z}_1, \ldots, \mathbf{Z}_t\}$), where $\tau = 6$ (corresponding to a forecast with 6-month forecast lead time). It is important to reiterate that in this application we are focused on *forecasting*; and since we are assuming that the dynamics are controlled by $\{\boldsymbol{\alpha}_t\}$, it is reasonable to consider only the smoothed process $\{\mathbf{Y}_t^P\}$. We note that if the goal was spatio-temporal prediction, then we would want to take into account the truncation error, $\boldsymbol{\gamma}_t$, and forecast $\mathbf{Y}_t \equiv \mathbf{Y}_t^P + \boldsymbol{\gamma}_t$ (e.g., see Wikle and Cressie, 1999; Cressie, Shi, and Kang, 2010).

Consider the data model,

$$\mathbf{Z}_t = \mathbf{Y}_t^P + \boldsymbol{v}_t, \qquad \boldsymbol{v}_t \sim iid\,Gau(\mathbf{0}, \boldsymbol{\Sigma}_v), \tag{9.1}$$

where $\mathbf{Y}_t^P$ (i.e., $\boldsymbol{\alpha}_t$) and not $\mathbf{Y}_t$ is featured, and the error process $\{\boldsymbol{v}_t\}$ includes both the SST measurement/representativeness error (Section 7.1.2) and the truncation error (Section 7.1.3). In this implementation of a linear DSTM, we assume $\boldsymbol{\Sigma}_v = \sigma_v^2 \mathbf{I}$.

The process model in this case is given by the p_α-dimensional process,

$$\boldsymbol{\alpha}_{t+\tau} = \mathbf{M}\boldsymbol{\alpha}_t + \boldsymbol{\eta}_t, \quad \boldsymbol{\eta}_t \sim iid\,Gau(\mathbf{0}, \boldsymbol{\Sigma}_\eta), \qquad t = 1, 2, \ldots, \tag{9.2}$$

where we note that the α-process at time $t + \tau$ is conditioned on the α-process at time t to obtain the long-lead forecast [see BWC for relevant discussion].

Since we are taking a BHM approach, the parameter model must be specified; here, we choose

$$\mathrm{vec}(\mathbf{M}) \sim Gau(\mathbf{0}, 100\,\mathbf{I}),$$

$$\boldsymbol{\Sigma}_\eta^{-1} \sim W((\mathbf{S}_\eta\,d_\eta)^{-1}, d_\eta), \qquad \text{with } \mathbf{S}_\eta = 100\,\mathbf{I}, d_\eta = p_\alpha - 1,$$

$$\sigma_v^2 \sim IG(q_v, r_v), \qquad \text{with } q_v = 0.1, r_v = 100,$$

where $W(\cdot, d_\eta)$ corresponds to a Wishart distribution with d_η degrees of freedom, and the choices for q_v and r_v correspond to an inverse gamma distribution with mean, 0.1 and variance, 100. These prior distributions were chosen to suggest relatively non-informative priors, and a sensitivity analysis showed that the results were not overly sensitive to these choices. Note that since we have SST data for quite a long time period ($T = 349$), we do not expect our results to be very sensitive to the initial conditions, so rather than specify prior distributions for the initial conditions, we simply fix $\boldsymbol{\alpha}_t = \boldsymbol{\Phi}'\mathbf{Z}_t$; $t = 1, \ldots, \tau = 6$.

For this BHM implementation, we use the basic Gibbs-sampler MCMC for linear DSTMs described in Section 8.3. However, rather than inferring a data-model error matrix that is left unspecified, recall we use $\sigma_v^2 \mathbf{I}$ here. Then, in the Gibbs sampler in Section 8.3, the full conditional distribution of σ_v^2 is given by

$$
\sigma_v^2 \sim IG\left(\left(\frac{1}{r_v} + (1/2)\sum_{t=1}^{T}(\mathbf{Z}_t - \boldsymbol{\Phi}\boldsymbol{\alpha}_t)'(\mathbf{Z}_t - \boldsymbol{\Phi}\boldsymbol{\alpha}_t)\right)^{-1}, \frac{mT}{2} + q_v\right).
$$

The algorithm was run for 6000 iterations, with the first 1000 iterations set aside as a period of "burn-in." From trace plots, the algorithm appears to converge quite rapidly.

BHM Results: Linear DSTM

For this example, we considered two separate long-lead forecasts with $p_\alpha = 10$, corresponding to the leading EOFs in the reduced-dimension linear DSTM given by (9.2). First, we forecasted the six-month-lead October 1997 smoothed SST anomalies (i.e., $\mathbf{Y}_{t+\tau}^P$), given data through t, which corresponds to April 1997. Then we performed an equivalent forecast for October 1998, given data through April 1998. These forecasts are shown in Figure 9.1. In particular, the first row of panels, (a) and (f), show the data (i.e., $\mathbf{Z}_{t+\tau}$) for the forecast target months, respectively. The second row of panels, (b) and (g), show the smoothed data (i.e., $\boldsymbol{\Phi}\boldsymbol{\Phi}'\mathbf{Z}_{t+\tau}$) for the forecast target months; the third row of panels, (c) and (h), show the corresponding smooth forecasts (i.e., $E(\mathbf{Y}_{t+\tau}^P|\mathbf{Z}_{1:t})$); the fourth row of panels, (d) and (i), show the pixelwise 2.5 percentiles of the posterior forecast distribution (i.e., $[\mathbf{Y}_{t+\tau}^P|\mathbf{Z}_{1:t}]$), and the fifth row of panels (e) and (j) show the corresponding pixelwise 97.5 percentiles of the posterior forecast distribution (i.e., $[\mathbf{Y}_{t+\tau}^P|\mathbf{Z}_{1:t}]$).

Additionally, Figure 9.2 shows the posterior forecast density for SST averages over the Niño 3.4 region (5° S–5° N, 120°–170° W) for (a) the forecast of October 1997 (onset of an El Niño event) given data up to April 1997 and (b) the forecast of October 1998 (onset of a La Niña event) given data up to April 1998. The posterior means for these distributions are shown with a blue "star" on the horizontal axis, and the calculated Niño 3.4 index from the actual observations (6 months after the forecast was made) are shown with a red "star." These forecast distributions are quite narrow, suggesting more accuracy than appears to be realistic, when compared to the observed values. In particular, although the forecast for October 1997 did indicate a higher (i.e., warmer) than average Niño 3.4 index, it did not come close to capturing the intensity of the actual warm (El Niño) event. In the case of the cool (La Niña) event in October 1998, the forecast distribution does contain

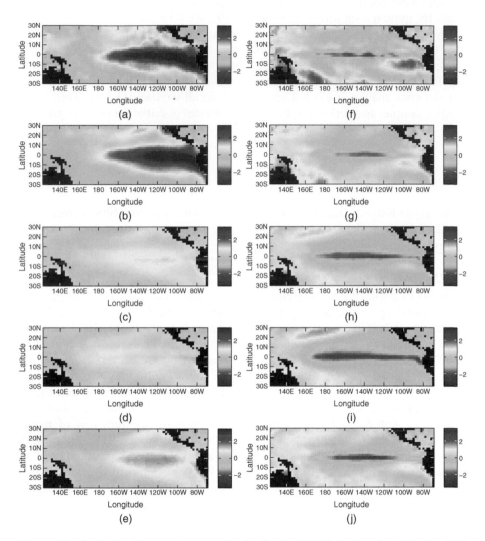

Figure 9.1 Sea Surface Temperature anomalies for October 1997 (left column) and October 1998 (right column). The first row of panels (**a, f**) show data for October 1997 and 1998, respectively. The second row of panels (**b, g**) show the smoothed data for October 1997 and 1998, respectively. The third row of panels (**c, h**) show the smooth forecast (mean of the posterior forecast distribution) from the reduced-dimension linear DSTM for October 1997 and October 1998, given data through April 1997 and April 1998, respectively. The fourth row of panels (**d, i**) show the pixelwise lower 2.5 percentiles from the posterior forecast distribution for October 1997 and 1998, respectively. The fifth row of panels (**e, j**) show the pixelwise upper 97.5 percentiles of the posterior forecast distribution for October 1997 and 1998, respectively.

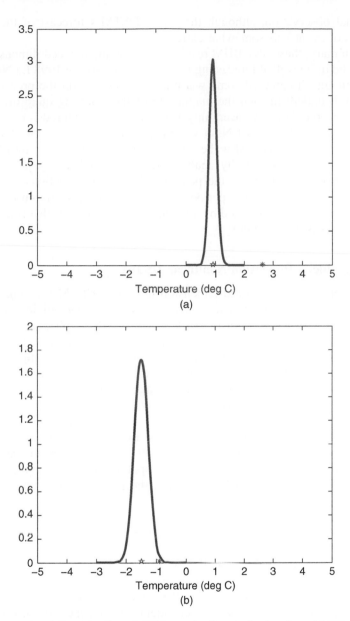

Figure 9.2 Reduced-dimension linear DSTM posterior forecast density of monthly Niño 3.4 region (5° S–5° N, 120°–170° W) SST averages. The top panel (**a**) shows the posterior forecast density for October 1997 given data up to April 1997. The bottom panel (**b**) shows the corresponding posterior forecast density for October 1998 given data up to April 1998. In each panel, the blue "star" shows the mean of the forecast distribution, and the red "star" shows the corresponding observed value (6 months later) of the Niño 3.4 region.

the actual observation, although the linear DSTM's forecast of the intensity of the cool event was somewhat extreme.

In summary, these SST BHM results show that the reduced-dimension linear DSTM did quite well at forecasting the onset of the strong 1998 La Niña. However, although it captured some warming associated with the preceding 1997 El Niño, it underestimated the magnitude of the warming quite dramatically. In addition, the forecast uncertainty was somewhat captured for the La Niña cooling, but not for the El Niño warming. One might question if the mixed success of the linear DSTM is the result of the (somewhat extreme) truncation to $p_\alpha = 10$ EOFs. Sensitivity analyses showed that keeping $p_\alpha = 20$ EOFs did not change substantially the posterior forecast distributions. This limited example for the 1997–1998 period suggests that at least the onset of the La Niña is reasonably represented by a linear DSTM; however, that is not the case for the onset of the El Niño.

9.1.2 Reduced-Dimension Nonlinear DSTM

BWC implemented a reduced-dimension nonlinear DSTM for long-lead forecasting of Pacific SST anomalies. The emphasis in that article was a model that allowed the dynamics of the El Niño and La Niña phenomena to be different (e.g., Hoerling, Kumar, and Zhong, 1997), due to a regime-switching model [e.g., see Section 7.3.2, equation (7.69)]. Given the complexity of this model, along with the fact that qualitative scientific knowledge was included in parameter specifications, it was natural to take a BHM approach. We reproduce the key elements of that analysis here.

The BHM in this context is similar to the reduced-dimension EOF model given in (9.1), with two major exceptions. First, rather than assuming $\Sigma_v = \sigma_v^2 \mathbf{I}$, we specify that v_t in the data model (9.1) is dependent in space; that is, $v_t \sim iid\, Gau(\mathbf{0}, \Sigma_v)$, where BWC used a spatial covariance matrix Σ_v based on higher-order EOFs. More importantly, the process model on the reduced-dimensional space is

$$\alpha_{t+\tau} = \mu_t + \mathbf{M}_t \alpha_t + \eta_{t+\tau}, \tag{9.3}$$

where $\eta_t \sim iid\, Gau(\mathbf{0}, \Sigma_\eta)$, for all t. We also need to specify prior distributions for initial values $\{\alpha_t : t = 1, \ldots, \tau\}$ in this framework (or, fix them as described in the linear DSTM given in Section 9.1.1.) The critical modeling assumption here is that we let $\mathbf{M}_t$ and μ_t be dependent on both the current (i.e., time t) and future (i.e., time $t + \tau$) climate regimes. That is,

$$\mathbf{M}_t = \mathbf{M}(I_t, J_t),$$

$$\mu_t = \mu(I_t, J_t),$$

where I_t classifies the current regime as "cool" (0), "normal" (1), or "warm" (2), and J_t anticipates a transition to one of the three regimes at time $t + \tau$.

Specifically, consider a threshold model for the index of the "current state":

$$I_t = \begin{cases} 0, & \text{if } SOI_t < \text{low threshold,} \\ 1, & \text{if } SOI_t \text{ in between,} \\ 2, & \text{if } SOI_t > \text{upper threshold,} \end{cases}$$

where SOI_t is the Southern Oscillation Index (i.e., the surface air pressure anomalies at Tahiti minus those at Darwin), which is related to the El Niño and La Niña phenomena, and the threshold values are chosen empirically as described in BWC. The "future" state index J_t is then defined by the following latent process model:

$$J_t = \begin{cases} 0, & \text{if } W_t < \text{low threshold,} \\ 1, & \text{if } W_t \text{ in between,} \\ 2, & \text{if } W_t > \text{upper threshold,} \end{cases}$$

where W_t is a latent process that anticipates the future climate regime, with the threshold values calibrated empirically to the threshold parameters for I_t. This latent process is modeled by

$$W_t | \boldsymbol{\beta}_w, \sigma_w^2 \sim Gau(\mathbf{X}_t' \boldsymbol{\beta}_w, \sigma_w^2),$$

where

$$\mathbf{X}_t \equiv (1, U_t, U_t \sin(2\pi b_t/12), U_t \cos(2\pi b_t/12), U_t^2)',$$

U_t is the low-pass filtered east–west component of the wind at 10 meters above the surface at $5°$ N and $157°$ E, and b_t is an index of month (i.e., $b_t = 0, 1, \ldots, 11$) at time t. Note that the use of the wind process at this location is motivated by known relationships between the atmospheric forcing and the ocean response in the Western Pacific ocean [see BWC for more discussion]. This relationship is evident empirically from Figure 5.8. However, there is recent evidence (SSES, 2009) to suggest that this relationship is changing.

The actual reduced-dimensional process model is somewhat more involved. In particular, we decompose the p_α-dimensional state process $\{\boldsymbol{\alpha}_t\}$ into large-scale and small-scale components: $\boldsymbol{\alpha}_t = (\boldsymbol{\alpha}_t^{(1)\prime}, \boldsymbol{\alpha}_t^{(2)\prime})'$, where $\boldsymbol{\alpha}_t^{(1)}$ is a p_1-dimensional vector corresponding to the first p_1 EOFs, and $\boldsymbol{\alpha}_t^{(2)}$ is a p_2-dimensional vector corresponding to the next p_2 EOFs (where $p_\alpha = p_1 + p_2$). Then, the evolution model,

$$\boldsymbol{\alpha}_{t+\tau} = \boldsymbol{\mu}(I_t, J_t) + \mathbf{M}(I_t, J_t)\boldsymbol{\alpha}_t + \boldsymbol{\eta}_{t+\tau},$$

is parameterized as

$$
\begin{pmatrix} \boldsymbol{\alpha}_{t+\tau}^{(1)} \\ \boldsymbol{\alpha}_{t+\tau}^{(2)} \end{pmatrix} = \begin{pmatrix} \boldsymbol{\mu}^{(1)}(I_t, J_t) \\ \mathbf{0} \end{pmatrix} + \begin{pmatrix} \mathbf{M}^{(1,1)}(I_t, J_t) & \mathbf{M}^{(1,2)} \\ \mathbf{M}^{(2,1)} & \mathbf{M}^{(2,2)} \end{pmatrix} \begin{pmatrix} \boldsymbol{\alpha}_t^{(1)} \\ \boldsymbol{\alpha}_t^{(2)} \end{pmatrix} + \begin{pmatrix} \boldsymbol{\eta}_{t+\tau}^{(1)} \\ \boldsymbol{\eta}_{t+\tau}^{(2)} \end{pmatrix},
$$

$$(9.4)$$

where

$$
\begin{pmatrix} \boldsymbol{\eta}_t^{(1)} \\ \boldsymbol{\eta}_t^{(2)} \end{pmatrix} \sim iid\, Gau \begin{pmatrix} \boldsymbol{\Sigma}_\eta^{(1,1)} & \boldsymbol{\Sigma}_\eta^{(1,2)} \\ (\boldsymbol{\Sigma}_\eta^{(1,2)})' & \boldsymbol{\Sigma}_\eta^{(2,2)} \end{pmatrix}.
$$

$$(9.5)$$

As discussed in BWC, these parameterizations are motivated by the desire to make the model more parsimonious (i.e., to achieve dimension reduction in the parameter space).

At the next level of the HM hierarchy, we specify distributions for the parameters in the data model and the process model. In some cases, data-based hyperparameters were selected, with the variances inflated in the direction of non-informativeness. Considerable detail on specification of the parameter distributions can be found in BWC. More generally, the covariance matrix $\boldsymbol{\Sigma}_\nu$ defined in (9.1) was parameterized in terms of some of the truncated EOFs, as suggested in BWC and given by equation (7.26). The initial state-process components and propagator matrices were given multivariate Gaussian prior distributions with data-driven hyperparameters. Covariance matrices in the process model were given Wishart distributions with data-driven hyperparameters, and the regression parameters $\boldsymbol{\beta}_w$ and σ_w^2 in the model for W_t were given (data-driven) Gaussian and inverse-gamma priors.

SST BHM Results: Nonlinear DSTM

The MCMC algorithm for this model is given in specific detail in Berliner, Wikle, and Cressie (2000b). Although somewhat tedious to derive, it is quite efficient and consists exclusively of Gibbs updates.

One advantage of the threshold formulation described above for the process model, is that we can look at the posterior probability of the forecast state being in a particular regime j, with the long-lead forecast maps for that regime, and the probability-weighted mixture (the weighted mean over $j = 0, 1, 2$) of these regimes. That is, we can obtain

$$
E(\boldsymbol{\alpha}_{t+\tau}|\mathbf{Z}_{1:t}) = \sum_{j=0}^{2} Pr\{J_t = j|\mathbf{Z}_{1:t}\} E(\boldsymbol{\mu}(I_t, j) + \mathbf{M}(I_t, j)\boldsymbol{\alpha}_t|\mathbf{Z}_{1:t}),
$$

where recall that $\mathbf{Z}_{1:t}$ corresponds to all of the data up to time t. Hence, $E(\mathbf{Y}_{t+\tau}^P|\mathbf{Z}_{1:t}) = \boldsymbol{\Phi} E(\boldsymbol{\alpha}_{t+\tau}|\mathbf{Z}_{1:t})$. We can also obtain pixelwise percentiles of the posterior distribution, $[\mathbf{Y}_{t+\tau}^P|\mathbf{Z}_{1:t}]$, as well as summary measures of El

Niño/La Niña (e.g., Niño 3.4 values: averages over the 5° N to 5° S and 170° W to 120° W) and their posterior distributions.

We consider the same long-lead forecasting application described above in Section 9.1.1. As in that example, we consider $p_\alpha = 10$ EOFs in (9.4), with $p_1 = 4$, $p_2 = 6$. In contrast to that example, Σ_ν in (9.1) used the next 20 EOFs to model spatial dependence. We ran the MCMC for 6000 iterations, the first 1000 of which we discarded as a period of "burn-in."

Figure 9.3 shows the forecasts of the smoothed SST anomalies (i.e., $Y_{t+\tau}^P$) for October 1997 and October 1998, given data through April 1997 and April 1998, respectively. As with the linear case shown in Figure 9.1, the first row of panels show the data (i.e., $Z_{t+\tau}$) for the forecast target months, the second row of panels show the smoothed data (i.e., $\Phi\Phi'Z_{t+\tau}$) for the forecast target months, the third row of panels show the corresponding smooth forecasts (i.e., $E[Y_{t+\tau}^P | Z_{1:t}]$), and the fourth and fifth rows of panels show the pixelwise 2.5 and 97.5 percentiles of the posterior forecast distribution (i.e., $[Y_{t+\tau}^P | Z_{1:t}]$).

Interestingly, when comparing these forecasts to those from the linear model, it is clear that the nonlinear model does a much better job of forecasting the intensity of the developing El Niño in October, 1997. However, the linear model seems to forecast the intensity of the developing La Niña better than the nonlinear model. Regarding variability, the spread of the nonlinear-model forecast distribution (as evidenced by the lower 2.5 and upper 97.5 percentiles) is quite a bit wider than that for the linear model, reflecting more realistic prediction uncertainty.

Aditionally, Figure 9.4 shows the posterior forecast density for the Niño 3.4 region (5° S–5° N, 120°–170° W) SST averages for (a) the forecast of October 1997, given data up to April 1997, and (b) the forecast of October 1998, given data up to April 1998. The posterior means for these distributions are shown with a blue "star" on the horizontal axis, and the calculated Niño 3.4 averages from the actual observations (6 months after the forecast was made) are shown with a red "star." As with the forecast fields, the nonlinear DSTM does a better job of forecasting the magnitude of the warm event than does the linear DSTM, but the nonlinear model does not forecast the cool event as well. However, the uncertainty bounds on the forecast are much wider for the nonlinear model, reflecting the fact that it accommodates more sources of uncertainty.

As mentioned above, the nonlinear DSTM allows forecasts to be considered that depend on the (unknown) regime of the hidden future state process. In addition, the posterior probability of each regime can be calculated. The predictions for each of these states (cool, normal, and warm) and their probabilities for the October 1997/October 1998 cases are included in Figure 9.5, along with their probability-weighted average. For the October 1997 (El Niño) forecast, the model assigned a 97% probability that the future state will be warm, thus weighting the prediction under that regime much more than the other two regimes (normal and cool). In contrast, the forecast for October 1998 (La Niña) assigned a 24% probability that the future state would be cool,

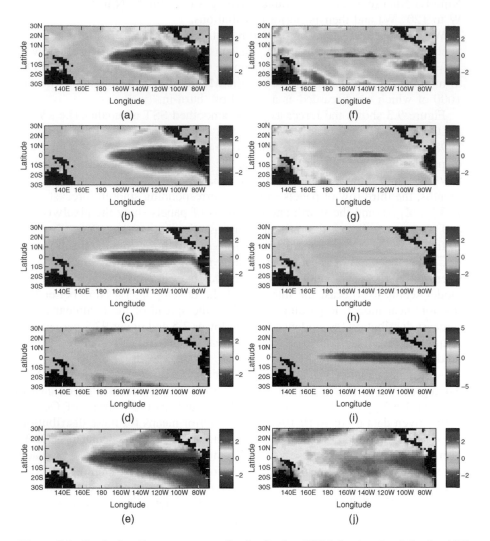

Figure 9.3 Sea Surface Temperature anomalies for October 1997 (left column) and October 1998 (right column). The first row of panels (**a, f**) show data for October 1997 and 1998, respectively. The second row of panels (**b, g**) show the smoothed data for October 1997 and 1998, respectively. The third row of panels (**c, h**) show the smooth forecast (mean of the posterior forecast distribution) from the reduced-dimension nonlinear DSTM for October 1997 and October 1998, given data through April 1997 and April 1998, respectively. The fourth row of panels (**d, i**) show the pixelwise lower 2.5 percentiles of the posterior forecast distribution for October 1997 and 1998, respectively. The fifth row of panels (**e, j**) show the pixelwise upper 97.5 percentiles of the posterior forecast distribution for October 1997 and 1998, respectively.

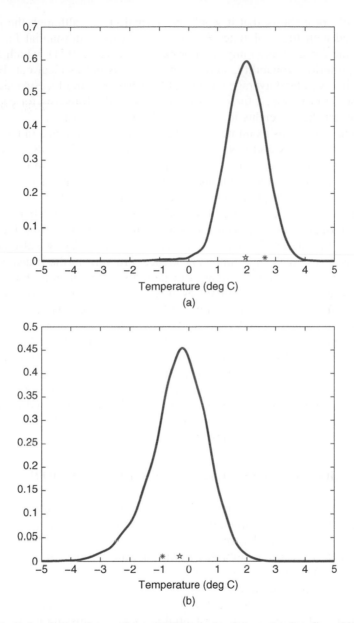

Figure 9.4 Reduced-dimension nonlinear DSTM posterior forecast density of monthly Niño 3.4 region (5° S–5° N, 120°–170° W) SST averages. The top panel (**a**) shows the posterior forecast distribution for October 1997, given data up to April 1997. The bottom panel (**b**) shows the corresponding forecast for October 1998, given data up to April 1998. In each panel, the blue "star" shows the mean of the forecast distribution and the red "star" shows the corresponding observed value (6 months later) of the Niño 3.4 region.

and a 74% probability that it would be normal. Thus, although the prediction associated with the cool state (Figure 9.5e) shows a substantial La Niña signature, the forecast assuming the normal state (Figure 9.5f), which has much higher posterior probability, shows that cooling is not as clear cut. Hence, the probability weighted average somewhat "washes out" the La Niña signature in this case. In principle, a forecaster could look at the forecasts for each regime and readjust these weights to produce a different forecast.

In conclusion, this example shows that there is a difference in the long-lead forecasts of the El Niño/La Niña phenomena during 1997–1998, as given by an SST BHM with a linear and a nonlinear DSTM. In addition to the differences in process dynamics, the linear and nonlinear implementations considered here differed in their assumptions about truncation-error variability: The linear BHM assumed truncation errors that were independent in time and space, while the nonlinear BHM assumed such errors were independent in time but spatially dependent (through additional EOF expansions). To be fair, we also considered the linear BHM with this same dependence structure in the truncation errors, and the forecasted results were not substantially different from those presented here, suggesting that the differences in model performance were due to the linear versus nonlinear dynamics in the DSTM. We note that many other types of nonlinear models could be considered for long-lead forecasting of SSTs. For example, Wikle and Hooten (2010) use the general quadratic nonlinear structure described in Section 7.3.3 to construct a BHM implementation of a nonlinear DSTM for long-lead forecasting of SSTs. Their results show that the 1997 El Niño can be forecasted quite well by such a model. (They did not implement their model to forecast the 1998 La Niña.) Wikle and Holan (2011) consider a quadratically nonlinear model for SST within the IDE framework. Their results corroborate the results presented here.

9.2 REMOTELY SENSED AEROSOL OPTICAL DEPTH

The National Aeronautics and Space Administration (NASA) has a remote-sensing program with a large array of satellites whose mission is earth-system science. To carry out this mission, NASA produces data at various levels: Level 2 data have been calibrated to the satellite's footprint at high temporal resolution, although there is often a lot of missing data. Level 3 data are produced on a regular latitude-longitude grid over the whole globe at a coarser spatial and temporal (such as a day, a month, or a repeat-cycle of the satellite) resolution, and there are still substantial amounts of missing data.

NASA's Terra satellite was launched on December 18, 1999, and the Multi-angle Imaging SpectroRadiometer (MISR) instrument on board collects global aerosol information; this includes aerosol optical depth, or AOD (a large value in a given pixel indicates a high aerosol content in the column of the atmosphere above that pixel), aerosol shapes, and aerosol sizes (Diner et al., 1999; Kaufman et al., 2000). MISR is one of the key instruments for long-term global aerosol monitoring. Since aerosol forcing is one of

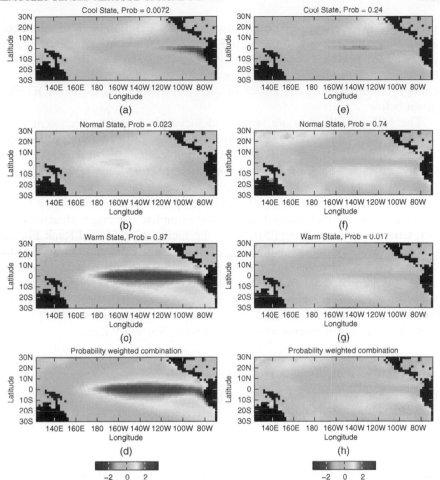

Figure 9.5 Nonlinear DSTM forecast of smooth SST anomalies for October 1997 (left column) and October 1998 (right column). Panels **(a)** and **(e)** show the forecast anomalies assuming that the future regime state in October 1997/1998 will be cold (regime 0); **(b)** and **(f)** show the forecast anomalies assuming the future regime state is normal (regime 1); **(c)** and **(g)** show the forecast anomalies assuming the future regime state is warm (regime 2). The title at the top of each panel gives the posterior probability, each to two significant figures, of these conditions. Panels **(d)** and **(h)** give the probability-weighted mixture of the images shown in the first three rows of panels for October 1997 and October 1998, respectively.

the major sources of uncertainty in climate models, accurate global aerosol records based on satellites play a vital role in calibrating the climate models. Consequently, complete-coverage aerosol values are needed.

Level 2 MISR data are collected at a spatial resolution of 17.6 km × 17.6 km. The satellite's orbit is repeated exactly, every 16 days. Level 3 data products are generated at a much coarser spatial resolution ($0.5° × 0.5°$), by averaging Level 2 observations falling in the Level 3 pixels in a given time period. In this section, we use a spatio-temporal EHM to analyze all Level 3 AOD data collected during the period July 1, 2001 through August 17, 2001, in a study region that consists of $128 \times 256 = 32{,}768$ Level 3 pixels. While the dataset is not massive, it involves about 120,000 observations and is large enough to demonstrate the power of dimension reduction in the AOD EHM given below.

The MISR AOD data are noisy and incomplete due to alignment of the satellite's orbit and failure of the instrument to retrieve (e.g., presence of clouds, hardware or software failures). In this section, we fit an EHM, where the dynamical spatial variation, the nondynamical fine-scale variation, and the measurement error are explicitly modeled. A reduced-dimension DSTM is used in the process model, and a rapid recursive updating procedure (i.e., a type of Kalman filter) is implemented to provide complete coverage of aerosol values. Cressie, Shi, and Kang (2010) call the methodology Fixed Rank Filtering (FRF); they study the computational complexity of FRF and compare it to a spatial-only version called Fixed Rank Kriging (FRK; Cressie and Johannesson, 2008). As part of the AOD EHM, data-model and process-model parameters have to be *estimated*. How this is done (e.g., likelihood based, loss-function based, moment based) is often determined by the practicalities of the problem; here, a method-of-moments approach is taken (Section 9.2.2).

9.2.1 AOD Data Model and Process Model

Assume that observations $Z_t(\cdot)$ are taken on $Y_t(\cdot)$, the difference being due to measurement error. That is, the *data model* is

$$Z_t(\mathbf{s}) = Y_t(\mathbf{s}) + \varepsilon_t(\mathbf{s}), \ \mathbf{s} \in D_s, t = 1, 2, \ldots, \tag{9.6}$$

where $Y_t(\cdot)$ is the underlying (true) spatio-temporal process that will be modeled at the process-model level of the HM; $\varepsilon_t(\cdot)$ is a mean-zero Gaussian process that is uncorrelated in space and time, and $\text{var}(\varepsilon_t(\mathbf{s})) = \sigma_\varepsilon^2 v_t(\mathbf{s}) > 0$. The only parameter in the data model is σ_ε^2, since $v_t(\mathbf{s})$ is assumed known for all $\mathbf{s} \in D_s$ (e.g., see Section 9.2.3).

The *process model* for $\{Y_t(\mathbf{s}): \mathbf{s} \in D_s, t = 1, 2, \ldots\}$ assumes that the true (hidden) spatio-temporal process $Y_t(\cdot)$ can be decomposed as follows:

$$Y_t(\mathbf{s}) = \mathbf{X}_t(\mathbf{s})'\boldsymbol{\beta} + \kappa_t(\mathbf{s}) + \xi_t(\mathbf{s}), \qquad \mathbf{s} \in D_s, t = 1, 2, \ldots, \tag{9.7}$$

where the first, second, and third components on the right-hand side of (9.7) represent the large-scale, small-scale, and fine-scale components, respectively, of spatial variability. Define the known covariate vector, $\mathbf{X}_t(\cdot) \equiv (X_{1,t}(\cdot), \ldots, X_{p,t}(\cdot))'$, and think of the p elements of $\boldsymbol{\beta}$ as parameters of the process model. That is, the large-scale component is assumed to be deterministic. In contrast, assume that $\kappa_t(\cdot)$ and $\xi_t(\cdot)$ are random processes that each have mean zero. Consequently, $E(Y_t(\mathbf{s})) \equiv \mu_t(\mathbf{s}) = \mathbf{X}_t(\mathbf{s})'\boldsymbol{\beta}; \mathbf{s} \in D_s$.

In the rest of this section, we assume that $\boldsymbol{\beta}$ and hence $\mu_t(\cdot)$ is known; in practice, this amounts to having a stable estimate of trend and then working with the detrended data. Although we lose a component of uncertainty due to estimation of the mean, the ultimate goal of a fast and efficient computational algorithm for very large data sets leads to this data/model/computing compromise (Section 2.5).

At any *fixed* time t, assume that $\kappa_t(\cdot)$ has mean zero and is written in terms of a basis function expansion (e.g., Cressie and Johannesson, 2008):

$$\kappa_t(\mathbf{s}) = \boldsymbol{\phi}(\mathbf{s})'\boldsymbol{\alpha}_t, \qquad \mathbf{s} \in D_s, \tag{9.8}$$

where $\boldsymbol{\phi}(\cdot) \equiv (\phi_1(\cdot), \dots, \phi_{p_\alpha}(\cdot))'$ is a vector of p_α known *spatial* basis functions and $\boldsymbol{\alpha}_t \equiv (\alpha_t(1), \dots, \alpha_t(p_\alpha))'$ is a mean-zero Gaussian random vector with $p_\alpha \times p_\alpha$ covariance matrix given by

$$\text{var}(\boldsymbol{\alpha}_t) \equiv \boldsymbol{\Sigma}_t,$$

where we have chosen *not* to write this as $\boldsymbol{\Sigma}_{\alpha,t}$, for ease of exposition. Notice that $\text{cov}(\kappa_t(\mathbf{s}), \kappa_t(\mathbf{x})) = \boldsymbol{\phi}(\mathbf{s})'\boldsymbol{\Sigma}_t\boldsymbol{\phi}(\mathbf{x})$, which is a positive-definite function (Section 6.1.1) for *any* set of spatial basis functions chosen.

As time t progresses, we assume that $\{\boldsymbol{\alpha}_t : t = 1, 2, \dots\}$ evolves as a first-order linear DSTM process (Section 6.4):

$$\boldsymbol{\alpha}_{t+1} = \mathbf{M}_{t+1}\boldsymbol{\alpha}_t + \boldsymbol{\xi}_{t+1}, \qquad t = 1, 2, \dots, \tag{9.9}$$

where $\mathbf{M}_{t+1}$ is a $p_\alpha \times p_\alpha$ propagator matrix that generally depends on time; and the p_α-dimensional Gaussian error vector, $\boldsymbol{\xi}_{t+1}$, is independent of $\boldsymbol{\alpha}_t$, has mean zero, and has covariance matrix, $\text{var}(\boldsymbol{\xi}_{t+1}) \equiv \mathbf{Q}_{t+1}$. Notice that in (9.9), we have chosen *not* to write the propagator matrix as $\mathbf{M}_{\alpha,t+1}$, nor the error covariance matrix as $\mathbf{Q}_{\xi,t+1}$, for ease of exposition. (The reason for this simplification in notation is that the model allows $\boldsymbol{\Sigma}_t$, $\mathbf{M}_t$, and $\mathbf{Q}_t$ to depend on t, and in the presentation that follows, double subscripts would be cumbersome.) Define the cross-covariances,

$$\boldsymbol{\Sigma}_{t,r} \equiv \text{cov}(\boldsymbol{\alpha}_t, \boldsymbol{\alpha}_r), \qquad t, r = 1, 2, \dots, \tag{9.10}$$

where we have already notated $\boldsymbol{\Sigma}_{t,t}$ as simply, $\boldsymbol{\Sigma}_t$. Recall from Section 6.4.1 that for $r > t$ we have

$$\boldsymbol{\Sigma}_{r,t} = \mathbf{M}_r\mathbf{M}_{r-1}\cdots\mathbf{M}_{t+1}\boldsymbol{\Sigma}_t, \tag{9.11}$$

and

$$\boldsymbol{\Sigma}_{t+1} = \mathbf{M}_{t+1}\boldsymbol{\Sigma}_t\mathbf{M}'_{t+1} + \mathbf{Q}_{t+1}. \tag{9.12}$$

If we put $r = t + 1$ in (9.11), the $p_\alpha \times p_\alpha$ *lag-1 cross-covariance* matrix is given by

$$\mathbf{\Sigma}_t^{(1)} \equiv \mathbf{\Sigma}_{t+1,t} = \mathbf{M}_{t+1} \mathbf{\Sigma}_t, \qquad t = 1, 2, \ldots. \qquad (9.13)$$

The cross-covariance matrix, $\mathbf{\Sigma}_t^{(1)}$, captures the lag-1 (in time) cross-covariances between $\boldsymbol{\alpha}_t$ and $\boldsymbol{\alpha}_{t+1}$, in the reduced-dimensional space.

The third component in (9.7), $\xi_t(\cdot)$, is assumed to be independent of $\{\boldsymbol{\alpha}_t\}$, to have mean zero, and *not* to have temporally dynamical structure (as $\{\boldsymbol{\alpha}_t\}$ does). Its role is to capture the fine-scale spatial structure, which in this application to AOD, is at the pixel scale. Here, we assume the simplest possible form for its covariance function, namely

$$E(\xi_t(\mathbf{s})\xi_r(\mathbf{x})) = \begin{cases} \sigma_\xi^2, & \text{if } \mathbf{s} = \mathbf{x} \text{ and } t = r, \\ 0, & \text{otherwise.} \end{cases} \qquad (9.14)$$

All together, the parameters of the *process* model are: σ_ξ^2, $\mathbf{\Sigma}_1$, and $\{\mathbf{M}_{t+1}, \mathbf{Q}_{t+1} : t = 1, 2, \ldots\}$.

Upon combining the parameters of the data model and the process model, we obtain

$$\mathbf{\Theta} \equiv \{\sigma_\varepsilon^2, \sigma_\xi^2, \mathbf{\Sigma}_1, \{\mathbf{M}_{t+1}, \mathbf{Q}_{t+1} : t = 1, 2, \ldots\}\},$$

which we assume are fixed but unknown. Their estimation is discussed in Section 9.2.2.

From (9.10), the covariance structure of the *spatio-temporal* process $Y_t(\cdot)$ is given by

$$\text{cov}(Y_t(\mathbf{s}), Y_r(\mathbf{x})) = \boldsymbol{\phi}(\mathbf{s})' \mathbf{\Sigma}_{t,r} \boldsymbol{\phi}(\mathbf{x}) + \sigma_\xi^2 I(\mathbf{s} = \mathbf{x} \text{ and } t = r), \qquad (9.15)$$

where $I(\cdot)$ denotes the indicator function. Furthermore, it is straightforward to see that the covariances between the process and the data are given by $\text{cov}(Y_t(\mathbf{s}), Z_r(\mathbf{x})) = \text{cov}(Y_t(\mathbf{s}), Y_r(\mathbf{x}))$, which is given by (9.15).

9.2.2 The AOD EHM: Implementation and Inference

Our principal interest is in inference on the process $\{Y_t(\mathbf{s}) : \mathbf{s} \in D_s\}$, given the data $\mathbf{Z} = (\mathbf{Z}_1', \ldots, \mathbf{Z}_t')'$, which includes all of the observations up through time t (i.e., there are m_t observations for each data vector $\mathbf{Z}_t$). This is in contrast to Section 9.1, where our principal interest was in inference on $\{\mathbf{\Phi}(\mathbf{s})' \boldsymbol{\alpha}_t : \mathbf{s} \in D_s\}$, given the data $\mathbf{Z}$. Another difference is that an EHM approach is taken in this section, which involves *estimating* the parameters $\mathbf{\Theta}$ and substituting them into the posterior distribution of $Y_t(\cdot)$.

Optimal Prediction

To make inference on $Y_t(\mathbf{s}_0)$, where $\mathbf{s}_0$ is a given location in D_s, we use the (estimated) posterior mean (Section 2.2.2), written here as $E(Y_t(\mathbf{s}_0)|\mathbf{Z}, \hat{\boldsymbol{\Theta}})$. At first glance, this would require calculating $(\text{var}(\mathbf{Z}|\boldsymbol{\Theta}))^{-1}$ and $\text{cov}(Y_t(\mathbf{s}_0), \mathbf{Z}|\boldsymbol{\Theta})$ in terms of $\boldsymbol{\Theta}$, and substituting $\hat{\boldsymbol{\Theta}}$ for $\boldsymbol{\Theta}$ in the formulas. These matrices are huge, due to both a large number of data locations, and because the latest time t is always increasing. The temporal aspect can be handled through jointly Kalman filtering $\{(\boldsymbol{\alpha}_t, \xi_t(\mathbf{s}_0)) : t = 1, 2, \dots\}$; the basic forecasting and filtering algorithm for $\{\boldsymbol{\alpha}_t : t = 1, 2, \dots\}$ is given in Section 8.2.1, and Cressie, Shi, and Kang (2010) extend this to jointly filtering $\{(\boldsymbol{\alpha}_t, \xi_t(\mathbf{s}_0)) : t = 1, 2, \dots\}$. The spatial aspect is handled through dimension reduction and the Kalman filter's implicit incorporation of the Sherman–Morrison–Woodbury identity, (8.18); then all matrix inverses used to calculate the optimal predictor are either $p_\alpha \times p_\alpha$ or (large) diagonal matrices. Cressie, Shi, and Kang (2010) show that the computational complexity of calculating $E(Y_t(\mathbf{s}_0)|\mathbf{Z}, \boldsymbol{\Theta})$ and its mean squared prediction error, $\text{var}(Y_t(\mathbf{s}_0)|\mathbf{Z}, \boldsymbol{\Theta})$, is $O\left(\left(\sum_{i=1}^t m_i\right)t\right)$.

In terms of the notation in (9.6) and (9.7), if $\hat{\boldsymbol{\alpha}}_{t|t}$ and $\hat{\xi}_{t|t}(\mathbf{s}_0)$ are the Kalman-filtered random effects, then the optimal predictor is

$$\hat{Y}_t(\mathbf{s}_0) = \mathbf{X}_t(\mathbf{s}_0)'\boldsymbol{\beta} + \boldsymbol{\Phi}_t(\mathbf{s}_0)'\hat{\boldsymbol{\alpha}}_{t|t} + \hat{\xi}_{t|t}(\mathbf{s}_0), \tag{9.16}$$

which is called the Fixed Rank Filtering (FRF) predictor by Cressie, Shi, and Kang (2010). An expression for the mean squared prediction error matrix of $(\hat{\boldsymbol{\alpha}}'_{t|t}, \hat{\xi}_{t|t}(\mathbf{s}_0))'$, and hence the mean squared prediction error of (9.16), is given by Cressie, Shi, and Kang (2010). They call the square root of this latter quantity, which we write as $\sigma_t(\mathbf{s}_0)$, the FRF standard error. Then, estimates $\hat{\boldsymbol{\Theta}}$ are substituted into $\hat{Y}_t(\mathbf{s}_0)$ and $\sigma_t(\mathbf{s}_0)$; as $\mathbf{s}_0$ varies over D_s, maps of predictions and associated prediction standard errors are generated. Since the variability of $\hat{\boldsymbol{\Theta}}$ has not been accounted for, an EHM approach tends to result in inferences that are liberal. Again, this is a data/model/computing compromise (Section 2.5) that is critical for the model to process very large datasets in a relatively short time (on the order of minutes).

Parameter Estimation

Choosing to estimate parameters rather than putting a prior on them leads to choices about the estimation method to employ. There are two common types of estimators, one based on maximum likelihood and the other based on the method of moments. It is this choice and its implementation that is often the most labor-intensive part of implementation and inference in an EHM. In the AOD EHM, $\boldsymbol{\Theta}$ is made up of scalar variance components, σ_ε^2 and σ_ξ^2, and $p_\alpha \times p_\alpha$ matrices that are related through the expressions (9.11), (9.12), and (9.13); recall that $\boldsymbol{\beta}$ is assumed known. In what follows, we shall present estimation via the method of moments (e.g., Wikle and Cressie, 1999), although it should be noted that the likelihood-based EM algorithm could have been tried (e.g., Xu and Wikle, 2007; Katzfuss and Cressie, 2011). The method-of-moments estimates we present have an advantage in that they are very fast to compute when datasets are very large.

We estimate σ_ε^2 and σ_ξ^2 separately, using empirical semivariograms for small spatial lags; the robust semivariogram estimator, $\hat{\gamma}(h)$, of Cressie and Hawkins (1980) was plotted against h, for h near the origin, and a straight line, $\tilde{\gamma}(h)$, was fitted by weighted least squares (Cressie, 1985). For regional data, Kang, Liu, and Cressie (2009) show that σ_ε^2 is estimated unbiasedly from the fitted line's intercept. Furthermore, σ_ξ^2 is estimated from another moment relation, this one involving the semivariogram at spatial lag 1 (Kang, Cressie, and Shi, 2010, Section 3).

Method-of-moments estimates of the $p_\alpha \times p_\alpha$ matrices, $\mathbf{\Sigma}_1$, $\{\mathbf{M}_{t+1}\}$, and $\{\mathbf{Q}_{t+1}\}$, are obtained by computing empirical covariance and cross-covariance matrices from the data $\mathbf{Z}_t$ and $\mathbf{Z}_{t+1}$ based on dividing D_s up into "bins" (spatial areas of larger support than the data). Each bin receives all the data in $\mathbf{Z}_t$ whose locations fall within the bin; likewise for $\mathbf{Z}_{t+1}$. The purpose of the bins is to average over them in order to decrease the variability of the estimated covariance matrix and lag-one cross-covariance matrix; hence, the number of bins will be considerably less than $\min\{m_t, m_{t+1}\}$. This suggests that the spatial basis matrix ($\mathbf{\Phi}$) must also be aggregated to account for the binning of the data. The details are given in Kang, Cressie, and Shi (2010), who show that the moment estimates can be obtained by minimizing appropriate Frobenius norms.

The estimation is done sequentially: Solve for $\hat{\mathbf{\Sigma}}_1$ first, based on $\mathbf{Z}_1$ and (9.15) with $t = r = 1$; then solve for $\hat{\mathbf{\Sigma}}_2$ and $\hat{\mathbf{M}}_2$, based on $\mathbf{Z}_2$ and $\mathbf{Z}_1$ and (9.15) and (9.13); then from (9.12) obtain

$$\hat{\mathbf{Q}}_2 \equiv \hat{\mathbf{\Sigma}}_2 - \hat{\mathbf{M}}_2 \hat{\mathbf{\Sigma}}_1 \hat{\mathbf{M}}_2' \, ; \tag{9.17}$$

then solve for $\hat{\mathbf{\Sigma}}_3$ and $\hat{\mathbf{M}}_3$ based on $\mathbf{Z}_3$ and $\mathbf{Z}_2$ and (9.15) and (9.13); and so forth. On occasions, there are difficulties encountered that involve estimates of positive-definite matrices that are *not* positive-definite. Kang, Cressie, and Shi (2010) give a method of "lifting" eigenvalues of such estimates in a way that total variability is preserved. Finally, the method-of-moments estimates, $\hat{\mathbf{\Sigma}}_1$, $\hat{\mathbf{M}}_2$, $\hat{\mathbf{Q}}_2$, $\hat{\mathbf{M}}_3$, $\hat{\mathbf{Q}}_3$, ..., are obtained, which together with the semivariogram-based estimates, $\hat{\sigma}_\varepsilon^2$ and $\hat{\sigma}_\xi^2$, result in the method-of-moments estimate, $\hat{\mathbf{\Theta}}$.

The last stage of the AOD EHM is to substitute $\hat{\mathbf{\Theta}}$ into the expressions for $\hat{Y}_t(\mathbf{s}_0)$ and $\sigma_t(\mathbf{s}_0)$ and to make the prediction and prediction standard error maps by allowing $\mathbf{s}_0$ to vary over (a fine grid of) D_s. We note that the computations to obtain $\hat{\mathbf{\Theta}}$ are extremely fast (Section 9.2.3).

9.2.3 Predictions for Aerosol Optical Depth

The study region D_s we chose is the rectangular area between longitudes $125°$ W and $3°$ E and between latitudes $20°$ S and $44°$ N, which covers North and

South America, the western part of the Sahara Desert in Africa, the Iberian Peninsula in Europe, and parts of the Atlantic and Pacific Oceans; a map of the region is given in Figure 9.6. Recall that the dataset consists of the MISR Level 3 AOD data collected between July 1 and August 17, and we chose eight days as the time unit; that is, time unit 1 corresponds to July 1–8, time unit 2 corresponds to July 9–16, ..., and time unit 6 corresponds to August 10–17. The number of data in each of these time units is, respectively, $m_1 = 20{,}970$, $m_2 = 19{,}398$, $m_3 = 20{,}819$, $m_4 = 20{,}167$, $m_5 = 21{,}759$, and $m_6 = 20{,}625$. The choice of 8 days allowed enough spatial coverage to estimate the parameters of the EHM. Although the evolutionary time scale of AOD is probably on the order of a day, there is still quite strong temporal dependence between eight-day time periods (Kang, Cressie, and Shi, 2010).

AOD data are highly (right) skewed, even when they are aggregated from Level 2 to Level 3. Hence, we used a logarithmic transformation, as described below. An individual datum in a given 8-day period is obtained by taking a *weighted average* of daily Level 3 log(AOD) values, where the corresponding weight is proportional to $N_d(\mathbf{s})$, the number of Level 2 observations in the Level 3 pixel $\mathbf{s}$ on day d. Henceforth, all analyses are done on this log(AOD) scale. The transformed data for $t = 1, 2, \ldots, 6$ are shown in Figure 9.7.

After considerable exploratory data analysis, we divided the study region D_s into three areas: the oceans, the Americas, and the rest (i.e., the land in the

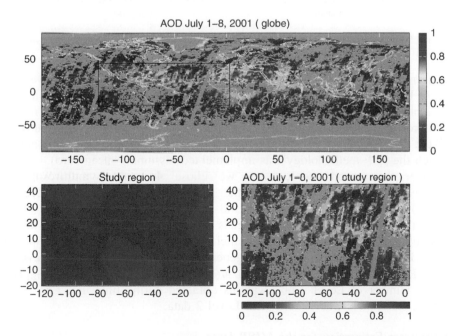

Figure 9.6 Data are retrieved Aerosol Optical Depth (AOD). **Top panel:** Global Level 2 data for $t = 1$ (July 1–8, 2001). **Bottom-left panel:** Study region D_s that includes the Americas and part of Africa (Sahara Desert). **Bottom-right panel:** AOD data in the study region, for $t = 1$.

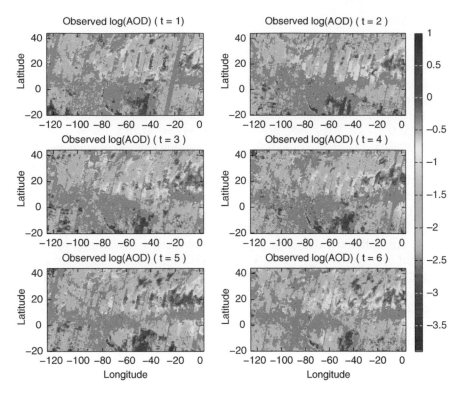

Figure 9.7 Data are (weighted average) log(AOD) at Level 3 ($0.5° \times 0.5°$), for time periods (8 days) $t = 1, 2, \ldots, 6$.

eastern part of D_s, which consists of the Sahara Desert and the southwestern tip of Europe). Then, using indicator functions of these regions as explanatory variables, we detrended the original dataset with a spatial-only linear model and ordinary-least-squares (OLS) estimation of the regression parameters from all the data. This created a spatio-temporal *detrended* dataset, $\mathbf{Z}_1, \ldots, \mathbf{Z}_6$, upon which the FRF methodology was implemented (assuming mean zero).

Over the period $t = 1, \ldots, 6$, we chose $\mathbf{\Phi}(\cdot)$ from multiresolution W-wavelet basis functions, using the strategy given by Shi and Cressie (2007), which is based on Huang and Cressie (2000). All 32 W-wavelets from the first scale and 62 W-wavelets from the second scale with "large" absolute coefficients were chosen, which resulted in $p_\alpha = 32 + 62 = 94$, for all t. Recall that Level 3 data are generally obtained by averaging Level 2 data. Hence, we assume in (9.6) that $v_t(\mathbf{s}) = 1/\widetilde{N}_t(\mathbf{s})$, where $\{\widetilde{N}_t(\mathbf{s}): \mathbf{s} \in D_s\}$ is the number of Level 2 observations obtained during time unit t in those $0.5° \times 0.5°$ pixels where there were Level 2 data.

Parameter Estimation for the MISR Data

Using the methodology described in Section 9.2.2, we obtained, $\hat{\sigma}_\varepsilon^2 = 0.0191$ and $\hat{\sigma}_\xi^2 = 0.0310$. Figure 9.8 shows the behavior of the robust semivariogram

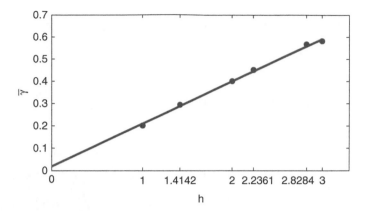

Figure 9.8 Empirical (robust) semivariogram versus spatial lag h, for h near 0. A weighted-least-squares, straight-line fit (Cressie, 1985), $\bar{\gamma}(h)$, is shown. Its intercept at $h = 0$ is $\hat{\sigma}_\varepsilon^2 = 0.0191$.

estimator (based on all data $\mathbf{Z}$) for small spatial lags h, from which $\hat{\sigma}_\varepsilon^2$ was derived.

The method-of-moments estimation of $\mathbf{\Sigma}_1$, $\{\mathbf{M}_{t+1}\}$, and $\{\mathbf{Q}_{t+1}\}$ is based on binned empirical covariance and lag-one cross-covariance matrices, as described in Section 9.2.2. The estimate, $\hat{\mathbf{\Sigma}}_1$, upon which all other estimates depend, has to be positive-definite. By "lifting" negative eigenvalues (and reducing some positive ones) and ensuring that the sum of the lifted eigenvalues is equal to the sum of the original eigenvalues (Kang, Cressie, and Shi, 2010), it was found that all method-of-moments estimates of the $p_\alpha \times p_\alpha$ matrices were in their respective parameter spaces and, by definition, total variability was preserved.

Upon substituting the estimates $\hat{\sigma}_\varepsilon^2$, $\hat{\sigma}_\xi^2$, $\hat{\mathbf{\Sigma}}_1$, $\{\hat{\mathbf{M}}_{t+1}\}$, and $\{\hat{\mathbf{Q}}_{t+1}\}$, into $\hat{Y}_t(\mathbf{s}_0)$ given by (9.16) and into $\sigma_t(\mathbf{s}_0)$, we obtain AOD EHM predictions of $Y_t(\mathbf{s}_0)$ and the predictor's standard error, respectively. An illustration of the results of these predictions is seen in Figure 9.9. Shown are the observed log(AOD) values (original data without the trend removed), the OLS trend, the final prediction maps produced by this FRF procedure *with the trend added back*, and the associated standard errors. Notice that the latter map displays the same pattern as seen in the map of the log(AOD) data, as expected.

Large log(AOD) values are observed/predicted in the region of the Sahara Desert, decreasing gradually farther to the west. From the prediction map in Figure 9.9, values for the gray regions, where no log(AOD) data were observed, have been inferred, and the associated standard errors shown in Figure 9.9 give larger values at locations where there were no data, as expected. Finally, the predictions are smoother than the observed data (again, as expected). The presence of the fine-scale variation, $\xi_t(\cdot)$, in the model, is meant to capture a possibly nonsmooth process, and filtering it jointly with α_t represents a departure from the usual filtering methodology (e.g., Section 7.2.1). The fine-scale process allows for "rougher" predictions and more conservative prediction

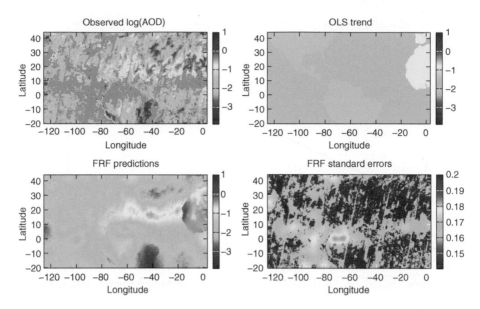

Figure 9.9 Fixed Rank Filtering (FRF) at $t = 6$. **Upper-left panel:** log(AOD) data at $t = 6$. **Upper-right panel:** Ordinary-least-squares (OLS) fitted trend for all $t = 1, 2, \ldots, 6$. **Lower-left panel:** Optimal FRF prediction based on data $\mathbf{Z}_1, \ldots, \mathbf{Z}_6$. **Lower-right panel:** FRF standard errors of prediction.

standard errors. Finally, back-transforming the log(AOD) predictions to the original AOD scale can be done using the results given in Cressie (1993, Section 3.2.2); this must be done if the predictions are to be used as input to climate models.

For this spatio-temporal dataset with $128 \times 256 = 32{,}768$ pixels and sample size around 120,000, the computation time for binning and fitting the parameters was about a minute on a 2010 vintage workstation. Furthermore, it took about another minute and a half to calculate the FRF predictions and standard errors, up to and including $t = 6$. It is also worth pointing out that the incremental time for updating the Kalman filter at time 6, based on the new data $\mathbf{Z}_6$ and the filtered results at time $t = 5$, was only about 20 seconds. For more details on the computational complexity of this procedure, see Cressie, Shi, and Kang (2010).

We did not give computation time for the other three examples in this chapter, which are based on BHMs and MCMC; implementation can take on the order of minutes to days. While the EHM gives uncertainty measures that are generally too liberal, its computations can be very fast, a factor that is definitely important as spatio-temporal datasets and implementation issues loom large. This is what we refered to as a data/model/computing compromise in Section 2.5.

9.3 MODELING AND FORECASTING THE EURASIAN COLLARED DOVE INVASION

Ecologists have long been interested in the growth and dispersal of biotic organisms. In particular, the dynamics of invasive species are important because the presence of nonnative animals and plants can lead to significant impacts on native biotic communities. Using DSTMs in a BHM is a natural framework for modeling invasive species, given the uncertainties in observations, process dynamics, and associated parameters. Wikle (2003b), Wikle and Hooten (2006), and Hooten and Wikle (2007) show how explicit nonlinear PDE dynamics for invasive species can be incorporated into a BHM.

Rather than employing PDE dynamics, Hooten et al. (2007) used a so-called "matrix model" (e.g., Caswell, 2001) for modeling the invasive Eurasian Collared Dove (*Streptopelia decaocto*). We describe their approach in this section. Critically, this example considers the non-Gaussian nature of the observations and the inherent uncertainty associated with the probability of detection. The dynamics are nonlinear (indeed, they are a special case of the generalized quadratic nonlinearity described in Section 7.3.3), and they are considered within a population model that includes density-dependent growth and dispersal. Another feature of this example is that it illustrates the importance of allowing the process-model parameters (e.g., dispersal rates) to vary spatially.

9.3.1 The Eurasian Collared Dove Invasion of North America

The Eurasian Collared Dove (ECD) was first observed in North America in the early 1980s (Romagosa and Labisky, 2000). Just as they spread through Europe in the early 1900s, they are spreading quickly through North America, and they are posing a potential threat to native ecosystems (e.g., Hengeveld, 1993).

As part of the North American Breeding Bird Survey (BBS; Robbins, Bystrak, and Geissler, 1986), each year, during the peak of the avian breeding season, skilled observers collect bird-population data along predetermined roadside survey routes. Each survey route is approximately 39.4 km in length, and an observer makes 50 stops over each route. At each stop, the observer counts and identifies, by sight or sound for a 3-minute period, all bird species observed within an approximate 0.4-km radius. Not surprisingly, this presents a fairly complicated spatial unit of measurement. In this example, we assume that the data collected along each route corresponds to a count at the route center. Given that our interest is on the invasion at a continental scale, the effects of such aggregation should be quite minimal; however, we note that this aggregation does influence how we should interpret model parameters. We also note that BBS data are subject to other sources of uncertainty (e.g., Link et al., 1994; Sauer, Peterjohn, and Link, 1994), which suggests that we should try to account for these data uncertainties in our BHM.

Figure 9.10 shows BBS observations of the ECD from 1986 through 2003 across a portion of the United States. This figure shows that the ECD occupied much of the southeastern United States by 2003, and that the invasion is ongoing. Hooten and Wikle (2007) showed that on continental scales, the ECD follows a fairly typical pattern of invasion. That is, after the species has established itself, the underlying dynamics are reasonably well characterized by density-dependent population growth and dispersal models. Indeed, Romagosa and Labisky (2000) suggested that the ECD would most likely colonize the entire United States within a few decades.

9.3.2 ECD Data Model

Animals are usually detected imperfectly in surveys. If one assumes that each animal is observed independently in space and time *given* that the animal is in fact present, then a binomial model is reasonable. That is,

$$Z_t(\mathbf{s}_i)|Y_t(\mathbf{s}_i), \theta \sim ind. Bin(Y_t(\mathbf{s}_i), \theta), \qquad i = 1, \ldots, m, \, t = 1, \ldots, T,$$

where $Z_t(\mathbf{s}_i)$ is the observed ECD count for route i and year t; $Y_t(\mathbf{s}_i)$ is the true (but unknown) number of ECDs for location $\mathbf{s}_i$ and year t, called the *population abundance*; and θ is the probability of detecting each ECD. Ideally, one would like to consider spatially and/or temporally varying detection probabilities, but neither the requisite data nor prior information is available for ecologically meaningful inference. In fact, even estimating the single parameter θ can be problematic. In general, $Y_t(\mathbf{s}_i)$ and θ are not identifiable without additional information (e.g., Royle, 2004). Replicate sampling approaches can be used to provide this information (e.g., see Royle and Dorazio, 2006, 2008), but such replicate information is not available for the operational BBS sample. However, Hooten et al. (2007) used results by Link et al. (1994), whereby replicate counts were taken on a different, but related species (Mourning Dove, *Zenaida macroura*) that was thought to share similar detectability characteristics with the ECD. This information was used to suggest hyperparameters, a_θ and b_θ, for an informative beta prior distribution for θ. Finally then, since no additional information about θ can be obtained from the ECD data, this detection parameter was treated as a nuisance parameter; integrating it out of the data model yields,

$$[Z_t(\mathbf{s}_i)|Y_t(\mathbf{s}_i)] = \int_0^1 [Z_t(\mathbf{s}_i)|Y_t(\mathbf{s}_i), \theta][\theta]\,d\theta, \qquad i = 1, \ldots, m, \, t = 1, \ldots, T.$$

Since $[\theta]$ is a $Beta(a_\theta, b_\theta)$ distribution, we obtain a beta-binomial data model:

$$Z_t(\mathbf{s}_i)|Y_t(\mathbf{s}_i), a_\theta, b_\theta \sim Beta\text{-}Bin(Y_t(\mathbf{s}_i), a_\theta, b_\theta),$$

$$i = 1, \ldots, m, \, t = 1, \ldots, T. \tag{9.18}$$

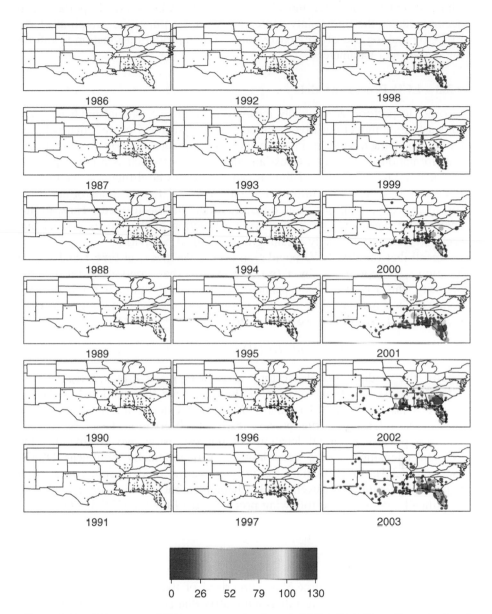

Figure 9.10 ECD counts at BBS route centers for the period 1986–2003. The radius and color of the circles are proportional to the ECD counts. Note that the small dots correspond to locations at which there were ECD counts at some time point in the record.

Thus, (9.18) is the data model used in the ECD BHM. Importantly, it accommodates the uncertainty associated with the imprecise sampling of the ECD, by making use of previously published empirical information to inform the data-model parameters.

9.3.3 ECD Process Model

In order to perform ecologically meaningful inference (spatial prediction and forecasting), a model must be specified for the dynamical process that is based on known characteristics of invasive species. Although it is possible to perform transformations on the non-Gaussian state process (which is a count process in this case) to simplify modeling, it can sometimes be difficult to incorporate scientifically meaningful information into a model for the transformed state (or, to extract such information, once the model has been fitted). Thus, in this analysis we consider a more intuitive construction of the process model that seeks to retain ecologically meaningful dynamical behavior.

Recall that the true ECD population (i.e., abundance) at time t and spatial location $\mathbf{s}_i$ is represented by $Y_t(\mathbf{s}_i)$. We assume that, conditional on the true intensity, this follows an independent Poisson distribution. Furthermore, we define the m-dimensional vector (corresponding to observation locations), $\mathbf{Y}_t \equiv (Y_t(\mathbf{s}_1), \ldots, Y_t(\mathbf{s}_m))'$, and we assume that,

$$\mathbf{Y}_t | \boldsymbol{\lambda}_t \sim \text{ind. } Poi(\mathbf{H}\boldsymbol{\lambda}_t), \qquad t = 1, 2, \ldots,$$

where the n-dimensional vector, $\boldsymbol{\lambda}_t \equiv (\lambda_t(\mathbf{s}_1), \ldots, \lambda_t(\mathbf{s}_m), \lambda_t(\mathbf{s}_{m+1}), \ldots, \lambda_t(\mathbf{s}_n))'$ corresponds to the observation locations *and* the additional prediction locations $\{\mathbf{s}_{m+1}, \ldots, \mathbf{s}_n\}$. The matrix $\mathbf{H}$ is an incidence matrix (see Section 7.1.2) that relates the true process $Y_t(\cdot)$ at observation locations, to the intensity process $\boldsymbol{\lambda}_t$ at all locations of interest. Now, we assume that the Poisson intensities evolve according to a quadratically nonlinear DSTM (Section 7.3.3). In particular, we use a "matrix model" framework from population dynamics (Caswell, 2001, Chapter 3), but with *random* parameters. Specifically, consider the following process model for the ECD intensities

$$\boldsymbol{\lambda}_t = \mathbf{M}\boldsymbol{\lambda}_{t-1}$$
$$= \mathbf{B}(\boldsymbol{\tau})\mathbf{G}(\boldsymbol{\lambda}_{t-1}; \boldsymbol{\theta}^G)\boldsymbol{\lambda}_{t-1}, \qquad t = 2, 3, \ldots, \qquad (9.19)$$

where the propagator matrix $\mathbf{M}$ is comprised of two distinct $n \times n$ matrices. Specifically, $\mathbf{G}(\boldsymbol{\lambda}_{t-1}; \boldsymbol{\theta}^G)$ is a diagonal matrix that accommodates growth over time and is dependent on the previous state $\boldsymbol{\lambda}_{t-1}$ and growth parameters $\boldsymbol{\theta}^G$; and $\mathbf{B}(\boldsymbol{\tau})$ accommodates dispersal of the population and is dependent on dispersal parameters $\boldsymbol{\tau}$. In this case, the initial condition $\boldsymbol{\lambda}_1$ must also be specified.

Notice the distinct lack of an error term in (9.19). Although this model is deterministic when conditioned on the parameters and initial state, it is random when the random nature of these quantities is considered. Additive error processes can be considered for latent invasive-species dynamics (e.g.,

Wikle, 2003b; Hooten and Wikle, 2007), but they can complicate the analysis computationally, as well as inferentially (in terms of parameter interpretation and the lack of "smoothness" in the forecasts). Hooten et al. (2007) show that allowing the initial state and parameters to be random alleviates these complications yet provides flexibility for the latent process to adapt to the data. One convenient feature of this parameterization is that, given an initial condition for a set of prediction locations (that may contain the observation locations), say λ_1, and the corresponding model parameters, θ^G and τ, one immediately obtains the predictions λ_t for any time t, by iterating the model (9.19) forward in time. This allows $\lambda_t(\cdot)$ (and, eventually, $Y_t(\cdot)$) to be predicted easily and to be forecasted at any spatial location of interest.

Here, we parameterize the diagonal matrix $\mathbf{G}$ in terms of a Ricker growth equation (e.g., see Turchin, 2003, Chapter 3). That is, the ith diagonal element of $\mathbf{G}$ is parameterized as follows:

$$G_{ii}(\theta_1^G, \theta_2^G, \lambda_t(\mathbf{s}_i)) \equiv \exp\left\{\theta_1^G\left(1 - \frac{\lambda_t(\mathbf{s}_i)}{\theta_2^G}\right)\right\}, \qquad i = 1, \ldots, n,$$

where θ_1^G and θ_2^G are the growth and carrying-capacity parameters, respectively. One could certainly imagine scenarios where one or both of these parameters could vary across space. However, it is difficult to estimate carrying capacities for populations that are still growing, and thus a spatially explicit carrying-capacity parameter would have to rely heavily on prior information. Similarly, in the presence of spatially varying dispersal, estimation of spatially varying growth rates for such a transient population would need strong prior information. In the absence of such prior information, we choose to focus on the spatially varying dispersal term (see below) and do not allow the growth and carrying capacities to vary spatially.

The dispersal in (9.19) is governed by the matrix $\mathbf{B}(\tau)$. Specifically, analogous to the IDE models presented in Section 7.2.5, we use a Gaussian kernel to characterize dispersal, such that the population at a specific location at time t is a weighted average of the population at surrounding locations at time $t - 1$. In this case, we suppose that the (i, j)th element of the $n \times n$ matrix $\mathbf{B}(\tau)$ is given by

$$B_{i,j}(\tau) \propto \exp\left\{-\frac{d_{i,j}^2}{\tau(\mathbf{s}_i)}\right\},$$

where $d_{i,j}$ is the distance between location $\mathbf{s}_i$ and $\mathbf{s}_j$, and $\tau \equiv (\tau(\mathbf{s}_1), \ldots, \tau(\mathbf{s}_n))'$ are spatially varying dispersal coefficients. In this formulation, it is assumed that each row of $\mathbf{B}(\tau)$ is constrained to sum to one. As noted by Hooten et al. (2007), other parameterizations are possible, but this particular parameterization corresponds to a discretized diffusion equation with a population that can pass through "open boundaries," something that is typical of invasive species.

9.3.4   ECD Parameter Model

Since we are interested in predicting at locations different from our observations, we specify a spatial model for λ_1 and τ. In both cases, we assume that the spatial processes are log-Gaussian with an exponential covariance function (see Section 4.1.1). In addition, the population-growth parameter, θ_1^G, and the carrying-capacity parameter, θ_2^G, are assumed to be independent and follow a Gaussian distribution and an inverse gamma distribution, respectively. As detailed in Hooten et al. (2007), considerable care went into the choice of the hyperparameters for these parameter models, as well as the hyperparameters for the spatial models associated with the initial condition and dispersal coefficients. Finally, recall from Section 9.3.2 that empirical results from Link et al. (1994) were used to specify the data-model parameters, a_θ and b_θ.

9.3.5   The ECD BHM: Implementation and Inference

The implementation details of the ECD BHM can be found in Hooten et al. (2007) and the associated online appendices cited therein. In summary, prediction and forecasting was implemented on a grid of points across the eastern two-thirds of the United States. The MCMC algorithm, which was a combination of Gibbs and Metropolis–Hastings steps, was run for 200,000 iterations, the first 20,000 of which were set aside for "burn-in."

The primary focus in this example is on spatial prediction and forecasting of ECD population abundance, $Y_t(\cdot)$, at various spatial locations in the United States. Summaries of these predictions can be shown as spatial maps. Figure 9.11 shows the maps of the posterior mean of the ECD abundance for each year from 1986 through 2003. Note that, although these maps are displayed as images, where the color of the grid cell is representative of the ECD abundance, the prediction actually corresponds to a *point* in the middle of the box. The image format is for clarity of presentation and is not meant to imply that prediction is for an areal spatial support. Note also that the white areas of the map were not considered in the analysis. These correspond to the ocean, Mexico, and the northeast United States, where there were no ECD data available during the 1986–2003 time period. This figure gives a large-scale perspective of the ECD invasion that was in progress through 2003. Additionally, Figure 9.12 shows the posterior mean of ECD-abundance forecasts through the year 2020. This figure suggests that the ECD is on track to successfully colonize this entire region of the United States by about 2016 (i.e., it is forecasted to be at, or near, its carrying capacity by this time).

Obviously, when making predictions or forecasts, one should examine the associated prediction and forecast uncertainties. The prediction and forecast uncertainty maps for ECD abundance look very much like the posterior mean maps shown in Figures 9.11 and 9.12; this is not surprising, given that we are assuming that the abundance follows a (conditional) Poisson distribution (for which the mean is equal to the variance). It is more informative to examine these distributions in the context of time series of abundance predictions for

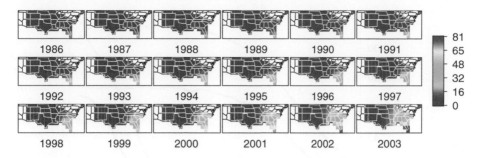

Figure 9.11 Posterior means of ECD abundance in the United States for the period 1986 to 2003 (corresponding to the sampling period considered in this analysis). Areas of the map shown as "white" were not included in the prediction grid.

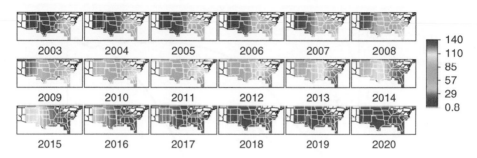

Figure 9.12 Posterior mean of the ECD-abundance forecast in the United States for the period 2003 to 2020 (where the years 2004–2020 correspond to out-of-sample forecasts). Areas of the map shown as "white" were not included in the prediction grid.

specific locations. For example, Figure 9.13 shows the posterior 95% credible intervals for ECD abundance at a location in south Florida, one in eastern Kansas, and one in northern Utah. Clearly, the population at the south Florida location likely reached its carrying capacity in the early 2000s, whereas the Kansas and Utah locations are forecasted to reach their carrying capacities in the middle and late 2010s, respectively.

Although the main goal for this analysis was to spatially predict and forecast abundance, gaining knowledge about the underlying process parameters that govern the population dynamics can also be useful. As described in Hooten et al. (2007), the posterior distributions for the growth parameters were substantially narrower than their prior distributions, which suggested that the data were informative for inference on these parameters. Furthermore, the posterior distribution associated with the spatially varying dispersal parameters also suggested "learning." Figure 9.14 shows the posterior mean of the dispersal parameters on the grid used for spatial prediction and forecasting. Note that the magnitudes of these dispersal parameters are directly related to the scale of the map-distance units; therefore, it is the overall pattern and relative magnitude that

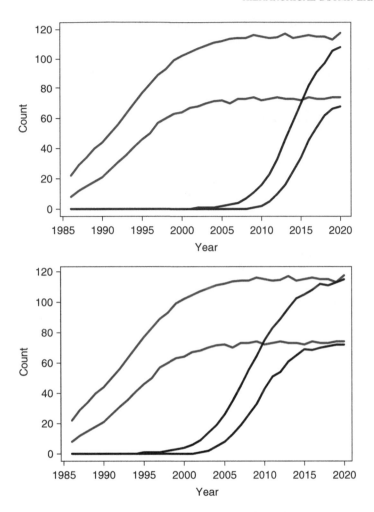

Figure 9.13 Comparisons of posterior credible intervals for the ECD population from 1986 to 2020. **Top panel:** Credible intervals for a location in south Florida (red) and for northern Utah (black). **Bottom panel:** Credible intervals for the south Florida location (red) and for eastern Kansas (black).

is important, not the actual value of the estimate. This map shows that there is clearly an area of lower dispersal in northern Florida, which would suggest that the ECD invasion was relatively slower to spread north and westward out of Florida. In addition, the dispersal in the western United States is likely to be faster than in the southeast. Hooten et al. (2007) show, using the deviance information criterion (DIC) measure (e.g., Spiegelhalter et al., 2002), that the model with spatially varying (heterogeneous) dispersal coefficients fits the data better than the model assuming constant (homogenous) dispersal.

The analysis shown here was originally performed in the mid-2000s, based on data through 2003. It is interesting to examine the state of the ECD invasion

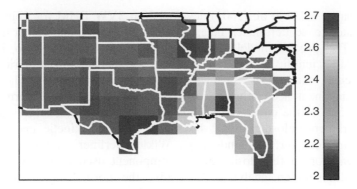

Figure 9.14 Posterior mean of the spatially varying dispersal coefficients (τ) in the ECD process model (9.19).

of North America in 2010. Maps of user-reported ECD sightings through the Spring of 2010 show relatively frequent ECD encounters throughout the continental United States, with the exception of the northeast (e.g., see the maps of ECD "checklist frequency" from the eBird project; eBird, 2010). Thus, the forecast shown in Figure 9.12 was quite reasonable, if somewhat conservative, in the speed of the invasion. Presumably, the forecast could have been improved if ecologically relevant covariates were used in the model for the dispersal parameters.

In summary, this approach for modeling invasive species was able to take into account uncertainty in the detection of ECDs in the North American BBS observations, within the context of a scientifically intuitive and useful nonlinear DSTM that could be used in a BHM to predict and forecast the ongoing ECD invasion. This illustrates the power of the BHM approach for combining observations and scientific information in the presence of uncertainty.

9.4 MEDITERRANEAN SURFACE VECTOR WINDS

Beginning in the late 1990s, a sequence of increasingly sophisticated BHMs for near-surface wind fields (so-called "surface vector winds," or SVWs) were developed using satellite scatterometer observations. In particular, Royle et al. (1999) derived a BHM for SVWs based on a single snapshot in time (i.e., a spatial model); data were made up of two swaths of satellite scatterometer SVWs in the Labrador Sea region. The process model in Royle et al. (1999) was based on a PDE representing a *geostrophic-ageostrophic* partition (e.g., Holton, 2004, Chapter 3) of the SVW field. Sea-level pressure (SLP) was represented by a latent spatial process model with random parameters. As described in Section 5.5, conditioning multivariate processes on a common process is a very effective approach for building dependence, especially if, as in this case, there is strong scientific motivation for the conditioning.

Similarly, Wikle et al. (2001) developed an SVW BHM for tropical winds using satellite scatterometer data, in addition to weather-center reanalysis winds. The process-model component of their BHM is also based on substantial scientific knowledge, both from theory and empirical study. In particular, the process is made up of three components: (1) a spatial mean component accounting for land–sea contrasts, (2) the normal modes (Section 5.5) of the equatorial shallow water equations (at large scales), and (3) a turbulence-closure model based on observed kinetic energy spectra for the tropical surface winds (e.g., Wikle, Berliner, and Cressie, 1998). Implementation of the closure-model component used nested wavelet bases (i.e., multiresolution analysis). Critically, the normal mode and wavelet coefficients were assumed to evolve according to a linear dynamical model, with hyperparameters suggested by independent empirical results from the literature (Wheeler and Kiladis, 1999). Realistic surface convergence features in the posterior wind distributions were shown to correspond well with intense atmospheric deep convection and rainband signatures in infrared cloud imagery during the mature phase of tropical cyclone Dale (Wikle et al., 2001). Hoar et al. (2003) extended this model to generate a multi-year dataset of 50 realizations from the SVW posterior distribution for the tropical Indian and western Pacific oceans. Mapes, Milliff, and Morzel (2009) combined the winds reported by Hoar et al. (2003) with cloud and precipitable-water datasets to identify lead-lag relationships in the life cycles of over 10,000 mesoscale convective systems (MCS) in the tropical Indian and western Pacific Oceans.

Berliner, Milliff, and Wikle (2003) demonstrated how a BHM could handle multi-platform observations in the data model, where the process model is based on an idealized coupled air–sea interaction model in a high-latitude, partially enclosed sea. A key feature of this study is the demonstration that a process model based on discretized quasi-geostrophic dynamics (see Section 7.4; Wikle and Hooten, 2010), with random parameters and additive error, is sufficient to fully capture the nonlinear dynamics from a simulated truth based on shallow-water equations. This is so, even with relatively sparse observations.

The latest SVW BHM in this series of models is due to Milliff et al. (2011), who extend the geostrophic–ageostrophic process model for the SVW to include explicit surface-friction effects. Data include satellite retrievals of SVW, as well as SVW and sea-level-pressure fields from weather-center analyses. The energy spectrum of the weather-center winds is not realistic at the spatial scales of interest here, but the scatterometer data do represent realistic energy content. Thus, one of the goals of this analysis was to merge systematically these two datasets, in order to obtain posterior realizations that have a realistic energy spectrum.

We focus on an extension of the model and analysis of Milliff et al. (2011) here, as discussed in detail in Bonazzi (2008). In particular, this example shows how a science-based framework can suggest a *conditional* multivariate model in the presence of multiple data sources. More importantly, the broader goal of this study is to provide SVW forcing fields for an operational, deterministic, ocean-forecast model for the Mediterranean Sea. These forcing winds have realistic spatio-temporal structure (in terms of means, variances, covariances, and energy spectra) relative to known regional wind regimes. Such realistic variation in the SVW leads to realistic uncertainties in the ocean fields used to intialize the forecast model and, thus, it leads to more realistic assessments of forecast accuracy (Milliff et al., 2011; Pinardi et al., 2011).

Before we describe the SVW BHM, we give a little background on how an ocean-forecast system works. In particular, we consider the Mediterranean Forecast System (MFS), which produces 10-day forecasts of the ocean state variables (e.g., three-dimensional fields of temperature, pressure, density, salinity, flow vectors, sea-surface height, etc.) every day (for details, see Pinardi et al., 2003; Dobricic et al., 2005; Pinardi et al., 2011). The forecast system is comprised of a data-assimilation part leading to a forecast of initial ocean conditions, along with a deterministic ocean-forecast model. The underlying ocean model in this system represents a discretization (in three dimensions) of the PDEs that govern ocean dynamics and thermodynamics. In the MFS, a *sequential* data assimilation method is used, in which the ocean state variables are adjusted daily from a first guess (prior forecast) by incorporating multivariate observations of the Mediterranean Sea. These observations accumulate over a 14-day period leading up to the initial time of the forecast. In this way, the forecast model launches from an initial state that includes the influence of the latest observations. During the data-assimilation step, the sequential procedure is forced by observed winds and, during the forecast step, the deterministic ocean-forecast-model integration is forced by forecasted SVW from a fitted BHM. One way to obtain uncertainty measures for such forecasts is to start with multiple initial conditions (so-called "ensembles") and generate an ensemble of forecasts. It is this component of the system, namely generating ensembles, that the SVW BHM is designed to address.

9.4.1 Scientific Motivation for the Process Model

The process model for SVW is motivated by an approximation to the full momentum and thermodynamic equations for the surface wind, known as the *Rayleigh friction equations* (RFE; e.g., Stevens et al., 2002):

$$
\begin{aligned}
\frac{\partial u}{\partial t} - fv &= -\frac{1}{\rho_0}\frac{\partial p}{\partial x} - \gamma u, \\
\frac{\partial v}{\partial t} + fu &= -\frac{1}{\rho_0}\frac{\partial p}{\partial y} - \gamma v,
\end{aligned}
\tag{9.20}
$$

where u and v are the east–west and north–south components of the surface winds (and are functions of time and space), respectively; f is the Coriolis parameter; ρ_0 is the reference atmospheric density; p is the sea-level pressure (also a function of time and space); and γ is the Rayleigh friction term. These equations are important in that they allow friction effects to be captured (which are important for surface winds, even over the ocean) with linear dynamics. Following an approach similar to Milliff et al. (2011), one can show that a reasonable low-order approximation to the RFE equations leads to the following representation of the velocity components (e.g., Bonazzai, 2008)

$$
\begin{aligned}
u \simeq &-\frac{f}{\rho_0(f^2+\gamma^2)}\frac{\partial p}{\partial y} - \frac{\gamma}{\rho_0(f^2+\gamma^2)}\frac{\partial p}{\partial x} \\
&-2\frac{\gamma}{\rho_0(f^2+\gamma^2)}\frac{\partial u}{\partial t} - \frac{1}{\rho_0(f^2+\gamma^2)}\frac{\partial^2 p}{\partial x\,\partial t}, \\
v \simeq &\frac{f}{\rho_0(f^2+\gamma^2)}\frac{\partial p}{\partial x} - \frac{\gamma}{\rho_0(f^2+\gamma^2)}\frac{\partial p}{\partial y} \\
&-2\frac{\gamma}{\rho_0(f^2+\gamma^2)}\frac{\partial v}{\partial t} - \frac{1}{\rho_0(f^2+\gamma^2)}\frac{\partial^2 p}{\partial y\,\partial t}.
\end{aligned}
\tag{9.21}
$$

If we consider centered differences to replace the spatial derivatives in (9.21), we can write a process model in vector form as

$$
\begin{aligned}
\mathbf{u}_t &= a_1^{(u)}\mathbf{D}_y\mathbf{p}_t + a_2^{(u)}\mathbf{D}_x\mathbf{p}_t + a_3^{(u)}\mathbf{u}_{t-1} + a_4^{(u)}\mathbf{D}_x\mathbf{p}_{t-1} + \boldsymbol{\eta}_t^{(u)}, \\
\mathbf{v}_t &= a_1^{(v)}\mathbf{D}_x\mathbf{p}_t + a_2^{(v)}\mathbf{D}_y\mathbf{p}_t + a_3^{(v)}\mathbf{v}_{t-1} + a_4^{(v)}\mathbf{D}_y\mathbf{p}_{t-1} + \boldsymbol{\eta}_t^{(v)},
\end{aligned}
\tag{9.22}
$$

where $\mathbf{u}_t$ and $\mathbf{v}_t$ represent a vectorization of the gridded wind components; $\mathbf{p}_t$ and $\mathbf{p}_{t-1}$ represent vectorizations of the gridded pressure field at time t and $t-1$, respectively; $\{a_i^{(\cdot)}: i=1,\dots,4\}$ are parameters corresponding to the respective coefficients in front of the partial derivative terms in (9.21); $\mathbf{D}_x$ and $\mathbf{D}_y$ are matrix operators that give the x-direction and y-direction centered differences, respectively; and $\boldsymbol{\eta}_t^{(u)}$ and $\boldsymbol{\eta}_t^{(v)}$ are additive error terms that represent the effects of the approximation used to obtain (9.21). These error processes are further decomposed in terms of wavelet basis functions, as described in Section 9.4.2.

9.4.2 The SVW BHM

As is customary with BHM implementations, we distinguish between the data-model, process-model, and parameter-model levels of the hierarchy.

Data Model

In this application, we consider two sources of wind data and one source of sea-level pressure data. In particular, we have satellite wind observations from the QuikSCAT scatterometer, along with surface winds and pressures from an analysis by the European Center for Medium range Weather Forecasting (ECMWF). The specific data models are

$$\mathbf{d}_t^{Qu}|\mathbf{u}_t, \sigma_Q^2 \sim ind. Gau(\mathbf{H}_t^Q \mathbf{u}_t, \sigma_Q^2 \mathbf{I}),$$

$$\mathbf{d}_t^{Qv}|\mathbf{v}_t, \sigma_Q^2 \sim ind. Gau(\mathbf{H}_t^Q \mathbf{v}_t, \sigma_Q^2 \mathbf{I}),$$

$$\mathbf{d}_t^{Eu}|\mathbf{u}_t, \sigma_E^2 \sim ind. Gau(\mathbf{H}_t^E \mathbf{u}_t, \sigma_E^2 \mathbf{I}),$$

$$\mathbf{d}_t^{Ev}|\mathbf{v}_t, \sigma_E^2 \sim ind. Gau(\mathbf{H}_t^E \mathbf{v}_t, \sigma_E^2 \mathbf{I}),$$

$$\mathbf{d}_t^{Ep}|\mathbf{p}_t, \sigma_{E_p}^2 \sim ind. Gau(\mathbf{H}_t^E \mathbf{p}_t, \sigma_{E_p}^2 \mathbf{I}),$$

where $\mathbf{d}_t^{Qu}$ and $\mathbf{d}_t^{Qv}$ are vectors of scatterometer u-wind and v-wind observations, respectively, within a specified time window indexed by t; and $\mathbf{d}_t^{Eu}$, $\mathbf{d}_t^{Ev}$, and $\mathbf{d}_t^{Ep}$ are ECMWF u-wind and v-wind component and pressure observations, respectively, within the same time window. In addition, recall that $\mathbf{u}_t$, $\mathbf{v}_t$, and $\mathbf{p}_t$ represent vectorizations of the gridded wind components and pressure, respectively, of the true processes. The mapping matrices (incidence matrices in this case; see Section 7.1.2) for the scatterometer and ECMWF observations are given by $\mathbf{H}_t^Q$ and $\mathbf{H}_t^E$, respectively. Finally, measurement errors are assumed to be independent in space and time, conditional upon the true process values; they have Gaussian distributions with mean zero and measurement-error variances, σ_Q^2, σ_E^2, and $\sigma_{E_p}^2$ (corresponding to scatterometer wind components, ECMWF wind components, and ECMWF pressures, respectively).

A sample of the wind data for February 2, 2005 is shown in Figure 9.15. These panels show the QuikSCAT scatterometer and ECMWF analysis observations available within a window of ± 3 h of $t = 00{:}00$, $06{:}00$, $12{:}00$, and $18{:}00$ UTC ("Coordinated Universal Time"). Note that the ECMWF-analysis winds and pressures are available on a $0.5° \times 0.5°$ spatial grid, and they are available at each time period for all locations. This grid is also used for the process vectors. In contrast, the QuikSCAT observations are available intermittently in space due to the polar orbit of the satellite, but at much higher spatial resolution (25 km) when they are available. In this sense, the mapping matrices for the scatterometer data $\mathbf{H}_t^Q$ are incidence matrices based on the assumption that all scatterometer observations within $0.25°$ of a process gridpoint, and within 3 hours of time t, are associated with the wind process at that gridpoint and time.

Process Model

The process model given by (9.22) is motivated by the RFE. The model can be rewritten in terms of the process distributions:

$$\mathbf{u}_t|\mathbf{p}_t, \boldsymbol{\beta}_t^{(u)}, \{a_i^{(u)} : i = 1, \ldots, 4\}, \sigma_u^2 \sim ind. Gau(\boldsymbol{\mu}_t^{(u)}, \sigma_u^2 \mathbf{I}),$$

$$\mathbf{v}_t|\mathbf{p}_t, \boldsymbol{\beta}_t^{(v)}, \{a_i^{(v)} : i = 1, \ldots, 4\}, \sigma_v^2 \sim ind. Gau(\boldsymbol{\mu}_t^{(v)}, \sigma_v^2 \mathbf{I}),$$

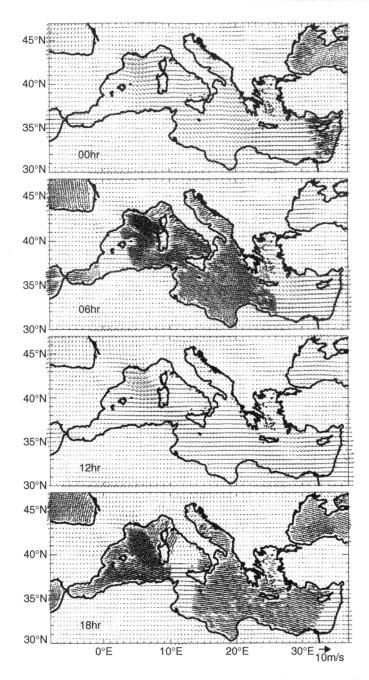

Figure 9.15 Wind observations from February 1, 2005. From top to bottom, the panels correspond to available data at 00:00, 06:00, 12:00, and 18:00 UTC. The red vectors over the Mediterranean Sea correspond to ECMWF-analysis winds on a $0.5° \times 0.5°$ grid. The black vectors correspond to the much-higher-resolution (25 km), but spatially intermittent, wind retrievals from the QuickSCAT scatterometer.

where

$$\boldsymbol{\mu}_t^{(u)} = a_1^{(u)}\mathbf{D}_y\mathbf{p}_t + a_2^{(u)}\mathbf{D}_x\mathbf{p}_t + a_3^{(u)}\mathbf{u}_{t-1} + a_4^{(u)}\mathbf{D}_x\mathbf{p}_{t-1} + \mathcal{W}\boldsymbol{\beta}_t^{(u)},$$
$$\boldsymbol{\mu}_t^{(v)} = a_1^{(v)}\mathbf{D}_x\mathbf{p}_t + a_2^{(v)}\mathbf{D}_y\mathbf{p}_t + a_3^{(v)}\mathbf{v}_{t-1} + a_4^{(v)}\mathbf{D}_y\mathbf{p}_{t-1} + \mathcal{W}\boldsymbol{\beta}_t^{(v)},$$

and we have assumed that the error processes, $\boldsymbol{\eta}_t^{(u)}$ and $\boldsymbol{\eta}_t^{(v)}$, are decomposed in terms of a wavelet-basis expansion plus white noise. That is, given $\boldsymbol{\beta}_t^{(u)}$ and $\boldsymbol{\beta}_t^{(v)}$, we have

$$\boldsymbol{\eta}_t^{(u)} = \mathcal{W}\boldsymbol{\beta}_t^{(u)} + \mathbf{v}_t^{(u)}; \quad \mathbf{v}_t^{(u)} \sim ind.\,Gau(\mathbf{0}, \sigma_u^2\mathbf{I}),$$
$$\boldsymbol{\eta}_t^{(v)} = \mathcal{W}\boldsymbol{\beta}_t^{(v)} + \mathbf{v}_t^{(v)}; \quad \mathbf{v}_t^{(v)} \sim ind.\,Gau(\mathbf{0}, \sigma_v^2\mathbf{I}),$$

where $\mathcal{W}$ is a matrix of wavelet basis functions, and $\boldsymbol{\beta}_t^{(u)}$ and $\boldsymbol{\beta}_t^{(v)}$ are the associated wavelet coefficients. This formulation is adapted from Wikle et al. (2001) to account for multiscale spatially correlated error processes that have been shown to be important after large-scale features were removed from the scatterometer data [see Milliff et al. (2011) for details].

Now, as in Milliff et al. (2011), we write the vector of gridded pressures as

$$\mathbf{p}_t = \mu_p\mathbf{1} + \boldsymbol{\Phi}\boldsymbol{\alpha}_t,$$

where μ_p represents the overall (known) mean sea-level pressure, $\boldsymbol{\Phi}$ is defined as a set of p_α EOF basis functions (where the EOFs were calculated based on historical sea-level pressure from the ECMWF reanalysis), and $\boldsymbol{\alpha}_t$ are the EOF spectral coefficients. Because the pressure field is deterministically related to the spectral coefficients (since the mean μ_p and the basis functions $\boldsymbol{\Phi}$ are assumed known), the pressure "process" is determined by $\boldsymbol{\alpha}_t$ on a reduced-dimensional space. Given that we have "complete" data fields for pressure data, a fairly simple model for $\boldsymbol{\alpha}_t$ can be specified:

$$\boldsymbol{\alpha}_t|\boldsymbol{\lambda} \sim iid\,Gau(\mathbf{0}, \mathrm{diag}(\boldsymbol{\lambda})),$$

where $\boldsymbol{\lambda}$ is a p_α-dimensional vector with positive entries.

In conclusion, the dynamics in the process model for SVW are not complicated, because the large-scale dynamics are already accounted for in the pressure data. This is an example of a model/data trade-off, in which a less complicated dynamical model is offset by fairly complete observations. It is the wavelet spectral coefficients, $\boldsymbol{\beta}_t^{(u)}$ and $\boldsymbol{\beta}_t^{(v)}$, that are dynamical; it is seen in the parameter models below that they evolve as univariate AR(1) processes.

Parameter Model

The process-model parameters associated with the pressure derivatives are given in (9.22). Their prior distributions are assumed to be

$$a_j^{(u)} \sim Gau(\tilde{\mu}_j^{(u)}, \sigma_{u,j}^2), \quad a_j^{(v)} \sim Gau(\tilde{\mu}_j^{(v)}, \sigma_{v,j}^2), \qquad j = 1, \dots, 4,$$

independently. Now, the theoretical relationship in (9.21) can be used to suggest the prior means:

$$\tilde{\mu}_1^{(u)} = -\tilde{\mu}_1^{(v)} = \frac{-f}{\rho_0(f^2 + \gamma^2 + 2\gamma/\Delta)}$$

$$\tilde{\mu}_2^{(u)} = \tilde{\mu}_2^{(v)} = \frac{-(1/\Delta + \gamma)}{\rho_0(f^2 + \gamma^2 + 2\gamma/\Delta)}$$

$$\tilde{\mu}_3^{(u)} = \tilde{\mu}_3^{(v)} = \frac{2\gamma}{\Delta(f^2 + \gamma^2 + 2\gamma/\Delta)}$$

$$\tilde{\mu}_4^{(u)} = \tilde{\mu}_4^{(v)} = \frac{1}{\rho_0\Delta(f^2 + \gamma^2 + 2\gamma/\Delta)},$$

where f, ρ_0, and γ take values that are physically realistic for the region under consideration and Δ is the time discretization constant [for details, see Milliff et al. (2011) and Bonazzi (2008)]. Furthermore, the wavelet spectral coefficients are dynamical and are assumed to evolve as univariate AR(1) processes. That is,

$$\beta_t^{(k)}(i) \sim Gau(m_k(i)\beta_{t-1}^{(k)}(i), \sigma_{\beta_k}^2(i)), \qquad \text{for } k = u, v \text{ and } i = 1, \dots, n_\beta,$$

where n_β is the dimension of $\boldsymbol{\beta}_t^{(u)}$ and $\boldsymbol{\beta}_t^{(v)}$. We then specify Gaussian priors for $m_k(i)$ for $k = u, v$ and $i = 1, \dots, n_\beta$; Gaussian priors for the initial conditions, $\boldsymbol{\beta}_0^{(u)}$ and $\boldsymbol{\beta}_0^{(v)}$; and independent inverse gamma priors for all variances and the elements of $\boldsymbol{\lambda}$. For details of the hyperparameter specifications, see Milliff et al. (2011).

9.4.3 The SVW BHM: Implementation and Inference

As discussed above, the eventual goal of this analysis is to use the SVW BHM to produce realistic realizations of wind fields to initialize the MFS operational ocean-forecast model. The BHM was implemented for various 24-day periods in 2005 and 2006, with the first 14 days in each corresponding to the "assimilation" period, where both scatterometer and ECMWF winds were available, and the last 10 days corresponding to a "forecast" period, where SVW observations and analyses are replaced by ECMWF surface-wind forecasts. That is, there are no "observations" in the forecast period, but the BHM treats the ECMWF forecasted SVWs as if they were data during this period. The wind component processes were considered on a grid with $0.5° \times 0.5°$ spatial resolution and a 6-h time resolution. For BHM-implementation details, see Milliff et al. (2011) and Bonazzi (2008).

Figure 9.16 shows posterior-distribution summaries for the wind process for February 2, 2005, over the western portion of the Mediterranean basin. The red vector shows the posterior mean, and the variation about that mean is illustrated by the spread (i.e., variation) in 10 samples from the posterior distribution (black vectors), taken at widely separated intervals in the MCMC iterations. Each of the 11 vectors in a grid cell emanates from a common vertex; therefore, the *direction* of a vector is *away* from its vertex. Note that at any given grid cell, there is considerable spread in the black vectors, which could be important when these winds are used to force an ocean model. In particular, note that the so-called *Mistral winds* (strong northerly winds blowing off the south coast of France into the Gulf of Lyon) are quite evident, as well as strong north–northwest winds in the region of the Sicily Straits. In general, although there is reasonable spread associated with these high wind speeds, the wind (direction and speed) uncertainty is larger in more sheltered regions, where the wind speeds are lower on average.

The atmospheric winds force the ocean primarily through the wind-stress curl (see Section 7.4; Milliff and Morzel, 2001). Figure 9.17 shows the posterior mean and posterior standard deviation for wind-stress curl for the four model times on February 2, 2005. In this case, we simply show the standard deviations calculated from the 10 realizations (i.e., ensembles) of wind fields taken from the posterior, which are shown in Figure 9.16. Note that relatively small differences in the wind fields can lead to large differences in the wind-stress curl,

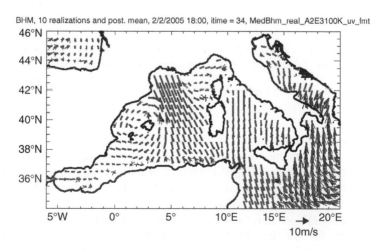

Figure 9.16 Posterior means (red vectors) and ten samples (black vectors) from the posterior distribution for SVW over the western Mediterranean basin for 18:00 UTC on February 2, 2005. Wind speed is proportional to the length of the vectors. The direction of a vector is away from the vertex at the center of its grid cell.

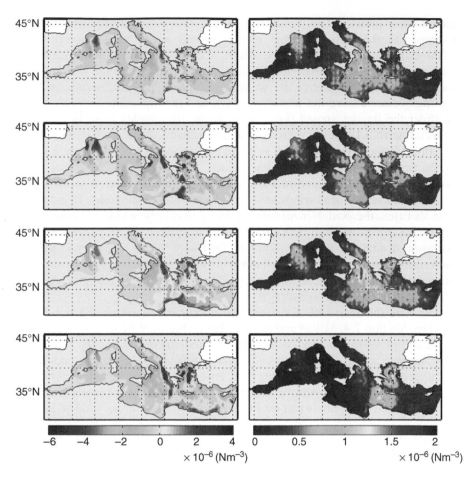

Figure 9.17 Wind stress curl maps for 00:00, 06:00, 12:00, and 18:00 UTC (from top to bottom) for February 2, 2005. The left panels show the posterior means obtained from the SVW BHM; the right panels show the corresponding standard deviations obtained from the 10 samples from the posterior distribution shown in Figure 9.16.

due to the nonlinear nature of the drag law used to derive this quantity. The dominant features in the wind-stress-curl posterior mean (e.g., corresponding to the Mistral event in the Gulf of Lyon) are at relatively large (i.e., "synoptic") spatial scales, whereas the areas of greatest standard deviations tend to be at smaller (i.e., "mesoscale") spatial scales.

The small-scale variations in wind forcing can have dramatic impacts on the ocean, in that they lead to uncertainties in the ocean state variables at comparable scales of spatial resolution. Uncertainties on these scales correspond to the scales of greatest uncertainty in the ocean-forecast system as well. This is exactly what the forecaster wants—knowledge in regions where the ocean model and analyses are least certain. The resulting uncertainties can then be propagated through the deterministic ocean model to produce realistic forecast uncertainties. In particular, the ensembles from the SVW BHM have a substantial and realistic impact on the ocean initial conditions, because they are incorporated throughout a 14-day sequential data assimilation system in the MFS. For example, to see how the uncertainties in the initial wind forcing, obtained from the BHM, impact the multivariate ocean state variables, consider the impact on sea surface temperature (SST) and sea surface height (SSH). Figure 9.18 shows the posterior mean and posterior standard deviation for the MFS-derived SST initial condition for March 14, 2006 at 12:00 UTC, based on the corresponding SVW posterior distributions used in the previous 14-day data-assimilation cycle. Similarly, Figure 9.19 shows the posterior mean and posterior standard deviation for the corresponding SSH. In both cases, the posterior means exhibit relatively large-scale features of the general ocean circulation and its response to wind forcing. Importantly, the posterior standard deviations show that the uncertainties are at much smaller, but coherent spatial scales. Remarkably, as discussed in Milliff et al. (2011), these features correspond to persistent "hot spots" in the mesoscale circulation of the Mediterranean Sea (e.g., the Algerian Current, the Atlantic-Ionian Stream, and the Mersa Matruh gyre). Thus, the uncertainty in the initial wind

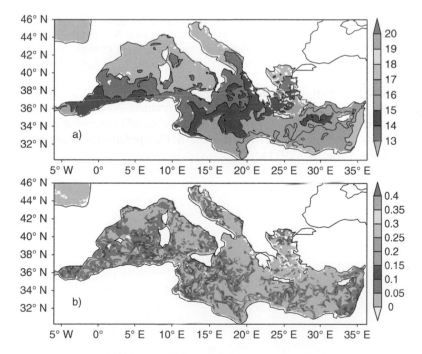

Figure 9.18   Sea surface temperature (SST, in units of °C) posterior means (top panel) and posterior standard deviations (bottom panel) at 12:00 UTC on March 14, 2006. Note that the posterior standard deviations were obtained from 10 realizations from the SST posterior distribution.

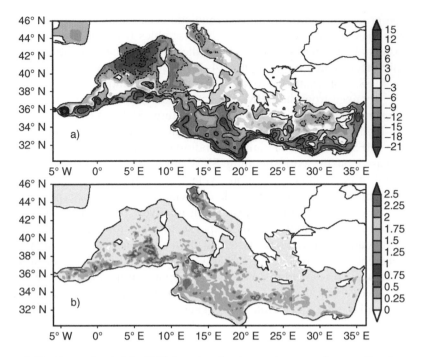

Figure 9.19 Sea surface height (SSH, in units of cm) posterior means (top panel) and posterior standard deviations (bottom panel) at 12:00 UTC on March 14, 2006. Note that the posterior standard deviations were obtained from 10 realizations from the SSH posterior distribution.

fields have provided a localization of forecast uncertainty in the oceanic state variables, which is essential for producing realistic forecast uncertainties in the operational ocean forecast system. Specific details regarding the impact of these winds from the SVW BHM, in the MFS operational ocean model, are given in Pinardi et al. (2011).

Epilogue

This book was about the statistical analysis of *spatio-temporal* data. Throughout our exploration of this topic, we have repeatedly come back to a few key themes: dividing a complex problem into simpler components by thinking conditionally (i.e., hierarchical modeling); accounting for uncertainty in data, process, and parameters; the use of scientific principles and findings to motivate each level of a hierarchical model; the dynamical specification of spatio-temporal models; and data/model/computing compromises. Perhaps the best way to summarize this book is that it provides a systematic approach for quantification of uncertainty in spatio-temporal data in a way that scientific information can be easily incorporated in support of inference.

Admittedly, our coverage of this topic has been far from complete. Some topics were covered in less depth than we would have liked (e.g., descriptive spatio-temporal models, multivariate spatio-temporal processes, nonlinear dynamical models, dynamical design, sequential Monte Carlo); some things were hardly covered (e.g., change-point detection, spatio-temporal point processes, dynamical modeling of objects, spatio-temporal field comparison); and some things were not considered at all (e.g., model selection, extremes). In the end, we made decisions and choices to emphasize certain topics for myriad reasons. One of them was that this is a big book that simply could not get any bigger; time and space were limited!

Ultimately, we chose topics that we thought were fundamental and some topics that were, in some sense, "dear to our hearts." We do feel that this book represents a fairly accurate snapshot of (a projection of) the state of statistical analysis of spatio-temporal data *circa* 2010. But this is a rapidly evolving field, and it is notoriously hard to hit a moving target. We have attempted to be scholarly, and we have tried to look beyond our own discipline for important contributions. We have almost certainly fallen short and unintentionally missed some useful and important papers. We offer our apologies for these oversights.

At the end of a long book like this, it is tempting to say something about the *future* of the field. As statisticians, we recognize that it is dangerous to extrapolate, but the opportunity to forecast is too great to resist.

We are certain that computational issues are always going to be linked closely with spatio-temporal statistical analysis. For most problems, the datasets are large, and they keep getting larger! In addition, as datasets grow, model complexity grows, and consequently there is a need for ever-increasing computing power and/or algorithms for efficient estimation and inference. Of course, there will always be trade-offs between what one would like a model to be and what the available tools will allow it to be, suggesting a modeling strategy of "dialing back" from what one would like to do, to what one is able to do. This is a "progressive" strategy that we expect will offer continual improvement of the state-of-the-art.

As for the field itself, we believe that we have only just begun to realize the potential of modeling complex spatio-temporal systems. Nonlinear interactions across many processes define the world in which we live. To address important scientific questions in the presence of uncertainty, we shall need to develop spatio-temporal statistical methodologies that can efficiently accommodate multivariate interactions in nonlinear and nonstationary environments. One promising avenue of research is the further development of individual-based (or, agent-based) models. We also believe that there will be increased use of a variety of deterministic "computer" models, and we see our topic playing a role in making such models more stochastic and more responsive to data. In addition, we believe there will be increased data on non-Euclidean spaces (such as networks, social or otherwise), that change with time. This will come as a result of our society becoming increasingly "connected." In some sense, cyber networks, in addition to being non-Euclidean, also tend to change our perception of time. That is, information may travel much faster than it would have in the past, resulting in processes with vastly different "clock speeds" that interact in nonstationary ways.

Finally, we believe that spatio-temporal statistics has a large, and mainly untapped role to play in public policy. That is, as the questions we are faced with (e.g., global climate change, water resources, hunger, economic stability) become more critical to society in general, we believe strongly that honest quantification and accounting of uncertainty must play a bigger role in decision making, which is the apex of the knowledge pyramid described at the beginning of the book. Here, a summary based on the posterior mean and the posterior variance will not be enough. Development of multivariate loss functions (or, better, utility functions that involve cost components) are needed to quantify policy questions. Many of these issues are indeed spatio-temporal, and it is important that we discover better ways to incorporate our understanding of data, processes, and parameters into a decision-support environment. Importantly, it should be acknowledged that this is not just a matter of scientific and statistical discovery, since there is increasingly less distinction between policy and politics. Nevertheless, we can and should continue to provide information and, better yet, knowledge, so that uncertainties and data/model issues are presented completely and openly. In this way, we shall do our part in contributing to "Science in the service of Society."

This book is finished, and now we can see what wasn't obvious before ...

We shall not cease from exploration
And the end of all our exploring
Will be to arrive where we started
And know the place for the first time
(T. S. Eliot)

References

K. Abend, T. J. Harley, and L. N. Kanal. Classification of binary random patterns. *IEEE Transactions on Information Theory*, **11**:538–544, 1965.

M. Abramowitz and I. A. Stegun. *Handbook of Mathematical Functions with Formulas, Graphs, and Mathematical Tables*. National Bureau of Standards, Washington DC, 1964.

R. J. Adler. *The Geometry of Random Fields*. John Wiley & Sons, Chichester, UK, 1981.

O. Aguilar and M. West. Bayesian dynamic factor models and variance matrix discounting for portfolio allocation. *Journal of Business & Economic Statistics*, **18**:338–357, 2000.

O. Ahlqvist, H. Ban, N. Cressie, and N. Zuniga-Shaw. Statistical counterpoint: Knowledge discovery of choreographic information using spatio-temporal analysis and visualization. *Applied Geography*, **30**:548–560, 2010.

J. Aitchison and J. A. C. Brown. *The Lognormal Distribution*. Cambridge University Press, London, 1957.

W. J. Aldworth and N. Cressie. Sampling designs and prediction methods for Gaussian spatial processes. In S. Ghosh, editor, *Multivariate Analysis, Design of Experiments and Survey Sampling*, pages 1–54. Marcel Dekker, New York, 1999.

W. J. Aldworth and N. Cressie. Prediction of nonlinear spatial functionals. *Journal of Statistical Planning and Inference*, **112**:3–41, 2003.

M. M. Ali. Analysis of stationary spatial-temporal processes: Estimation and prediction. *Biometrika*, **66**:513–518, 1979.

D. J. Allcroft and C. A. Glasbey. A latent Gaussian Markov random-field model for spatiotemporal rainfall disaggregation. *Applied Statistics*, **52**:487–498, 2003.

B. Anderson and J. Moore. *Optimal Filtering*. Prentice-Hall, Englewood Cliffs, NJ, 1979.

C. Andrieu, A. Doucet, and R. Holenstein. Particle Markov chain Monte Carlo methods. *Journal of the Royal Statistical Society, Series B*, **72**:1–33, 2010.

L. Anselin. *Spatial Econometrics: Methods and Models*. Kluwer, Dordrecht, NL, 1988.

523

L. Anselin. Local indicators of spatial association—LISA. *Geographical Analysis*, **27**:93–115, 1995.

A. Antoulas. *Approximation of Large-Scale Dynamical Systems*. SIAM, Philadelphia, 2005.

A. Arab. *Hierarchical Spatio-temporal Models for Environmental Processes*. Ph.D. Dissertation, University of Missouri, Columbia, MO, 2007.

G. Arbia. *Spatial Data Configuration in Statistical Analysis of Regional Economics and Related Problems*. Kluwer, Dordrecht, NL, 1989.

M. S. Arulampalam, S. Maskell, N. Gordon, and T. Clapp. A tutorial on particle filters for online nonlinear/non-Gaussian Bayesian tracking. *IEEE Transactions on Signal Processing*, **50**:174–188, 2002.

F. G. A. Asselbergs. *Conquered Conquistadors: The Lienzo De Quauhquechollan: A Nahua Vision of the Conquest of Guatamala*. University Press of Colorado, Boulder, CO, 2008.

R. M. Assunção and T. Correa. Surveillance to detect emerging space–time clusters. *Computational Statistics and Data Analysis*, **53**:2817–2830, 2009.

R. M. Assunção, I. A. Reis, and C. Oliveira. Diffusion and prediction of Leishmaniasis in a large metropolitan area in Brazil with a Bayesian space–time model. *Statistics in Medicine*, **20**:2319–2335, 2001.

K. J. Aström. *Introduction to Stochastic Control Theory*. Academic Press, New York, 1970.

N. Aubry, W.-Y. Lian, and E. S. Titi. Preserving symmetries in the proper orthogonal decomposition. *SIAM Journal of Scientific Computing*, **14**:483–505, 1993.

N. H. Augustin, M. Musio, K. von Wilpert, E. Kublin, S. N. Woods, and M. Schumacher. Modeling spatiotemporal forest health monitoring data. *Journal of the American Statistical Association*, **104**:899–911, 2009.

G. J. Babu and E. D. Feigelson. Spatial point processes in astronomy. *Journal of Statistical Planning and Inference*, **50**:311–326, 1996.

A. J. Baddeley and E. B. V. Jensen. *Stereology for Statistics*. Chapman & Hall/CRC, Boca Raton, FL, 2005.

A. J. Baddeley and J. Møller. Nearest-neighbor Markov point processes and random sets. *International Statistical Review*, **57**:89–121, 1989.

A. J. Baddeley, J. Møller, and R. Waagepetersen. Non- and semi-parametric estimation of interaction in inhomogeous point patterns. *Statistica Neerlandica*, **54**:329–350, 2000.

A. J. Baddeley, G. Nair, and N. Cressie. Directed Markov point processes—characterization and construction. Department of Statistics Preprint No. 693, The Ohio State University, Columbus, OH, 2002.

A. J. Baddeley and R. Turner. Practical maximum pseudolikelihood for spatial point patterns. *Australian and New Zealand Journal of Statistics*, **42**:283–322, 2000.

A. J. Baddeley and R. Turner. Modelling spatial point patterns in R. In A. Baddeley, P. Gregori, J. Mateu, R. Stoica, and D. Stoyan, editors, *Case Studies in Spatial Point Process Modeling, Springer Lecture Notes in Statistics, No. 185*, pages 183–195. Springer, New York, 2006.

A. J. Baddeley, R. Turner, J. Møller, and N. Hazelton. Residual analysis for spatial point process. *Journal of the Royal Statistical Society, Series B*, **67**:617–666, 2005.

A. J. Baddeley and M. N. M. van Lieshout. Area-interaction point processes. *Annals of the Institute of Statistical Mathematics*, **47**:601–619, 1995.

T. C. Bailey and A. C. Gatrell. *Interactive Spatial Data Analysis*. Longman Scientific & Technical, New York, 1992.

S. Banerjee. On geodetic distance computations in spatial modeling. *Biometrics*, **61**:617–625, 2005.

S. Banerjee, B. P. Carlin, and A. E. Gelfand. *Hierarchical Modeling and Analysis for Spatial Data*. Chapman & Hall/CRC, Boca Raton, FL, 2004.

S. Banerjee and A. E. Gelfand. Bayesian wombling: Curvilinear gradient assessment under spatial process models. *Journal of the American Statistical Association*, **101**:1487–1501, 2006.

S. Banerjee, A. E. Gelfand, A. O. Finley, and H. Sang. Gaussian predictive process models for large spatial data sets. *Journal of the Royal Statistical Society, Series B*, **70**:825–848, 2008.

S. Banerjee, M. M. Wall, and B. P. Carlin. Frailty modeling for spatially correlated survival data, with application to infant mortality in Minnesota. *Biostatistics*, **4**:123–142, 2003.

A. Bárdossy and J. Li. Geostatistical interpolation using copulas. *Water Resources Research*, **44**:W07412, doi:10.1029/2007WR006115, 2008.

O. E. Barndorff-Nielsen, D. R. Cox, and C. Kluppelberg. *Complex Stochastic Systems*. Chapman & Hall/CRC, Boca Raton, FL, 2001.

T. P. Barnett. The principal time and space scales of the Pacific trade wind fields. *Journal of the Atmospheric Sciences*, **34**:221–236, 1977.

T. P. Barnett. Interaction of the monsoon and Pacific trade wind system at interannual time scales. Part I: The equatorial zone. *Monthly Weather Review*, **11**:756–773, 1983.

T. P. Barnett and R. W. Preisendorfer. Origins and levels of monthly and seasonal forecast skill for United States surface air temperature determined by canonical correlation analysis. *Monthly Weather Review*, **115**:1825–1850, 1987.

A. G. Barnston. Linear statistical short-term climate predictive skill in the Northern Hemisphere. *Journal of Climate*, **7**:1513–1564, 1994.

A. G. Barnston, M. H. Glantz, and Y. He. Predictive skill of statistical and dynamical climate models in forecasts of SST during the 1998–97 El Niño episode and the 1998 La Niña onset. *Bulletin of the American Meteorological Society*, **80**:217–244, 1999.

A. G. Barnston and C. F. Ropelewski. Prediction of ENSO episodes using canonical correlation analysis. *Journal of Climate*, **5**:1316–1345, 1992.

R. Barry and J. Ver Hoef. Blackbox kriging: Spatial prediction without specifying variogram models. *Journal of Agricultural, Biological and Environmental Statistics*, **1**:297–322, 1996.

M. S. Bartlett. The approximate recovery of information from replicated field experiments with large blocks. *Journal of Agricultural Science (Cambridge)*, **28**:418–427, 1938.

M. S. Bartlett. Smoothing periodograms from time series with continuous spectra. *Nature*, **161**:686–687, 1948.

M. S. Bartlett. The spectral analysis of two-dimensional point processes. *Biometrika*, **51**:299–311, 1964.

M. S. Bartlett. *The Statistical Analysis of Spatial Pattern*. Chapman & Hall, London, 1975.

M. S. Bartlett. Change or chaos? *Journal of the Royal Statistical Society, Series A*, **153**:321–347, 1990.

M. J. Bayarri and J. Berger. *p*-values for composite null models. *Journal of the American Statistical Society*, **95**:1127–1142, 2000.

T. Bayes. An essay towards solving a problem in the doctrine of chances. *Philosophical Transactions of the Royal Society of London*, **53**:370–418, 1763. Reprinted in *Biometrika*, **45**:293–315, 1958.

A. F. Bennett. *Inverse Modeling of the Ocean and Atmosphere*. Cambridge University Press, Cambridge, 2002.

R. J. Bennett. *Spatial Time Series: Analysis-Forecasting-Control*. Pion, London, UK, 1979.

J. O. Berger, V. De Oliveira, and B. Sansó. Objective Bayesian analysis of spatially correlated data. *Journal of the American Statistical Association*, **96**:1361–1374, 2001.

P. G. Bergmann. *Introduction to the Theory of Relativity*. Dover, New York, 1976.

L. M. Berliner. Statistics, probability and chaos (with discussion). *Statistical Science*, **7**:69–122, 1992.

L. M. Berliner. Hierarchical Bayesian time-series models. In *Maximum Entropy and Bayesian Methods*, pages 15–22. Kluwer Academic Publishers, Dordrecht, NL, 1996.

L. M. Berliner. Physical–statistical modeling in geophysics. *Journal of Geophysical Research*, **108**(D24): STS 3–1–STS 3–10, 2003. doi:10.1029/2002JD002865.

L. M. Berliner, K. Jezek, N. Cressie, Y. Kim, C. Q. Lam, and C. J. van der Veen. Modeling dynamic controls on ice streams: A Bayesian statistical approach. *Journal of Glaciology*, **54**:705–714, 2008.

L. M. Berliner, R. A. Levine, and D. J. Shea. Bayesian climate change assessment. *Journal of Climate*, **13**:3805–3820, 2000.

L. M. Berliner, Z.-Q. Lu, and C. Snyder. Statistical design for adaptive weather observations. *Journal of Atmospheric Sciences*, **56**:2536–2552, 1999.

L. M. Berliner, R. F. Milliff, and C. K. Wikle. Bayesian hierarchical modeling of air–sea interaction. *Journal of Geophysical Research—Oceans*, **108**(C4): 3104–:doi:10.1029/2002Jbref1413, 2003.

L. M. Berliner and C. K. Wikle. Approximate importance sampling Monte Carlo for data assimilation. *Physica D*, **230**:37–49, 2007.

L. M. Berliner, C. K. Wikle, and N. Cressie. Long-lead prediction of Pacific SSTs via Bayesian dynamic modeling: Gibbs sampler. (http://www.stat.ous.edu/~sses/ps_and_pdf/ sampler.pdf).

L. M. Berliner, C. K. Wikle, and N. Cressie. Long-lead prediction of Pacific SSTs via Bayesian dynamic modeling. *Journal of Climate*, **13**:3953–3968, 2000.

L. M. Berliner, C. K. Wikle, and R. F. Milliff. Multiresolution wavelet analyses in hierarchical Bayesian turbulence models. In P. Mueller and B. Vidakovic, editors,

Bayesian Inference in Wavelet Based Models, a Springer Lecture-Notes Volume, pages 341–359. Springer, New York, 1999.

V. J. Berrocal, A. E. Gelfand, and D. M. Holland. A spatio-temporal downscaler for output from numerical models. *Journal of Agriculutral, Biological, and Environmental Statistics*, 2010. doi: 10.1007/s13253-009-0004-z.

K. K. Berthelsen and J. Møller. Non-parametric Bayesian inference for inhomogeneous Markov point processes. *Australian and New Zealand Journal of Statistics*, **50**:257–272, 2008.

C. Berzuini, N. Best, W. Gilks, and C. Larizza. Dynamic conditional independence models and Markov chain Monte Carlo methods. *Journal of the American Statistical Association*, **92**:1403–1412, 1997.

J. E. Besag. On a system of two-dimensional recurrence equations. *Journal of the Royal Statistical Society, Series B*, **43**:302–309, 1981.

J. E. Besag. Spatial interaction and the statistical analysis of lattice systems. *Journal of the Royal Statistical Society, Series B*, **36**:192–225, 1974.

J. E. Besag. Discussion of "Markov chains for exploring posterior distributions" by L. J. Tierney. *Annals of Statistics*, **22**:1734–1741, 1994.

J. E. Besag and C. Kooperberg. On conditional and intrinsic autoregression. *Biometrika*, **82**:733–746, 1995.

J. Besag, R. K. Milne, and S. Zachary. Point process limits of lattice processes. *Journal of Applied Probability*, **19**:210–216, 1982.

J. E. Besag, J. C. York, and A. Mollié. Bayesian image restoration, with two applications in spatial statistics (with discussion). *Annals of the Institute of Statistical Mathematics*, **43**:1–59, 1991.

N. Best, S. Cockings, J. Bennett, J. Wakefield, and P. Elliott. Ecological regression analysis of environmental benzene exposure and childhood leukaemia: Sensitivity to data inaccuracies, geographical scale and ecological bias. *Journal of the Royal Statistical Society, Series A*, **164**:155–174, 2001.

N. G. Best, K. Ickstadt, and R. L. Wolpert. Spatial Poisson regression for health and exposure data measured at disparate resolutions. *Journal of the American Statistical Association*, **95**:1076–1088, 2000.

D. Bhattacharjya, J. Eidsvik, and T. Mukerji. The value of information in spatial decision making. *Mathematical Geosciences*, **42**:141–163, 2010.

D. Billheimer, T. Cardoso, E. Freeman, P. Guttorp, H. Ko, and M. Silkey. Natural variability of benthic species composition in the Delaware Bay. *Environmental and Ecological Statistics*, **4**:95–115, 1997.

R. A. Bilonick. The space-time distribution of sulfate deposition in the Northeastern United States. *Atmospheric Environment*, **19**:1829–1845, 1985.

R. S. Bivand, E. J. Pebesma, and V. Gómez-Rubio. *Applied Statistical Data with R*. Springer, New York, 2008.

P. Bloomfield. *Fourier Analysis of Time Series*, second edition. John Wiley & Sons, New York, 2000.

P. Bloomfield, G. Oehlert, M. L. Thompson, and S. L. Zeger. A frequency domain analysis of trends in Dobson total ozone records. *Journal of Geophysical Research*, **88**:8512–8522, 1983.

B. Blumenthal. Predictability of a coupled ocean-atmosphere model. *Journal of Climate*, **4**:766–784, 1991.

S. Bochner. *Harmonic Analysis and the Theory of Probability*. University of California Press, Berkeley, CA, 1955.

O. Bodnar and W. Schmid. Nonlinear locally weighted kriging prediction for spatio-temporal environmental processes. *Environmetrics*, **21**:365–381, 2010.

J. B. Boisvert, J. G. Manchuk, and C. V. Deutsch. Kriging in the presence of locally varying anisotropy using non-Euclidean distances. *Mathematical Geosciences*, **41**:585–601, 2009.

A. Bonazzi. *Ensemble Forecasting in the Mediterranean Sea*. Ph.D. Dissertation, University of Bologna, 156 pages, 2008.

G. E. P. Box. Sampling and Bayes' inference in scientific modelling and robustness. *Journal of the Royal Statistical Society, Series A*, **143**:383–430, 1980.

G. E. P. Box and D. R. Cox. An analysis of transformations. *Journal of the Royal Statistical Society, Series B*, **26**:211–252, 1964.

G. E. P. Box and G. M. Jenkins. *Time Series Analysis, Forecasting, and Control*. Holden-Day, Oakland, CA, 1970.

G. E. P. Box, G. M. Jenkins, and G. C. Reinsel. *Time Series Analysis, Forecasting, and Control*, fourth edition. John Wiley & Sons, Hoboken, NJ, 2008.

G. Branstator, A. Mai, and D. Baumhefner. Identification of highly predictable flow element for spatial filtering of medium- and extended-range numerical forecasts. *Monthly Weather Review*, **121**:17860–1802, 1993.

R. L. Bras and I. Rodriguez-Iturbe. *Random Functons and Hydrology*. Addison-Wesley, Reading, MA, 1985.

I. Braud and C. Obled. On the use of empirical orthogonal function (EOF) analysis in the simulation of random fields. *Stochastic Hydrology and Hydraulics*, **5**:125–134, 1991.

N. E. Breslow and D. G. Clayton. Approximate inference in generalized linear mixed models. *Journal of the American Statistical Association*, **88**:9–25, 1993.

C. S. Bretherton, C. Smith, and J. M. Wallace. An intercomparison of methods for finding coupled patterns in climate data. *Journal of Climate*, **5**:541–560, 1992.

W. M. Briggs and R. A. Levine. Wavelets and field forecast verification. *Monthly Weather Review*, **125**:1329–1341, 1997.

D. R. Brillinger. *Time Series Data Analysis and Theory*. SIAM, Philadelphia, PA, 2001.

A. Brix and P. J. Diggle. Spatiotemporal prediction for log-Gaussian Cox processes. *Journal of the Royal Statistical Society, Series B*, **63**:823–841, 2001.

A. Brix and J. Moller. Space–time multi-type log Gaussian Cox processes with a view of modelling weeds. *Scandinavian Journal of Statistics*, **28**:471–488, 2001.

P. J. Brockwell and R. A. Davis. *Time Series: Theory and Methods*, second edition. Springer-Verlag, New York, 1991.

D. Brook. On the distinction between the conditional probability and the joint probability approaches in the specification of nearest-neighbour systems. *Biometrika*, **51**:481–483, 1964.

P. I. Brooker. *A Geostatistical Primer*. World Scientific Publishing, Singapore, 1991.

P. E. Brown, K. F. Kåresen, G. O. Roberts, and S. Tonellato. Blur-generated non-separable space–time models. *Journal of the Royal Statistical Society, Series B*, **62**:847–860, 2000.

P. J. Brown, N. D. Le, and J. V. Zidek. Multivariate spatial interpolation and exposure to air pollutants. *Canadian Journal of Statistics*, **22**:489–510, 1994.

W. J. Browne and D. Draper. A comparison of Bayesian and likelihood-based methods for fitting multilevel models. *Bayesian Analysis*, **1**:473–514, 2006.

C. Brownie and M. L. Gumpertz. Validity of spatial analyses for large field trials. *Journal of Agriculture, Biological and Environmental Statistics*, **2**:1–23, 1997.

D. J. Brus and J. J. de Gruijter. Random sampling or geostatistical modeling? Choosing between design-based and model-based sampling strategies for soil (with discussion). *Geoderma*, **60**:1–44, 1997.

C. E. Buell. Integral equation representation for factor analysis. *Journal of the Atmospheric Sciences*, **28**:1502–1505, 1972.

C. E. Buell. The topography of empirical orthogonal functions. In *Preprints Fourth Conference on Probability and Statistics in Atmospheric Science*, pages 188–193. American Meteorological Society, Boston, MA, 1975.

J. M. Bueso, J. M. Angulo, and F. J. Alonso. A state-space model approach to optimum spatial sampling design based on entropy. *Environmental and Ecological Statistics*, **5**:29–44, 1998.

G. Bürger. Complex principal oscillation pattern analysis. *Journal of Climate*, **6**:1972–1986, 1993.

G. Burgers and D. B. Stephenson. The "normality" of El Niño. *Geophysical Research Letters*, **26**:1027–1030, 1999.

P. Burrough and R. A. McDonnell. *Principles of Geographical Information Systems*, second edition. Oxford University Press, Oxford, UK, 1998.

C. A. Calder. Dynamic factor process convolution model for multivariate space–time data with application to air quality. *Environmental and Ecological Statistics*, **14**:229–247, 2007.

C. A. Calder, C. Holloman, and D. Higdon. Exploring space–time structure in ozone concentration using a dynamic process convolution model. In *Case Studies in Bayesian Statistics 6*, pages 165–176. Springer-Verlag, New York, 2002.

A. R. Cangelosi and M. B. Hooten. Models for bounded systems with continuous dynamics. *Biometrics*, **65**:850–856, 2009.

B. P. Carlin and S. Banerjee. Hierarchical multivariate CAR models for spatio-temporally correlated survival data. In J. M. Bernardo, M. J. Bayarri, J. O. Berger, A. P. Dawid, D. Heckerman, A. F. M. Smith, and M. West, editors, *Bayesian Statistics 7*, pages 45–63. Oxford University Press, Oxford, UK, 2003.

B. P. Carlin and T. A. Louis. *Bayes and Empirical Bayes Methods for Data Analysis*, second edition. Chapman & Hall/CRC, Boca Raton, FL, 2000.

B. P. Carlin, N. G. Polson, and D. S. Stoffer. A Monte Carlo approach to nonnormal and nonlinear state-space modeling. *Journal of the American Statistical Association*, **87**:493–500, 1992.

D. B. Carr and L. W. Pickle. *Visualizing Data Patterns with Micromaps*. Chapman & Hall/CRC, Boca Raton, FL, 2010.

C. K. Carter and R. Kohn. On Gibbs sampling for state space models. *Biometrika*, **81**:541–553, 1994.

C. M. Carvalho, M. S. Johannes, H. F. Lopes, and N. G. Polson. Particle learning and smoothing. *Statistical Science*, **25**:88–106, 2010.

H. Caswell. *Matrix Population Models*. Sinauer Associates, Sunderland, MA, 2001.

K. Chaloner and I. Verdinelli. Bayesian experimental designs: A review. *Statistical Science*, **10**:273–304, 1995.

K.-S. Chan and H. Tong. *Chaos: A Statistical Perspective*. Springer-Verlag, New York, 2001.

R. E. Chandler and E. M. Scott. *Statistical Methods for Trend Detection and Analysis in the Environmental Sciences*. John Wiley & Sons, Hoboken, NJ, 2011.

C.-T. Chao and S. K. Thompson. Optimal adaptive selection of sampling sites. *Environmetrics*, **12**:517–538, 2001.

C. R. Charig, D. R. Webb, S. R. Payne, and J. E. A. Wickham. Comparison of treatment of renal calculi by open surgery; percutaneous nephroilthotomy, and extracorporeal shockwave lithotripsy. *British Medical Journal (Clinical Research Edition)*, **292**:879–882, 1986.

C. Chatfield. *The Analysis of Time Series, An Introduction*, fourth edition. Chapman & Hall, London, UK, 1989.

C. Chatfield. *The Analysis of Time Series: An Introduction*, sixth edition. Chapman & Hall/CRC, Boca Raton, FL, 2004.

C. Chen, W. Härdle, and A. Unwin. *Handbook of Data Visualization*. Springer-Verlag, Berlin, 2008.

L. Chen, M. Fuentes, and J. M. Davis. Spatial-temporal statistical modeling and prediction of environmental processes. In J. S. Clark and A. E. Gelfand, editors, *Hierarchical Modelling for the Environmental Sciences*, pages 121–144. Oxford University Press, New York, 2006.

Z. Chen and D. B. Dunson. Random effects selection in linear mixed models. *Biometrics*, **59**:762–769, 2003.

S. Cherry. Some comments on singular value decomposition analysis. *Journal of Climate*, **10**:1759–1761, 1997.

J.-P. Chiles and P. Delfiner. *Geostatistics: Modeling Spatial Uncertainty*. John Wiley & Sons, New York, 1999.

S. N. Chiu and M. P. Quine. Central limit theorem for germination-growth models in $\mathbb{R}^d$ with non-Poisson locations. *Advances in Applied Probability*, **33**:751–755, 2001.

E. Choi and P. Hall. Nonparametric analysis of earthquake point-process data. In *State of the Art in Probability and Statistics*, pages 324–344. Institute of Mathematical Statistics, Beechwood, OH, 2001.

S. Choi, A. Cichocki, H.-M. Park, and S.-Y. Lee. Blind source separation and independent component analysis: A review. *Neural Information Processing—Letters and Reviews*, **6**:1–57, 2005.

K. C. Chou, A. S. Willsky, and R. Nikoukhah. Multiscale systems, Kalman filters, and Riccati equations. *IEEE Transactions on Automatic Control*, **39**:479–492, 1994.

G. Christakos. *Random Field Models in Earth Sciences*. Academic Press, San Diego, CA, 1992.

G. Christakos. *Modern Spatiotemporal Geostatistics*. Oxford University Press, Oxford, UK, 2000.

J. A. Christen and C. Fox. A general purpose sampling algorithm for continuous distributions (the t-walk). *Bayesian Analysis*, **5**:1–20, 2010.

O. F. Christensen, G. O. Roberts, and M. Skold. Robust Markov chain Monte Carlo method for spatial generalized linear mixed models. *Journal of Computational and Graphical Statistics*, **15**:1–17, 2006.

R. Christensen. *Linear Models for Multivariate, Time Series, and Spatial Data*. Springer-Verlag, New York, 1991.

O. F. Christensen and R. P. Waagepetersen. Bayesian prediction of spatial count data using generalized linear mixed models. *Biometrics*, **58**:280–286, 2002.

W. I. Christensen and R. A. Bryson. An investigation of the potential of component analysis for weather classification. *Monthly Weather Review*, **94**:697–709, 1966.

A. B. Clark and A. B. Lawson. Spatio-temporal cluster modelling for small area health data. In *Spatial Cluster Modelling*, pages 235–258. Chapman & Hall/CRC, Boca Raton, FL, 2002.

I. Clark. *Practical Geostatistics*. Applied Science Publishers, London, UK, 1979.

J. S. Clark. *Models for Ecological Data, An Introduction.* Princeton University Press, Princeton, NJ, 2007.

J. S. Clark and A. E. Gelfand. *Hierarchical Modelling for the Environmental Sciences: Statistical Methods and Applications*. Oxford University Press, New York, 2006.

D. Clayton and J. Kaldor. Empirical Bayes estimates of age-standardized relative risks for use in disease mapping. *Biometrics*, **43**:671–681, 1987.

A. D. Cliff and J. K. Ord. *Spatial Processes: Models and Applications*. Pion, London, UK, 1981.

P. Clifford. Markov random fields in statistics. In *Disorder in Physical Systems*, pages 20–32. Oxford University Press, Oxford, UK, 1990.

A. Cohen and R. H. Jones. Regression on a random field. *Journal of the American Statistical Association*, **64**:1172–1182, 1969.

C. Comas P. Delicado, and J. Mateu, A second order approach to analyse spatial point patterns with functional marks. *Test*, **20**:503–523, 2011.

R. D. Cook and C. J. Nachtsheim. A comparison of algorithms for constructing exact D-optimal designs. *Technometrics*, **22**:315–324, 1980.

D. Cooley, D. Nychka, and P. Naveau. Bayesian spatial modeling of extreme precipitation return levels. *Journal of the American Statistical Association*, **102**:824–840, 2007.

J. W. Cooley and J. W. Tukey. An algorithm for the machine calculation of complex Fourier series. *Mathematics of Computation*, **19**:297–301, 1965.

D. R. Cox. Some statistical methods related with series of events. *Journal of the Royal Statistics Society, Series B*, **17**:129–157, 1955.

D. R. Cox and V. Isham. *Point Processes*. Chapman & Hall, London, UK, 1980.

P. F. Craigmile, C. A. Calder, H. Li, R. Paul, and N. Cressie. Hierarchical model building, fitting, and checking: A behind-the-scenes look at a Bayesian analysis of arsenic exposure pathways (with discussion). *Bayesian Analysis*, **4**:1–62, 2009.

C. M. Crainiceanu, P. J. Diggle, and B. Rowlingson. Bivariate binomial spatial modeling of Loa Loa prevalence in tropical Africa. *Journal of the American Statistical Association*, **103**:21–47, 2008.

N. Cressie. A central limit theorem for random sets. *Zeitschrift fur Wahrscheinlichkeitstheorie und verwandte Gebiete*, **49**:37–47, 1979.

N. Cressie. Fitting variogram models by weighted least squares. *Journal of the International Society for Mathematical Geology*, **17**:563–586, 1985.

N. Cressie. Spatial prediction and ordinary kriging. *Mathematical Geology*, **20**:405–421, 1988. Erratum, *Mathematical Geology*, **21**:493–494, 1989.

N. Cressie. The origins of kriging. *Mathematical Geology*, **22**:239–252, 1990.

N. Cressie. *Statistics for Spatial Data*. John Wiley & Sons, New York, 1991.

N. Cressie. Smoothing regional maps using emperical Bayes predictors. *Geographical Analysis*, **24**:75–95, 1992.

N. Cressie. *Statistics for Spatial Data*, revised edition. John Wiley & Sons, New York, 1993.

N. Cressie. Change of support and the modifiable areal unit problem. *Geographical Systems*, **3**:159–180, 1996.

N. Cressie. Aggregation and interaction issues in statistical modeling of spatiotemporal processes. *Geoderma*, **85**:133–140, 1998a.

N. Cressie. Transect-spacing design of ice cores on the Antarctic continent. *Canadian Journal of Statistics*, **26**:405–418, 1998b.

N. Cressie. Geostatistical methods for mapping environmental exposures. In P. Elliott, J. Wakefield, N. Best, and D. Briggs, editors, *Spatial Epidemiology: Methods and Applications*, pages 185–204. Oxford University Press, Oxford, UK, 2000.

N. Cressie. Block kriging for lognormal spatial processes. *Mathematical Geology*, **38**:413–443, 2006.

N. Cressie, C. A. Calder, J. S. Clark, J. M. Ver Hoef, and C. K. Wikle. Accounting for uncertainty in ecological analysis: The strengths and limitations of hierarchical statistical modeling (with discussion). *Ecological Applications*, **19**:553–570, 2009.

N. Cressie and N. H. Chan. Spatial modeling of regional variables. *Journal of the American Statistics Association*, **84**:393–401, 1989.

N. Cressie and L. B. Collins. Analysis of spatial point patterns using bundles of product density LISA functions. *Journal of Agriculture, Biological, and Ecological Statistics*, **6**:118–135, 2001.

N. Cressie and J. L. Davidson. Image analysis with partially ordered Markov models. *Computational Statistics and Data Analysis*, **29**:1–26, 1998a.

N. Cressie and J. L. Davidson. Image processing. In *Encyclopedia of Statistical Sciences*, Updated Volume 2, pages 314–328. John Wiley & Sons, New York, 1998b.

N. Cressie, J. Frey, B. Harch, and M. Smith. Spatial prediction on a river network. *Journal of Agricultural, Biological, and Environmental Statistics*, **11**:127–150, 2006.

N. Cressie, C. A. Gotway, and M. O. Grondona. Spatial prediction from networks. *Chemometrics and Intelligent Laboratory Systems*, **7**:251–271, 1990.

N. Cressie and M. N. Hartfield. Conditionally specified Gaussian models for spatial statistical analysis of field trials. *Journal of Agricultural, Biological, and Environmental Statistics*, **1**:60–77, 1996.

N. Cressie and D. M. Hawkins. Robust estimation of the variogram, I. *Journal of the International Association of Mathematical Geology*, **12**:115–125, 1980.

N. Cressie and J. D. Helterbrand. Multivariate spatial statistical models. *Geographical Systems*, **1**:179–188, 1994.

N. Cressie and H.-C. Huang. Classes of nonseparable, spatio-temporal stationary covariance functions. *Journal of the American Statistical Association*, **94**:1330–1340, 1999.

N. Cressie and F. L. Hulting. A spatial statistical analysis of tumor grouth. *Journal of the American Statistical Association*, **87**:272–283, 1992.

N. Cressie and G. Johannesson. Spatial prediction for massive datasets. In *Mastering the Data Explosion in the Earth and Environmental Sciences: Proceedings of the Australian Academy of Science Elizabeth and Frederick White Conference*, pages 1–11, Australian Academy of Science, Canberra, Australia, 2006.

N. Cressie and G. Johannesson. Fixed rank kriging for very large spatial data sets. *Journal of the Royal Statistical Society, Series B*, **70**:209–226, 2008.

N. Cressie and P. Kapat. Some diagnostics for Markov random fields. *Journal of Computational and Graphical Statistics*, **17**:726–749, 2008.

N. Cressie and J. Kornak. Spatial statistics in the presence of location error with an application to remote sensing of the environment. *Statistical Science*, **18**:436–456, 2003.

N. Cressie and G. M. Laslett. Random set theory and problems of modeling. *SIAM Review*, **29**:557–574, 1987.

N. Cressie and A. B. Lawson. Hierarchical probability models and Bayesian analysis of mine locations. *Advances in Applied Probability*, **32**:315–330, 2000.

N. Cressie and C. Liu. Binary Markov mesh models and symmetric Markov random fields: Some results on their equivalence. *Methodology and Computing in Applied Probability*, **3**:5–34, 2001.

N. Cressie and J. J. Majure. Spatio-temporal statistical modeling of livestock waste in streams. *Journal of Agricultural, Biological, and Environmental Statistics*, **2**:24–47, 1997.

N. Cressie and M. Pavlicova. Calibrated spatial moving average simulations. *Statistical Modeling*, **2**:267–279, 2002.

N. Cressie, O. Perrin, and C. Thomas-Agnan. Likelihood-based estimation for Gaussian MRFs. *Statistical Methodology*, **2**:1–16, 2005.

N. Cressie, S. Richardson, and I. Jaussent. Ecological bias: Use of maximum-entropy approximations. *Australian and New Zealand Journal of Statistics*, **46**:233–255, 2004.

N. Cressie, T. Shi, and E. L. Kang. Fixed Rank Filtering for spatio-temporal data. *Journal of Computational and Graphical Statistics*, **19**:724–745, 2010.

N. Cressie and N. Verzelen. Conditional-mean least-squares fitting of Gaussian Markov random fields to Gaussian fields. *Computational Statistics and Data Analysis*, **52**:2794–2807, 2008.

N. Cressie, D. A. Wendt, G. Johannesson, A. S. Mugglin, and B. Hrafnkelsson. A spatial–temporal statistical approach to problems in command and control. In B. A. Bodt and E. J. Wegman, editors, *Proceedings of the Sixth Annual U.S. Army*

Conference on Applied Statistics, pages 170–190, Aberdeen Proving Ground, MD, Army Research Laboratory, 2000a.

N. Cressie and C. K. Wikle. Strategies for dynamic space–time statistical modeling: Discussion of "The Kriged Kalman filter" by K. V. Mardia et al. *Test*, 7:257–264, 1998a.

N. Cressie and C. K. Wikle. The variance-based cross-variogram: You can add apples and oranges. *Mathematical Geology*, 30:789–799, 1998.

N. Cressie and C. K. Wikle. Space-time Kalman filter. In A. H. El-Shaarawi and W. W. Piegorsch, editors, *Encyclopedia of Environmetrics*, pages 2045–2049. John Wiley & Sons, New York, 2002.

N. Cressie, J. Zhu, A. J. Baddeley, and M. G. Nair. Directed Markov point processes as limits of partially ordered Markov models. *Methodology and Computing in Applied Probability*, 2:5–21, 2000b.

D. T. Crommelin and A. J. Majda. Strategies for model reduction: Comparing different optimal bases. *Journal of the Atmospheric Sciences*, 61:2206–2217, 2004.

R. M. Crujeiras, R. Fernandez-Casal, and W. González-Manteiga. Nonparametric test for separability of spatio-temporal processes. *Environmetrics*, 21:382–399, 2010.

F. C. Curriero. On the use of non-Euclidean distance measures in geostatistics. *Mathematical Geology*, 38:907–926, 2006.

D. J. Daley and D. Vere-Jones. *Introduction to the Theory of Point Process*. Springer, New York, 1988.

D. J. Daley and D. Vere-Jones. *Introduction to the Theory of Point Process*, second edition. Springer, New York, 2003.

R. Daley. *Atmospheric Data Analysis*. Cambridge University Press, Cambridge, UK, 1991.

P. J. Daniell. Discussion of "On the theoretical specification and sampling properties of autocorrelated time-series". *Journal of the Royal Statistical Society, Series B*, 8:88–90, 1946.

M. J. Daniels and N. Cressie. A hierarchical approach to covariance-function estimation for time series. *Journal of Time Series Analysis*, 22:253–266, 2001.

M. J. Daniels, Z. Zhou, and H. Zou. Conditionally specified space–time models for multivariate processes. *Journal of Computational and Graphical Statistics*, 15:157–177, 2006.

S. Darby, H. Deo, and R. Doll. A parallel analysis of individual and ecological data on residential radon and lung cancer in south-west England. *Journal of the Royal Statistical Society, Series A*, 164:193–203, 2001.

M. David. *Geostatistical Ore Reserve Estimation*. Elsevier, Amsterdam, NL, 1977.

R. C. Davis. On the theory of prediction of nonstationary stochastic processes. *Journal of Applied Physics*, 23:1047–1053, 1952.

L. De Cesare, D. E. Myers, and D. Posa. Estimating and modeling space–time correlation structures. *Statistics and Probability Letters*, 51:9–14, 2001.

S. De Iaco, D. E. Myers, and D. Posa. Space–time analysis using a general product-sum model. *Statistics and Probability Letters*, 52:21–28, 2001.

S. De Iaco, D. E. Myers, and D. Posa. Nonseparable space–time covariance models: Some parametric families. *Mathematical Geology*, 34:23–42, 2002.

X. de Luna and M. G. Genton. Predictive spatio-temporal models for spatially sparse environmental data. *Statistica Sinica*, **15**:547–568, 2005.

V. De Oliveira and M. D. Ecker. Bayesian hot spot detection in the presence of a spatial trend: Application to total nitrogen concentration in Chesapeake Bay. *Environmetrics*, **13**:85–101, 2002.

M. H. DeGroot. *Optimal Statistical Decisions*. McGraw-Hill, New York, 1970.

R. J. Deland. Traveling planetary waves. *Tellus*, **16**:271–273, 1964.

R. J. Deland. On the spectral analysis of traveling waves. *Journal of the Meteorological Society of Japan*, **50**:104–109, 1972.

P. Delicado, R. Giraldo, C. Comas, and J. Mateu. Statistics for spatial functional data: Some recent contributions. *Environmetrics*, **21**:224–239, 2010.

E. Demidenko. *Mixed Models: Theory and Applications*. John Wiley & Sons, Hoboken, NJ, 2004.

A. P. Dempster, N. M. Laird, and D. B. Rubin. Maximum likelihood from incomplete data via the EM algorithm. *Journal of the Royal Statistical Society, Series B*, **39**:1–38, 1977.

C. V. Deutsch and A. G. Journel. *GSLIB: Geostatistical Software Library and User's Guide*. Oxford University Press, Oxford, UK, 1992.

R. L. Devaney. *An Introduction to Chaotic Dynamical Systems*, second edition. Westview Press, Boulder, CO, 2003.

M. Dewar, K. Scerri, and V. Kadirkamanathan. Data-driven spatio-temporal modeling using the integro-difference equation. *IEEE Transactions on Signal Processing*, **57**:83–91, 2009.

P. J. Diggle. *Statistical Analysis of Spatial Point Patterns*. Academic Press, London, UK, 1983.

P. J. Diggle. A kernel method for smoothing point process data. *Applied Statistics*, **34**:138–147, 1985.

P. J. Diggle. Point process modeling in environmental epidemiology. In *Statistics for the Environment*, pages 89–110. John Wiley & Sons, Chichester, UK, 1993.

P. J. Diggle. *Statistical Analysis of Spatial Point Patterns*, second edition. Arnold, London, UK, 2003.

P. J. Diggle. Spatio-temporal point processes, partial likelihood, foot and mouth disease. *Statistical Methods in Medical Research*, **15**:325–336, 2006.

P. J. Diggle. Spatio-temporal point processes: Methods and applications. In *Statistical Methods for Spatio-Temporal Systems*, pages 1–45. Chapman & Hall/CRC, London, UK, 2007.

P. J. Diggle and S. Lophaven. Bayesian geostatistical design. *Scandinavian Journal of Statistics*, **33**:53–64, 2006.

P. J. Diggle, R. Menezes, and T.-L. Su. Geostatistical inference under preferential sampling (with discussion). *Applied Statistics*, **59**:191–232, 2010.

P. J. Diggle and P. J. Ribeiro, Jr. *Model-Based Geostatistics*. Springer, New York, 2007.

P. J. Diggle, B. Rowlingson, and T.-L. Su. Point process methodology for on-line spatio-temporal disease surveillance. *Environmetrics*, **16**:423–434, 2005.

P. J. Diggle, J. A. Tawn, and R. A. Moyeed. Model-based geostatistics (with discussion). *Applied Statistics*, **47**:299–350, 1998.

D. J. Diner, G. P. Asner, R. Davies, Y. Knyazikhin, J. Muller, A. W. Nolin, B. Pinty, C. B. Schaaf, and J. Stroeve. New directions in earth observing scientific applications of multiangle remote sensing. *Bulletin of the American Meteorological Society*, **80**:2209–2228, 1999.

M. J. Dobbie, B. L. Henderson, and D. L. Stevens. Sparse sampling: Spatial design for monitoring stream networks. *Statistical Surveys*, **2**:113–153, 2008.

S. Dobricic, N. Pinardi, M. Adani, A. Bonazzi, C. Fratianni, and M. Tonani. Mediterranean forecasting system: A new assimilation scheme for sea level anomaly and its validation. *Quarterly Journal of the Royal Meteorological Society*, **131**:3627–3642, 2005.

R. L. Dobrushin. On Poisson laws for distributions of particles in space. *Ukrains'kyi Matematychnyl Zhurnal*, **8**:127–134, 1963.

A. Doucet, N. de Freitas, and N. Gordon, editors. *Sequential Monte Carlo Methods in Practice*. Springer-Verlag, New York, 2001.

I. L. Dryden and K. V. Mardia. *Statistical Shape Analysis*. John Wiley & Sons, Chichester, UK, 1998.

J. Durbin and S. J. Koopman. *Time Series Analysis by State Space Methods*. Oxford University Press, New York, 2001.

E. E. Ebert and K. McBride. Verification of precipitation in weather systems: Determination of systematic errors. *Journal of Hydrology*, **239**:179–202, 2000.

eBird. eBird: An online database of bird distribution and abundance. (http://ebird.org), 2010.

M. D. Ecker and A. E. Gelfand. Bayesian variogram modeling for an isotropic spatial process. *Journal of Agricultural, Biological, and Environmental Statistics*, **2**:347–369, 1997.

R. M. Edsall. The parallel coordinate plot in action: Design and use for geographic visualization. *Computational Statistics and Data Analysis*, **43**:605–619, 2003.

B. Efron and R. J. Tibshirani. *An Introduction to the Bootstrap*. Chapman & Hall, New York, 1993.

A. Einstein. On the method of theoretical physics. *Philosophy of Science*, **1**:163–169, 1934.

P. Elliott, J. C. Wakefield, N. G. Best, and D. J. Briggs. *Spatial Epidemiology: Methods and Applications*. Oxford University Press, Oxford, UK, 2000.

J. B. Elsner and A. A. Tsonis. *Singular Spectrum Analysis: A New Tool in Time Series Analysis*. Plenum Press, New York, 1996.

X. Emery. Conditional simulation of random fields with bivariate isofactorial distribution. *Mathematical Geology*, **37**:419–445, 2005.

R. L. Eubank. *A Kalman Filter Primer*. Chapman & Hall/CRC, Boca Raton, FL, 2006.

G. Evensen. Sequential data assimilation with a nonlinear quasi-geostrophic model using Monte Carlo methods to forecast error statistics. *Journal of Geophysical Research*, **99**:10143–10162, 1994.

G. Evensen. *Data Assimilation: The Ensemble Kalman Filter*, second edition. Springer, New York, 2009.

G. Evensen and P. J. van Leeuwen. Assimilation of Geosat altimeter data for the Agulhas Current using the ensemble Kalman filter with a quasigeostrophic model. *Monthly Weather Review*, **124**:85–96, 1996.

L. Fahrmeir. Posterior mode estimation by extended Kalman filtering for a multivariate dynamic generalized linear models. *Journal of the American Statistical Association*, **87**:501–509, 1992.

L. Fahrmeir and H. Kaufmann. On Kalman filtering, posterior mode estimation and Fisher scoring in dynamic exponential family regression. *Metrika*, **38**:37–60, 1991.

L. Fahrmeir, T. Kneib, and S. Lang. Penalized structured additive regression for space–time data: A Bayesian perspective. *Statistica Sinica*, **14**:731–761, 2004.

H. Fairfield Smith. An empirical law describing heterogeneity in the yields of agricultural crops. *Journal of Agricultural Science*, **28**:1–23, 1938.

J. Fan and Q. Yao. *Nonlinear Time Series*. Springer, New York, 2005.

T. R. Fanshawe and P. J. Diggle. Spatial prediction in the presence of positional error. *Environmetrics*, **22**:109–122, 2011.

B. F. Farrell and P. J. Ioannou. Accurate low-dimensional approximation of the linear dynamics of fluid flow. *Journal of the Atmospheric Sciences*, **58**:2771–2789, 2001.

W. T. Federer, E. A. Newton, and N. S. Altman. Combining standard block analyses with spatial analyses under a random effects model. In *Modelling Longitudinal and Spatially Correlated Data*, pages 374–386. Springer, New York, 1997.

V. V. Fedorov. *Theory of Optimal Experiments*. Academic Press, New York, 1972.

T. S. Ferguson. *Mathematical Statistics: A Decision Theoretic Approach*. Academic Press, New York, 1967.

R. Fernandez-Casal, W. González-Manteiga, and M. Febrero-Bande. Flexible spatio-temporal stationary variogram models. *Statistics and Computing*, **13**:127–136, 2003.

M. A. R. Ferreira and V. De Oliveira. Bayesian reference analysis for Gaussian Markov random fields. *Journal of Multivariate Analysis*, **98**:789–812, 2007.

M. A. R. Ferreira and H. K. H. Lee. *Multiscale Modeling: A Bayesian Perspective*. Springer, New York, 2007.

R. M. Fewster. A spatiotemporal stochastic process model for species spread. *Biometrics*, **59**:640–649, 2003.

P. W. Fieguth, W. C. Karl, A. S. Willsky, and C. Wunsch. Multiresolution optimal interpolation and statistical analysis of TOPEX/POSEIDON satellite altimetry. *IEEE Transactions on Geoscience Remote Sensing*, **33**:280–292, 1995.

B. Finkenstädt, L. Held, and V. Isham, editors. *Statistical Methods for Spatio-Temporal Systems*. Chapman & Hall/CRC, Boca Raton, FL, 2007.

A. O. Finley, S. Banerjee, A. R. Ek, and R. E. McRoberts. Bayesian multivariate process modeling for prediction of forest attributes. *Journal of Agricultural, Biological and Environmental Statistics*, **13**:1–24, 2008.

A. O. Finley, H. Sang, S. Banerjee, and A. E. Gelfand. Improving the performance of predictive process modeling for large datasets. *Computational Statistics and Data Analysis*, **53**:2873–2884, 2009.

R. A. Fisher. *The Design of Experiments*. Oliver and Boyd, Edinburgh, UK, 1935.

P. M. Fishman and D. L. Snyder. The statistical analysis of space–time point processes. *IEEE Transactions on Information Theory*, **IT-22**:257–274, 1976.

M. Forni, M. Hallin, M. Lippi, and L. Reichlin. The generalized dynamic factor model: One-sided estimation and forecasting. *Journal of the American Statistical Association*, **100**:830–480, 2005.

M.-J. Fortin and M. R. T. Dale. *Spatial Analysis: A Guide for Ecologists*. Cambridge University Press, Cambridge, UK, 2009.

A. S. Fotheringham, C. Brunsdon, and M. Charlton. *Geographically Weighted Regression: The Analysis of Spatially Varying Relationships*. John Wiley & Sons, Chichester, UK, 2002.

B. Frcalová, V. Beneš, and D. Klement. Spatio-temporal point process filtering methods with an application. *Environmetrics*, **21**:240–252, 2010.

W. Freiberger and U. Grenander. On the formulation of statistical meteorology. *Review of the International Statistical Institute*, **33**:59–86, 1965.

S. Frühwirth-Schnatter. Data augmentation and dynamic linear models. *Journal of Time Series Analysis*, **15**:183–202, 1994.

M. Fuentes. Spectral methods for nonstationary spatial processes. *Biometrika*, **89**: 197–210, 2002.

M. Fuentes. Testing for separability of spatial temporal covariance functions. *Journal of Statistical Planning and Inference*, **136**:447–466, 2006.

M. Fuentes. Approximate likelihood for large irregularly spaced spatial data. *Journal of the American Statistical Association*, **102**:321–331, 2007.

M. Fuentes, L. Chen, and J. M. Davis. A class of nonseparable and nonstationary spatial temporal covariance functions. *Environmetrics*, **19**:487–507, 2008.

M. Fuentes, P. Guttorp, and P. D. Sampson. Using transforms to analyze space–time processes. In *Statistical Methods for Spatio-Temporal Systems*, pages 78–147. Chapman & Hall/CRC, Boca Raton, FL, 2007.

W. A. Fuller. *Introduction to Statistical Time Series*, second edition. John Wiley & Sons, New York, 1996.

R. Furrer, M. Genton, and D. Nychka. Covariance tapering for interpolation of large spatial datasets. *Journal of Computational and Graphical Statistics*, **15**:502–523, 2005.

E. Gabriel and P. J. Diggle. Second-order analysis of inhomogeneous spatio-temporal point process data. *Statistica Neerlandica*, **63**:43–51, 2009.

C. Gaetan and X. Guyon. *Spatial Statistics and Modeling*. Springer, New York, 2010.

D. Gamerman. Markov chain Monte Carlo for dynamic generalized linear models. *Biometrika*, **85**:215–227, 1998.

D. Gamerman and H. F. Lopes. *Markov Chain Monte Carlo—Stochastic Simulation for Bayesian Inference*. Chapman & Hall/CRC, Boca Raton, FL, 2006.

L. S. Gandin. *Objective Analysis of Meteorological Fields*. Gidrometeorologicheskoe Izdatel'stvo (GIMIZ), Leningrad, 1963. (Translated by Israel Program for Scientific Translations, Jerusalem, 1965.).

A. E. Gelfand. Model determination using sampling based methods. In W. R. Gilks, S. Richardson, and D. J. Spiegelhalter, editors, *Markov Chain Monte Carlo in Practice*, pages 145–161. Chapman and Hall, London, UK, 1996.

A. E. Gelfand, S. Banerjee, and D. Gamerman. Spatial process modelling for univariate and multivariate dynamic spatial data. *Environmetrics*, **16**:465–479, 2005.

A. E. Gelfand, D. K. Dey, and H. Chang. Model determination using predictive distributions with implementation via sampling-based methods. In J. M. Bernardo, J. O. Berger, A. P. Dawid, and A. F. M. Smith, editors, *Bayesian Statistics 4*, pages 147–167. Oxford University Press, Oxford, UK, 1992.

A. E. Gelfand, P. J. Diggle, M. Fuentes, and P. Guttorp, editors. *Handbook of Spatial Statistics*. Chapman and Hall/CRC, Boca Raton, FL, 2010.

A. E. Gelfand, H.-J. Kim, C. F. Sirmans, and S. Banerjee. Spatial modeling with spatially varying coefficient processes. *Journal of the American Statistical Association*, **98**:387–396, 2003.

A. E. Gelfand, A. Kottas, and S. MacEachern. Bayesian non-parametric spatial modeling with Dirichlet process mixing. *Journal of the American Statistical Association*, **100**:1021–1035, 2005.

A. E. Gelfand, A. M. Schmidt, S. Banerjee, and C. F. Sirmans. Nonstationary multivariate process modeling through spatially varying coregionalization (with discussion). *Test*, **13**:263–312, 2004.

A. E. Gelfand and A. F. M. Smith. Sampling based approaches to calculating marginal densities. *Journal of the American Statistical Association*, **85**:398–409, 1990.

A. E. Gelfand and P. Vounatsou. Proper multivariate conditional autoregressive models for spatial data analysis. *Biostatistics*, **4**:11–15, 2003.

A. E. Gelfand, L. Zhu, and B. P. Carlin. On the change of support problem for spatio-temporal data. *Biostatistics*, **2**:31–45, 2001.

A. Gelman. Prior distributions for variance parameters in hierarchical models. *Bayesian Analysis*, **1**:515–533, 2006.

A. Gelman, F. Bois, and J. Jiang. Physiological pharmacokinetic analysis using population modeling and informative prior distributions. *Journal of the American Statistical Association*, **91**:1400–1412, 1996.

A. Gelman, J. B. Carlin, H. S. Stern, and D. B. Rubin. *Bayesian Data Analysis*, second edition. Chapman & Hall/CRC, Boca Raton, FL, 2003.

A. Gelman, X.-L. Meng, and H. S. Stern. Posterior predictive assessment of model fitness via realized discrepancies (with discussion). *Statistica Sinica*, **6**:733–807, 1996.

V. Gelpke and H. R. Künsch. Estimation of motion from sequences of images: Daily variability of total ozone mapping spectrometer ozone data. *Journal of Geophysical Research*, **106**: 11825–11834, 2001.

S. Geman and D. Geman. Stochastic relaxation, Gibbs distributions and the Bayesian restoration of images. *IEEE Transactions on Pattern Analysis and Machine Intelligence*, **PAMI-6**:721–741, 1984.

M. G. Genton. Separable approximations of space-time covariance matrices. *Environmetrics*, **18**:681–695, 2007.

E. George and R. McCulloch. Variable selection via Gibbs sampling. *Journal of the American Statistical Association*, **85**:398–409, 1993.

A. Getis, J. Mur, and H. Zoller. *Spatial Econometrics and Spatial Statistics*. Palgrave-Macmillan, New York, 2004.

C. Geyer. Likelihood inference for spatial point processes. In *Stochastic Geometry: Likelihood and Computation*, pages 79–140. Chapman & Hall/CRC, Boca Raton, FL, 1999.

C. J. Geyer and E. A. Thompson. Constrained Monte Carlo maximum likelihood for dependent data. *Journal of the Royal Statistical Society, Series B*, **54**:657–699, 1992.

M. Ghil and P. Malanotte-Rizzoli. Data assimilation in meteorology and oceanography. In *Avances in Geophysics*, Vol. 33, pages 141–266. Academic Press, San Diego, CA, 1991.

M. Ghosh. Constrained Bayes estimation with applications. *Journal of the American Statistics Association*, **87**:533–540, 1992.

S. K. Ghosh, P. V. Bhave, J. M. Davis, and H. Lee. Spatio-temporal analysis of total nitrate concentrations using dynamic statistical models. *Journal of the American Statistical Association*, **105**:538–551, 2010.

D. C. Giancoli. *Physics: Principles with Applications*, fifth edition. Prentice Hall, Upper Saddle River, NJ, 1998.

J. W. Gibbs. *Elementary Principles in Statistical Mechanics, Developed with Especial Reference to the Rational Foundation of Thermodynamics*. Charles Scribner's Sons, New York, 1902.

W. R. Gilks, S. Richardson, and D. J. Spiegelhalter. *Markov Chain Monte Carlo in Practice*. Chapman & Hall, New York, 1996.

R. Giraldo, P. Delicado, and J. Mateu. Continuous time-varying kriging for spatial prediction of functional data: An environmental application. *Journal of Agricultural, Biological, and Environmental Statistics*, **15**:66–82, 2010.

H. R. Glahn. Canonical correlation and its relationship to discriminant analysis and multiple regression. *Journal of the Atmospheric Sciences*, **25**:23–31, 1968.

P. Glasserman. *Monte Carlo Methods in Financial Engineering*. Springer, New York, 2004.

J. Gleick. *Chaos: Making a New Science*. Viking Press, New York, 1987.

T. Gneiting. Nonseparable, stationary covariance functions for space–time data. *Journal of the American Statistical Association*, **97**:590–600, 2002.

T. Gneiting, M. G. Genton, and P. Guttorp. Geostatistical space–time models, stationarity, separability and full symmetry. In B. Finkenstädt, L. Held, and V. Isham, editors, *Statistical Methods for Spatio-Temporal Systems*, pages 151–175. Chapman & Hall/CRC, Boca Raton, FL, 2007.

T. Gneiting, W. Kleiber, and M. Schlather. Matérn cross-covariance functions for multivariate random fields. *Journal of the American Statistical Association*, **105**:1167–1177, 2010.

S. Godsill and T. Clapp. Improvement strategies for Monte Carlo particle filters. In *Sequential Monte Carlo Methods in Practice*, pages 139–158. Springer-Verlag, New York, 2001.

A. S. Goldberger. Best linear unbiased prediction in the generalized linear regression model. *Journal of the American Statistical Association*, **57**:369–375, 1962.

P. Goovaerts. *Geostatistics for Natural Resources Evaluation*. Oxford University Press, New York, 1997.

N. Gordon, J. Salmond, and A. Smith. A novel approach to nonlinear/non-Gaussian Bayesian state estimation. *IEEE Proceedings on Radar and Signal Processing*, **140**:107–113, 1993.

C. Gotway and N. Cressie. A spatial analysis of variance applied to soil water infiltration. *Water Resources Research*, **26**:2695–2703, 1990.

C. Gotway and N. Cressie. Improved multivariate prediction under a general linear model. *Journal of Multivariate Analysis*, **45**:56–72, 1993.

C. Gotway and L. J. Young. Combining incompatible spatial data. *Journal of the American Statistical Association*, **97**:632–648, 2002.

J. Goutsias. Mutually compatible Gibbs random fields. *IEEE Transactions on Information Theory*, **35**:1233–1249, 1989.

N. E. Graham and J. Michaelsen. An investigation of the El Niño-Southern Oscillation cycle with statistical models. 1. Predictor field characteristics. *Journal of Geophysical Research*, **92**:14251–14270, 1987.

R. B. Gramacy and H. K. H. Lee. Bayesian treed Gaussian process models with an application to computer modeling. *Journal of the American Statistical Association*, **103**:1119–1130, 2008.

M. Gray. On the stability of temperature eigenvector patterns. *Journal of Climate*, **1**:273–281, 1981.

T. G. Gregoire, D. R. Brillinger, P. J. Diggle, E. Russek-Cohen, W. G. Warren, and R. D. Wolfinger, editors. *Modelling Longitudinal and Spatially Correlated Data*. Springer, New York, 1997.

U. Grenander. *Elements of Pattern Theory*. The Johns Hopkins University Press, Baltimore, MD, 1996.

U. Grenander and M. Miller. *Pattern Theory: From Representation to Inference*. Oxford University Press, New York, 2007.

M. S. Grewal and A. P. Andrews. *Kalman Filtering, Theory and Practice*. Prentice-Hall, Englewood Cliffs, NJ, 1993.

D. A. Griffith. *Advanced Spatial Statistics: Special Topics in the Exploration of Quantitative Spatial Data*. Kluwer Academic Press, Dordrecht, NL, 1988.

D. A. Griffith. *Spatial Autocorrelation and Spatial Filtering: Gaining Understanding Through Theory and Scientific Visualization*. Springer-Verlag, Berlin, DE, 2003.

D. A. Griffith and L. J. Layne. *A Casebook for Spatial Statistical Data Analysis: A Compilation of Analyses of Different Thematic Data Sets*. Oxford University Press, New York, 1999.

V. Grimm and S. F. Railsback. *Individual-Based Modeling and Ecology*. Princeton University Press, Princeton, NJ, 2005.

M. O. Grondona and N. Cressie. Using spatial considerations in the analysis of experiments. *Technometrics*, **33**:381–392, 1991.

M. O. Grondona and N. Cressie. Efficiency of block design under stationary second-order autoregressive errors. *Sankhyā A*, **55**:267–284, 1993.

Y. Guan. A composite likelihood approach in fitting spatial point process models. *Journal of the American Statistical Association*, **101**:1502–1512, 2006.

Y. Guan. On consistent nonparametric intensity estimation for inhomogeneous spatial point processes. *Journal of the American Statistical Association*, **103**:1238–1247, 2008.

Y. Guan and J. M. Loh. A thinned block bootstrap variance estimation procedure for inhomogeneous spatial point patterns. *Journal of the American Statistical Association*, **102**:1377–1386, 2007.

Y. Guan and M. Sherman. On least squares fitting for stationary spatial point processes. *Journal of the Royal Statistical Society, Series B*, **69**:31–49, 2007.

Y. Guan, M. Sherman, and J. A. Calvin. A nonparametric test for spatial isotropy using subsampling. *Journal of the American Statistical Association*, **99**:810–821, 2004.

N. K. Gupta and R. K. Mehra. Computational aspects of maximum likelihood estimation and reduction in sensitivity function calculations. *IEEE Transactions on Automatic Control*, **AC-19**:774–783, 1974.

V. K. Gupta and E. C. Waymire. A stochastic kinematic study of subsynoptic space–time rainfall. *Water Resources Research*, **15**:637–644, 1979.

P. Guttorp, W. Meiring, and P. D. Sampson. A space–time analysis of ground-level ozone data. *Environmetrics*, **5**:241–254, 1994.

X. Guyon. *Random Fields on a Network: Modeling, Statistics, and Applications*. Springer-Verlag, New York, 1995.

H. Haario, M. Laine, A. Mira, and E. Saksman. DRAM: Efficient adaptive MCMC. *Statistical Computing*, **16**:339–354, 2006.

T. C. Haas. Local prediction of a spatio-temporal process with an application to wet sulfate deposition. *Journal of the American Statistical Association*, **90**:1189–1199, 1995.

T. C. Haas. New systems for modeling, estimating, and predicting a multivariate spatio-temporal process. *Environmetrics*, **13**:311–332, 2002.

R. Haberman. *Elementary Applied Partial Differential Equations*, second edition. Prentice-Hall, Engelwood Cliffs, NJ, 1987.

R. Haining. *Spatial Data Analysis in the Social and Environmental Sciences*. Cambridge University Press, Cambridge, UK, 1990.

R. Haining. *Spatial Data Analysis: Theory and Practice*. Cambridge University Press, Cambridge, UK, 2003.

R. P. Haining. Space-time processes and spatial interaction models. In R. L. Martin, N. Thrift, and R. J. Bennett, editors, *Towards the Dynamic Analysis of Spatial Systems*, pages 91–103. Pion, London, UK, 1978.

J. M. Hammersley and P. Clifford. Markov fields on finite graphs and lattices. Unpublished manuscript, 1971.

M. S. Handcock and J. R. Wallis. An approach to statistical spatial–temporal modeling of meteorological fields. *Journal of the American Statistical Association*, **89**:368–378, 1994.

R. Hare. *The Birth of Penicillin*. Allen & Unwin, London, UK, 1970.

M. I. Hartfield and R. F. Gunst. Identification of model components for a class of continuous spatiotemporal models. *Journal of Agricultural, Biological, and Environmental Statistics*, **8**:105–121, 2003.

A. C. Harvey. *Time Series Models*, second edition. The MIT Press, Cambridge, MA, 1993.

J. L. Harvill and B. K. Ray. Functional coefficient autoregressive models for vector time series. *Computational Statistics and Data Analysis*, **50**:3547–3566, 2006.

J. Haslett, M. Whiley, S. Bhattacharya, M. Salter-Townshend, S. P. Wilson, J. R. M. Allen, B. Huntley, and F. J. G. Mitchell. Bayesian paleoclimate reconstruction. *Journal of the Royal Statistical Society, Series A*, **169**:395–438, 2006.

K. Hasselmann. On the signal-to-noise problem in atmospheric response studies. In *Meteorology of Tropical Oceans*, pages 251–259. Royal Meteorological Society, Reading, UK, 1979.

K. Hasselmann. PIPs and POPs: The reduction of complex dynamical systems using principal interaction and oscillation patterns. *Journal of Geophysical Research*, **93**:11015–11021, 1988.

K. Hasselmann. Optimal fingerprinting for the detection of time-dependent climate change. *Journal of Climate*, **6**:1957–1969, 1993.

Y. Hayashi. A generalized method of resolving disturbances into progressive and regressive waves by space Fourier and time cross-spectral analysis. *Journal of the Meteorological Society of Japan*, **49**:125–128, 1971.

Y. Hayashi. Interpretations of space–time spectral energy equations. *Journal of the Atmospheric Sciences*, **39**:685–688, 1982a.

Y. Hayashi. Space–time spectral analysis and its applications to atmospheric waves. *Journal of the Meteorological Society of Japan*, **60**:156–171, 1982b.

J. Heikkinen and A. Penttinen. Bayesian smoothing in the estimation of the pair potential function of Gibbs point processes. *Bernoulli*, **5**:1119–1136, 1999.

M. Heine. Models for two-dimensional stationary stochastic processes. *Biometrika*, **42**:170–178, 1955.

H. V. Henderson and S. R. Searle. On deriving the inverse of a sum of matrices. *SIAM Review*, **23**:53–60, 1981.

R. Henderson, S. Shimakura, and D. Gorst. Modeling spatial variation in leukemia survival data. *Journal of the American Statistical Association*, **97**:965–972, 2002.

G. M. Henebry. Spatial model error analysis using autocorrelation indices. *Ecological Modelling*, **82**:75–91, 1995.

R. Hengeveld. What to do about North American invasion by the Collard Dove. *Journal of Field Ornithology*, **64**:477–489, 1993.

M. Hénon. A two-dimensional mapping with a strange attractor. *Communications in Mathematical Physics*, **50**:69–77, 1976.

P. A. Henrys and P. E. Brown. Inference for clustered inhomogeneous spatial point processes. *Biometrics*, **65**:423–430, 2009.

A. S. Hering and M. G. Genton. Powering up with space-time wind forecasting. *Journal of the American Statistical Association*, **105**:92–104, 2010.

D. M. Higdon. A process-convolution approach to modeling temperatures in the North Atlantic ocean. *Journal of Ecological and Environmental Statistics*, **5**:173–190, 1998.

D. M. Higdon. A primer on space-time modeling from a Bayesian perspective. In B. Finkenstädt, L. Held, and V. Isham, editors, *Statistical Methods for Spatio-Temporal Systems*, pages 217–279. Chapman and Hall/CRC, Boca Raton, FL, 2007.

D. M. Higdon, C. S. Reese, J. D. Moulton, J. A. Vrugt, and C. Fox. Posterior exploration for computationally intensive forward models. Technical report LA-UR 08-05905, Statistical Sciences Group, Los Alamos National Laboratory, Los Alamos, NM, 2008. In S. Brooks, A. Gelman, G. L. Jones, and X.-L. Meng, editors, *The Handbook of Markov Chain Monte Carlo*, forthcoming. CRC Press, Boca Raton, FL, 2011.

D. M. Higdon, J. Swall, and J. Kern. Non-stationary spatial modeling. In *Bayesian Statistics 6*, pages 761–768. Oxford University Press, Oxford, UK, 1999.

N. L. Hjort and H. Omre. Topics in spatial statistics. *Scandinavian Journal of Statistics*, **21**:289–357, 1994.

T. J. Hoar, R. F. Milliff, D. Nychka, C. K. Wikle, and L. M. Berliner. Winds from a Bayesian hierarchical model: Computation for atmosphere–ocean research. *Journal of Computational and Graphical Statistics*, **12**:781–807, 2003.

J. S. Hodges and B. J. Reich. Adding spatially-correlated errors can mess up the fixed effect you love. *The American Statistician*, **64**:325–334, 2010.

M. P. Hoerling, A. Kumar, and M. Zhong. El Niño, La Niña, and the nonlinearity of their teleconnections. *Journal of Climate*, **10**:1769–1786, 1997.

J. A. Hoeting, R. A. Davis, A. A. Merton, and S. E. Thompson. Model selection for geostatistical models. *Ecological Applications*, **16**:87–98, 2006.

R. N. Hoffman, Z. Liu, J.-F. Louis, and C. Grassotti. Distortion representation of forecast errors. *Monthly Weather Review*, **123**:2758–2770, 1995.

M. E. Hohn. *Geostatistics and Petroleum Geology*, second edition. Kluwer, Dordrecht, NL, 1999.

J. R. Holton. *An Introduction to Dynamic Meteorology*, fourth edition. Academic Press, Boston, MA, 2004.

M. B. Hooten, J. Anderson, and L. A. Waller. Assessing North American influenza dynamics with a statistical SIRS model. *Spatial and Spatio-temporal Epidemiology*, **1**:177–185, 2010.

M. B. Hooten, D. R. Larsen, and C. K. Wikle. Predicting the spatial distribution of ground flora on large domains using a hierarchical Bayesian model. *Landscape Ecology*, **18**:487–502, 2003.

M. B. Hooten and C. K. Wikle. Shifts in the spatio-temporal growth dynamics of shortleaf pine. *Environmental and Ecological Statistics*, **14**:207–227, 2007.

M. B. Hooten and C. K. Wikle. A hierarchical Bayesian non-linear spatio-temporal model for the spread of invasive species with applicaton to the Eurasian Collared Dove. *Environmental and Ecological Statistics*, **15**:59–70, 2008.

M. B. Hooten and C. K. Wikle. Statistical agent-based models for discrete spatio-temporal systems. *Journal of the American Statistical Association*, **105**:236–248, 2010.

M. B. Hooten, C. K. Wikle, R. M. Dorazio, and J. A. Royle. Hierarchical spatio-temporal matrix models for characterizing invasions. *Biometrics*, **63**:558–567, 2007.

M. B. Hooten, C. K. Wikle, S. L. Sheriff, and J. W. Rushin. Optimal spatio-temporal hybrid sampling designs for ecological monitoring. *Journal of Vegetation Science*, **20**:639–649, 2009.

A. C. A. Hope. A simplified Monte Carlo significance test procedure. *Journal of the Royal Statistical Society, Series B*, **30**:582–598, 1968.

J. D. Horel. Complex principal component analysis: Theory and examples. *Journal of Climate and Applied Meteorology*, **23**:1660–1673, 1984.

H. Hotelling. Differential equations subject to error, and population estimates. *Journal of the American Statistical Association*, **22**:283–314, 1927.

H. Hotelling. Analysis of a complex of statistical variables into principal components. *Journal of Educational Psychology*, **24**:417–441 and 498–520, 1933.

H. Hotelling. Relations between two sets of variables. *Biometrika*, **28**:321–377, 1936.

P. L. Houtekamer and H. L. Mitchell. Data assimilation using an ensemble Kalman filter technique. *Monthly Weather Review*, **126**:796–811, 1998.

E. Hovmöller. The trough and ridge diagram. *Tellus*, **1**:62–66, 1949.

B. Hrafnkelsson and N. Cressie. Hierarchical modeling of count data with application to nuclear fall-out. *Environmental and Ecological Statistics*, **10**:179–200, 2003.

C. Huang, T. Hsing, and N. Cressie. Spectral density estimation through a regularized inverse function. *Statistica Sinica*, **21**:1115–1124, 2011.

C. Huang, Y. Yao, N. Cressie, and T. Hsing. Multivariate intrinsic random functions for cokriging. *Mathematical Geosciences*, **41**:887–904.

H.-C. Huang and C.-S. Chen. Optimal geostatistical model selection. *Journal of the American Statistical Association*, **102**:1009–1024, 2007.

H.-C. Huang and N. Cressie. Spatio-temporal prediction of snow water equivalent using the Kalman filter. *Computational Statistics and Data Analysis*, **22**:159–175, 1996.

H.-C. Huang and N. Cressie. Deterministic/stochastic wavelet decomposition for recovery of signal from noisy data. *Technometrics*, **42**:262–276, 2000.

H.-C. Huang and N. Cressie. Multiscale graphical modeling in space: Applications to command and control. In M. Moore, editor, *Spatial Statistics: Methodological Aspects and Some Applications*, pages 83–113. Springer Lecture Notes in Statistics, Vol. 159. Springer, New York, 2001.

H.-C. Huang, N. Cressie, and J. Gabrosek. Fast, resolution-consistent spatial prediction of global processes from satellite data. *Journal of Computational and Graphical Statistics*, **11**:63–88, 2002.

H.-C. Huang and N.-J. Hsu. Modeling transport effects on ground-level ozone using a nonstationary space–time model. *Environmetrics*, **15**:251–268, 2004.

Y. Huang, D. Liu, and H. Wu. Hierarchical Bayesian methods for estimation of parameters in a longitudinal HIV dynamical system. *Biometrics*, **62**:413–423, 2006.

J. P. Hughes and P. Guttorp. A class of stochastic models for relating synoptic atmospheric patterns to regional hydrologic phenomena. *Water Resources Research*, **30**:1535–1546, 1994.

A. Hyvärinen, J. Karhunen, and E. Oja. *Independent Component Analysis*. John Wiley & Sons, New York, 2001.

J. Illian, A. Penttinen, H. Stoyan, and D. Stoyan. *Statistical Analysis and Modelling of Spatial Point Patterns*. John Wiley & Sons, Chichester, UK, 2008.

H. K. Im, M. L. Stein, and Z. Zhu. Semiparametric estimation of spectral density with irregular observations. *Journal of the American Statistical Association*, **102**:726–735, 2007.

A. Inselberg. The plane with parallel coordinates. *Visual Computer*, **1**:69–91, 1985.

K. M. Irvine, A. I. Gitelman, and J. A. Hoeting. Spatial designs and properties of spatial correlation: Effects on covariance estimation. *Journal of Agricultural, Biological, and Environmental Statistics*, **12**:450–469, 2007.

M. E. Irwin, N. Cressie, and G. Johannesson. Spatial–temporal nonlinear filtering based on hierarchical statistical models. *Test*, **11**:249–302, 2002.

E. H. Isaaks and R. M. Srivastava. *An Introduction to Applied Geostatistics*. Oxford University Press, Oxford, UK, 1989.

E. Ising. Beitrag zur theorie des ferromagnetismus. *Zeitschrift für Physik*, **31**:253–258, 1925.

A. V. Ivanov and N. N. Leonenko. *Statistical Analysis of Random Fields*. Kluwer Academic Publishers, Dordrecht, NL, 1989.

M. Jansen, G. P. Nason, and B. W. Silverman. Multiscale methods for data on graphs and irregular multidimensional situations. *Journal of the Royal Statistical Society, Series B*, **71**:97–125, 2009.

A. H. Jazwinski. *Stochastic Processes and Filtering Theory*. Academic Press, New York, 1970.

E. B. V. Jensen, K. Y. Jónsdóttir, J. Schmiegel, and O. E. Barndorff-Nielsen. Spatio-temporal modelling—with a view to biological growth. In *Statistical Methods for Spatio-Temporal Systems*, pages 47–75. Chapman & Hall/CRC, Boca Raton, FL, 2007.

J. L. Jensen and J. Møller. Pseudolikelihood for exponential family models of spatial point processes. *Annals of Applied Probability*, **3**:445–461, 1991.

X. Jin, B. P. Carlin, and S. Banerjee. Generalized hierarchical multivariate CAR models for areal data. *Biometrics*, **61**:950–961, 2005.

X. Jin, S. Banerjee, and B. P. Carlin. Order-free co-regionalized areal data models with application to multiple-disease mapping. *Journal of the Royal Statistical Society, Series B*, **69**:817–838, 2007.

G. Johannesson and N. Cressie. Variance-covariance modeling and estimation for multi-resolution spatial models. In X. Sanchez-Villa, J. Carrera, and J. Gomez-Hernandez, editors, *geoENV IV—Geostatistics for Environmental Applications*, pages 319–330. Kluwer Academic Publishers, Dordrecht, NL, 2004.

G. Johannesson, N. Cressie, and H.-C. Huang. Dynamic multi-resolution spatial models. *Environmental and Ecological Statistics*, **14**:5–25, 2007.

R. A. Johnson and D. W. Wichern. *Applied Multivariate Statistical Analysis*, third edition. Prentice-Hall, Englewood Cliffs, NJ, 1992.

R. A. Johnson and D. W. Wichern. *Applied Multivariate Statistical Analysis*, sixth edition. Pearson Prentice-Hall, Upper Saddle River, NJ, 2007.

I. T. Jolliffe. *Principal Component Analysis*, second edition. Springer-Verlag, New York, 2002.

R. H. Jones. An experiment in non-linear prediction. *Journal of Applied Meteorology*, **4**:701–705, 1965.

R. H. Jones. Nonlinear autoregressive processes. *Proceedings of the Royal Society of London, Series A*, **360**:71–95, 1978.

R. H. Jones and Y. Zhang. Models for continuous stationary space–time processes. In *Modelling Longitudinal and Spatially Correlated Data*, pages 289–298. Lecture Notes in Statistics, Springer, New York, Vol. **159**. 1997.

K. Y. Jónsdóttir, J. Schmiegel, and E. B. V. Jensen. Levy-based growth models. *Bernoulli*, **14**:62–90, 2008.

A. G. Journel. Geostatistics for conditional simulation of ore bodies. *Economic Geology*, **69**:673–687, 1974.

A. G. Journel and C. J. Huijbregts. *Mining Geostatistics*. Academic Press, London, UK, 1978.

G. H. Jowett. The accuracy of systematic sampling from coveyer belts. *Applied Statistics*, **1**:50–59, 1952.

M. Jun and M. L. Stein. An approach to producing space–time covariance functions on spheres. *Technometrics*, **49**:468–479, 2007.

M. Jun and M. L. Stein. Nonstationary covariance models for global data. *Annals of Applied Statistics*, **2**:1271–1289, 2008.

B. Jungbacker and S. J. Koopman. Monte Carlo estimation for nonlinear non-Gaussian state space models. *Biometrika*, **94**:827–839, 2007.

C. Jutten, J. Herault, and A. Guerin. IN.C.A.: An independent components analyser based on an adaptive neuromimetic network. In *Proceedings in Nonlinear Science, Artificial Intelligence and Cognitive Sciences*, pages 231–248. Manchester University Press, Manchester, 1988.

T. Kailath. *Linear Systems*. Prentice-Hall, NJ, 1980.

M. S. Kaiser and N. Cressie. Modeling Poisson variables with positive spatial dependence. *Statistics and Probability Letters*, **35**:423–432, 1997.

M. S. Kaiser and N. Cressie. The construction of multivariate distributions from Markov random fields. *Journal of Multivariate Analysis*, **73**:199–220, 2000.

R. E. Kalman. A new approach to linear filtering and prediction problems. *Transactions of the ASME—Journal of Basic Engineering, Series D*, **82**:35–45, 1960.

E. Kalnay. *Atmospheric Modeling, Data Assimilation and Predictability*. Cambridge University Press, Cambridge, UK, 2003.

E. L. Kang and N. Cressie. Bayesian inference for the Spatial Random Effects model. *Journal of the American Statistical Association*, **106**:972–983. 2011.

E. L. Kang, N. Cressie, and T. Shi. Using temporal variability to improve spatial mapping with application to satellite data. *The Canadian Journal of Statistics*, **38**:271–289, 2010.

E. L. Kang, D. Liu, and N. Cressie. Statistical analysis of small-area data based on independence, spatial, non-hierarchical, and hierarchical models. *Computational Statistics and Data Analysis*, **53**:3016–3032, 2009.

W. Kaplan. *Advanced Calculus*. Addison-Wesley Publishing, Redwood City, CA, 1991.

T. R. Karl, A. J. Koscielny, and H. F. Diaz. Potential errors in the application of principal component (eigenvector) analysis to geophysical data. *Journal of Applied Meteorology*, **21**:1183–1186, 1982.

R. E. Kass and A. E. Raftery. Bayes factors. *Journal of the American Statistical Association*, **90**:773–795, 1995.

M. Katzfuss and N. Cressie. Spatio-temporal smoothing and EM estimation for massive remote-sensing data sets. *Journal of Time Series Analysis*, **32**:430–446, 2011.

C. G. Kaufman, M. J. Schervish, and D. W. Nychka. Covariance tapering for likelihood-based estimation in large spatial data sets. *Journal of the American Statistical Association*, **103**:1545–1555, 2008.

Y. J. Kaufman, B. N. Holben, D. Tanre, I. Slutsker, and A. Smirnov. Will aerosol measurements from Terra and Aqua polar orbiting satellites represent the daily aerosol abundance and properties? *Geophysical Research Letters*, **27**:3861–3864, 2000.

J. W. Kay and D. M. Titterington, editors. *Statistics and Neural Networks: Advances at the Interface*. Oxford University Press, New York, 2000.

F. P. Kelly and B. D. Ripley. A note on Strauss's model for clustering. *Biometrika*, **63**:357–360, 1976.

D. G. Kendall. Foundations of a theory of random sets. In E. F. Harding and D. G. Kendall, editors, *Stochastic Geometry*, pages 322–376. John Wiley & Sons, New York, 1974.

J. T. Kent and K. V. Mardia. The link between kriging and thin-plate splines. In F. P. Kelly, editor, *Statistics and Optimization*, pages 325–339. John Wiley & Sons, New York, 1994.

H. Kim, D. Sun, and R. K. Tsutakawa. A bivariate Bayes method for improving the estimates of mortality rates with a twofold conditional autoregressive model. *Journal of the American Statistical Association*, **96**:1506–1521, 2001.

G. King. *A Solution to the Ecological Inference Problem: Reconstructing Individual Behavior from Aggregate Data*. Princeton University Press, Princeton, NJ, 1997.

G. Kitagawa. An algorithm for solving the matrix equation $x = fxf^t + s$. *The International Journal of Control*, **25**:745–753, 1977.

G. Kitagawa. Non-Gaussian state-space modeling of non-stationary time series. *Journal of the American Statistical Association*, **82**:1032–1041, 1987.

G. Kitagawa. *Introduction to Time Series Modeling*. Chapman and Hall/CRC, Boca Raton, FL, 2010.

P. K. Kitanidis. Parameter uncertainty in estimation of spatial functions: Bayesian analysis. *Water Resources Research*, **22**:499–507, 1986.

P. K. Kitanidis. *Introduction to Geostatistics: Applications in Hydrology*. Cambridge University Press, New York, 1997.

L. Knorr-Held. Bayesian modelling of inseparable space-time variation in disease risk. *Statistics in Medicine*, **19**:2555–2567, 2000.

L. Knorr-Held and J. Besag. Modelling risk from a disease in time and space. *Statistics in Medicine*, **17**:2045–2060, 1998.

K. H. Knuth. A Bayesian approach to source separation. In J.-F. Cardoso, C. Jutten, and P. Loubaton, editors, *Proceedings of the First International Workshop on Independent Component Analysis and Signal Separation*, pages 283–288, Aussois, France, 1999.

K. H. Knuth. Informed source separation: A Bayesian tutorial. In B. Sanjur, E. Cetin, E. Tekalp, and E. Kuruoglu, editors, *Proceedings of the European Signal Processing Conference*, Antalya, Turkey, 2005.

E. D. Kolaczyk. Bayesian multiscale models for Poisson processes. *Journal of the American Statistical Association*, **94**:920–933, 1999.

E. D. Kolaczyk and R. D. Nowak. Multiscale, generalized linear models for nonparametric function estimation. *Biometrika*, **92**:119–133, 2004.

A. N. Kolmogorov. The local structure of turbulence in an incompressible fluid at very large reynolds numbers. *Doklady Akademii Nauk SSSR*, **30**:301–305, 1941. Reprinted in S. K. Friedlander and L. Topping, editors, *Turbulence: Classic Papers on Statistical Theory*, pages. 151–155. Interscience Publishers, New York, 1961

D. Kondrashov, S. Kravtsov, A. W. Robertson, and M. Ghil. A hierarchy of databased ENSO models. *Journal of Climate*, **18**:4425–4444, 2005.

C. Kooperberg and F. O'Sullivan. Predictive oscillation patterns: A synthesis of methods for spatial-temporal decomposition of random fields. *Journal of the American Statistical Association*, **91**:1485–1496, 1996.

J. Kornak, M. E. Irwin, and N. Cressie. Spatial point process models of defensive strategies: Detecting changes. *Statistical Inference for Stochastic Processes*, **9**:31–46, 2006.

M. Kot. Discrete-time travelling waves: Ecological examples. *Journal of Mathematical Biology*, **30**:413–436, 1992.

M. Kot, M. Lewis, and P. van den Driessche. Dispersal data and the spread of invading organisms. *Ecology*, **77**:2027–2042, 1996.

A. Kottas and B. Sansó. Bayesian mixture modeling for spatial Poisson process intensities, with applications to extreme value analysis. *Journal of Statistical Planning and Inference*, **137**:3151–3163, 2007.

S. Koyama, L. Castellanos Péez-Bolde, C. R. Shalizi, and R. E. Kass. Approximate methods for state-space models. *Journal of the American Statistical Association*, **105**:170–180, 2010.

M. Kulldorff. A spatial scan statistic. *Communications in Statistics. Theory and Methods*, **26**:1481–1496, 1997.

M. Kulldorff, R. Heffernan, J. Hartman, R. M. Assunção, and F. Mostashari. A space time permutation scan statistic for disease outbreak detection. *PLoS Medicine*, **2**:216–224, 2005.

H. R. Künsch, A. Papritz, and F. Bassi. Generalized cross-covariances and their estimation. *Mathematical Geology*, **29**:779–799, 1997.

J. E. Kutzbach. Empirical eigenvectors of sea level pressure, surface temperature and precipitation complexes over North America. *Journal of Applied Meteorology*, **6**:791–802, 1967.

P. C. Kyriakidis. A geostatistical framework for area to point spatial interpolation. *Geographical Analysis*, **36**:259–289, 2004.

P. C. Kyriakidis and A. G. Journel. Geostatistical space–time models: A review. *Mathematical Geology*, **31**:651–684, 1999.

C. Lagazio, E. Dreassi, and A. Biggeri. A hierarchical Bayesian model for space–time variaton of disease risk. *Statistical Modelling*, **1**:17–29, 2001.

S. N. Lahiri. On inconsistency of estimators under infill asymptotics for spatial data. *Sankhya, Series A*, **58**:403–417, 1996.

S. N. Lahiri. *Resampling Methods for Dependent Data*. Springer, New York, 2003.

S. N. Lahiri, M. S. Kaiser, N. Cressie, and N.-J. Hsu. Prediction of spatial cumulative distribution functions using subsampling. *Journal of the American Statistical Association*, **94**:86–110, 1999.

S. N. Lahiri, Y.-D. Lee, and N. Cressie. Asymptotic distribution and asymptotic efficiency of least squares estimators of variogram parameters. *Journal of Statistical Planning and Inference*, **103**:65–85, 2002.

C. Lantuéjoul. *Geostatistical Simulation: Models and Algorithms*. Springer, Berlin, DE, 2002.

S. L. Lauritzen. *Graphical Models*. Clarendon Press, Oxford, UK, 1996.

M. Lavine and S. Lozier. A Markov random field spatio-temporal analysis of ocean temperature. *Environmental and Ecological Statistics*, **6**:249–273, 1999.

D. N. Lawley. Tests of significance for the latent roots of covariance and correlation matrices. *Biometrika*, **43**:128–136, 1956.

A. B. Lawson. *Statistical Methods in Spatial Epidemiology*. John Wiley & Sons, Chichester, UK, 2001.

A. B. Lawson. *Bayesian Disease Mapping: Hierarchical Modeling in Spatial Epidemiology*. Chapman and Hall/CRC, Boca Raton, FL, 2009.

A. B. Lawson and N. Cressie. Spatial statistical methods for environmental epidemiology. In *Handbook of Statistics*, Vol. 18: *Bioenvironmental and Public Health Statistics*, pages 357–396. Elsevier, Amsterdam, NL, 2000.

N. D. Le and J. V. Zidek. *Statistical Analysis of Environmental Space Time Processes*. Springer, New York, 2006.

H. Lee and S. K. Ghosh. A reparameterization approach for dynamic space-time models. *Journal of Statistical Theory and Practice*, **2**:1–14, 2008.

J. Lee, M. S. Kaiser, and N. Cressie. Multiway dependence in exponential family conditional distributions. *Journal of Multivariate Analysis*, **79**:171–190, 2001.

Y. C. Lee, S. Qian, R. D. Jones, C. W. Barnes, G. W. Flake, M. K. O'Rourke, K. Lee, H. H. Chen, G. Z. Sun, Y. Q. Zhang, and D. Chen. Adaptive stochastic cellular automata: Theory. *Physica D*, **45**:159–180, 1990.

Y.-D. Lee and S. N. Lahiri. Least squares variogram fitting by spatial subsampling. *Journal of the Royal Statistical Society, Series B*, **64**:837–854, 2002.

P. Legendre, M. R. T. Dale, M.-J. Fortin, P. Casgrain, and J. Gurevitch. Effects of spatial structures on the results of field experiments. *Ecology*, **85**:3202–3214, 2004.

E. L. Lehmann. *Theory of Point Estimation*. John Wiley & Sons, New York, 1983.

R. T. Lemos and B. Sansó. A spatio-temporal model for mean, anomaly, and trend fields of North Atlantic sea surface temperature. *Journal of the American Statistical Association*, **104**:5–18, 2009.

S. S. Leroy. Detecting climate signals: Some Bayesian aspects. *Journal of Climate*, **11**:640–651, 1998.

J. LeSage and R. K. Pace. *Introduction to Spatial Econometrics*. Chapman & Hall/CRC, Boca Raton, FL, 2009.

M. Lesieur. *Turbulance in Fluids*, fourth edition. Springer, Dordrecht, NL, 2008.

S. A. Levin. The problem of pattern and scale in ecology. *Ecology*, **73**:1943–1967, 1992.

M. A. Lewis. Spread rate for a nonlinear stochastics invasion. *Journal of Mathematical Biology*, **41**:430–454, 2000.

H. Li, C. A. Calder, and N. Cressie. Beyond Moran's I: Testing for spatial dependence based on the SAR model. *Geographical Analysis*, **39**:357–375, 2007.

B. Li, M. G. Genton, and M. Sherman. A non-parametric assessment of properties of space-time covariance functions. *Journal of the American Statistical Association*, **102**:736–744, 2007.

F. Lindgren, H. Rue, and J. Lindström. An explicit link between Gaussian fields and Gaussian Markov random fields: the stochastic partial differential equation approach. *Journal of the Royal Statistical Society, Series B*, **73**:423–498, 2011.

W. A. Link, R. J. Barker, J. R. Sauer, and S. Droege. Within-site variability in surveys of wildlife populations. *Ecology*, **74**:1097–1108, 1994.

J. Liu and M. West. Combined parameter and state estimation in simulation-based filtering. In *Sequential Monte Carlo Methods in Practice*, pages 197–223. Springer, New York, 2001.

J. S. Liu. *Monte Carlo Strategies in Scientific Computing*. Springer, New York, 2004.

C. D. Lloyd. *Local Models for Spatial Analysis*. Chapman & Hall/CRC, Boca Raton, FL, 2007.

M. Loéve. *Probability Theory*. Van Nostrand Company, Princeton, NJ, 1963.

M. Loéve. *Probability Theory I*, fourth edition. Springer-Verlag, New York, 1977.

M. Loéve. *Probability Theory II*, fourth edition. Springer-Verlag, New York, 1978.

P. Longley, M. F. Goodchild, D. J. Maguire, and D. W. Rhind. *Geographical Information Systems and Science*, second edition. John Wiley & Sons, New York, 2005.

H. F. Lopes, E. Salazar, and D. Gamerman. Spatial dynamic factor models. *Bayesian Analysis*, **3**:1–34, 2008.

S. Lophaven, J. Carstensen, and H. Rootzen. Space-time modeling of environmental monitoring data. *Environmental and Ecological Statistics*, **11**:237–256, 2004.

E. N. Lorenz. Empirical orthogonal functions and statistical weather prediction. Scientific Report No. 1, Statistical Forecasting Project, MIT, Cambridge, MA, 1956.

E. N. Lorenz. Deterministic non-periodic flow. *Journal of the Atmospheric Sciences*, **20**:130–141, 1963.

E. N. Lorenz. *The Essence of Chaos*. University of Washington Press, Seattle, WA, 1993.

T. A. Louis. Estimating a population of parameter values using Bayes and empirical Bayes methods. *Journal of the American Statistical Association*, **79**:393–398, 1984.

Z. Lu, D. J. Steinskog, D. Tjostheim, and Q. Yao. Adaptively varying-coefficient spatiotemporal models. *Journal of the Royal Statistical Society, Series B*, **71**:859–880, 2009.

R. B. Lund, H. L. Hurd, P. Bloomfield, and R. Smith. Climatological time series with periodic correlation. *Journal of Climate*, **8**:2787–2809, 1995.

H. Lütkepohl. *Introduction to Multiple Time Series: Theory and Methods*, second edition. Springer-Verlag, Berlin, DE, 1993.

H. Lütkepohl. *New Introduction to Multiple Time Series Analysis*. Springer-Verlag, Berlin, DE, 2005.

C. Ma. Families of spatio-temporal stationary covariance models. *Journal of Statistical Planning and Inference*, **116**:489–501, 2003.

C. Ma. Linear combinations of space-time covariance functions and variograms. *IEEE Transactions on Signal Processing*, **53**:857–864, 2005.

Y. Z. Ma. Simpson's Paradox in natural resource evaluation. *Mathematical Geosciences*, **41**:193–213, 2009.

S. N. MacEachern, M. Clyde, and J. Liu. Sequential importance sampling for nonparametric Bayes models: The next generation. *Canadian Journal of Statistics*, **27**:251–267, 1999.

A. J. Majda, R. V. Abramov, and M. J. Grote. *Information Theory and Stochastics for Multiscale Nonlinear Systems*. American Mathematical Society, Providence, RI, 2005.

A. J. Majda and X. Wang. *Nonlinear Dynamics and Statistical Theories for Basic Geophysical Flows*. Cambridge University Press, Cambridge, 2006.

A. J. Majda, C. Franzke, and D. Crommelin. Normal forms for reduced stochastic climate models. *Proceedings of the National Academy of Sciences*, **106**:3649–3653, 2009.

A. Majumdar and A. E. Gelfand. Multivariate spatial modeling for geostatistical data using convolved covariance functions. *Mathematical Geology*, **39**:225–245, 2007.

S. Mallat. A theory of multiresolution signal decomposition: The wavelet representation. *IEEE Transactions on Pattern Analysis and Machine Intelligence*, **11**:674–693, 1989.

A. Malmberg, A. Arellano, D. P. Edwards, N. Flyer, D. Nychka, and C. K. Wikle. Interpolation fields of carbon monoxide data using a hybrid statistical-physical model. *Annals of Applied Statistics*, **2**:1231–1248, 2008.

B. B. Mandelbrot. *The Fractal Geometry of Nature*. W. H. Freeman, San Francisco, CA, 1982.

B. E. Mapes, R. F. Milliff, and J. Morzel. Composite life cycle of maritime tropical mesoscale convective systems in scatterometer and microwave satellite observations. *Journal of the Atmospheric Sciences*, **66**:199–208, 2009.

B. P. Marchant and R. M. Lark. Optimized sample schemes for geostatistical surveys. *Mathematical Geology*, **39**:113–134, 2007.

K. V. Mardia. Multi-dimensional multivariate Gaussian Markov random fields with application to image processing. *Journal of Multivariate Analysis*, **24**:265–284, 1988.

K. V. Mardia, C. Goodall, E. J. Redfern, and F. J. Alonso. The kriged Kalman filter (with discussion). *Test*, **7**:217–285, 1998.

J.-M. Marin and C. P. Robert. *Bayesian Core: A Practical Approach to Computational Bayesian Statistics*. Springer, New York, 2007.

S. L. Marple, Jr. *Digital Spectral Analysis with Applications*. PTR Prentice-Hall, Englewood Cliffs, NJ, 1987.

R. J. Martin. Comparing and contrasting some environmental and experimental design problems. *Environmetrics*, **12**:273–287, 2001.

S. Martino and H. Rue. The R-INLA Project, 2009 (http://www.r-inla.org/home/).

O. Martius, C. Schwierz, and H. C. Davies. A refined Hovmüller diagram. *Tellus*, **58A**:221–226, 2006.

J. Mateu. Discussion of the paper: "A general science-based framework for dynamical spatio-temporal models" by C. K. Wikle and M. B. Hooten. *Test*, **19**:452–455, 2010.

B. Matérn. *Spatial Variation*. Meddelanden fran Statens Skogsforskningsinstitut, Vol. 49, No. 5, 1960. Second edition: Lecture Notes in Statistics, No. 36, Springer, New York, 1986.

G. Matheron. *Traité de Géostatistique Appliquée, Tome I*. Memoires du Bureau de Recherches Géologiques et Minières, No. 14, Editions Technip, Paris, 1962.

G. Matheron. *Traité de Géostatistique Appliquée, Tome II: le Krigeage*. Memoires du Bureau de Recherches Géologiques et Minières, No. 24, Paris, 1963.

G. Matheron. Principles of geostatistics. *Economic Geology*, **58**:1246–1266, 1963.

G. Matheron. Random sets theory and its application to stereology. *Journal of Microscopy*, **95**:15–23, 1971.

G. Matheron. The intrinsic random functions and their applications. *Advances in Applied Probability*, **5**:439–468, 1973.

G. Matheron. *Random Sets and Integral Geometry*. John Wiley & Sons, New York, 1975.

T. Matsuno. Quasi-geostrophic motions in the equatorial area. *Journal of the Meteorological Society of Japan*, **41**:25–42, 1966.

P. McCullagh and D. Clifford. Evidence for conformal invariance of crop yields. *Proceedings of the Royal Society of London, Series A*, **462**:2119–2143, 2006.

P. McCullagh and J. A. Nelder. *Generalized Linear Models*, second edition. Chapman & Hall, New York, 1989.

C. E. McCulloch and S. R. Searle. *Generalized, Linear, and Mixed Models*. John Wiley & Sons, New York, 2001.

G. J. McLachlan and T. Krishnan. *The EM Algorithm and Extensions*. John Wiley & Sons, New York, 1997.

R. J. Meinhold and N. D. Singpurwalla. Understanding the Kalman filter. *The American Statistician*, **37**:123–127, 1983.

X.-L. Meng. Statistics: Your chance for happiness (or misery). *The Harvard Undergraduate Research Journal*, **2**:21–27, 2009.

A. C. Micheas, N. I. Fox, S. A. Lack, and C. K. Wikle. Cell identification and verification of QPF ensembles using shape analysis techniques. *Journal of Hydrology*, **343**:105–116, 2007.

A. C. Micheas and C. K. Wikle. A Bayesian hierarchical non-overlapping random disc growth model. *Journal of the American Statistical Association*, **194**:274–283, 2009.

R. F. Milliff, A. Bonazzi, C. K. Wikle, N. Pinardi, and L. M. Berliner. Ocean ensemble forecasting, Part I: Ensemble Mediterranian winds from a Bayesian hierarchical model. *Quarterly Journal of the Royal Meteorological Society*, **137**:858–878, 2011.

R. F. Milliff and J. Morzel. The global distribution of the time-average wind-stress curl from NSCAT. *Journal of the Atmospheric Sciences*, **58**:109–131, 2001.

M. Mitchell, M. G. Genton, and M. Gumpertz. Testing for separability of space-time covariances. *Environmetrics*, **16**:819–831, 2005.

I. S. Molchanov. *Limit Theorems for Unions of Random Closed Sets*. Springer-Verlag, Berlin, DE, 1993.

I. S. Molchanov. *Theory of Random Sets*. Springer, New York, 2005.

J. Møller. Markov chain Monte Carlo spatial point processes. In O. E. Barndorff-Nielsen, W. S. Kendall, and M. M. van Lieshout, editors, *Stochastic Geometry: Likelihood and Computations*, pages 141–172. Chapman & Hall/CRC, Boca Raton, FL, 1999.

J. Møller. *Spatial Statistics and Computational Methods*. Springer Lecture Notes in Statistics, No. 173. Springer, New York, 2003.

J. Møller and C. Díaz-Avalos. Structured spatio-temporal shot-noise Cox point process models, with a view to modelling forest fires. *Scandinavian Journal of Statistics*, **37**:2–25, 2010.

J. Møller and K. Helisova. Likelihood inference for unions of intersecting discs. *Scandinavian Journal of Statistics*, **37**:365–381, 2009.

J. Møller, A. N. Pettitt, R. W. Reeves, and K. K. Berthelsen. An efficient Markov chain Monte Carlo method for distributions with intractable normalising constants. *Biometrika*, **93**:451–458, 2006.

J. Møller and E. Rubak. A model for positively correlated count variables. *International Statistical Review*, **78**:65–80, 2010.

J. Møller, A. R. Syversveen, and R. P. Waagepetersen. Log Gaussian Cox processes. *Scandinavian Journal of Statistics*, **25**:451–482, 1998.

J. Møller and R. P. Waagepetersen. *Statistical Inference and Simulation for Spatial Point Processes*. Chapman & Hall/CRC, Boca Raton, FL, 2004.

J. Møller and R. P. Waagepetersen. Modern statistics for spatial point processes. *Scandinavian Journal of Statistics*, **34**:643–711, 2007.

P. Monestiez, L. Dubroca, E. Bonnin, J. Durbec, and C. Guinet. Comparison of model based geostatistical method in ecology: Application to fin whale spatial distribution in Northwestern Mediterranean Sea. In O. Leuangthong and C. V. Deutsch, editors, *Geostatistics Banff 2004*, Volume 2, pages 777–786. Springer, Dordrecht, NL, 2005.

P. Monestiez, L. Dubroca, E. Bonnin, J.-P. Durbec, and C. Guinet. Geostatistical modelling of spatial distribution of *Balaenoptera physalus* in the Northwestern Mediterranean Sea from sparse count data and heterogeneous observation efforts. *Ecological Modeling*, **193**:615–628, 2006.

B. C. Moore. Principal component analysis in linear systems: Controllability, observability, and model reduction. *IEEE Transactions on Automatic Control*, **26**:17–32, 1981.

M. Moore, editor. *Spatial Statistics: Methodological Aspects and Applications*. Springer, New York, 2001.

P. A. P. Moran. Notes on continuous stochastic phenomena. *Biometrika*, **37**:17–23, 1950.

J. Moussouris. Gibbs and Markov random systems with constraints. *Journal of Statistical Physics*, **10**:11–33, 1974.

A. S. Mugglin, B. P. Carlin, and A. E. Gelfand. Fully model-based approaches for spatially misaligned data. *Journal of the American Statistical Association*, **95**:877–887, 2000.

A. S. Mugglin, N. Cressie, and I. Gemmell. Hierarchical statistical modeling of influenza epidemic dynamics in space and time. *Statistics in Medicine*, **21**:2703–2721, 2002.

P. Müller. Simulation based optimal design. In *Bayesian Statistics 6*, pages 459–474. Oxford University Press, Oxford, UK, 1999.

W. G. Müller. *Collecting Spatial Data: Optimum Design of Experiments for Random Fields*. Physica-Verlag, New York, 1998.

W. G. Müller. *Collecting Spatial Data: Optimum Design of Experiments for Random Fields*, second edition. Physica-Verlag, Heidelberg, DE, 2000.

W. G. Müller. A comparison of spatial design methods for correlated observations. *Environmetrics*, **16**:495–505, 2005.

W. G. Müller and M. Stehlík. Compound optimal spatial designs. *Environmetrics*, 21:354–364, 2010.

B. Munoz, V. M. Lesser, and F. L. Ramsey. Design-based empirical orthogonal function model for environmental monitoring data analysis. *Environmetrics*, 19:805–817, 2008.

A. H. Murphy. The coefficients of correlation and determination as measures of performance in forecast verification. *Weather and Forecasting*, 10:681–688, 1995.

M. Musio, N. H. Augustin, and K. von Wilpert. Geoadditive Bayesian model for forestry defoliation data: A case study. *Environmetrics*, 19:630–642, 2008.

D. E. Myers. Matrix formulation of cokriging. *Mathematical Geology*, 14:249–257, 1982.

D. E. Myers. Cokriging, radial basis functions and positive definiteness. *Computers and Mathematics with Applications*, 24:139–148, 1992.

V. F. Nettles, J. H. Shaddock, R. K. Sikes, and C. R. Reyes. Rabies in translocated racoons. *American Journal of Public Health*, 69:601–602, 1979.

H. T. Nguyen. *An Introducton to Random Sets*. Chapman & Hall/CRC, Boca Raton, FL, 2006.

N. Nicholls. The use of canonical correlation to study teleconnections. *Monthly Weather Review*, 115:393–399, 1987.

D. J. Nordman. A blockwise empirical likelihood for spatial data. *Statistica Sinica*, 18:1111–1129, 2008a.

D. J. Nordman. Empirical likelihood for spatial regression. *Metrika*, 68:351–363, 2008b.

D. J. Nordman and P. C. Caragea. Point and interval estimation of variogram models using spatial empirical likelihood. *Journal of the American Statistical Association*, 103:350–361, 2008.

G. R. North, T. L. Bell, R. F. Calahan, and F. J. Moeng. Sampling errors in the estimation of empirical orthogonal functions. *Monthly Weather Review*, 110:699–706, 1982.

J. D. Norton and X.-F. Niu. Intrinsically autoregressive spatiotemporal models with application to aggregated birth outcomes. *Journal of the American Statistical Association*, 104:638–649, 2009.

D. J. Nott and W. T. Dunsmuir. Estimation of nonstationary spatial coverance structure. *Biometrika*, 89:819–829, 2002.

W. Nowak. Measures of parameter uncertainty in geostatistical estimation and geostatistical optimal design. *Mathematical Geosciences*, 42:199–221, 2010.

D. Nychka, C. K. Wikle, and J. A. Royle. Multiresolution models for nonstationary spatial covariance functions. *Statistical Modelling*, 2:315–331, 2002.

D. Nychka, Q. Yang, and J. A. Royle. Constructing spatial designs using regression subset selection. In *Statistics for the Environment 3: Pollution Assessment and Control*, pages 131–154. John Wiley & Sons, New York, 1997.

C. Obled and J. D. Creutin. Some developments in the use of empirical orthogonal functions for mapping meteorological fields. *Journal of Applied Meteorology*, 25:1189–1204, 1986.

G. W. Oehlert. Regional trends in sulfate wet deposition. *Journal of the American Statistical Association*, 88:390–399, 1993.

Y. Ogata. Space–time point-process models for earthquake occurrences. *Annals of the Institute of Statistical Mathematics*, **50**:379–402, 1998.

Y. Ogata. Space-time model for regional seismicity and detection of crustal stress changes. *Journal of Geophysical Research*, **109**:1–16, 2004.

Y. Ogata, A. Kobayashi, N. Mikami, Y. Murata, and K. Katsura. Correction of earthquake location estimation in a small-seismic-array system. *Bernoulli*, **4**:167–184, 1998.

H. Omre and K. B. Halvorsen. The Bayesian bridge between simple and universal kriging. *Mathematical Geology*, **21**:767–786, 1989.

H. Omre and H. Tjelmeland. Petroleum geostatistics. In E. Y. Baafi and N. A. Schofield, editors, *Geostatistics Wollongong '96*, Vol. 1, pages 41–52. Kluwer Academic Publishers, Dordrecht, NL, 1997.

S. Openshaw and P. Taylor. A million or so correlation coefficients. In N. Wrigley, editor, *Statistical Methods in the Spatial Sciences*, pages 127–144. Pion, London, UK, 1979.

R. Osserman. *Poetry of the Universe*. Random House, New York, 1995.

W. S. Overton and S. V. Stehman. Desirable design considerations for long-term monitoring of ecological variables. *Environmental and Ecological Statistics*, **3**:349–361, 1996.

C. J. Paciorek. Computational techniques for spatial logistic regression with large datasets. *Computational Statistics and Data Analysis*, **51**:3631–3653, 2007.

C. J. Paciorek. The importance of scale for spatial-confounding bias and precision of spatial regression estimators. *Statistical Science*, **25**:107–125, 2010.

C. J. Paciorek and M. J. Schervish. Spatial modelling using a new class of nonstationary covariance functions. *Environmetrics*, **17**:483–506, 2006.

J. H. P. Paelinck and L. H. Klaassen. *Spatial Econometrics*. Saxon House, Farnborough, UK, 1979.

M. Palacios and M. Steel. Non-Gaussian Bayesian geostatistical modeling. *Journal of the American Statistical Association*, **101**:604–618, 2006.

J. S. Papadakis. Méthode statistique pour des expériences sur champ. Bulletin Scientifique No. 23, Institut d'Amélioration des Plantes à Salonique, Greece, 1937.

A. Papoulis. *Probability, Random Variables, and Stochastic Processes*. McGraw-Hill, New York, 1965.

B. U. Park, T. Y. Kim, J.-S. Park, and S. Y. Hwang. Practical applicable central limit theorem for spatial statistics. *Mathematical Geosciences*, **41**:555–569, 2009.

L. Pasanen and L. Holmström. Bayesian scale space analysis of image differences. In *Proceedings of the Joint Statistical Meetings*, American Statistical Association, Alexandria, VA, 1786–1793, 2008.

R. Paulo. Default priors for Gaussian processes. *Annals of Statistics*, **33**:556–582, 2005.

J. M. Pavía, B. Larraz, and J. M. Montero. Election forecasts using spatiotemporal models. *Journal of the American Statistical Association*, **103**:1050–1059, 2008.

M. Pavlicová, T. J. Santner, and N. Cressie. Detecting signals in FMRI data using powerful FDR procedures. *Statistics and Its Interface*, **1**:231–321, 2008.

J. N. Peagle and R. B. Haslam. Statistical prediction of 500mb height field using eigenvectors. *Journal of Applied Meteorology*, **21**:127–138, 1982.

J. Pedlosky. *Geophysical Fluid Dynamics*, second edition. Springer-Verlag, New York, 1987.

R. D. Peng, F. P. Schoenberg, and J. A. Woods. A space–time conditional intensity model for evaluating a wildfire hazard index. *Journal of the American Statistical Association*, **100**:26–35, 2005.

C. Penland and T. Magorian. Prediction of Niño 3 sea surface temperatures using linear inverse modeling. *Journal of Climate*, **6**:1067–1076, 1993.

A. Penttinen, D. Stoyan, and H. M. Henttonen. Marked point processes in forest statistics. *Forest Science*, **38**:806–824, 1992.

D. B. Percival and A. T. Walden. *Spectral Analysis for Physical Applications: Multitaper and Conventional Univariate Techniques*. Cambridge University Press, Cambridge, UK, 1993.

A. N. Pettitt, I. S. Weir, and A. G. Hart. A conditional autoregressive Gaussian process for irregularly spaced multivariate data with application to modeling large sets of binary data. *Statistics and Computing*, **12**:353–367, 2002.

P. E. Pfeifer and S. J. Deutsch. A three-stage iterative procedure for space–time modeling. *Technometrics*, **22**:35–47, 1980.

S. G. Philander. *El Niño, La Niña, and the Southern Oscillation*. Academic Press, San Diego, CA, 1990.

D. K. Pickard. Inference for discrete Markov fields: The simplest nontrivial case. *Journal of the American Statistical Association*, **82**:90–96, 1987.

E. C. Pielou. *Mathematical Ecology*. John Wiley & Sons, London, UK, 1977.

N. Pinardi, I. Allen, E. Demirov, P. DeMey, G. Kores, A. Lascaratos, P.-Y. LeTraon, C. Maillard, G. Manzella, and C. Tziavos. The Mediterranean Ocean forecasting system: First phase of implementation (1998–2001). *Annales Geophysicae*, **21**:3–20, 2003.

N. Pinardi, A. Bonazzi, S. Dobricic, R. F. Milliff, C. K. Wikle, and L. M. Berliner. Ocean ensemble forecasting. Part II: Mediterranean forecast system response. *Quarterly Journal of the Royal Meterological Society*, **137**:879–893, 2011.

M. K. Pitt and N. Shephard. Filtering via simulation: Auxiliary particle filters. *Journal of the American Statistical Association*, **94**:590–599, 1999.

W. J. Platt, G. W. Evans, and S. L. Rathbun. The population dynamics of a long-lived conifer (*Pinus palustris*). *The American Naturalist*, **131**:491–525, 1988.

N. G. Polson, J. R. Stroud, and P. Müller. Particle filtering with sequential parameter learning. *Journal of the Royal Statistical Society, Series B*, **70**:413–428, 2008.

E. Porcu P. Gregori, and J. Mateu. Nonseparable stationary anisotropic space–time covariance functions. *Stochastic Environmental Research and Risk Assessment*, **21**:113–122, 2006.

E. Porcu, J. Mateu, and F. Saura. New classes of covariance and spectral density functions for spatio-temporal modeling. *Stochastic Environmental Research and Risk Assessment*, **22** (Supplement 1): S65–S79, 2008.

A. Possolo, editor. *Spatial Statistics and Imaging*. Institute of Mathematical Statistics, Hayward, CA, 1991.

M. Pourahmadi. Joint mean-covariance models with applications to longitudinal data: Unconstrained parameterisation. *Biometrika*, **86**:677–690, 1999.

R. Prado and M. West. *Time Series Modeling, Computation, and Inference*. Chapman and Hall/CRC, Boca Raton, FL, 2010.

R. W. Preisendorfer. *Principal Component Analysis in Meteorology and Oceanography*. Elsevier, Amsterdam, NL, 1988.

R. W. Preisendorfer and T. P. Barnett. Numerical model-reality intercomparison test using small-sample statistics. *Journal of the Atmospheric Sciences*, **40**:1884–1896, 1983.

S. J. Press. *Bayesian Statistics: Principles, Models, and Applications*. John Wiley & Sons, New York, 1989.

C. E. Priebe, T. Olson, and D. M. Healy, Jr. A spatial scan statistic for stochastic scan partitions. *Journal of the American Statistical Association*, **92**:1476–1484, 1997.

M. B. Priestley. *Non-linear and Non-stationary Time Series*. Academic Press, London, UK, 1988.

B. Prum and J. C. Fort. *Stochastic Processes on a Lattice and Gibbs Measures*. Kluwer Academic Publishers, Dordrecht, NL, 1991.

H. Putter and G. A. Young. On the effect of covariance function estimation on the accuracy of kriging predictors. *Bernoulli*, **7**:421–438, 2001.

T. Raiko and M. Tornio. Variational Bayesian learning of nonlinear hidden statespace models for model predictive control. *Neurocomputing*, **72**:3704–3712, 2009.

T. Raiko, H. Valpola, M. Harva, and J. Karhunen. Building blocks for variational Bayesian learning of latent variable models. *Journal of Machine Learning Research*, **8**:155–201, 2007.

J. O. Ramsay, G. Hooker, D. Campbell, and J. Cao. Parameter estimation for differential equations: A generalized smoothing approach. *Journal of the Royal Statistical Society, Series B*, **69**:741–796, 2007.

C. R. Rao. *Linear Statistical Inference and Its Applications*. John Wiley & Sons, New York, 1965.

J. N. K. Rao. *Small Area Estimation*. John Wiley & Sons, New York, 2003.

J. G. Rasmussen, P. A. Arkin, and W. Y. Chen. Biennial variation in surface temperature over the United States as revealed by singular decomposition. *Monthly Weather Review*, **109**:587–598, 1981.

S. L. Rathbun and N. Cressie. A space–time survival point process for a longleaf pine forest in Southern Georgia. *Journal of the American Statistical Association*, **89**:1164–1174, 1994.

B. J. Reich, J. S. Hodges, and V. Zadnik. Effects of residual smoothing on the posterior of the fixed effects in disease-mapping models. *Biometrics*, **62**:1197–1206, 2006.

G. Reinsel, G. C. Tiao, N. M. Wang, R. Lewis, and D. Nychka. Statistical analysis of stratospheric ozone data for the detection of trend. *Atmospheric Environment*, **15**:1569–1577, 1981.

N. Remy, A. Boucher, and J. Wu. *Applied Geostatistics with SGeMS: A User's Guide*. Cambridge University Press, Cambridge, UK, 2009.

A. C. Rencher. *Methods of Multivariate Analysis*, second edition. John Wiley & Sons, New York, 2002.

E. Renshaw. *Modelling Biological Populations in Space and Time*. Cambridge University Press, Cambridge, UK, 1991.

E. Renshaw. Spatial-temporal marked point processes: a spectrum of stochastic models. *Environmetrics*, **21**:253–269, 2010.

E. Renshaw and E. D. Ford. The interpretation of process from pattern using two-dimensional spectral analysis: Methods and problems of intepretation. *Applied Statistics*, **32**:51–63, 1983.

H. R. Richardson and L. D. Stone. Operations analysis during the underwater search for *Scorpion*. *Naval Research Logistics Quarterly*, **2**:141–157, 1971.

M. B. Richman. Obliquely rotated principal components: An improved meteorological map tying technique? *Journal of Applied Meteorology*, **20**:1145–1159, 1981.

M. B. Richman. Review article: Rotation of principal components. *International Journal of Climatology*, **6**:293–335, 1986.

B. D. Ripley. The second-order analysis of stationary point processes. *Journal of Applied Probability*, **13**:255–266, 1976.

B. D. Ripley. *Spatial Statistics*. John Wiley & Sons, New York, 1981.

B. D. Ripley. *Statistical Inference for Spatial Processes*. Cambridge University Press, Cambridge, UK, 1988.

J. Rivoirard. Concepts and methods of geostatistics. In M. Bilodeau, F. Meyer, and M. Schmitt, editors, *Space, Structure and Randomness*, pages 17–37. Springer, New York, 2005.

C. Robbins, D. Bystrak, and P. Geissler. *The breeding bird survey: Its first fifteen years, 1965–1979*. Fish and Wildlife Service Resource Publication 157, USDOI, Washington, DC, 1986.

C. P. Robert and G. Casella. *Introducing Monte Carlo Methods with R*. Springer, New York, 2010.

C. P. Robert and G. Casella. *Monte Carlo Statistical Methods*, second edition. Springer, New York, 2004.

W. S. Robinson. Ecological correlation and the behavior of individuals. *American Sociological Review*, **15**:351–357, 1950.

A. Rodrigues and P. J. Diggle. A class of convolution-based models for spatio-temporal processes with non-separable covariance structure. *Scandinavian Journal of Statistics*, **37**:553–567, 2010.

I. Rodriguez-Iturbe, D. R. Cox, and V. Isham. A point process model for rainfall: Further developments. *Proceedings of the Royal Society of London, Series A*, **417**:283–298, 1988.

I. Rodriguez-Iturbe and P. S. Eagleson. Mathematical models of rainstorm events in space and time. *Water Resources Research*, **23**:181–190, 1987.

A. Rogers. *Statistical Analysis of Spatial Dispersion*. Pion, London, UK, 1974.

C. Romagosa and R. Labisky. Establishment and dispersal of the Eurasian Collared Dove in Florida. *Journal of Field Ornithology*, **71**:159–166, 2000.

S. Rouhani and T. J. Hall. Space-time kriging of groundwater data. In M. Armstrong, editor, *Geostatistics: Proceedings of the Third International Geostatistics Congress (1988)*, pages 639–650. Kluwer Academic Publishers, Dordrecht, NL, 1989.

S. Rouhani and H. Wackernagel. Multivariate geostatistical approach to space–time data analysis. *Water Resources Research*, **26**:585–591, 1990.

J. A. Royle. *n*-mixture model for estimating population size for spatially replicated counts. *Biometrics*, **60**:108–115, 2004.

J. A. Royle and L. M. Berliner. A hierarchical approach to multivariate spatial modeling and prediction. *Journal of Agricultural, Biological, and Environmental Statistics*, **4**:1–28, 1999.

J. A. Royle, L. M. Berliner, C. K. Wikle, and R. Milliff. A hierarchical spatial model for constructing wind fields from scatterometer data in the Labrador Sea. In G. Gatsonis, B. Carlin, A. Gelman, M. West, R. E. Kass, A. Carriquiry, and I. Verdinelli, editors, *Case Studies in Bayesian Statistics IV*, pages 367–382. Springer-Verlag, New York, 1999.

J. A. Royle and R. M. Dorazio. Hierarchical models of animal abundance or occurrence. *Journal of Agricultural, Biological, and Environmental Statistics*, **11**:249–263, 2006.

J. A. Royle and R. M. Dorazio. *Hierarchical Modeling and Inference in Ecology: The Analysis of Data from Populations, Metapopulations and Communities*. Elsevier, Amsterdam, NL, 2008.

J. A. Royle and M. Kery. A Bayesian state-space formulation of dynamic occupancy models. *Ecology*, **88**:1813–1823, 2007.

J. A. Royle and C. K. Wikle. Efficient statistical mapping of avian count data. *Environmental and Ecological Statistics*, **12**:225–243, 2005.

D. B. Rubin. Bayesianly justifiable and relevant frequency calculations for the applied statistician. *Annals of Statistics*, **12**:1151–1172, 1984.

H. Rue and L. Held. *Gaussian Markov Random Fields: Theory and Applications*. Monographs on Statistics and Applied Probability, Vol. 104. Chapman & Hall/CRC, London, UK, 2005.

H. Rue, S. Martino, and N. Chopin. Approximate Bayesian inference for latent Gaussian models by using integrated nested Laplace approximations (with discussion). *Journal of the Royal Statistical Society, Series B*, **71**:319–392, 2009.

H. Rue, I. Steinsland, and S. Erland. Approximating hidden Gaussian Markov random fields. *Journal of the Royal Statistical Society, Series B*, **66**:877–892, 2004.

H. Rue and H. Tjelmeland. Fitting Gaussian Markov random fields to Gaussian fields. *Scandinavian Journal of Statistics*, **29**:31–50, 2002.

R. Ruiz-Cárdenas, E. T. Krainski, and H. Rue. Fitting dynamic models using integrated nested Laplace approximations—INLA. Preprint Statistics No. 12/2010. Norwegian University of Science and Technology, Trondheim, Norway, 2010.

J. Sacks, W. J. Welch, T. J. Mitchell, and H. P. Wynn. Design and analysis of computer experiments. *Statistical Science*, **4**:409–423, 1989.

T. Sáfadi and D. Peña. Bayesian analysis of dynamic factor models: An application to air pollution and mortality in São Paulo, Brazil. *Environmetrics*, **19**:582–601, 2008.

S. K. Sahu and P. Challenor. A space–time model for joint modeling of ocean temperature and salinity levels as measured by Argo floats. *Environmetrics*, **19**:509–528, 2008.

S. K. Sahu, A. E. Gelfand, and D. M. Holland. Fusing point and areal level space-time data with application to wet deposition. *Applied Statistics*, **59**:77–103, 2009.

S. Sain and N. Cressie. A spatial model for multivariate lattice data. *Journal of Econometrics*, **140**:226–259, 2007.

S. Sain, R. Furrer, and N. Cressie. A spatial analysis of multivariate output from regional climate models. *Annals of Applied Statistics*, **5**:150–175, 2011.

P. D. Sampson and P. Guttorp. Nonparametric estimation of nonstationary spatial covariance structure. *Journal of the American Statistical Association*, **87**:108–119, 1992.

J. T. Sandefur. *Discrete Dynamical Systems: Theory and Applications*. Clarendon Press, New York, 1990.

B. Sansó and L. Guenni. Venezuelan rainfall data analysed by using a Bayesian space–time model. *Applied Statistics*, **48**:345–362, 1999.

B. Sansó, A. Schmidt, and A. Nobre. Spatio-temporal models based on discrete convolutions. *Canadian Journal of Statistics*, **36**:239–258, 2008.

T. J. Santner, W. Notz, and B. J. Williams. *The Design and Analysis of Computer Experiments*. Springer, New York, 2003.

A. Särkkä and E. Renshaw. The analysis of marked point patterns evolving through space and time. *Computational Statistics and Data Analysis*, **51**:1698–1718, 2006.

J. R. Sauer, B. G. Peterjohn, and W. A. Link. Observer difference in the North American Breeding Bird Survey. *Auk*, **111**:50–62, 1994.

L. Scaccia and R. J. Martin. Testing axial symmetry and separability of lattice process. *Journal of Statistical Planning and Inference*, **131**:19–39, 2005.

K. Scerri, M. Dewar, and K. Kadirkamanathan. Estimation and model selection for an IDE-based spatio-temporal model. *IEEE Transactions on Signal Processing*, **57**:482–492, 2009.

O. Schabenberger and C. A. Gotway. *Statistical Methods for Spatial Data Analysis*. Chapman & Hall/CRC, Boca Raton, FL, 2005.

H. Scheffé. *The Analysis of Variance*. John Wiley & Sons, New York, 1959.

L. Schelin and S. Sjostedt-de Luna. Kriging prediction intervals based on semiparametric bootstrap. *Mathematical Geosciences*, **42**:985–1000, 2010.

M. Schlather. On the second order characteristics of marked point processes. *Bernoulli*, **7**:99–117, 2001.

M. Schlather, P. J. Ribeiro, Jr., and P. J. Diggle. Detecting dependence between marks and locations of marked point processes. *Journal of the Royal Statistical Society, Series B*, **66**:79–93, 2004.

A. Schmidt and A. E. Gelfand. A Bayesian coregionalization model for multivariate pollutant data. *Journal of Geophysics Research—Atmospheres*, **108(D24)**: 8783, doi:10.1029/2002JD002905, 2003.

F. P. Schoenberg. Multidimensional residual analysis of point process models for earthquake occurrences. *Journal of the American Statistical Society*, **98**:789–795, 2003.

F. P. Schoenberg. Consistent parametric estimation of the intensity of a spatial-temporal point process. *Journal of Statistical Planning and Inference*, **128**:79–93, 2005.

F. P. Schoenberg, C. Barr, and J. Seo. The distribution of Voronoi cells generated by Southern California earthquake epicenters. *Environmetrics*, **19**:1–14, 2008.

J. Serra. *Image Analysis and Mathematical Morphology*. Academic Press, London, UK, 1982.

G. Shaddick and J. Wakefield. Modelling daily multivariate pollutant data at multiple sites. *Applied Statistics*, **51**:351–372, 2002.

D. E. Shapiro and P. Switzer. Extracting time trends from multiple monitoring sites. Technical Report No. 132, Department of Statistics, Stanford University, Stanford, CA, 1989.

X. Shen, H.-C. Huang, and N. Cressie. Nonparametric hypothesis testing for a spatial signal. *Journal of the American Statistical Association*, **97**:1122–1140, 2002. Correction, **100**:716–718, 2005.

M. Sherman. *Spatial Statistics and Spatio-Temporal Data: Covariance Functions and Directional Properties*. John Wiley & Sons, Hoboken, NJ, 2011.

T. Shi and N. Cressie. Global statistical analysis of MISR aerosol data: A massive data product from NASA's Terra satellite. *Environmetrics*, **18**:665–680, 2007.

L. Shlain. *Art and Physics*. Harper Collins, New York, 1991.

R. H. Shumway and D. S. Stoffer. An approach to time series smoothing and forecasting using the EM algorithm. *Journal of Time Series Analysis*, **3**:253–264, 1982.

R. H. Shumway and D. S. Stoffer. *Time Series Analysis and its Applications*. Springer-Verlag, New York, 2000.

R. H. Shumway and D. S. Stoffer. *Time Series Analysis and its Applications, With R Examples*, second edition. Springer, New York, 2006.

R. A. Silverman. Locally stationary processes. *IEEE Transactions on Information Theory*, **IT-3**:183–187, 1957.

E. H. Simpson. The interpretation of interaction in contingency tables. *Journal of the Royal Statistical Society, Series B*, **13**:238–241, 1951.

D. L. Smith, B. Lucey, L. A. Waller, J. E. Childs, and L. A. Real. Predicting the spatial dynamics of rabies epidemics on heterogeneous landscapes. *Proceedings of the National Academy of Sciences*, **99**:3668–3672, 2002.

J. A. Smith and A. F. Karr. Parameter estimation for a model of space–time rainfall. *Water Resources Research*, **21**:1251–1257, 1985.

M. K. P. So. Posterior mode estimation for nonlinear and non-Gaussian state space models. *Statistica Sinica*, **13**:255–274, 2003.

H. Solomon. *Geometric Probability*. Society for Industrial and Applied Mathematics, Philadelphia, PA, 1978.

A. R. Solow. Detecting change in the composition of a multispecies community. *Biometrics*, **50**:556–565, 1994.

H.-R. Song, M. Fuentes, and S. Ghosh. A comparative study of Gaussian geostatistical models and Gaussian Markov random field models. *Journal of Multivariate Analysis*, **99**:1681–1697, 2008.

J. Sparks. *The Works of Benjamin Franklin*, Vol. 10. Hilliard, Gray & Company, Boston, MA, 1840.

P. Speth and R. A. Madden. A space–time spectral analysis of Northern hemisphere geopotential heights. *Journal of the Atmospheric Sciences*, **40**:1086–1100, 1983.

D. Spiegelhalter, D. Lunn, A. Thomas, and N. Best. *Bayesian Analysis Using BUGS*. Chapman & Hall/CRC, Boca Raton, FL, 2010.

D. J. Spiegelhalter, N. G. Best, B. P. Carlin, and A. van der Linde. Bayesian measures of model complexity and fit (with discussion). *Journal of the Royal Statistical Society, Series B*, **64**:583–639, 2002.

F. Spitzer. Markov random fields and Gibbs ensembles. *American Mathematical Monthly*, **78**:142–154, 1971.

S. K. Srinivasan and R. Vasudevan. *Introduction to Random Differential Equations and Their Applications*. Elsevier, New York, 1971.

SSES. ENSO Web Project: Niño 3.4 Region Time Series. *Program in Spatial Statistics and Environmental Statistics*, The Ohio State University, Columbus, OH, 2009 (http://www.stat.osu.edu/~sses/collab_enso_nino34_timeseries.php).

J. L. Stanford and J. R. Ziemke. Field (map) statistics. In *Statistical Methods for Physical Science*, pages 457–479. Academic Press, San Diego, CA, 1994.

M. L. Stein. A simple model for spatial–temporal processes. *Water Resources Research*, 22:2107–2110, 1986.

M. L. Stein. *Interpolation of Spatial Data*. Springer, New York, 1999.

M. L. Stein. Space–time covariance functions. *Journal of the American Statistical Association*, 100:310–321, 2005.

M. L. Stein. Statistical methods for regular monitoring data. *Journal of the Royal Statistical Society, Series B*, 67:667–787, 2005.

M. L. Stein, Z. Chi, and L. J. Welty. Approximating likelihoods for large spatial data sets. *Journal of the Royal Statistical Society, Series B*, 66:275–296, 2004.

H. Stern and N. Cressie. Inference for extremes in disease mapping. In A. Lawson, A. Biggeri, D. Böhning, E. Lesaffre, J.-F. Viel, and R. Bertollini, editors, *Disease Mapping and Risk Assessment for Public Health*, pages 63–84. John Wiley & Sons, Chichester, UK, 1999.

H. S. Stern and N. Cressie. Posterior predictive model checks for disease mapping models. *Statistics in Medicine*, 19:2377–2397, 2000.

B. Stevens, J. Duan, J. C. McWilliams, M. Munnich, and J. D. Neelin. Entrainment, Rayleigh friction, and boundary layer winds over the tropical Pacific. *Journal of Climate*, 15:30–44, 2002.

D. L. Stevens and A. R. Olsen. Spatially balanced sampling of natural resources. *Journal of the American Statistical Association*, 99:262–278, 2004.

D. Stoffer and K. Wall. Bootstrapping state-space models: Gaussian maximum likelihood estimation and the Kalman filter. *Journal of the American Statistical Association*, 86:1024–1033, 1991.

G. Storvik, A. Frigessi, and D. Hirst. Stationary space-time Gaussian fields and their time autoregressive representation. *Statistical Modelling*, 2:139–161, 2002.

D. Stoyan, W. S. Kendall, and J. Mecke. *Stochastic Geometry and its Applications*. John Wiley & Sons, Chichester, UK, 1987.

D. Stoyan and A. Penttinen. Recent applications of point process methods in forestry statistics. *Statistical Science*, 15:61–78, 2000.

D. Stoyan and H. Stoyan. *Fractals, Random Shapes and Point Fields: Methods of Geometrical Statistics*. John Wiley & Sons, Chichester, UK, 1994.

S. Strebelle. Conditional simulation of complex geological structures using multiple-point statistics. *Mathematical Geology*, 34:1–21, 2002.

C. M. Strickland, D. P. Simpson, I. W. Turner, R. Denham, and K. L. Mengersen. Fast Bayesian analysis of spatial dynamic factor models for multitemporal remotely sensed imagery. *Applied Statistics*, 60:109–124, 2011.

J. R. Stroud, P. Müller, and B. Sansó. Dynamic models for spatiotemporal data. *Journal of the Royal Statistical Society, Series B*, 63:673–689, 2001.

J. R. Stroud, M. L. Stein, B. M. Lesht, D. J. Schwab, and D. Beletsky. An ensemble Kalman filter and smoother for satellite data assimilation. *Journal of the American Statistical Association*, 105:978–990, 2010.

G. Sugihara, and R. M. May. Nonlinear forecasting as a way of distinguishing chaos from measurment error in time series. *Nature*, **344**:734–741, 1990.

F. Takens. *Detecting Strange Attractors in Turbulence*. Lecture Notes in Mathematics, Vol. 898, Dynamical Systems and Turbulence. Springer-Verlag, Berlin, DE, 1981.

F. Takens. *On the Numerical Determination of the Dimension of an Attractor*. Lecture Notes in Mathematics, Vol. 1125, Dynamical Systems and Bifurcations. Springer-Verlag, Berlin, DE, 1985.

O. Talagrand. Assimilation of observations, an introduction. *Journal of the Meteorological Society of Japan*, **75**:191–209, 1997.

B. Y. Tang, W. W. Hsieh, A. H. Monahan, and F. t. Tangang. Skill comparisions between neural networks and canonical correlation analysis in predicting the equatorial Pacific sea surface temperatures. *Journal of Climate*, **13**:287–293, 2000.

F. T. Tangang, B. Tang, A. H. Monahan, and W. W. Hsieh. Forecasting ENSO events: A neural network-extended EOF approach. *Journal of Climate*, **11**:29–41, 1998.

M. A. Tanner. *Tools for Statistical Inference: Methods for the Exploration of Posterior Distributions and Likelihood Functions*. Springer, New York, 1996.

G. I. Taylor. The spectrum of turbulance. *Proceedings of the Royal Society of London*, **164**:476–490, 1938.

C. F. J. ter Braak. A Markov chain Monte Carlo version of the genetic algorithm differential evolution: Easy Bayesian computing for real parameter spaces. *Statistics and Computing*, **16**:239–249, 2006.

S. K. Thompson. On sampling and experiments. *Environmetrics*, **13**:429–436, 2002.

D. J. Thomson. Spectrum estimation and harmonic analysis. *Proceedings of the IEEE*, **70**:1055–1096, 1982.

M. Tiefelsdorf. *Modeling Spatial Processes: The Identification and Analysis of Spatial Relationships in Regression Residuals by Means of Moran's I*. Springer, Berlin, DE, 2000.

L. Tierney. Markov chains for exploring posterior distributions (with discussion). *Annals of Statistics*, **22**:1701–1762, 1994.

A. Timmermann, H. U. Voss, and R. Pasmanter. Empirical dynamic system modeling of ENSO using nonlinear inverse techniques. *Journal of Physical Oceanography*, **31**:1579–1598, 2001.

D. M. Titterington. Aspects of optimal design in dynamic systems. *Technometrics*, **22**:287–299, 1980.

D. Tjostheim. Statistical spatial series modelling II: Some further results on unilateral lattice processes. *Advances in Applied Probability*, **15**:562–584, 1983.

W. R. Tobler. A computer movie simulating urban growth in the Detroit region. *Economic Geography*, **46**:234–240, 1970.

S. F. Tonellato. A multivariate time series model for the analysis and prediction of carbon monoxide atmospheric concentrations. *Applied Statistics*, **50**:187–200, 2001.

H. Tong. *Non-Linear Time Series: A Dynamical System Approach*. Oxford University Press, Oxford, UK, 1990.

R. Tsay. *Analysis of Financial Time Series*, second edition. John Wiley & Sons, New York, 2005.

P. Turchin. *Complex Population Dynamics*. Princeton University Press, Princeton, NJ, 2003.

S. L. Tzeng, H.-C. Huang, and N. Cressie. A fast, optimal spatial-prediction method for massive datasets. *Journal of the American Statistical Association*, **100**:1343–1357, 2005.

M. D. Ugarte, T. Goicoa, and A. F. Militino. Spatio-temporal modeling of mortality risks using penalized splines. *Environmetrics*, **21**:270–289, 2010.

G. J. G. Upton and B. Fingleton. *Spatial Data Analysis by Example*, Volume 1: *Point Pattern and Quantitative Data*. John Wiley & Sons, Chichester, UK, 1985.

G. J. G. Upton and B. Fingleton. *Spatial Data Analysis by Example*, Volume 2: *Categorical and Directional Data*. John Wiley & Sons, Chichester, UK, 1989.

J. van den Berg. A uniqueness condition for Gibbs measures, with application to the 2-dimensional Ising antiferromagnet. *Communications in Mathematical Physics*, **152**:161–166, 1993.

M. N. M. van Lieshout. *Markov Point Processes and Their Applications*. Imperial College Press, London, UK, 2000.

G. J. van Oldenborgh, M. A. Balmaseda, L. Ferranti, T. N. Stockdale, and D. L. T. Anderson. Did the ECMWF seasonal forecast model outperform statistical ENSO forecast models over the last 15 years? *Journal of Climate*, **18**:3240–3249, 2005.

A. V. Vecchia. Estimation and model identification for continuous spatial processes. *Journal of the Royal Statistical Society, Series B*, **50**:297–312, 1988.

A. Veen and F. P. Schoenberg. Estimation of space-time branching process models in seismology using an EM-type algorithm. *Journal of the American Statistical Association*, **103**:614–624, 2008.

T. Velghe, P. A. Troch, F. P. De Troch, and J. van de Velde. Evaluation of cluster-based rectangular pulses point process models for rainfall. *Water Resources Research*, **30**:2847–2857, 1994.

J. M. Ver Hoef. Sampling and geostatistics for spatial data. *Ecoscience*, **9**:152–161, 2002.

J. M. Ver Hoef and R. P. Barry. Constructing and fitting models for cokriging and multivariable spatial prediction. *Journal of Statistical Planning and Inference*, **69**:275–294, 1998.

J. M. Ver Hoef and N. Cressie. Multivariable spatial prediction. *Mathematical Geology*, **25**:219–240, 1993. Errata: **26**, 273–275, 1994.

J. M. Ver Hoef, N. Cressie, and R. P. Barry. Flexible spatial models based on the Fast Fourier Transform (FFT) for cokriging. *Journal of Computational and Graphical Statistics*, **13**:265–282, 2004.

J. M. Ver Hoef and E. E. Peterson. A moving average approach for spatial statistical models of stream networks (with discussion). *Journal of the American Statistical Association*, **105**:6–24, 2010.

J. M. Ver Hoef, E. E. Peterson, and D. Theobald. Spatial statistical models that use flow and stream distance. *Environmental and Ecological Statistics*, **3**:449–464, 2006.

A. Villagran, G. Huerta, C. S. Jackson, and M. K. Sen. Computational methods for parameter estimation in climate models. *Bayesian Analysis*, **3**:823–850, 2008.

H. von Storch, T. Bruns, I. Fisher-Bruns, and K. H. Hasselmann. Principal oscillation pattern analysis of the 30 and 60 day oscillation in a GCM. *Journal of Geophysical Research*, **93**:11022–11036, 1988.

H. von Storch, G. Büger, R. Schnur, and J.-S. von Storch. Principal oscillation patterns: A review. *Journal of Climate*, **8**:377–400, 1995.

H. von Storch and G. Hannoschöck. Comment on "Empirical Orthogonal Function analysis of wind vectors over the tropical Pacific region". *Bulletin of the American Meteorological Society*, **65**: 162, 1984.

H. von Storch and G. Hannoschöck. Statistical aspects of estimated principal vectors (EOFs) based on small sample sizes. *Journal of Climate and Applied Meteorology*, **24**:716–724, 1985.

H. von Storch and F. W. Zwiers. *Statistical Analysis in Climate Research*. Cambridge University Press, Cambridge, UK, 1999.

J. A. Vrugt, C. J. F. ter Braak, C. G. H. Dilks, B. A. Robinson, J. M. Hyman, and D. Higdon. Accelerating Markov chain Monte Carlo simulation by differential evolution with self-adaptive randomized subspace sampling. *International Journal of Nonlinear Sciences and Numerical Simulation*, **10**:273–290, 2009.

R. Waagepetersen and Y. Guan. Two-step estimation for inhomogeneous spatial point processes. *Journal of the Royal Statistical Society, Series B*, **71**:685–702, 2009.

H. Wackernagel. *Multivariate Geostatistics*. Springer, Berlin, DE, 1995.

H. Wackernagel. *Multivariate Geostatistics: An Introduction with Applications*, third edition. Springer, Berlin, DE, 2003.

G. Wahba. Bayesian "confidence intervals" for the cross-validated smoothing spline. *Journal of the Royal Statistical Society, Series B*, **45**:133–150, 1983.

G. Wahba. *Spline Models for Observational Data*. Society for Industrial and Applied Mathematics, Philadelphia, PA, 1990.

J. C. Wakefield, J. E. Kelsall, and S. E. Morris. Clustering, cluster detection, and spatial variation in risk. In *Spatial Epidemiology: Methods and Applications*, pages 128–152. Oxford University Press, Oxford, UK, 2000.

J. C. Wakefield and R. Salway. A statistical framework for ecological and aggregate studies. *Journal of the Royal Statistical Society, Series A*, **164**:119–137, 2001.

J. C. Wakefield, A. F. M. Smith, A. Racine-Poon, and A. E. Gelfand. Bayesian analysis of linear and non-linear population models by using the Gibbs sampler. *Applied Statistics*, **43**:201–221, 1994.

K. Wall and D. Stoffer. A state space approach to bootstrapping conditional forecasts in ARMA models. *Journal of Time Series Analysis*, **23**:733–751, 2002.

J. M. Wallace. Empirical orthogonal representation of time series in the frequency domain. Part II: Application to the study of tropical wave disturbances. *Journal of Applied Meteorology*, **11**:893–900, 1972.

J. M. Wallace and R. E. Dickinson. Empirical orthogonal representation of time series in the frequency domain. Part I: Theoretical considerations. *Journal of Applied Meteorology*, **11**:887–892, 1972.

L. A. Waller, B. P. Carlin, H. Xia, and A. E. Gelfand. Hierarchical spatio-temporal mapping of disease rates. *Journal of the American Statistical Association*, **92**:607–617, 1997.

L. A. Waller and C. A. Gotway. *Applied Spatial Statistics for Public Health Data*. John Wiley & Sons, Hoboken, NJ, 2004.

G. G. Walter. *Wavelets and Other Orthogonal Systems with Applications*. Chapman & Hall/CRC, Boca Raton, FL, 1994.

F. Wang and M. M. Wall. Generalized common spatial factor model. *Biostatistics*, **4**:569–582, 2003.

B. C. Weare and J. S. Nasstrom. Examples of extended empirical orthogonal function analysis. *Monthly Weather Review*, **110**:481–485, 1982.

R. Webster, O. Atteia, and J. P. Dubois. Coregionalization of trace metals in the soil in the Swiss Jura. *European Journal of Soil Science*, **45**:205–218, 1994.

R. Webster and M. Oliver. *Geostatistics for Environmental Scientists*. John Wiley & Sons, Chichester, UK, 2001.

E. J. Wegman. Hyperdimensional data analysis using parallel coordinates. *Journal of the American Statistical Association*, **85**:664–675, 1990.

E. J. Wegman and D. B. Carr. Statistical graphics and visualization. In C. R. Rao, editor, *Handbook of Statistics: Computational Statistics*, pages 857–958. North Holland/Elsevier Science Publishers, Amsterdam, NL, 1993.

P. D. Welch. The use of fast Fourier transform for estimation of power spectra: A method based on time averaging over short modified periodograms. *IEEE Transactions on Audio Electroacoustics*, **AU-15**:70–73, 1967.

D. A. Wendt, M. E. Irwin, and N. Cressie. Waypoint analysis for command and control. *Naval Research Logistics*, **51**:1045–1067, 2004.

M. West. Bayesian model monitoring. *Journal of the Royal Statistical Society, Series B*, **48**:70–78, 1986.

M. West and J. Harrison. *Bayesian Forecasting and Dynamic Models*. Springer-Verlag, New York, 1997.

M. Wheeler and G. N. Kiladis. Convectively-coupled equatorial waves: Analysis of clouds and temperature in the wavenumber–frequency domain. *Journal of the Atmospheric Sciences*, **56**:374–399, 1999.

P. Whittle. On stationary processes in the plane. *Biometrika*, **41**:434–449, 1954.

P. Whittle. Topographic correlation, power-law covariance functions, and diffusion. *Biometrika*, **49**:305–314, 1962.

P. Whittle. Stochastic processes in several dimensions. *Bulletin of the International Statistical Institute*, **40**:974–994, 1963.

P. Whittle. *Systems in Stochastic Equilibrium*. John Wiley & Sons, Chichester, UK, 1986.

B. Widom and J. S. Rowlinson. New model for the study of liquid-vapor phase transitions. *Journal of Chemical Physics*, **52**:1670–1684, 1970.

T. M. L. Wigley and B. D. Santer. Statistical comparison of spatial fields in model validation, perturbation, and predictability experiments. *Journal of Geophysical Research*, **95**:851–865, 1990.

C. K. Wikle. *Spatio-temporal Statistical Models with Applications to Atmospheric Processes*. Ph.D. Dissertation, Iowa State University, Ames, IA, 1996.

C. K. Wikle. A kernel-based spectral model for non-Gaussian spatio-temporal processes. *Statistical Modelling*, **2**:299–314, 2002a.

C. K. Wikle. Spatial modeling of count data: A case study in modelling breeding bird survey data on large spatial domains. In *Spatial Cluster Modelling*, pages 199–209. Chapman & Hall/CRC, Boca Raton, FL, 2002b.

C. K. Wikle. Hierarchical models in environmental science. *International Statistical Review*, **71**:181–199, 2003a.

C. K. Wikle. Hierarchical Bayesian models for predicting the spread of ecological processes. *Ecology*, **84**:1382–1394, 2003b.

C. K. Wikle. Hierarchical modeling with spatial data. In A. E. Gelfand, P. J. Diggle, M. Fuentes, and P. Guttorp, editors, *Handbook of Spatial Statistics*, pages 89–106, Chapman & Hall/CRC, Boca Raton, FL, 2010a.

C. K. Wikle. Low rank representations as models for spatial processes. In A. E. Gelfand, P. J. Diggle, M. Fuentes, and P. Guttorp, editors, *Handbook of Spatial Statistics*, pages 107–118, Chapman & Hall/CRC, Boca Raton, FL, 2010b.

C. K. Wikle and C. K. Anderson. Climatological analysis of tornado report counts using a hierarchical Bayesian spatio-temporal model. *Journal of Geophysical Research—Atmospheres*, **108(D24)**: 9005, STS 20-1-12-15, 2003. doi:10.1029/2002JD002806.

C. K. Wikle and L. M. Berliner. Combining information across spatial scales. *Technometrics*, **47**:80–91, 2005.

C. K. Wikle and L. M. Berliner. A Bayesian tutorial for data assimilation. *Physica D*, **230**:1–16, 2007.

C. K. Wikle, L. M. Berliner, and N. Cressie. Hierarchical Bayesian space-time models. *Environmental and Ecological Statistics*, **5**:117–154, 1998.

C. K. Wikle, L. M. Berliner, and R. F. Milliff. Hierarchical Bayesian approach to boundary value problems with stochastic boundary conditions. *Monthly Weather Review*, **131**:1051–1062, 2003.

C. K. Wikle and N. Cressie. A dimension-reduced approach to space-time Kalman filtering. *Biometrika*, **86**:815–829, 1999.

C. K. Wikle and S. H. Holan. Polynomial nonlinear spatio-temporal integro-difference equation models. *Journal of Time Series Analysis*, **32**:339–350, 2011.

C. K. Wikle and M. B. Hooten. Hierarchical Bayesian spatio-temporal models for population spread. In J. S. Clark and A. E. Gelfand, editors, *Applications of Computational Statistics in the Environmental Sciences: Hierarchical Bayes and MCMC Methods*, pages 145–169. Oxford University Press, Oxford, UK, 2006.

C. K. Wikle and M. B. Hooten. A general science-based framework for dynamical spatio-temporal models (with discussion). *Test*, **19**:417–468, 2010.

C. K. Wikle, R. A. Madden, and T.-C. Chen. Seasonal variation of upper tropospheric lower stratospheric equatorial waves over the tropical Pacific. *Journal of the Atmospheric Sciences*, **54**:1895–1909, 1997.

C. K. Wikle, R. F. Milliff, D. Nychka, and L. M. Berliner. Spatiotemporal hierarchical Bayesian modeling: Tropical ocean surface winds. *Journal of the American Statistical Association*, **96**:382–397, 2001.

C. K. Wikle and J. A. Royle. Space-time dynamic design of environmental monitoring networks. *Journal of Agricultural, Biological, and Environmental Statistics*, **4**:489–507, 1999.

C. K. Wikle and J. A. Royle. Dynamic design of ecological monitoring networks for non-Gaussian spatio-temporal data. *Environmetrics*, **16**:507–522, 2005.

D. S. Wilks. *Statistical Methods in the Atmospheric Sciences*, second edition. Elsevier/Academic Press, Boston, MA, 2006.

P. Wilmott, S. Howison, and J. Dewynne. *The Mathematics of Financial Derivatives, A Student Introduction*. Cambridge University Press, Cambridge, UK, 1995.

L. Wittgenstein. *Philosophical Investigations*. Translated by G. E. M. Anscombe. Macmillan, New York, 1958.

R. C. L. Wolff. Chaos. In P. Armitage, editor, *Encyclopedia of Biostatistics, 1*, pages 600–604. John Wiley & Sons, Chichester, UK, 1998.

S. Wolfram. Cellular automata as models for complexity. *Nature*, **311**:419–424, 1984.

R. Wolpert and K. Ickstadt. Poisson/gamma random field models for spatial statistics. *Biometrika*, **85**:251–267, 1998.

D. L. Wright, H. L. Stern, and N. Cressie. Loss functions for estimation of extrema with an application to disease mapping. *Canadian Journal of Statistics*, **31**:251–266, 2003.

K. Xu and C. K. Wikle. Estimation of parameterized spatio-temporal dynamic models. *Journal of Statistical Planning and Inference*, **137**:567–588, 2007.

K. Xu, C. K. Wikle, and N. I. Fox. A kernel-based spatio-temporal dynamical model for nowcasting radar precipitation. *Journal of the American Statistical Association*, **100**:1133–1144, 2005.

M. I. Yadrenko. *Spectral Theory of Random Fields*. Optimization Software Inc., New York, 1983.

A. M. Yaglom. Some classes of random fields in *n*-dimensonal space, related to stationary random processes. *Theory of Probability and its Applications*, **2**:273–320, 1957.

A. M. Yaglom. *An Introduction to the Theory of Stationary Random Functions*. Translated and edited by R. A. Silverman. Dover, New York, 1962.

A. M. Yaglom. *Correlation Theory of Stationary and Related Random Functions*, Vol. II: *Supplementary Notes and References*. Springer, New York, 1987.

J. Yan, M. Cowles, S. Wang, and M. Armstrong. Parallelizing MCMC for Bayesian spatiotemporal geostatistical models. *Statistics and Computing*, **17**:323–335, 2007.

M. Yanai and T. Maruyama. Stratospheric wave disturbances propagating over the equatorial Pacific. *Journal of the Meteorological Society of Japan*, **44**:291–294, 1966.

F. Yao, and H.-G. Müller. Functional quadratic regression. *Biometrika*, **97**:49–64, 2010.

P. Young. Stochastic, dynamic modelling and signal processing: Time variable and state dependent parameter estimation. In *Nonlinear and Nonstationary Signal Processing*, pages 74–114. Cambridge University Press, Cambridge, UK, 2000.

Y. Yue and P. L. Speckman. Nonstationary spatial Gaussian Markov random fields. *Journal of Computational and Graphical Statistics*, **19**:96–116, 2010.

H. Zhang. On estimation and prediction for spatial generalized linear mixed models. *Biometrics*, **58**:129–136, 2002.

H. Zhang. Optimal interpolation and the appropriateness of cross-validating variogram in spatial generalized linear mixed models. *Journal of Computational and Graphical Statistics*, **12**:1–16, 2003.

H. Zhang. Inconsistent estimation and asymptotically equal interpolations in model-based geostatistics. *Journal of the American Statistical Association*, **99**:250–261, 2004.

H. Zhang and D. L. Zimmerman. Hybrid estimation of semivariogram parameters. *Mathematical Geology*, **39**:247–260, 2007.

J. Zhang, P. F. Craigmile, and N. Cressie. Loss function approaches to predict a spatial quantile and its exceedance region. *Technometrics*, **50**:216–227, 2008.

Y. Zhang and J. Zhu. Markov chain Monte Carlo for spatial–temporal autologistic regression. *Journal of Computational and Graphical Statistics*, **17**:123–137, 2008.

Y. Zheng and B. H. Aukema. Hierarchical dynamic modeling of outbreaks of mountain pine beetle using partial differential equations. *Environmetrics*, **21**:801–816, 2010.

H. Zhu, M. Gu, and B. Peterson. Maximum likelihood from spatial random effects models via the stochastic approximation expectation maximization algorithm. *Statistics and Computing*, **17**:163–177, 2007.

J. Zhu, H.-C. Huang, and C.-T. Wu. Modeling spatial-temporal binary data using Markov random fields. *Journal of Agriculutral, Biological, and Environmental Statistics*, **10**:212–225, 2005.

J. Zhu, J. G. Rasmussen, J. Møller, B. H. Aukema, and K. F. Raffa. Spatial-temporal modeling of forest gaps generated by colonization from below- and above-ground bark beetle species. *Journal of the American Statistical Association*, **103**:162–177, 2008.

L. Zhu, and B. P. Carlin. Comparing hierarchical models for spatio-temporally misaligned data using the deviance information criterion. *Statistics in Medicine*, **19**:2265–2278, 2000.

D. L. Zimmerman. Optimal network design for spatial prediction, covariance parameter estimation, and empirical prediction. *Environmetrics*, **17**:635–652, 2006.

Index

Statistics for Spatio-Temporal Data, by Noel Cressie and Christopher K. Wikle
Copyright © 2011 John Wiley & Sons, Inc.

571